THE FUTURE OF
DISABILITY
IN AMERICA

Committee on Disability in America

Board on Health Sciences Policy

Marilyn J. Field and Alan M. Jette, *Editors*

INSTITUTE OF MEDICINE
OF THE NATIONAL ACADEMIES

THE NATIONAL ACADEMIES PRESS
Washington, D.C.
www.nap.edu

THE NATIONAL ACADEMIES PRESS   500 Fifth Street, N.W.   Washington, DC 20001

NOTICE: The project that is the subject of this report was approved by the Governing Board of the National Research Council, whose members are drawn from the councils of the National Academy of Sciences, the National Academy of Engineering, and the Institute of Medicine. The members of the committee responsible for the report were chosen for their special competences and with regard for appropriate balance.

This study was supported by Contract No. 223-01-2460, Task Order 26, between the National Academy of Sciences and the Centers for Disease Control and Prevention; Contract No. ED-06-CO-0105 between the National Academy of Sciences and the U.S. Department of Education; and Contract No. N01-OD-4-2139, Task Order 164, between the National Academy of Sciences and the National Institutes of Health. Any opinions, findings, conclusions, or recommendations expressed in this publication are those of the authors and do not necessarily reflect the view of the organizations or agencies that provided support for the project.

Library of Congress Cataloging-in-Publication Data

The future of disability in America / Committee on Disability in America, Board on Health Sciences Policy ; Marilyn J. Field and Alan M. Jette, editors.
   p. ; cm.
   Includes bibliographical references and index.
   ISBN-13: 978-0-309-10472-2 (hardback : alk. paper)
   ISBN-10: 0-309-10472-6 (hardback : alk. paper) 1. People with disabilities--United States. 2. People with disabilities—Services for—United States. 3. Sociology of disability—United States. I. Field, Marilyn J. (Marilyn Jane) II. Jette, Alan M. III. Institute of Medicine (U.S.). Committee on Disability in America: a New Look.
   [DNLM: 1. Disabled Persons—United States. 2. Age Factors—United States. 3. Chronic Disease—prevention & control—United States. 4. Comorbidity—United States. 5. Health Services Accessibility—trends—United States. 6. Insurance Coverage—United States.]
   HV1553.F87 2007
   362.40973—dc22
                                        2007019908

Additional copies of this report are available from the National Academies Press, 500 Fifth Street, N.W., Lockbox 285, Washington, DC 20055; (800) 624-6242 or (202) 334-3313 (in the Washington metropolitan area); Internet, http://www.nap.edu.

For more information about the Institute of Medicine, visit the IOM home page at: www.iom.edu.

The serpent has been a symbol of long life, healing, and knowledge among almost all cultures and religions since the beginning of recorded history. The serpent adopted as a logotype by the Institute of Medicine is a relief carving from ancient Greece, now held by the Staatliche Museen in Berlin.

Suggested citation: Institute of Medicine (IOM). 2007. *The Future of Disability in America*. Washington, DC: The National Academies Press.

"Knowing is not enough; we must apply.
Willing is not enough; we must do."
—Goethe

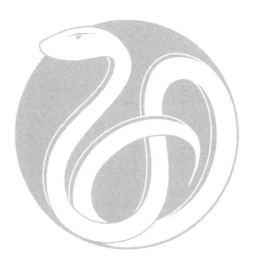

INSTITUTE OF MEDICINE
OF THE NATIONAL ACADEMIES

Advising the Nation. Improving Health.

THE NATIONAL ACADEMIES
Advisers to the Nation on Science, Engineering, and Medicine

The **National Academy of Sciences** is a private, nonprofit, self-perpetuating society of distinguished scholars engaged in scientific and engineering research, dedicated to the furtherance of science and technology and to their use for the general welfare. Upon the authority of the charter granted to it by the Congress in 1863, the Academy has a mandate that requires it to advise the federal government on scientific and technical matters. Dr. Ralph J. Cicerone is president of the National Academy of Sciences.

The **National Academy of Engineering** was established in 1964, under the charter of the National Academy of Sciences, as a parallel organization of outstanding engineers. It is autonomous in its administration and in the selection of its members, sharing with the National Academy of Sciences the responsibility for advising the federal government. The National Academy of Engineering also sponsors engineering programs aimed at meeting national needs, encourages education and research, and recognizes the superior achievements of engineers. Dr. Charles M. Vest is president of the National Academy of Engineering.

The **Institute of Medicine** was established in 1970 by the National Academy of Sciences to secure the services of eminent members of appropriate professions in the examination of policy matters pertaining to the health of the public. The Institute acts under the responsibility given to the National Academy of Sciences by its congressional charter to be an adviser to the federal government and, upon its own initiative, to identify issues of medical care, research, and education. Dr. Harvey V. Fineberg is president of the Institute of Medicine.

The **National Research Council** was organized by the National Academy of Sciences in 1916 to associate the broad community of science and technology with the Academy's purposes of furthering knowledge and advising the federal government. Functioning in accordance with general policies determined by the Academy, the Council has become the principal operating agency of both the National Academy of Sciences and the National Academy of Engineering in providing services to the government, the public, and the scientific and engineering communities. The Council is administered jointly by both Academies and the Institute of Medicine. Dr. Ralph J. Cicerone and Dr. Charles M. Vest are chair and vice chair, respectively, of the National Research Council.

www.national-academies.org

COMMITTEE ON DISABILITY IN AMERICA

ALAN M. JETTE (*Chair*), Director, Health & Disability Research Institute and Professor of Health Policy and Management, Boston University School of Public Health

ELENA M. ANDRESEN, Professor and Chair, Department of Epidemiology and Biostatistics, College of Public Health and Health Professions, University of Florida and Research Health Scientist, Department of Veterans Affairs, Gainesville

MICHAEL CHERNEW, Professor, Department of Health Care Policy, Harvard Medical School (formerly at the University of Michigan)

DUDLEY S. CHILDRESS, Professor of Biomedical Engineering and Physical Medicine and Rehabilitation, McCormick School of Engineering and Feinberg School of Medicine, Northwestern University

VICKI A. FREEDMAN, Professor, Department of Health Systems and Policy, School of Public Health, University of Medicine and Dentistry of New Jersey

PATRICIA HICKS, Associate Professor of Pediatrics and Director, Continuity of Care Clinic, University of Texas Southwestern Medical School, University of Texas Southwestern Medical Center at Dallas

LISA I. IEZZONI, Professor of Medicine, Harvard Medical School, and Associate Director, Institute for Health Policy, Massachusetts General Hospital

JUNE ISAACSON KAILES, Associate Director and Adjunct Professor, Center for Disability Issues and the Health Professions, Western University of Health Sciences

LAURA MOSQUEDA, Director of Geriatrics and Professor of Family Medicine, University of California at Irvine School of Medicine

P. HUNTER PECKHAM, Donnell Professor of Biomedical Engineering and Orthopaedics, Case Western Reserve University

JAMES MARC PERRIN, Professor of Pediatrics, Harvard Medical School and Massachusetts General Hospital

MARGARET A. TURK, Professor, Physical Medicine and Rehabilitation, State University of New York Upstate Medical University

GREGG VANDERHEIDEN, Professor of Industrial and Biomedical Engineering and Director, Trace Research and Development Center, University of Wisconsin at Madison

JOHN WHYTE, Director, Moss Rehabilitation Research Institute

Committee Consultants and Background Paper Authors

SCOTT BURRIS, James E. Beasley Professor of Law, Temple University Beasley School of Law

H. STEPHEN KAYE, Associate Adjunct Professor, Institute for Health & Aging, University of California at San Francisco

DAVID J. KNUTSON, Director, Health Systems Studies, Park Nicollet Institute

GREGORY S. LIPTAK, Professor of Pediatrics, State University of New York Upstate Medical University Hospital

KATHRYN MOSS, Research Fellow and Head, Disability Research Section, The University of North Carolina at Chapel Hill

SARA ROSENBAUM, Hirsh Professor and Chair, Department of Health Policy, George Washington University School of Public Health and Health Services

SANDRA ROSENBLOOM, Professor of Planning, University of Arizona

KAREN PELTZ STRAUSS, Principal, KPS Consulting

IOM Project Staff

MARILYN J. FIELD, Study Director

FRANKLIN BRANCH, Research Assistant

AFRAH J. ALI, Senior Program Assistant

LINDA MARTIN, IOM Scholar in Residence

---

*IOM Boards do not review or approve individual reports and are not asked to endorse conclusions and recommendations. The responsibility for the content of the report rests with the authoring committee and the institution.

Reviewers

This report has been reviewed in draft form by individuals chosen for their diverse perspectives and technical expertise, in accordance with procedures approved by the National Research Council's Report Review Committee. The purpose of this independent review is to provide candid and critical comments that will assist the institution in making its published reports as sound as possible and to ensure that the report meets institutional standards for objectivity, evidence, and responsiveness to the study charge. The review comments and draft manuscript remain confidential to protect the integrity of the deliberative process. We wish to thank the following individuals for their review of this report:

Barbara Altman, Disability Statistics Consultant, Rockville, Maryland
Michael L. Boninger, University of Pittsburgh School of Medicine
Howard Brody, University of Texas Medical Branch Institute for Medical Humanities
Cliff Brubaker, University of Pittsburgh School of Health and Rehabilitation Sciences
Gerben DeJong, National Rehabilitation Hospital
Linda P. Fried, Johns Hopkins Medical Institutions and Bloomberg School of Public Health
Walter R. Frontera, University of Puerto Rico School of Medicine
Laura N. Gitlin, Thomas Jefferson University College of Health Professions

Andrew J. Houtenville, Employment and Disability Institute, Cornell University

Corinne Kirchner, Consultant, New York, New York

Gloria Krahn, Oregon Institute on Disability and Development, Oregon Health and Science University

Richard Kronick, University of California at San Diego Division of Health Care Sciences

John L. Melvin, Jefferson Medical College of Thomas Jefferson University

Paul Newacheck, University of California at San Francisco Institute for Health Policy Studies and Department of Pediatrics

Judith Palfrey, Harvard Medical School and Children's Hospital of Boston

Michelle Putnam, George Warren Brown School of Social Work, Washington University

Amy K. Rosen, Boston University Schools of Medicine and Public Heath and Bedford Veterans Affairs Medical Center

Jack Winters, Marquette University College of Engineering

Although the reviewers listed above have provided many constructive comments and suggestions, they were not asked to endorse the conclusions or recommendations, nor did they see the final draft of the report before its release. The review of this report was overseen by **George W. Rutherford,** University of California at San Francisco School of Medicine, and **Elena O. Nightingale,** Institute of Medicine. Appointed by the National Research Council and the Institute of Medicine, these individuals were responsible for making certain that an independent examination of this report was carried out in accordance with the institutional procedures and that all review comments were carefully considered. Responsibility for the final content of this report rests entirely with the authoring committee and the institution.

Acknowledgments

In preparing this report, the committee and project staff benefited greatly from the assistance of many individuals and groups. Important information and insights came from a public workshop and two public meetings that the committee organized to obtain information and perspectives from groups and individuals knowledgeable and concerned about disability and the factors that contribute to it. Appendix A includes the public meeting agendas. Appendix B lists the authors of papers presented at the public workshop in August 2005. The committee also appreciates the work of the project consultants and the authors of background papers that are included as appendixes to this report.

Our project officers and other staff at our sponsoring agencies were always helpful and supportive. We particularly appreciate the assistance of John Crews, Don Betts, and Sandra Coulberson of the Disability and Health Team at the Centers for Disease Control and Prevention; Arthur Sherwood, Ruth Brannon, Connie Pledger, and Steven James Tingus (National Institute on Disability and Rehabilitation Research) and Robert Jaeger (now at the National Science Foundation); and Michael Weinrich (National Center on Medical Rehabilitation Research).

In addition, the committee and staff received useful information and guidance on data, policy, and other issues from staff in a number of agencies, including Barbara Altman, Ellen Kramarow, Susan Jack, and Jennifer Madans at the National Center for Health Statistics; David Bacquis at the Access Board; Kenneth Curley at the U.S. Army's Telemedicine and Advanced Technologies Research Center; Gil Devy at the National Science

Foundation; Patricia Dorn and Dennis Hancher at the U.S. Department of Veterans Affairs; Pamela Klein at the U.S. Census Bureau; Geoffrey Ling at the Defense Advanced Research Project Agency; Bill Long and Hongji Liu at the Centers for Medicare and Medicaid Services; Terence McMenamin at the Bureau of Labor Statistics; and Jeffrey Rhoades at the Agency for Health Care Policy and Research. An undoubtedly incomplete list of others whose assistance benefited the committee includes Mindy Aisen, United Cerebral Palsy Foundation; Susan Allen, Brown University; Rory Cooper and Mark Schmeler, University of Pittsburgh Medical Center; Marilyn Golden, Disability Rights Education and Defense Fund; Judy Hawkins, Gallaudet University; Karen Hendricks, American Academy of Pediatrics; Clayton Lewis, University of Colorado; Molly Follett Story, Human Spectrum Design; and Wendy Strobel, State University of New York at Buffalo.

The committee and project staff also appreciate the work of copy editor Michael Hayes. Within the Institute of Medicine, Michael McGeary was especially helpful, reflecting the work he has done as study director for projects on the social security disability decision-making process and the evaluation of veterans for disability benefits. We would also like to acknowledge the assistance of Lara Andersen, Judy Estep, Amy Haas, Bethany Hardy, Linda Kilroy, Bronwyn Schrecker, Sally Stanfield, Tyjen Tsai, and Gary Walker.

Preface

The 1991 Institute of Medicine (IOM) report *Disability in America: Toward a National Agenda for Prevention* identified disability as a significant social, public health, and moral issue that affects every individual, family, and community across America. This seminal volume articulated a series of comprehensive changes necessary to prevent disability in American society. Its recommendations included, for example, the development of new public and private leadership in disability prevention, the adoption of a unified conceptual framework to guide collaborative research, a national disability surveillance system, a comprehensive research program, coordinated approaches to delivering health and social services, and professional and public education to promote enlightened attitudes about disability. In 1997, the IOM followed with a second report, entitled *Enabling America: Assessing the Role of Rehabilitation Science and Engineering*, which critically evaluated the current federal programmatic efforts in science and engineering related to rehabilitation and disability. The 1997 IOM report called attention to the major shortcomings in the organization and administration of federal research programs pertinent to disability and rehabilitation. In doing so, it set forth a series of specific recommendations for more research, improved coordination, and a need for enhanced visibility of rehabilitation-related research within federal research programs.

Beginning in the fall of 2005, a dedicated group of clinicians, researchers, and consumers have collaborated in reviewing the nation's progress on disability since 1991 and 1997. As chair, I have had the privilege of working with an outstanding group of individuals who, despite their diverse backgrounds and disparate perspectives, listened, probed, and discussed to reach a consensus around our major findings and recommendations presented in this report. Let me thank each of them, along with our IOM staff, particularly Marilyn Field, the project director, who did an outstanding job of guiding us in our work. I also wish to extend my gratitude to numerous other individuals and organizations (listed in Appendix A) who provided us with information, background papers, and other assistance in our work.

Our conclusions, as detailed in this report, entitled *The Future of Disability in America*, document the sobering reality that far too little progress has been made in the last two decades to prepare for the aging of the baby boom generation and to remove the obstacles that limit what too many people with physical and cognitive impairments can achieve. Disturbingly, many of the major recommendations contained in the two earlier reports have received little or no serious consideration, and they remain as germane today as they were in 1991 and 1997. This report therefore reiterates several still pertinent goals from the earlier reports and offers new recommendations that, if enacted promptly, could create a future in which Americans of all abilities and ages can participate fully in society.

After reviewing the state of disability in America, the committee concluded that although important progress has been made over the past 17 years in our understanding of disability, its causes, and strategies that can prevent its onset and progression, society must do more now before a crisis is upon us. The chapters in this report cover a broad range of critical topics, including the prevention of secondary conditions, the role of technology and universal design, selected issues in health care organization and financing, as well as the environmental context of disability.

Our society faces several fundamental challenges, which are highlighted within this report. Will this country commit to actions that will limit the progression of physical and mental impairments into disabilities and prevent the development of secondary conditions? Will society provide affordable and accessible health care and technological aids that promote good health and maximize societal participation for people with disability? Will society reduce environmental barriers for people with existing impairments? And will society demand that all levels of government invest in more research, the improved coordination of research, and the need for the enhanced visibility of disability-related research within our public research programs? The answers to these questions will undoubtedly define the future of disability in America and leave lasting legacies for future generations.

The poet Archibald MacLeish once wrote, "America was always promises." There is still much work to do, but never have America's promises been within closer reach for people with disabilities, if only we harness the innovative spirit of American science and industry, promote and assist compliance with existing civil rights legislation, and remove outdated restrictions in public and private health plans. Working together, I know that we can transform the future of disability in America.

Alan M. Jette, *Chair*
April 2007

Contents

Boxes, Figures, and Tables

BOXES

FIGURES

TABLES

Summary

Today, between 40 million and 50 million people in the United States report some kind of disability. That number will likely grow significantly in the next 30 years as the baby boom generation enters late life, when the risk of disability is the highest. If one considers people who now have disabilities (at least one in seven Americans), people who are likely to develop disabilities in the future, and people who are or who will be affected by the disabilities of family members and others close to them, then disability affects today or will affect tomorrow the lives of most Americans. Clearly, disability is not a minority issue.

In considerable measure, the future of disability in America will depend on how this country prepares for and manages a complex array of demographic, fiscal, medical, technological, and other developments that will unfold in the next several decades. Much can be done now to make this future one that enables people with disabilities to lead full and productive lives. Inaction will lead to individual and societal costs—avoidable dependency, diminished quality of life, increased stress on individuals and families, and lost productivity.

DEVELOPMENTS SINCE PUBLICATION OF THE
1991 AND 1997 IOM DISABILITY REPORTS

The 1991 Institute of Medicine (IOM) report *Disability in America* and the 1997 IOM report *Enabling America* highlighted disability as a topic of public health action and scientific inquiry. The reports also offered recommendations on the prevention of disability and the role of rehabilitation science and engineering.

For this report, which was supported by the Centers for Disease Control and Prevention (CDC), the U.S. Department of Education, and the National Institutes of Health, a new IOM committee was charged with reviewing developments since the publication of the earlier IOM reports. As agreed upon with the study's sponsors, the review focused on several topics, including

- methodological and policy issues related to the definition, measurement, and monitoring of disability;
- trends in the amount, types, and causes of disability;
- secondary health conditions and aging with disability;
- transitions for young people with disabilities from pediatric to adult health care services;
- assistive technologies and supportive physical environments;
- coverage of assistive technologies and risk adjustment of payments to health plans; and
- directions for research.

The committee concluded that the United States has seen some progress since the publication of the earlier IOM reports. This progress includes a growing understanding that disability is not an inherent attribute of individuals. Rather, it results from interactions between individuals and their physical and social environments. Continuing advances in science and engineering have brought better assistive technologies that make these interactions with the environment easier. Likewise, advances in mainstream electronic and information technologies—combined with regulatory requirements for accessibility features—have been liberating for many people with disabilities.

In public health and clinical medicine, a range of new or improved preventive measures continue to reduce the incidence of certain kinds of injuries, developmental disorders, and other health conditions that can contribute to disability. Among older adults the chance of having an activity limitation has declined during the last two decades, although data suggest that younger adults and children have an increased chance of having an activity limitation. Most state Medicaid programs have increased the resources that they provide for community and home services that help people with serious disabilities to avoid institutional care. Programs for children with disabilities and other special health care needs have expanded.

At the same time, little progress has been made in adopting a number of the public policy and practice recommendations made in 1991 and 1997. For example, the 1997 IOM report bluntly stated that the federal research effort in the area of disability was inadequate. Despite modest increases in funding during the late 1990s, research spending on disability is miniscule in relation to current and future needs. Medicare, Medicaid, and private health plans continue to apply outdated policies that restrict access to assistive technologies and services. Other significant environmental barriers remain, for example, in hospitals and clinics that lack buildings, equipment, and services suitable for people with mobility, sensory, and other impairments. In 1991, the newly enacted Americans with Disabilities Act (ADA) was a source of great hope for those concerned about such barriers. Although the legislation has helped to increase awareness of the barriers in health care facilities, transportation, workplaces, and elsewhere, its implementation and enforcement have often been disappointing. These and other areas of inaction raise serious questions about how individuals, families, and society will cope with the challenges of disability in America during the coming decades.

This report argues that concerted action—taken sooner rather than later—is essential for this nation to avoid a future of harm and inequity and, instead, to improve the lives of people with disabilities. Its main themes and recommendations can be summarized and grouped around four general topics—disability monitoring, disability research, access to health care and other support services, and public and professional education—and 10 key points. Table S-1 presents an overview of the recommendations by showing the topic areas, the key points within these areas, the relevant actors, and the related recommendations. The complete list of 18 recommendations appears at the end of this summary.

DISABILITY MONITORING

Adopt and refine the *International Classification of Functioning, Disability and Health* as the conceptual framework for disability monitoring and research.

Since publication of the 1991 IOM report, many organizations have taken significant steps to improve disability monitoring, but further improvements are needed. These further improvements include adoption of the *International Classification of Functioning, Disability and Health* (ICF) of the World Health Organization (WHO) as the conceptual framework for

TABLE S-1 Report Recommendations in Overview

Actions Needed: Key Points	Primary Actors	Recommendation Number
Disability Monitoring		
Adopt and refine the *International Classification of Functioning, Disability and Health*.	CDC, U.S. Census Bureau, BLS, ICDR	2.1
Create a comprehensive disability monitoring system.	CDC, U.S. Census Bureau, BLS	2.2
Disability Research		
Fund a program of disability research that is commensurate with the need.	U.S. Congress, NIDRR, NIH, VHA, CDC	6.1 7.1 10.1 10.2
Increase the visibility and coordination of disability research.	U.S. Congress, CDC, U.S. Department of Education, ICDR	10.2 10.3
Access to Health Care and Support Services		
Improve accessibility in health care facilities and strengthen implementation of the Americans with Disabilities Act.	U.S. Congress, U.S. Department of Justice, accrediting agencies, Access Board	6.2 6.3
Reduce barriers to health insurance for people with disabilities.	U.S. Congress	8.1 8.2
Make needed assistive services technologies more available.	Research agencies U.S. Congress, DHHS	7.2 9.1
Promote models of coordinated chronic care and other strategies to support the transition of young people to adult health care.	Policy makers, professional societies, public and private payers Congress, SSA, CDC, Department of Education; MCHB	4.1 4.2
Public and Professional Education		
Develop evidence reviews and other tools to support health professionals in caring for people with disabilities.	AHRQ, professional societies, educators, others	4.2 5.1 5.2
Launch a campaign to increase public and professional awareness of assistive and accessible technologies.	CDC, NIDRR	7.3

NOTE: CDC = Centers for Disease Control and Prevention; BLS = Bureau of Labor Statistics, NIH = National Institutes of Health; NIDRR = National Institute on Disability and Rehabilitation Research; AHRQ = Agency for Healthcare Research and Quality; VHA = Veterans Health Administration; DHHS = U.S. Department of Health and Human Services; ICDR = Interagency Committee on Disability Research; MCHB = Maternal and Child Health Bureau; Access Board = Architectural and Transportation Barriers Compliance Board; SSA = Social Security Administration.

disability monitoring and research, promoting improvements in the framework, and working to align measures of disability with the ICF. Achieving agreement on concepts for describing and measuring different aspects of disability should increase the comparability of research findings and make research more useful for decision makers. Directions for improving the ICF framework include further development of the classification of environmental and personal factors that contribute to disability.

Although national and international efforts to develop these refinements are important and although it would be desirable to achieve resolution of these and other issues through WHO, U.S. agencies and researchers can act—as many are already doing—to apply the ICF concepts and terminology. This report follows the ICF by using "disability" as an umbrella term for physical or mental impairments (e.g., limitations in joint mobility), activity limitations (e.g., limitations in dressing), and participation restrictions (e.g., restrictions in working).

Create a comprehensive disability monitoring system.

The lack of a comprehensive disability monitoring program, highlighted in the 1991 IOM report, remains a serious shortcoming in the nation's health statistics system. Today, disability statistics must be patched together from multiple, often inconsistent surveys. The committee's review suggests that, overall, monitoring efforts continue to fall short of providing the nation with the basic data that it needs to monitor disability and manage for the future.

DISABILITY RESEARCH

Fund a program of clinical, health services, social, behavioral, and other disability research that is commensurate with the need.

Since 1997, rehabilitation and disability research has made some gains at the federal level. Funding has increased modestly for the National Institute on Disability and Rehabilitation Research (NIDRR), the National Center for Medical Rehabilitation Research (NCMRR), and the Rehabilitation Research and Development Service of the Veterans Health Administration. Overall, however, disability research continues to be funded at levels inconsistent with the current and projected impact of disability on individuals, families, and communities. Spending remains highly skewed toward basic and clinical research, with inadequate support for research on the physical, social, and other environmental contributors to disability and insufficient attention to the evaluation of interventions to minimize activity limitations and participation restrictions. In addition to further research in these areas, another priority is the identification of better strategies to develop and bring to market improved assistive technologies and accessible mainstream technologies.

Increase the visibility and coordination of federally supported disability research.

Disability research continues to lack adequate visibility and recognition within federal research agencies. This report reiterates the call for actions to address this problem made in the 1997 report. Among other steps, it proposes that the U.S. Congress consider making NCMRR a full institute or freestanding center within the National Institutes of Health. A similar step would be the creation of an Office of Disability and Health in the director's office at CDC to work with and support the Disability and Health Team in the Center for Birth Defects and Developmental Disabilities and to more fully integrate disability issues into CDC programs.

Inadequate coordination of disability research, highlighted in the 1997 IOM report, also remains a problem. With tighter federal budgets, the advantages of coordination—to avoid an insufficient emphasis on important issues as well as wasteful duplication—are even more important today than they were in 1997. The report recommends a more active role for the existing Interagency Committee on Disability Research in coordinating the identification and administration of high-priority, multiagency research.

ACCESS TO HEALTH CARE AND SUPPORT SERVICES

Improve the accessibility of health care facilities and strengthen implementation of the provisions of the ADA related to health care facilities.

Accessible environments are a matter of equity for adults and children with disabilities. People with mobility, sensory, or other impairments should expect that health care facilities will be accessible. Instead, these facilities often present significant barriers to the receipt of timely, high-quality health care.

Both public and private groups can act to improve access to health care facilities and equipment and strengthen the levels of awareness of and compliance with the relevant provisions of the ADA. The U.S. Department of Justice should continue to vigorously pursue and publicize effective settlements and, if necessary, the litigation of complaints of accessibility violations by major health care institutions. It should also issue and widely disseminate guidelines for health care professionals and executives that describe the government's expectations for compliance with the ADA. Likewise, the Joint Commission and other organizations that accredit health care organizations or that set federal program participation conditions should consider a facility's level of compliance with federal accessibility standards and guidelines in their accreditation and participation decisions. In addition, the Architectural and Transportation Barriers Compliance Board (Access Board) should develop standards for accessible medical equipment to be supported with technical assistance, dissemination, and enforcement by appropriate federal agencies.

Reduce barriers to health insurance for people with disabilities.

Although people with disabilities are slightly more likely than others to have health insurance, especially through public programs, access to insurance is not universal, especially among working-age individuals. To reduce the hardships facing many working-age people who have newly qualified for Social Security Disability Insurance (SSDI), the U.S. Congress should reduce or eliminate the waiting period between the time SSDI benefits start and eligibility for Medicare. The U.S. Congress and federal administrative agencies should also continue to test modifications in SSDI and Supplemental Security Income rules that would encourage people who are able to return to work to do so without losing Medicare or Medicaid coverage.

One persistent problem with government efforts to promote competition among managed care and other health plans and to enroll people with disabilities in such plans is that the methods that Medicare and Medicaid use to pay health plans have overpaid for individuals with few health conditions and underpaid for people with serious health conditions or disabilities. Despite recent improvements in Medicare's method for the risk adjustment of health plan payments, it remains financially more attractive for health plans to seek low-risk beneficiaries than to provide efficient, high-quality care to people with chronic health conditions and disabilities. The U.S. Congress should continue to support the research needed to improve risk adjustment methods.

Make needed assistive services and technologies more available to people with disabilities.

Research suggests that assistive technologies are playing important and increasingly prevalent roles in the lives of people with disabilities. Research agencies should further investigate strategies that can counter the current weak incentives for developing better assistive technologies and bringing them to market.

The committee recommends that policy makers eliminate or modify the "in-home-use" requirement for Medicare coverage of durable medical equipment and revise coverage criteria to consider the contribution of a technology to an individual's independence and participation in community life, including work. Policy makers should also investigate new approaches for supplying covered technologies and providing timely and appropriate repairs to equipment that is damaged or not working.

Promote models of coordinated chronic care and other strategies for improving the transition of young people from pediatric to adult health care.

For many young people with disabilities, the transition from pediatric to adult health care brings many challenges. These challenges include the fragmented organization and financing of health care, dysfunctional provider reimbursement methods, and the limited adoption of sophisticated information technology to support information exchange among the generalists and the specialists who care for young people with complex health conditions.

The convergence of the medical home model of care for children with special health care needs and the chronic care model designed primarily with adults in mind offers great promise. If the principles and practices underlying these models were widely adopted, young people would be much more likely to receive the comprehensive assessments, guidance, and services that correspond to the recommendations of professional societies for managing the transition from pediatric to adult health care. Among other steps needed to support the successful movement of young people from pediatric to adult care, the U.S. Congress should extend Medicaid and State Children's Health Insurance Program coverage through age 21 for all beneficiaries with chronic conditions or disabilities and should specify that program benefits cover appropriate transition assessment, coordination, and management services for these young people.

PUBLIC AND PROFESSIONAL EDUCATION

Develop educational programs, evidence-based reviews, practice guidelines, and other materials to support health professionals in caring for people with disabilities.

Health care professionals are not necessarily well informed about the primary health care needs of people with disabilities, the prevention and management of secondary health conditions, the challenges that adults face in aging with disabilities, and the transition of young people with disabilities from pediatric to adult services. Among other actions, this report recommends strengthening education in chronic illness and disability management in curricula for health care professionals, including education on the specific topics of secondary conditions and aging with disability.

To increase awareness of the secondary conditions and premature aging associated with many chronic health conditions and disabilities, the report also encourages the development of systematic reviews of existing evidence, and the identification of knowledge gaps. These reviews can be used as the basis for collaborative efforts by professional societies, people with disabilities, and others to formulate evidence-based guidelines clinical practice guidelines, guides for consumers, and other educational materials.

Launch a national public health campaign to increase public and health care professional awareness of assistive and accessible technologies.

Health care professionals also face difficulties in keeping abreast of developments in assistive technologies and their effective use. People with disabilities may themselves be unaware of technologies that could help them lead easier and more independent lives. The report recommends that the CDC collaborate with other public and private groups to launch a national campaign to increase public and health care professional awareness and acceptance of assistive and accessible technologies that can benefit people with disabilities.

CHOOSING THE FUTURE FOR DISABILITY IN AMERICA

Given the demographic, societal, and disability trends outlined above and discussed in detail within this report, a critical question is: how will Americans individually and collectively make the choices that will help define the future of disability? That is, will the country commit to actions to limit the development and progression of physical and mental impairments in late life, promote good health for children and young adults with early-onset disability, and reduce environmental barriers for people with existing impairments? The record of the past 17 years offers reasons for serious concern, especially given the cost projections for public programs that are critical to people with disabilities.

The trade-offs or choices that Americans make about future spending will reflect their fundamental values about the balance between community and individual responsibility. Still, it should be recognized that health, social, and other policies that assist people with disabilities do not only represent current transfers of resources from those without disabilities to those with disabilities—or from mostly younger people to mostly older people. Over their life spans, the majority of Americans will experience disabilities or will have family members who do. People may not realize it, but the support that they give today for policies that affect future funding for disability-related programs is a statement about the level of support that they can expect at later stages in their own lives.

This report underscores the growing evidence that disability is not an unavoidable consequence of injury and chronic disease but is substantially affected by the actions that society takes—in the public arena and in commerce and other private domains. Ultimately, the future of disability in America rests with Americans.

COMPLETE LIST OF RECOMMENDATIONS

Disability Monitoring

Recommendation 2.1: The National Center for Health Statistics, the U.S. Census Bureau, the Bureau of Labor Statistics, and other relevant government units involved in disability monitoring should adopt the *International Classification of Functioning, Health and Disability* (ICF) as their conceptual framework and should actively promote continued refinements to improve the framework's scope and utility for disability monitoring and research. The Interagency Subcommittee on Disability Statistics of the Interagency Committee on Disability Research should coordinate the work of these agencies to develop, test, validate, and implement new measures of disability that correspond to the components of the ICF, consistent with public policy priorities.

Recommendation 2.2: The National Center for Health Statistics, in collaboration with other relevant federal agencies, should continue to improve the scope and quality of data—including longitudinal or panel data—on disability, its causes, and its consequences. These improved data sources should serve as the cornerstone of a new national disability monitoring system.

Health Care Transitions, Secondary Conditions, and Aging with Disability

Recommendation 4.1: To improve the transition of young people with disabilities from pediatric to adult health care, policy makers, professional societies, public and private payers, and educators should work to
- align and strengthen incentives in public and private health care programs to support coordinated care and transition planning;
- expand the use of integrated electronic medical records for chronic disease management and during the transition of young people with disabilities from pediatric to adult health care; and
- expand chronic care education in pediatric and internal medicine

residency programs and add skills in the management of individuals with chronic health care needs to specialty board requirements.

Recommendation 4.2: To support the successful transition of young people with disabilities from pediatric to adult health care and independent living, the U.S. Congress should

• extend Medicaid and State Children's Health Insurance Program (SCHIP) coverage through age 21 for children with disabilities and specify that Medicaid and SCHIP benefits cover transition assessments, coordination, and management services for these young people;

• fund the U.S. Maternal and Child Health Bureau to expand its work to develop and implement medical home and other services for young people with special health care needs who are over age 21 and who need continued transition support;

• revise the Ticket to Work program by lowering the eligibility age to 16 years and directing the U.S. Department of Education and the Social Security Administration to develop guidance for the coordination of Ticket to Work services with the transition services and supports provided under the Individuals with Disabilities Education Act; and

• direct the Centers for Disease Control and Prevention to work with other relevant agencies to examine opportunities for the monitoring of transitions through additions to state and national youth surveys or other cross-sectional and longitudinal data collection efforts.

Recommendation 5.1: The U.S. Congress should direct and fund the Agency for Healthcare Research and Quality so that it may take the lead in

• evaluating the evidence base to support the development of clinical practice guidelines, quality goals, and monitoring standards for the prevention and management of secondary health conditions among people with disabilities and for the monitoring and management of people aging with disability;

• evaluating the evidence base about environmental contributors to secondary health conditions; and

• identifying research gaps and directions for further research on secondary health conditions and aging with disability.

Recommendation 5.2: As part of broader efforts to improve the quality of care provided to people with disabilities, health care professionals, educators, people with disabilities, and their family members should work together to

• develop, disseminate, and apply guidelines for the prevention and management of secondary conditions and for the monitoring and care of people aging with disability;

- design educational modules and other curriculum tools for all relevant types of health care professionals and all levels of education; and
- develop competency standards for these educational programs.

Environmental Barriers

Recommendation 6.1: Given the limited research on the effects of environmental factors on disability, the National Institute on Disability and Rehabilitation Research, the National Institutes of Health, the Veterans Health Administration, the Centers for Disease Control and Prevention, and other relevant agencies should collaborate to develop a program of research in this area. As part of developing such a program, these agencies should

- organize a symposium to engage people with disabilities, relevant governmental agencies, researchers, methodologists, and other interested parties in a collaborative process to recommend priorities for research on environmental factors, as defined in the *International Classification of Functioning, Disability and Health*;
- apply these priorities in a plan for outcomes research to investigate the relative effects of different aspects of the environment on disability; and
- intensify current efforts to improve epidemiological, observational, and experimental measures and methods to assess the effects of specific environmental features on independence, participation, and quality of life over the short term and long term for people with disabilities.

Recommendation 6.2: To improve the accessibility of health care facilities and equipment and to strengthen the awareness of and compliance with the provisions of the Americans with Disabilities Act related to accessible health care facilities,

- the U.S. Department of Justice should continue to vigorously pursue and publicize effective settlements and litigation (if necessary) of complaints of accessibility violations in major health care institutions;
- the U.S. Department of Justice should issue and widely disseminate guidelines for health care providers that describe expectations for compliance with the accessibility provisions of the act; and
- the Joint Commission and other organizations that accredit or set federal program participation conditions for health care organizations should explicitly consider compliance with federal accessibility standards and guidelines in making their accreditation and participation decisions.

Recommendation 6.3: The U.S. Congress should direct the Architectural and Transportation Barriers Compliance Board (the Access Board)

- to develop standards for accessible medical equipment to be supported with technical assistance and with dissemination and enforcement efforts by the appropriate federal agencies and

- to collaborate with the U.S. Department of Veterans Affairs, groups representing people with disabilities, and other relevant experts to assess whether the accessibility standards developed by the Access Board are appropriate for health care facilities serving people with disabilities and an aging population.

Assistive and Accessible Technologies

Recommendation 7.1: Federal agencies that support research on assistive technologies should collaborate on a program of research to improve strategies to identify, develop, and bring to market new or better assistive technologies for people with disabilities. Such research should involve consumers, manufacturers, medical and technical experts, and other relevant agencies and stakeholders.

Recommendation 7.2: To extend the benefits of accessibility provided by existing federal statutes and regulations, the U.S. Congress should direct the Architectural and Transportation Barriers Compliance Board (the Access Board) to collaborate with relevant public and private groups to develop a plan for establishing accessibility standards for important mainstream and general use products and technologies. The plan should

- propose criteria and processes for designating high-priority product areas for standard setting;
- identify existing public or private standards or guidelines that might be useful in setting standards; and
- include medical equipment as an initial priority area.

Recommendation 7.3: The Centers for Disease Control and Prevention, working with the National Institute on Disability and Rehabilitation Research, should launch a major public health campaign to increase public and health professional awareness and acceptance of assistive technologies and accessible mainstream technologies that can benefit people with different kinds of disabilities.

Recommendation 8.1: The U.S. Congress should support continued research and data collection efforts to

- evaluate and improve the accuracy and fairness of methods of risk adjusting payments to health plans serving Medicare and Medicaid beneficiaries with disabilities;
- assess how these methods affect the quality of care for people with disabilities, including those enrolled in special needs plans; and

- evaluate differences in the risk adjustment methods that state Medicaid programs use to pay health plans that enroll people with disabilities.

Recommendation 8.2: To improve access to health insurance for people with disabilities, the U.S. Congress should
- adopt a plan to reduce or eliminate the 24-month waiting period for Medicare eligibility for people who have newly qualified for Social Security Disability Insurance;
- encourage continued testing of methods to reduce disincentives in public insurance programs for people with disabilities to return to work; and
- direct states to limit recertification and reenrollment for the State Children's Health Insurance Program to no more than once a year for children with disabilities.

Recommendation 9.1: The U.S. Congress and the U.S. Department of Health and Human Services should begin a process of revising Medicare and Medicaid laws and regulations and other relevant policies to make needed assistive services and technologies more available to people with disabilities and to put more emphasis on beneficiaries' functional capacities, quality of life, and ability to participate in work, school, and other areas of community life. Priorities include
- eliminating or modifying Medicare's "in-home-use" requirement for durable medical equipment and revising coverage criteria to consider the contribution of these devices and equipment to an individual's independence and participation in community life;
- evaluating new approaches for supplying assistive technologies (such as time-limited rentals and recycling of used equipment) and providing timely and appropriate equipment repairs; and
- continuing research to assess and improve the appropriateness, quality, and cost-effectiveness of the assistive services and technologies provided to people with disabilities.

Organizing and Financing Disability Research

Recommendation 10.1: Federal agencies should invest in a coordinated program to develop, test, and disseminate promising interventions, practices, and programs to minimize activity limitations and participation restrictions and improve the quality of life of people with disabilities.

Recommendation 10.2: To support a program of disability research that is commensurate with the need for better knowledge about all aspects of disability at the individual and the societal levels, the U.S. Congress should increase the total amount of public funding provided for disability research. To strengthen the management and raise the profile of this research, the U.S. Congress should also consider

- elevating the National Center for Medical Rehabilitation Research to the status of a full institute or freestanding center within the National Institutes of Health with its own budget;
- creating an Office of Disability and Health in the Director's Office at the Centers for Disease Control and Prevention (CDC) to promote the integration of disability issues into all CDC programs; and
- directing the U.S. Department of Education to support the National Institute on Disability and Rehabilitation Research in continuing to upgrade its research review process and grants program administration.

Recommendation 10.3: To facilitate cross-agency strategic planning and priority setting around disability research and to expand efforts to reduce duplication across agencies engaged in disability research, the U.S. Congress should authorize and fund the Interagency Committee on Disability Research to

- undertake a government-wide inventory of disability research activities using the *International Classification of Functioning, Disability and Health*;
- identify underemphasized or duplicative areas of research;
- develop priorities for research that would benefit from multiagency collaboration;
- collaborate with individual agencies to review, fund, and administer this research portfolio; and
- appoint a public-private advisory committee that actively involves people with disabilities and other relevant stakeholders to provide advice on the activities described above.

1

Introduction

Having a disability shapes a person's life, but it is not their total destiny.

Senator Robert Dole (1999)

Disability is not destiny for either individuals or the communities in which they live. Rather, disability is shaped by personal and collective choices. Positive choices made today not only can prevent the onset of many potentially disabling conditions but also can mitigate their effects and help create more supportive physical and social environments that promote a future of increased independence and integration for people with disabilities.

The future of disability in America is not a minority issue. If one considers people who now have disabilities, people who are likely to develop disabilities in the future, and people who are or who will be affected by the disabilities of those close to them, then disability affects today or will affect tomorrow the lives of most Americans. Current statistics suggest that the number of people with disabilities living in the community or in institutional settings now totals more than 40 million (between 13 and 14 percent of the population) and perhaps as many as 50 million if a more expansive definition of disability is used (see Chapter 3). In addition, in 1999, nearly 18 million adults had an older spouse or parent with a disability, and almost 4 million provided care to such a family member living

16

in the community (Spillman and Black, 2005a). Millions more people have children, siblings, or other younger family members with disabilities; and many provide informal care to these family members or to younger or older friends (Pandya, 2005).

DISABILITY AND RELATED SOCIETAL TRENDS

What was a real—but still decades off—demographic projection in 1991 when the Institute of Medicine (IOM) report *Disability in America* was published is now a much more urgent concern as the initial movement of the post-World War II baby boom generation into late life is about to begin. People born in 1946 will turn age 65 in 2011. The future of disability in America will, in considerable measure, depend on the country's response to this demographic shift, which will substantially increase the numbers of people and the proportion of the population most at risk for disability. For people age 65 and over who live in the community, the percentage of individuals with disabilities is now approximately 40 percent, a figure that is three times that for younger people. A majority of those over age 85 experience disabilities.

The percentage of the population ages 65 years and over will increase from approximately 12 percent in 2000 to almost 20 percent in 2030—or from almost 35 million people to more than 71 million (U.S. Census Bureau, 2004). The number of people age 85 or over is expected to grow from approximately 4.3 million (1.5 percent of the population) to approximately 9.6 million (2.6 percent of the population). Chapter 3 provides projections for the rates of disability among those ages 65 and over.

Although older age is a major risk factor for disability, millions of younger people also live with disabilities. In 2004, more than 4 million children and young people between the ages of 5 and 20 years (6.5 percent) had disabilities (U.S. Census Bureau, 2005a). In the same year, some 20 million people ages 21 to 64 years, or approximately 12.1 percent of the total population in that age group, reported disabilities. Although the risk of an individual experiencing disability is lower in this age group than it is in the older age group, the total number of younger adults with disabilities currently exceeds the total for the population ages 65 and over. The younger group includes many people who have conditions that were once fatal in childhood and who are now experiencing premature or atypical aging related to their condition, its management, or other environmental factors. As discussed in Chapter 5, these individuals are moving into uncharted territory.

Another concern for the future is that the prevalence of health problems and disabilities for American adults who are now in early and midlife may be increasing. The percentage of Americans ages 18 to 64 with reported activity limitations grew during the 1990s (NCHS, 2005a). In addition, the prevalence of certain conditions that contribute to disability—notably, physical inactivity, diabetes, and obesity—is increasing in this age group; and surveys also show a worrisome increase in overweight or obesity among children (Federal Interagency Forum on Child and Family Statistics, 2005; NCHS, 2005a). These trends raise concerns that when people now in early or midlife enter late life, they may experience more disability than the current cohort of people over age 65.

Beyond a substantial increase in the number of people in the American population most at risk of disability, the changing age distribution of the American population has other important implications for the future of disability in America. The Social Security Administration estimates that in 2031 the United States will have 2.1 workers for each Social Security beneficiary, compared to approximately 3.3 today (SSA, 2007b; see also SSA [2006c]). This projected decrease in the worker-to-beneficiary ratio underlies well-publicized concerns about the long-term financial future of Social Security, Medicare, and other programs that assist older Americans and that also aid many younger Americans who have serious physical or mental impairments. To the extent that impairments and limitations re-lated to aging can be delayed or reduced, the expectation that many older individuals may need to work beyond the ages now specified for full Social Security benefits (age 67 for those born after 1959) will more easily be met (SSA, 2005b).

The changing age distribution of the population likewise explains con-cerns about ability of the future workforce to provide paid long-term care services for the growing numbers of older and younger people with serious disabilities. One estimate is that this workforce would need to grow at an annual rate of 2 percent to maintain the current ratio of long-term care workers for the population age 85 or older, a growth rate that is almost seven times the 0.3 percent rate of growth projected for the working-age population overall (Friedland, 2004). Recent years have seen a rapid in-crease in the number of workers providing personal care services and a less sharp increase in the number of nursing home and residential care aides, but data suggest that only one worker is available for every 10 potential consumers (Kaye et al., 2006).

As essential as paid caregivers are, family members—primarily wives, mothers, daughters, and daughters-in-law—have traditionally provided the great majority of care for older and younger people with disabilities. This source of support is under pressure from the post-baby boom reduction in family size, decreases in marriage rates and increases in divorce rates, and growth in the participation of women in the paid workforce during recent decades.

The average size of the American family dropped from 3.58 in 1970 to 3.14 in 2000, and the drop would have been even larger without the country's young immigrant families (Day, 1996; Simmons and O'Neill, 2001). In addition, the percentage of people who have no children has grown. For example, among women ages 40 to 44, the percentage with no children rose from 10.2 percent in 1976 to 19.3 percent in 2004 (U.S. Census Bureau, 2005b). Elderly people in the future will have fewer children to rely on for assistance, and lower rates of marriage and higher rates of divorce will limit the availability of spouses as caregivers (DHHS/U.S. Department of Labor, 2003).

Informal caregiving is also under pressure from the increases in the rates of female workforce participation. Between 1970 and 2000, the percentage of women who were in the labor force grew from 43 to 61 percent, although this trend seems to be leveling off (Population Reference Bureau, 2005). Paid employment, even full-time employment, certainly does not preclude a caregiving role, but it can make the role more difficult. One survey indicated that almost half of informal caregivers ages 50 to 64 who provided care for someone age 18 or over were employed full time (Pandya, 2005).

A 2004 survey reported that 61 percent of family caregivers for people ages 18 and over were women, down from a reported 73 percent in a 1997 survey (NAC/AARP, 1997, 2004). Women, however, represented a higher proportion of those providing the most intense levels of care. At the same time that they disproportionately provide care, women who themselves need care are the most vulnerable to the lack of family caregivers, in part because many women outlive their older husbands. Almost three-quarters of long-term nursing home residents are female (NCHS, 2005a).

In the future, assistive technology—from advanced technologies that monitor individuals in their homes to memory aids to relatively simple devices such as canes and walkers—likely will play an important role in supporting independence for older adults and reducing their need for personal caregiving. Researchers have reported that between 1984 and 1999 the use of formal or informal caregiving for older adults with disabilities declined, with especially steep drops from 1995 to 1999 (Spillman and Black, 2005a; see also Freedman et al. [2006]). They concluded that the decline is associated with an increase in the reported use of walkers, shower seats, and other assistive technologies, especially among older people who had neither a spouse nor children to provide informal caregiving.

ORIGIN OF STUDY TASKS AND OVERVIEW OF REPORT

The idea for this study emerged from discussions with the Centers for Disease Control and Prevention (CDC) about an examination of developments since the publication of *Disability in America* (IOM, 1991) and the subsequent 1997 IOM report *Enabling America*. The study began with a workshop in 2005 and a workshop report that included the papers presented at the workshop (IOM, 2006b). For the study's second phase, CDC enlisted support from the National Institute on Disability and Rehabilitation Research (U.S. Department of Education) and the National Center for Medical Rehabilitation Research (National Institutes of Health). As part of an examination of the developments that have taken place since the publication of the 1991 and 1997 reports and as agreed upon with the study's sponsors, the study focused on several topics, including

- Methodological and policy issues related to the definition, measurement, and monitoring of disability
- Trends in the amount, types, and causes of disability
- Secondary health conditions and aging with disability
- Transitions for young people from pediatric to adult health care services
- Assistive technologies and supportive physical environments
- Coverage of assistive technologies and risk adjustment of payments to health plans by Medicare and other payers
- Directions for research

To undertake this study, the IOM, which is the health policy arm of the National Academy of Sciences, appointed a 14-member committee of experts. As wide-ranging as the study topics are, they could not include many issues important to people with disabilities, policy makers, clinicians, researchers, and others interested in the future of disability in America. For example, to have investigated the financial dimensions of each of the study topics would have required a report in itself (perhaps more than one). Assessing just the public and private financing of assistive services and technologies proved a remarkably time-consuming task. To cite another example, a number of aspects of long-term care that are important to people with disabilities are not examined in depth; long-term care was, however, the focus of another IOM report, *Improving the Quality of Long-Term Care* (2001c). Also, when the present study was being planned, another project to examine formal and informal caregiving for people needing personal assistance was planned, so that topic was not included in this study. (That project has not, however, been funded.) Furthermore, during the course of its work, the committee found that the time and resources available to it would not allow a comprehensive review of certain issues, in particular, the broad range of environmental factors that contribute to disability.

One intended audience for this report includes administrative and legislative policy makers and those who advise them about programs, policies, and research priorities that affect people with disabilities and their families. Other audiences include health care professionals, researchers, and advocacy groups. Although this report and its recommendations are aimed at these groups, the committee has tried to make the discussion relevant and understandable to a broader public.

This report focuses on the United States. However, consistent with discussions with the project's sponsors, the next chapter selectively considers concepts of disability developed as part of an international consensus-building process. It endorses the use of those concepts as the basis for a common conceptual framework for disability research and policy.

The remainder of this chapter provides a brief overview of encouraging and disappointing developments since the publication of the 1991 IOM report and the choices ahead. It also places disability in public health and policy contexts. Chapter 2 examines different definitions of disability, presents the conceptual framework adopted by the committee, and provides an assessment of the system for monitoring disability in America. Chapter 3 describes trends in disability in early, middle, and late life. Chapter 4 emphasizes the importance of considering disability across the life span as the context for a discussion of one important health care transition: the transition for young people from pediatric health care to adult health care. Chapter 5 discusses secondary health conditions and aging with disability.

The focus of Chapters 6 and 7 is how the physical environment and technologies contribute to disability or to independence and participation in the community. Chapters 8 and 9 examine several issues related to the financing of health care for people with disabilities, including coverage of assistive technologies and services and methods for adjusting payments to health insurance plans so that they fairly reflect the expected costliness of the plan enrollees. Chapter 10 discusses the organization and financing of disability-related research.

Appendix A includes more information about the committee's charge and activities. Appendix B includes the table of contents for the committee's 2006 workshop report, and Appendix H includes short biographies of the committee members. The report also includes several substantive appendixes. Appendix C supplements Chapter 8 with a detailed discussion of the methods of risk adjustment of payments to health plans. Appendixes D through G provide supplementary information about the policy environment relevant to people with disabilities in the areas of employment, health, transportation, and telecommunications.

DEVELOPMENTS SINCE PUBLICATION OF
THE 1991 AND 1997 IOM REPORTS

The 1991 and 1997 IOM reports highlighted disability as a topic of scientific inquiry and public health action.[1] A significant feature of the 1991 IOM report was its advocacy for a comprehensive national approach to disability prevention based on a more environmentally focused and less individually and medically focused model of the processes that create or reverse disability. It also called for new collaborations among researchers and public and private health care groups and for innovations in the organization and delivery of health care services. The 1997 IOM report stressed the importance of recognizing rehabilitation science and rehabilitation engineering as legitimate scientific fields of study. It recommended a range of efforts aimed at strengthening the science base and the transfer of technology to prevent disability and improving the health, productivity, and quality of life for individuals with disabilities. In discussing developments since the earlier reports, the current report focuses more on developments since publication of the 1991 report and less on those since publication of the 1997 report, which was narrower in focus.

The nation has seen important progress since 1991. Studies indicate that the incidence of certain types of late-life disability has declined during the last two decades, although the reasons for these decreases and their implications have generated debate (see Chapter 3). As noted earlier, however, data for younger populations raise concerns that this trend of declining disability in late life may not continue.

In addition, advances in science and engineering increasingly allow people to overcome or compensate for physical or mental impairments through medical interventions, assistive technologies, or environmental modifications. Scientists and clinicians know more today about the nature, extent, and management of many secondary health conditions such as pressure ulcers that can—if they are not prevented or successfully treated—become more limiting and dangerous than the initial, primary health condition. Diverse preventive measures have contributed to reductions in the incidence of certain kinds of injuries, developmental disabilities, and other health

---

[1]Earlier, in 1976, the National Research Council of the National Academy of Sciences issued the report *Science and Technology in the Service of the Physically Handicapped* (NRC, 1976). In transmitting the report to the Congress, the president of the Academy said, "The concern of the National Academy of Sciences for the needs of the disabled and handicapped members of our society has deep roots, dating back to World War II when the Academy undertook a program to improve the quality and availability of prosthetic and orthotic devices for military amputees" (p. iii). Subsequent work extended that concern from veterans to all people with disabilities. The 1976 report dealt with children as well as adults and with many issues similar to those addressed in the present report, especially strengthening research and development and making assistive technologies more available.

conditions that can contribute to disability. Although the amounts invested in disability research are very modest compared with the amounts invested in biomedical research and are quite small given the impact of disability on individuals and communities, more social and behavioral research is available to guide understanding of how physical and social environments shape disability and how environments can be made more supportive. In addition to continuing efforts to prevent potentially disabling injuries and illnesses, continuing efforts to minimize the unwanted consequences of such conditions on people's lives are critical. Strategies for doing so are discussed in the report chapters devoted to discussions of secondary conditions, environmental barriers, assistive and accessible technologies, and financing of assistive services and equipment.

Many technological advances that affect consumers and workers overall have had liberating consequences for people with disabilities. For example, improvements in computer technology and electronic communications (combined with reductions in the costs of these technologies) make it much more feasible—if not common—for many people with disabilities to telecommute, which relieves employees of both the physical challenges and the time demands of traveling to workplaces. In the future, technological innovations and employment policies that provide additional work flexibility and accommodations at work should make it easier for both younger and older people with disabilities to be employed. For older workers with chronic health conditions, such accommodation could reduce the impact of the scheduled and potential future increases in the age at which full Social Security benefits are available.

Despite advances in science and technology, a critical question is whether the research gains achieved since 1991 have been translated into public and private policy and practice in the United States. Has society—in the form of government officials, clinicians, employers, and others—possessed the awareness, the resources, and the will to apply existing knowledge? This report describes a number of areas in which the application of existing knowledge is limited, and it discusses more generally the very modest progress made over the past two decades toward the adoption of several public policy and practice recommendations made in the 1991 and 1997 IOM reports.

For example, Medicare, Medicaid, and other health plans still significantly restrict access to the health care services, assistive technologies, and personal care services that can enhance independence and make it easier for people with physical and cognitive impairments to be productive and active members of their communities. Nonetheless, changes in the federal-state Medicaid program have—with some impetus from the U.S. Supreme Court—have reduced the imbalance between resources allocated for institutional care and resources for home- and community-based services for people of limited means who are seriously limited in their self-care abilities.

Even when services are covered by Medicare or other plans, physicians and others may lack the knowledge, motivation, and organizational or system support to appropriately assist individuals with disabilities with maintaining and improving their health and well-being and in managing age-related physical and cognitive changes. Some of the shortcomings in professional practice reflect the shortcomings in health care professions education.

During the past 40 years and more, the creation of accessible environments that promote independence and community participation has become a focal point of advocacy by and for people with disabilities. The 1991 IOM report particularly stressed the interaction between individual characteristics and environmental barriers in creating disability. Despite progress, significant environmental barriers remain, sometimes in places where one would not expect them, for example, in hospitals and health care professional offices that lack buildings, equipment, and services suitable for people with physical mobility, sensory, and other impairments. Outside the health care sphere, many public transportation systems, buildings, and neighborhoods still present barriers and even hazards to people with disabilities. As discussed in Chapter 7 and Appendix F, policies requiring accessibility are not always updated to cover new technologies, such as certain Internet communication tools. High rates of unemployment—and disincentives to employment—are a continuing problem for people with disabilities.

In 1991, the Americans with Disabilities Act (ADA) was new and a source of great hope. This law—in combination with other antidiscrimination policies and some state and local policies—has helped to increase the recognition of environmental obstacles to full participation in community life by people with disabilities. At the same time, as described in Appendixes D and E, limited resources for enforcement and several restrictive judicial interpretations of the law make the ADA one source among many of the missed opportunities that have left the future of disability in doubt.

The 1991 report noted that disability (in the form of activity limitations) was associated with lower income, although it noted different possible explanations for this relationship. Differences in survey questions make direct comparisons difficult, but disparities clearly remain. For example, based on census data for 2005, 25 percent of working-age people with disabilities and 9 percent of people without disabilities live in poverty (Houtenville, 2006). Seventy percent of working-age people without disabilities live in owner-occupied housing, whereas 62 percent of people with disabilities do so. The data reported in Chapter 3 show an increasing gap between the levels of employment for people with and people without activity limitations.

The 1997 report bluntly stated that the combined federal research effort in the area of disability was not adequate to address the current and future needs of people with disabilities and that more funding would be required to expand research to meet those needs. Notwithstanding modest increases in funding during the late 1990s, the situation remains essentially the same 10 years later. Disability research is a miniscule item in the federal government's research budget that is not in line with either the current or the projected future impact of disability on individuals, families, and American society.

Despite the important conceptual contributions achieved by the time of publication of the 1991 and 1997 reports, the absence of universally accepted and understood terminology and concepts with which to describe and discuss disability continues to hamper clear communication. Responding to these ongoing concerns and to increasing interest worldwide in monitoring and measuring disability, the World Health Organization released the *International Classification of Functioning, Disability and Health* (ICF) in 2001. The ICF was a major revision of the organization's 1980 classification, and it involved an international process of consultation and consensus building (WHO, 2001). As discussed further in Chapter 2, this report employs the language and concepts of the ICF framework and recommends the widespread adoption and further development of the framework to provide a common, international language for data collection and research to inform policies and programs that promote the independence and integration into the community of people with disabilities.

CHOOSING THE FUTURE OF DISABILITY IN AMERICA

The shortcomings just summarized raise serious questions about how individuals, families, and society in general will cope in coming decades when these deficiencies are combined with projections of significant increases in the population most at risk of disability; possible shortages in the caregiving workforce; and escalating costs for programs such as Medicare, and Medicaid. This report argues that further actions—taken sooner rather than later—can help this nation avoid the most harmful and inequitable outcomes and achieve positive improvements in the ability of people with disabilities to lead independent, fulfilling, and productive lives. Doing so will require more intensive efforts to build on past successes, for example, by more fully developing and taking advantage of research and technological advances to promote healthy aging and prevent or limit health conditions and environmental barriers that contribute to disability. It will also require a greater societal commitment to fulfilling the promise of the ADA and ending discrimination against people with disabilities.

Given the demographic, societal, and disability trends outlined above and discussed in detail in this report, how will U.S. society make the choices that will help define the future of disability? Will the country commit to actions to limit the development and progression of physical and mental impairments in late life, promote good health for children and young adults with early-onset disabilities, and reduce environmental barriers for people with existing impairments? The record of the past 16 years offers some basis for hope but also provides reason for serious concern about the future.

In the coming decades, as the number of Americans living with disabilities continues to increase, costs for health care and other services will increase. Concurrently, the nation will face pressure from other sources of increasing health care costs, which have consistently grown faster than the gross domestic product (Chernew et al, 2005a). Although individuals and families will bear a significant share of the increasing costs (and the noneconomic costs as well), rising costs will stress federal and state governments, which are responsible for Medicare, Medicaid, and other critical programs.

Medicare, Medicaid, and other public health care programs that benefit people with and without disabilities are supported by taxes. Projections of future spending increases for these programs and for income support programs such as Social Security have raised the prospect of difficult trade-offs, such as reduced spending for other purposes or higher taxes, or both. Reducing inefficiency and the inappropriate use of health care services will help, but such reductions are unlikely to eliminate the need for the difficult choices that policy makers recognize need to be made but are, in large measure, delaying.

How Americans make trade-offs or choices about future spending will reflect their fundamental values about the balance between community and individual responsibility. Still, it should be recognized that health, social, and other policies that assist people with disabilities do not represent only current transfers of resources from those without disabilities to those with disabilities or from mostly younger people to mostly older people. Over their life spans, the majority of Americans will experience disabilities or will have a family member who does. People may not realize it, but the support that they give today for policies that affect future funding for disability-related programs is a statement about the level of support that they can expect to receive at later stages in their own lives. These policies will help define the future of disability in America.

This report argues that Americans as a people should take explicit responsibility for defining the future of disability based on a commitment to fully integrating people with disabilities into community life and to developing the knowledge, policies, technologies, and public understanding to support that goal. This report underscores the growing evidence that disability is not an unavoidable consequence of injury and chronic disease but results, in considerable measure, from societal decisions and actions in the public arena as well as in commerce and other private domains. Actions that prevent or reduce rather than create disability include making products and places more accessible to people with disabilities, eliminating policy disincentives for work, financing equitable access to assistive services and technologies, preparing health care professionals to provide appropriate care to people with disabilities, and investing in research to guide the design of policies and practices that promote independence and participation. Ultimately, the future of disability in America rests with Americans.

THE FUTURE OF DISABILITY IN A PUBLIC HEALTH CONTEXT

The future of disability is part of the future of public health because public health initiatives are important to monitor disability trends, prevent primary and secondary disability, and reduce disparities in health and well-being in the population. In a 1988 report, *The Future of Public Health*, another IOM committee noted concerns that "this nation has lost sight of its public health goals" and concluded that "we have slackened our public health vigilance nationwide" and thereby unnecessarily threatened the public's health (IOM, 1988, pp. 1–2). The report cited chronic diseases among the "enduring" problems of public health, but it did not really anticipate *Disability in America*, which labeled disability as "the nation's largest public health problem, affecting not only people with disabilities and their immediate families, but also society at large" (IOM, 1991, p. 32).

During the past century and more, public health policies and programs have contributed to major decreases in mortality. In 1900, the age-adjusted death rate in the United States was an estimated 2,518 per 100,000 population (Hoyert and Anderson, 2001), whereas in 2003 the rate was an estimated 831 per 100,000 population (Hoyert et al., 2005). With this success in reducing premature mortality, the public health focus on preventing and reducing morbidity has increased, as has the emphasis on the more positively expressed goal of promoting health.

Specific attention to disability and the health and well-being of people with disabilities has taken more time to evolve. This evolution, which is still incomplete, is illustrated in the history of the Healthy People initiative, which was created by the U.S. Surgeon General in 1979 to establish, promote, and monitor national health objectives. The initial Healthy People objectives focused "primarily on premature death with little attention to premature disability" (Michael Marge, as quoted in a previous IOM report [IOM, 1990b, p. 64]). A few objectives did refer to disability, such as this goal: "To improve the health and quality of life for older adults and, by 1990, to reduce the average annual number of days of restricted activity due to acute and chronic conditions by 20 percent to fewer than 30 days per year for people aged 65 and older" (U.S. Public Health Service, 1979, p. 7-1). *Healthy People 2000* (DHHS, 1990), which was released in 1990, included objectives related to the prevention of certain disabling conditions and the collection of information about disabilities, but the number of such objectives was substantially short of the 32 proposed by an interagency group organized for that purpose (Marge, 1998). (Some objectives were omitted because baseline data with which to measure progress did not exist, and the availability of baseline data was a criterion for the inclusion of an objective.) It was only 2 years before publication of the 1990 report that CDC had emerged (after some hesitation) as the congressionally designated lead agency for a federal disability prevention initiative (Marge, 1999).

The increased awareness of disability as a public health issue is evident in *Healthy People 2010* (DHHS, 2000b). In addition to attention to disability throughout the document, the report devotes a chapter to disability and secondary conditions. That chapter sets forth specific goals, such as increasing the proportion of adults with disabilities who participate in social activities or who report satisfaction with life (Box 1-1). It takes aim at the notion that people with disabilities are necessarily in poor health and that public health should concern itself only with preventing disability rather than also promoting health and well-being among people with disabilities.

In 2005, the U.S. Surgeon General further underscored disability as an important public health concern in his *Call to Action to Improve the Health and Wellness of Persons with Disabilities* (U.S. Public Health Service, 2005). That statement appealed for action to improve the quality of life for people with disabilities and increase their access to disease prevention and health promotion services. It set forth four broad statements describing goals to be achieved (p. 2):

1.   People nationwide understand that persons with disabilities can lead long, healthy, productive lives.

2.   Health care providers have the knowledge and tools to screen, diagnose, and treat the whole person with a disability with dignity.

3.   Persons with disabilities can promote their own good health by developing and maintaining healthy lifestyles.

4.   Accessible health care and support services promote independence for persons with disabilities.

Despite these and other signs of progress since 1991 in the understanding of disability as a public health issue, policy and research on this dimen-

BOX 1-1
Public Health Objectives in *Healthy People 2010*

6-1   Include in the core of all relevant *Healthy People 2010* surveillance in-struments a standardized set of questions that identify "people with disabilities."

6-2   Reduce the proportion of children and adolescents with disabilities who are reported to be sad, unhappy, or depressed.

6-3   Reduce the proportion of adults with disabilities who report feelings such as sadness, unhappiness, or depression that prevent them from being active.

6-4   Increase the proportion of adults with disabilities who participate in social activities.

6-5   Increase the proportion of adults with disabilities reporting sufficient emo-tional support.

6-6   Increase the proportion of adults with disabilities reporting satisfaction with life.

6-7   Reduce the number of people with disabilities in congregate care facilities, consistent with permanency planning principles.

6-8   Eliminate disparities in employment rates between working-aged adults with and without disabilities.

6-9   Increase the proportion of children and youth with disabilities who spend at least 80 percent of their time in regular education programs.

6-10 (In development) Increase the proportion of health and wellness and treatment programs and facilities that provide full access for people with disabilities.*

6-11 (In development) Reduce the proportion of people with disabilities who report not having the assistive devices and technology needed.*

6-12 (In development) Reduce the proportion of people with disabilities reporting environmental barriers to participation in home, school, work, or community activities.*

6-13 Increase the number of Tribes, States, and the District of Columbia that have public health surveillance and health promotion programs for people with disabilities.

---

*As part of ongoing implementation activities to maintain the accuracy and relevance of *Healthy People 2010*, the U.S. Department of Health and Human Services has proposed that Objectives 6-10, 6-11, and 6-12 no longer be described as "developmental." It has also proposed revising the text of Objective 6-10 so that it would read "Increase the proportion of people with disabilities who report having access to health and wellness programs" (http://www.healthypeople.gov/data/midcourse/comments/facontents.asp?id=6).

SOURCE: DHHS (2000b).

sion of disability are still limited. Recommendations later in this report call for CDC to give disability issues more prominence in its oversight of public health programs, surveillance, and research and to help lead a campaign to increase public and professional awareness of technologies that promote independence and productivity.

THE POLICY ENVIRONMENT OF DISABILTY

Both *Disability in America* and *Enabling America* argued for fundamental changes in how policy makers think about disability. The two reports called for increased attention to the critical roles that the physical and social environments—for example, work and school arrangements, building design, and transportation—play in determining the extent to which individuals with chronic physical and mental conditions can function independently and participate fully in community life. The 1997 report stressed that federal investment in disability and rehabilitation research was seriously inadequate, given the potential for clinical, engineering, social, and other research to improve the health, productivity, and quality of life of people with disabilities.

As in the past, the future of disability in America will depend in important ways on government policies in many areas in addition to public health. This report raises questions about the content of some policies (e.g., the Medicare statute's narrow and sometimes counterproductive definition of "medically necessary care"), the implementation of other policies (e.g., the restrictive judicial interpretations of the ADA), and the timely adaptation of policies in response to changing circumstances (e.g., rapid innovation in communications technologies). Several chapters include policy recommendations.

Government policies related specifically and directly to disability—which reflect decades of advocacy by and on behalf of people with disabilities—are a source of both support and frustration. For example, although they are sometimes criticized for emphasizing welfare dependency over civil rights and distorting incentives for work, the Social Security Disability Insurance (SSDI) and Supplemental Security Income programs serve as important social safety nets for people with serious chronic health problems and impairments. At the end of 2004, almost 8 million "disabled workers and dependents" received income under the provisions of the Social Security Act, and that number increased significantly during the 1990s (SSA, 2006e). Still, features of SSDI, including the link between SSDI benefits and Medicare coverage, discourage people who might be able to do so from returning to work. As discussed in Chapter 8, the federal government has attempted to devise and test programs that reduce this disincentive for work by allow-

TABLE 1-1 Timeline of Milestones in U.S. Disability Policy

1857	Congress created the Columbia Institution for the Instruction of the Deaf and the Dumb and the Blind (now Gallaudet University)
1862	Congress established veterans' pensions based on war-related disability
1890	Disability Act of 1890 provided veterans' pensions whether or not a disability was war related
1918	Soldiers Disability Act created vocational rehabilitation program for veterans
1920	Civilian Vocational Rehabilitation Act expanded the program to civilians
1935	Social Security legislation did not include disability insurance but created state-federal assistance programs that covered certain adults and children with disabilities
1943	Barden-Lafollette Act expanded eligibility for vocational rehabilitation services to people with cognitive and psychiatric impairments
1950	Social Security Act amendments extended state-federal assistance program to include "needy disabled"
1956	Social Security Act amendments created Social Security Disability Insurance to provide cash benefits to eligible workers ages 50 to 64 and adult children of deceased or retired workers if the child was disabled before age 18; later amendments expanded eligibility to younger workers
1961	American National Standards Institutes (a private group) set first minimum standards for making buildings accessible for "the physically handicapped"
1961	President's Panel on Mental Retardation was created; in 1963 it called for the deinstitutionalization of people with mental illness
1965	Developmentally Disabled Assistance and Bill of Rights Act passed; Medicare and Medicaid programs established; Older Americans Act included provisions related to frail or homebound older people
1968	Architectural Barriers Act required accessibility in construction or alteration of federally owned or leased buildings
1970	Urban Mass Transportation Act required local authorities to design mass transit systems to be accessible to people with "handicaps"
1972	Supplemental Security Income (SSI) program established a federal needs-based income support program for "aged, blind, and disabled" to replace state-federal assistance program; SSI recipients became eligible for Medicaid in most states
1972	Medicare coverage extended to eligible adults under age 65 with disabilities
1973	Rehabilitation Act shifted priority for vocational rehabilitation to severely disabled individuals, provided civil rights protections (including nondiscrimination in federal programs and in hiring by federal agencies and most federal contractors), and created the Architectural and Transportation Compliance Board (now the Access Board) to set facility design criteria and improve compliance with accessibility standards
1975	Education for All Handicapped Children Act required free, appropriate public education for children with disabilities and authorized financial incentives to promote compliance

continued

TABLE 1-1 Continued

1978 National Institute on Disability and Rehabilitation Research and National Council on Disability created

1984 Voting Accessibility for the Elderly and Handicapped Act passed

1985 Amendments to Title V of the Social Security Act changed terminology related to block grant programs from "crippled children" to "children with special health care needs"

1986 Air Carriers Access Act passed

1986 Electronic Equipment Accessibility amendment (Section 508) to the Rehabilitation Act of 1973 provided guidelines for federal agency procurement

1988 Technology-Related Assistance for Individuals with Disabilities Act provided state grants to promote assistive technology

1988 Fair Housing Amendments Act prohibited discrimination in housing against people with disabilities

1990 Americans with Disabilities Act provided for inclusion and nondiscrimination based on disability in several areas: employment (Title I); government services (Title II); public accommodations, including medical facilities (Title III); telecommunications (Title IV); and certain other services, such as insurance (Title V)

1990 Education for All Handicapped Children Act renamed as Individuals with Disabilities Education Act (IDEA)

1991 National Center for Medical Rehabilitation Research created in the National Institute of Child Health and Human Development, National Institutes of Health (1990 legislation)

1996 Telecommunications Act of 1996 required that broadcast and cable television provide closed captions to improve accessibility for people with hearing loss

1997 Amendments to IDEA supported initiatives for transition services for young people moving from school to adult living

1998 Assistive Technology Act established grant program for states

1998 Amendments to the Rehabilitation Act required electronic and information technology acquired by federal agencies to meet accessibility standards (regulations issued in 2001)

1999 Ticket to Work and Work Incentives Improvement Act provided health benefits and other encouragements for people to work rather than rely on cash benefits and reinforced requirements for federal agency purchase of accessible electronic equipment

2001 New Freedom Initiative announced by executive order with a focus on access to assistive technologies, work, education, and other opportunities for people with disabilities

2004 Amendments to IDEA called for every state to develop a transition monitoring plan

NOTE: This table does not include important U.S. Supreme Court cases, negotiated settlements, or other outcomes of litigation. See Appendixes D, E, and F.
SOURCES: U.S. House of Representatives, Committee on Ways and Means (1974), Welch and Palames (1995), Berkowitz (2000), U.S. Department of Education (2000), Kaiser Commission (2002, Appendix 1), Blanck and Song (2003), Murray (2003), SSA, (2003a, 2005a), NCLD (2006), and Rasch (2006).

ing people who have qualified for SSDI and Medicare to retain health care benefits, under certain circumstances, if they become able to work.

Table 1-1 presents a capsule summary of historical milestones in federal legislative and administrative policies that were intended specifically to benefit people with disabilities. Early policies often emphasized income support. Many significant policies were adopted in the 1960s, and the pace of policy development accelerated through the 1970s as a civil rights perspective was embraced by and for people with physical or mental impairments. In addition, other policies that were not narrowly aimed at people with disabilities have brought substantial benefits to this group. Notable examples include the initial Social Security Act (1935) and the initial Medicare legislation (1965), both of which encompassed the age group at the highest risk for disability and made benefits available without regard to health or disability status or economic need.

The diverse targets of the policies listed above—education, employment, health, voting, transportation, telecommunications, housing, and more—underscore the breadth and depth of disadvantage and discrimination that people with disabilities experience. Today, much of the focus of advocates is on interpreting, refining, and fully implementing existing policies related to disability while defending against policy changes or interpretations that could directly or indirectly threaten people with disabilities. Examples of the latter include some potentially harmful changes in Medicaid, as described in Chapters 8 and 9.

Table 1-1 does not include decisive U.S. Supreme Court decisions that have affected—sometimes positively and sometimes negatively—the scope and application of federal disability statutes and regulations. For example, several decisions have significantly limited the scope and potential impact of the ADA as it affects discriminatory actions by state governments and discrimination in private employment (see, e.g., the discussion of *Murphy v. United Parcel Service*, *Toyota v. Williams*, and other cases in Appendix E). In contrast, the Supreme Court expanded the reach of the ADA in *Olmstead v. L.C.*, when it concluded that the ADA required states to provide community-based rather than institutional services for people with mental disabilities when it was medically appropriate and acceptable to the individual in question (see Appendix D). This decision reinforced and accelerated policies and programs already in place to promote home and community-based services as an alternative to institutional care (see Chapter 9).

Much of the foundation for the ADA, including key definitions and prohibitions, was laid by the Rehabilitation Act of 1973. This legislation, which remains in force, prohibits discrimination on the basis of disability in programs conducted by federal agencies, in programs receiving federal financial assistance, in federal employment, and in the employment practices of federal contractors.

The five titles of the ADA extended and expanded the protections of the Rehabilitation Act in important ways. They banned discrimination against qualified individuals with disabilities in any aspect of public- or private-sector employment; prohibited discrimination by public institutions, including state and local governments (whether federal funding is involved or not); and prohibited discrimination in the provision of goods or services by commercial facilities and places of public accommodation, including private health care facilities. The legislation also directed improvements in the availability of certain interstate and intrastate telecommunications services for people with hearing and speech impairments (see Appendix F).

One critical feature of the ADA is that enforcement is, for the most part, reactive. It depends substantially on federal agency responses to complaints by or on behalf of individuals who have encountered violations of the law. The U.S. Congress has been criticized for providing insufficient funding for enforcement, and agencies have been cited for not developing coherent strategies and priorities for enforcement of antidiscrimination laws (see, e.g., NCD [2000c]). The discussion of health care facilities in Chapter 6 illustrates some of the strengths and limitations of the ADA and other laws and regulations in achieving accessible physical environments.

As is true for many other public policies, the effectiveness of the ADA and other policies very much depends on voluntary action by regulated entities, informal pressure by advocates, and the creation of a supportive cultural environment. A supportive and aware public will be vitally important in the years to come as critical choices continue to be made about policies that affect people with disabilities.

2

Definition and Monitoring of Disability

> [D]isability no longer means a condition, an incapacity, or lack that be-
> longs to a body, but rather a product of the interactions between self,
> society, body, and the variety of interactions (from political economies to
> personal commitments) that they engender.
>
> Sharon Snyder (2006)

In the last half century, the understanding of disability and the language that has been used to describe it have changed dramatically. Certain
language—for example, "handicapped worker"—has largely disappeared.
More important, the point that Snyder made in the quotation presented
above—that disability is not an individual attribute but an interaction between the individual and the environment—increasingly informs discussions
of disability and disability policy. The Americans with Disabilities Act and
other public policies that are intended to eliminate or reduce environmental
barriers to independence and community integration illustrate the point.

Nonetheless, the absence of universally accepted and understood terms
and concepts with which to describe and discuss disability continues to be a
major barrier to consolidating scientific knowledge about the circumstances
that contribute to disability and the interventions that can prevent, mitigate,
or reverse it. Its absence hampers clear communication and complicates systematic comparisons across research studies, among groups with different
conditions, across nations and different cultures, and over time.

This chapter begins with an examination of concepts of disability.

35

It endorses the adoption of the conceptual framework published by the World Health Organization (WHO) in 2001 as a means of promoting clear communication and building a coherent base of national and international research findings to inform public and private decision making. At the same time, it identifies several directions for refining and improving that framework to better serve monitoring (surveillance), research, and public policy purposes. The chapter also reviews current disability monitoring activities, evaluates progress since publication of the 1991 and 1997 Institute of Medicine (IOM) reports on disability, and sets forth recommendations for further improvements in monitoring programs.

TOWARD A COMMON CONCEPTUAL FRAMEWORK

A significant feature of the 1991 IOM report *Disability in America* was the conceptual framework that it set forth for understanding disability not only as a series of consequences of disease or injury but as a consequence of people's relationship with their environments—environments that might be supportive of participation in society or that might present obstacles to such participation. Building in particular on the work of Saad Nagi (1965, 1991), it attempted to define a common language for describing and understanding disability and related concepts. The report used the following definitions of stages in the process by which people acquire disabilities or improve their functioning in the context of a particular social and physical environment:

- *Pathology:* "interruption or interference of normal bodily processes or structures caused by disease, trauma, or other conditions"
- *Impairment:* "loss and/or abnormality of mental, emotional, physiological, or anatomical structure or function; includes all losses or abnormalities, not just those attributable to active pathology; also includes pain"
- *Functional limitation:* "restriction or lack of ability to perform an action or activity in the manner or within the range considered normal that results from impairment"
- *Disability:* "inability or limitation in performing socially defined activity and roles expected of individuals within a social and physical environment;" also, a "gap between a person's capacities and the demands of relevant, socially defined roles and tasks in a particular physical and social environment" (IOM, 1991, pp. 79–81)

The 1997 IOM report *Enabling America* relied on the 1991 IOM conceptual framework but made some refinements related, in particular, to clarifying the interaction between the person and the environment and the dynamics of the "enabling/disabling" process. The two reports also pointed to secondary health conditions as important and potentially preventable contributors to the progression of health conditions to disability. (As defined in Chapter 5 of this report, secondary conditions are potentially preventable health conditions for which individuals with a primary health condition are at increased risk.) In addition, the two reports included quality of life as an important concept in understanding the impact of health conditions, impairments, functional limitations, and disabilities on people's sense of well-being in relation to their personal goals and expectations.

Although many researchers in the United States adopted the IOM framework, others, particularly in international circles, relied on the World Health Organization's *International Classification of Impairments, Disability and Handicaps* (ICIDH) (WHO, 1980). Responding to concerns that the ICIDH was outdated and inadequate to meet current needs for an international classification standard to describe disability, WHO developed a new *International Classification of Functioning, Disability and Health* (ICF), which was released in 2001 (WHO, 2001).

To encourage worldwide acceptance and cultural applicability, WHO developed the ICF framework using a global consensus-building process that involved multiple stakeholders, including people with disabilities. Unlike the ICIDH, the ICF was endorsed in May 2001 by the World Health Assembly as a member of the family of International Classifications, the best known of which is the International Classification of Diseases (ICD). Among the most promising aspects of the ICF framework is its potential to provide a standardized, internationally accepted language and conceptual framework that will facilitate communication across national and disciplinary boundaries and thereby help build a coherent and consistent body of scientific knowledge to inform policies and programs that promote the well-being, independence, and integration of people with disabilities.

Consistent with previous disability frameworks, the ICF attempts to provide a comprehensive view of health-related states from biological, personal, and social perspectives (Box 2-1). It describes human functioning and disability as the product of a dynamic interaction between various health conditions and environmental and personal contextual factors. In contrast to earlier frameworks and as reflected in its title, the ICF framework has components that can be "expressed in both positive and negative terms" (WHO, 2001, p. 10). The term "handicap" is no longer used in the English version of the revised classification.[1]

As in the frameworks presented in the 1991 and 1997 IOM reports and the earlier ICIDH framework, the ICF identifies multiple levels of hu-

---

[1]The French language version of ICF is, however, called the Classification Internationale du Fonctionnement, du Handicap et de la Santé.

BOX 2-1
Major Concepts in the *International Classification*
of Functioning, Disability and Health

Health condition: umbrella term for disease, disorder, injury, or trauma
Functioning: umbrella term for body functions and structures, activities, and participation
Disability: umbrella term for impairments, activity limitations, and participation restrictions

Body function: physiological functions of body systems (including psychological functions)
Body structure: anatomical parts of the body such as organs, limbs, and their components
Impairment: problems in body function or structure, such as a significant deviation or loss

Activity: execution of a task or action by an individual
Activity limitations: difficulties that an individual may have in executing activities

Participation: involvement in a life situation
Participation restriction: problems that an individual may experience in involvement in life situations

Environment: the physical, social, and attitudinal environment in which people live and conduct their lives

Personal factors: contextual factors that relate to the individual, such as age, gender, social status, and life experiences

SOURCE: WHO (2001, pp. 10, 211–214).

---

man functioning and disability: at the level of the body or body parts, at the level of the whole person, and at the level of the whole person who is functioning in his or her environment. These levels, in turn, involve three aspects of human functioning that the ICF terms *body functions and structures*, *activities*, and *participation*. One significant difference in the ICF framework in comparison with earlier frameworks is that the *function* and *disability* become generic or umbrella terms in the ICF framework. Thus, the term *disability* serves—and is used in this report—as an umbrella term for *impairments*, *activity limitations*, and *participation restrictions*.

The ICF framework starts with the concept of a *health condition*, a general term for a disease, disorder, injury, trauma, congenital anomaly, or genetic characteristic. ICF specifically includes aging as a health condition

(WHO, 2001, p. 212). A health condition is the starting point for the possible development of an impairment, activity limitation, or participation restriction. It usually has a diagnosis as defined and coded either in WHO's ICD (ICD-10, for its current 10th revision [WHO, 2006]) or in the American Psychiatric Association's Diagnostic and Statistical Manual of Mental Disorders (DSM IV TR, for its current fourth edition [APA, 2000]).[2]

The ICF concept of impairment is similar to that of the IOM. The IOM concept of functional limitations shares elements with the ICF concepts of impairment (e.g., for limitations in hearing) and activity limitation (e.g., for limitations in mobility).

In contrast, the definition of disability presented in the 1991 and 1997 IOM reports is more specific than that of the ICF. It highlights social roles—the expectations of a society or culture for its members—and the gap that may exist between individuals' capacities and their performance of social roles in given physical and social environments. The ICF component that most nearly corresponds to this conceptualization is *participation restriction*, which is defined as "problems an individual may experience in involvement in life situations" (WHO, 2001, p. 10). Restriction is explained as the "discordance between the observed and expected performance," in which *expected performance* refers to a "population norm" or standard based on the "experience of people without the specific health condition" (p. 15). Performance is described as "what an individual does in his or her current environment" (p. 15). *Life situation* is not explicitly defined; but the ICF domains of participation include categories of "domestic life" (e.g., acquiring a place to live and managing a household); "major life areas" (e.g., education and employment); and "community, social, and civic life" (e.g., attending religious services, voting, and participating in professional organizations).

Two other concepts defined in the ICF framework as contextual elements are environmental and personal factors. *Environmental factors* are "all aspects of the external or extrinsic world" that form "the physical, social, and attitudinal circumstances in which people live and conduct their lives" (pp. 10, 213). The domains for environmental factors cover specific features of the person's actual environment (e.g., the attitudes of community members) that facilitate or hinder a person's functioning. *Personal factors* include gender, race, age, lifestyle, habits, social background, and other individual characteristics or experiences that are not classified elsewhere in

---

[2]For example, spinal cord injury has 11 ICD-10 codes that distinguish different types of injury (e.g., fracture of the lumbar spine, fracture of the neck, or the sequelae of a spinal cord injury), whereas multiple sclerosis has a single ICD-10 code. ICD-10 includes codes for mental disorders, and these codes are used in many countries instead of the American Psychiatric Association's DSM.

the ICF. Although they are not characterized in this way by the ICF, the negative aspects of certain contextual elements could be included among the risk factors for disability, as defined in the 1991 and 1997 IOM reports.

The ICF categorizes most of its major concepts or components into domains (Box 2-2), which are further subdivided into chapter headings and more detailed classifications and codes. The exception is that the ICF includes neither domains nor codes for personal factors. Thus it does not provide a uniform scheme for classifying individual characteristics that may affect the outcome of a potentially disabling condition.

To capture more detailed descriptive information about functioning or disability, the framework includes qualifiers that identify the presence and severity of a decrement of functioning.[3] Within the activity and participation areas, the ICF advocates the use of qualifiers to assess performance and capacity.[4] In essence, the performance qualifiers capture what people actually do in their usual environments, whereas the capacity qualifiers describe the person's inherent ability to function without assistance.

In the ICF manual, WHO acknowledges that the developers of the ICF could not agree on what individual situations should be coded as activities and what individual situations should be coded as participation. Its explanation cites "international variation and differences in the approaches of professionals and theoretical frameworks" (WHO, 2001, p. 16). As a result, the ICF presents a single list of domains for activities and participation and invites users, if they so wish, to differentiate them in their own operational way. Thus some researchers might consider difficulty in preparing meals to be an activity limitation, whereas others might categorize it as a participation restriction. As discussed below, this lack of conceptual specificity is one of the shortcomings in the ICF.

---

[3]In the domain of body function, the qualifier is the presence and degree or severity of a specific impairment rated on a five-point scale: no, mild, moderate, severe, or complete impairment. For body structures, in addition to this severity qualifier, an additional qualifier is used to indicate the nature of a structural change (e.g., partial absence). To cite examples, b1678.3 is the code for "severe impairment in specific mental functions of language" (WHO, 2001, p. 59), and code s730.32 indicates "a severe impairment involving the partial absence of the upper extremity."

[4]A *performance qualifier* is used to describe what an individual does in his or her current environment, which may present barriers (e.g., the absence of personal help) or supports (e.g., the availability of assistive devices). In contrast, *capacity qualifiers* describe an individual's inherent ability to execute a task or an action. The capacity qualifier identifies a person's highest probable level of functioning without assistance at a given time. Ideally, capacity would be assessed in a standardized or uniform environment that would allow comparisons across research or assessment settings. The same five-point scale used for impairments is used to record the severity of performance or capacity limitations. For example, code d5100.1_ indicates "mild difficulty with bathing parts of the body with the use of assistive devices available to the person." Code d5100._2 indicates moderate difficulty in the same task without the use of assistive devices or person help.

BOX 2-2
Components and Domains of Human
Functioning in the *International Classification*
of Functioning, Disability and Health

Body Function and Structure

Body Function:
Mental functions
Sensory functions and pain
Voice and speech functions

Functions of the cardiovascular,
   hematological, immunological, and
   respiratory systems
Functions of the digestive, metabolic,
and endocrine systems
Genitourinary and reproductive
   functions
Neuromusculoskeletal and movement-
   related functions
Functions of the skin and related
   structures

Body Structure:
Structure of the nervous system
Eye, ear, and related structures
Structures involved in voice and
   speech
Structure of the cardiovascular, immu-
   nological, and respiratory systems

Structures related to the digestive,
   metabolic, and endocrine systems
Structure related to genitourinary and
   reproductive systems
Structures related to movement

Skin and related structures

Activities and Participation

Learning and applying knowledge
General tasks and demands
Communication
Mobility
Self-care
Domestic life
Interpersonal interactions and relationships
Major life areas
Community, social, and civic life

Environmental Factors

Products and technology
Natural environment and human-made changes to the environment
Support and relationships
Attitudes
Services, systems, and policies

Personal Factors

Not categorized

SOURCE: WHO (2001, pp. 29–30).

ADOPTING AND IMPROVING THE ICF

The international consensus process used to develop the ICF and its growing use worldwide have provided a significant opportunity to achieve agreement on an international taxonomy for defining, classifying, and measuring function, disability, and health with standard concepts and terminologies. As noted above, an important innovation provided by the ICF is that the nomenclature includes positive descriptions of human functioning and not just the negative consequences of disease or injury, a feature that is very important to the disability advocacy community. The development of standardized measurement instruments based on the ICF would contribute to their adoption in disability research, which would, in turn, help improve data comparability over time and across studies, cultures, and nations. This would aid analyses of the causes and consequences of disability and help guide the development of public policy to benefit people with disabilities, their families, and society at large. In addition, the ICF conceptual framework and classification scheme will support needed research on the contribution of environmental factors to disability. For these reasons, this report uses the ICF conceptual framework and supports its worldwide adoption and use as a standard terminology and classification system, although at times the use of other language employed in laws and policy discussions will be necessary.

At the same time, the committee has identified directions for improving and refining the ICF conceptual framework. These directions include developing activity-participation distinctions and measures, adding quality of life as a key concept in understanding disability, developing domains for personal factors, recognizing secondary health conditions related to a primary health condition, further developing environmental factors, and incorporating a dynamic model of the enabling/disabling process. (These areas for improvement are summarized in Box 2-7 in the Recommendations section at the end of this chapter.) Several of these topics are being considered by WHO, United States government agencies, and other groups around the world as part of conferences, working groups, and other activities to refine and apply the ICF.

Clarifying Activity Limitations and Participation Restrictions

A first and well-recognized aspect of the ICF that needs further development involves the interpretation and categorization of the concepts of activity and participation. Reflecting the difficulty that the ICF developers encountered in differentiating the two concepts, the final ICF document presents them as conceptually distinct with different definitions, but the actual classification scheme provides a single combined list of life areas that are not specifically linked to one concept or the other (as displayed earlier in Box 2-1). In an appendix (called an annex), the ICF manual describes how users could, if they so wished, develop operational measures that differentiated between activity and participation. Among the suggestions is the use of the qualifiers of performance and capacity to differentiate among these concepts at an operational level, but the usefulness of this approach has not been confirmed empirically.

Several researchers have criticized the lack of a clear operational differentiation between the concepts of activity and participation in the ICF as theoretically confusing and a step backward from earlier disability frameworks (see, e.g., the work of Jette et al. [2003], Nordenfelt [2003], Simeonsson et al. [2003], Barral [2004], Schuntermann [2005], and Whiteneck [2006]). Operational differentiation among concepts and the ability to measure each concept precisely and distinctly is important for clear communication, monitoring, and research. If the differences between these two concepts are not clarified or otherwise resolved in some coherent fashion and if different users distinguish these core concepts in different ways, the goal of a universal and standard language for classifying individuals with respect to the burden of health conditions will remain unfulfilled.

For example, Schuntermann (2005), who has worked on implementing the ICF in Germany, notes that severe problems have been encountered with the measurement of activity and participation using capacity and performance qualifiers. He also notes a fear that the lack of an agreed-upon way of differentiating activity and participation may undermine efforts to make valid international and cross-cultural comparisons.[5]

Researchers are beginning to examine the boundaries of the activity and participation domains of the ICF and exploring ways in which the ICF concepts might be reconceptualized (Nordenfelt, 2003; Perenboom and Chorus, 2003; Okochi et al., 2005; Schuntermann, 2005; Whiteneck, 2006). For example, Whiteneck (2006) has argued that activity is primarily individual (performed alone) and that participation is primarily social (performed with others). Also, activities tend to be somewhat less environmentally dependent and to be a primary focus of medical rehabilitation,

---

[5]With respect to international comparisons, Kapteyn and colleagues (2004) caution that categorization options (e.g., whether an impairment or limitation is mild or severe) may be interpreted differently in different cultures (see also Banks et al. [in press]). They cite Dutch and U.S. data showing quite different distributions of self-reported health status; for example, 6 percent of Dutch respondents categorized themselves in excellent health, whereas 25 percent of Americans did so. This suggests that the "circumspect Dutch appear to run to the center . . . while the ever optimistic Americans are four times more likely to state that they are in excellent health" (p. 7). Potentially, a process of cultural "norming" could compensate for some cultural and cross-national differences.

whereas participation restrictions, including discrimination in employment and other areas, offer clear targets for public policy.

Nordenfelt (2003) has offered a radical, yet simplifying, suggestion to resolve the current confusion between the activity and the participation domains of the ICF by combining the two domains into a single domain of *action*. He further proposes that action be qualified in ways that are relevant in the context of rehabilitation or health care but not exclusively so. In contrast to qualifiers contained in the current version of the ICF, he argues that actions could be subdivided in terms of their *simplicity* and *complexity*. (Climbing stairs would be a simple action, whereas working would be a complex action.[6]) Nordenfelt's analysis has some elements in common with that of Whiteneck, but it lacks the stress on community involvement or social role performance that Whiteneck's approach maintains, unless some of the subcategories of action could be formulated to re-create it.

Although this committee does not endorse any particular approach to resolving the problem, it believes that the lack of operational differentiation between the concepts of activity and participation is a significant deficit in the ICF. Developing the conceptual base for such differentiation or substituting some alternative conceptualization is a key step that needs to be taken to clarify and refine the ICF so that it provides a better foundation for disability monitoring and research.

Adding Quality of Life to the Framework

The committee is also concerned that the concept of quality of life is not explicitly named or defined as an ICF component or element, although "establishing links" with this concept is mentioned as a future direction in the ICF manual.[7] In other documents, WHO has defined quality of life as "the perception of individuals of their position in life, in the context of the culture and value systems in which they live and in relation to their goals, expectations, standards, and concerns" (WHOQOL, 1993, p. 153).

Conceptually, quality of life is much broader than the *health-related* quality of life. Indeed, some measures of health-related quality of life overlap with some measures of impairments or activity limitations. For ex-

---

[6]Nordenfelt also suggests that there are three preconditions for the types of actions that are now included within the activity and participation domains of the ICF. For any action to occur, the individual must have the capacity (i.e., inherent potential) to perform the action. The individual must also have the opportunity to transform inherent potential into action in his or her actual environment. Finally, the person must have the will to perform the action. All actions, whether they are defined as activity or participation, are performed in physical, social, and cultural contexts.

[7]A taxonomic annex to the ICF manual depicts a universe of "well-being" as part of the context of the ICF. Well-being is defined as "encompassing the total universe of human life domains . . . that make up what can be called 'a good life'" (WHO, 2001, p. 211).

ample, the Centers for Disease Control and Prevention (CDC) has a 14-item set of questions on health-related quality-of-life, one of which is, "Are you limited in any way in any activities because of any impairment or health problem?" (CDC, 2005a), which is similar to U.S. Census Bureau and other survey questions used to identify people with disabilities. A WHO instrument asks some similar questions, for example, "How well are you able to get around?" Unlike the CDC instrument, however, the WHO instrument also asks, "How much do any difficulties in mobility bother you?" as well as other more general questions such as "How satisfied are you with your abilities?" and "How satisfied are you with your quality of life?" (WHO, 1995; see also WHOQOL [1993] and Bonomi et al. [2000]). These additional questions tap the critical subjective dimension of perceptions and preferences that distinguish quality of life from other concepts.

In a paper prepared for an IOM workshop and workshop report (IOM, 2006b), Whiteneck (2006) identified quality of life as a key missing component of the ICF framework, and this committee agrees.[8] In addition to refining the ICF conceptual framework to include quality of life, a related area for conceptual and empirical work is clarification of the relationship between quality of life and the existing ICF concepts (see Jette and Badley [2002] for a discussion of conceptual issues).

Categorizing Personal Factors

An additional area for improvement in the ICF is the categorization of personal factors, which the ICF includes as a concept without a corresponding classification. Personal factors often have an environmentally influenced component (e.g., literacy may be limited by economic, cultural, or other constraints), which complicates the task but which does not eliminate the need for further development of the ICF in this area. This need is recognized in the ICF manual.

To the extent that personal factors, such as adherence to treatment recommendations or personality characteristics, are perceived as potentially "blaming the victim" or suggesting that a problem exists with the individual, then they will be controversial (Whiteneck, 2006). To deal with this realistic apprehension, the process of developing categorizations of personal factors should include, in particular, people with disabilities and others who are sensitive to this issue.

---

[8]Whiteneck suggests that qualify of life be added to the ICF as an additional domain. Excluding it from the framework would negate the importance of the individual's self-evaluation as part of any comprehensive assessment of disability. Treatment of qualify of life as another qualifier would add to the ICF's conceptual confusion and would, like excluding the concept, diminish its importance.

Recognizing Secondary Conditions

Another concern of the committee is that, although secondary conditions are stressed in both the 1991 and 1997 IOM reports and are the subject of a chapter in this report, they are not explicitly recognized in the ICF conceptual framework. As defined in Chapter 5 of this report, secondary conditions are potentially preventable health conditions for which individuals with a primary health condition are at increased risk. The contribution of such conditions to disability and the interactions of individual and environmental characteristics as they affect the development or prevention of secondary conditions should be incorporated into future refinements of the ICF framework. Such recognition would not require modifications to the coding structure of the ICF because these conditions can be coded by using the ICD, as is done for primary health conditions.

Further Developing Environmental Factors

Considerable attention is being paid to the further conceptual development of the environmental component in the ICF. As summarized earlier in Box 2-2, environmental factors include elements of the physical, societal, and attitudinal environments in which people live and conduct their lives. Sanford and Bruce (2006) have argued that the ICF lacks measurement constructs for important dimensions or characteristics of the environment. For example, it treats certain characteristics such as wheelchair ramps as either present or absent, without any provision for the rating of a ramp's slope, surface, length, or other features that could affect ease of use.

In another review of the ICF, Steinfeld and Danford (2006) noted that the ICF classification of environmental factors needs further development before it can be used as a tool to assess the outcomes of Universal Design applications (see discussions of Universal Design in Chapters 6 and 7). For example, although the ICF has a code for sound intensity, more guidance is needed on how to code or rate specific auditory aspects of the physical environment (and its design), such as background noise or the presence of a public address system. Thus, another direction for improving the ICF is the further evaluation and improvement of the environment coding scheme to allow more complete and accurate specification of environmental factors that may affect functioning (see also Keysor [2006]).

Depicting Functioning and Disability as Dynamic Processes

The committee notes that the ICF is a classification scheme. Unlike the Nagi and 1991 and 1997 IOM frameworks, it does not present a model of disability—or enablement/disablement—as a dynamic process. In this respect, even if a definitional "crosswalk" between these models and ICF concepts is required, process models and their elaborations remain important (see, e.g., Verbrugge and Jette [1994], Fougeyrollas et al. [1998], and Jette and Badley [2002]). Such models help focus research on identifying and understanding interactions among health conditions, other personal characteristics, and environmental factors that contribute to the movement of individuals from one health or disability state to another. One important obstacle to the development of a conceptually useful, testable model is the lack of agreement on these different states, that is, on what qualifies as an activity limitation or as a participation restriction.

A NATIONAL DISABILITY MONITORING SYSTEM

The lack of a national disability monitoring (surveillance) program, highlighted in the 1991 IOM report, remains a serious shortcoming in the country's health statistics system. The current program falls significantly short of providing key information that can be used to guide public and private action to improve opportunities and remove barriers to independence and community participation for people with disabilities. As demonstrated in Chapter 3, disability statistics must be patched together from multiple surveys to cover people of all ages and in all living situations, and gaps often remain. Surveys may exclude young children or adults younger than retirement age, and individuals with disabilities living in institutional settings or assistive living environments are excluded altogether or are not easily identified. Although panel studies that monitor disability trajectories and risk factors in the older population exist, they are much less complete for children and nonelderly adults. They thus offer few opportunities to study questions related to aging with disabilities for younger adults (see Chapter 5). Existing surveys are also particularly weak in terms of their ability to help evaluate progress in the removal of environmental barriers to participation. The committee's assessment is based on a review of national periodic or ongoing surveys that include measures of disability (Table 2-1).

The committee identified several key components of a comprehensive disability monitoring system that are consistent with the ICF framework. Ideally, core measures for such a system should include aspects of impairments in body structures and functions, activity limitations, participation restrictions, and key features of the environment as well as personal factors. (Note that certain important personal factors, such as race and ethnicity, education, and income, are already collected in most surveys.) Data collection and monitoring should cover individuals of all ages and in all living situations (including the community, group residential care settings, and institutions). It should provide information that can be used to monitor the

TABLE 2-1 Overview of National Surveys That Include Measures of Disability

Survey Type and Survey (Years of Data)	Ages (Years)	Institutional Population Included?
Cross-Sectional Surveys		
National Survey of Children with Special Health Care Needs (2000–2001, 2005–2006)	0-17	No
National Survey of Children's Health (2003–2004)	0-17	No
Behavioral Risk Factor Surveillance System Modules (1993–2005), Core (2001, 2003–present)	18+[a]	No
American Community Survey (1999–present)	All	Yes, beginning in 2006
National Health and Nutrition Examination Survey (1971–1975, 1976–1980, 1999–2003)	All	No
National Health Interview Survey (NHIS), (1957–present)	All	No
NHIS Disability Supplement (1994–1995)	All	No
Panel Surveys		
Current Population Survey (1942–present)	15+	No
Medicare Current Beneficiary Survey (1992–present), for elderly and disabled individuals	18+ (with disability) and 65+	Yes
Health and Retirement Study (1992–present)	50+	Yes
National Long-Term Care Survey (1982, 1984, 1989, 1994, 1999, 2004)	65+	Yes
NHIS Supplements on Aging/Longitudinal Study on Aging (1984–1990 and 1994–2000)	70+	No
National Longitudinal Survey of Labor Market Experience, Youth Cohort (NLSY79) (1979–present); NLSY79 Children (1986–present)	Youth cohort: 14–22 in 1979 Children: 0–14	No
Medical Expenditure Panel Survey (1996–present)	All	No
Panel Study of Income Dynamics (1968–present) Child Development Supplement (1997, 2002–2003)	All 0–12	No
Survey of Income and Program Participation (1983–present) Adult Disability Topical Module Child Disability Topical Module	All	No

[a]The Behavioral Risk Factor Surveillance System has had occasional childhood modules under its Child Health Assessment and Monitoring Program.

incidence, prevalence, severity, and duration of the various components of disability. In addition, it should help analysts and policy makers learn more about risk factors for disability, including the contribution of environmental and personal factors to the development or reversal of activity limitations and participation restrictions.[9]

Progress in Disability Monitoring

The 1991 IOM report proposed that "a national disability surveillance system should be developed to monitor over the life course the incidence and prevalence of (1) functional limitations and disabilities; (2) specific developmental disabilities, injuries, and diseases that cause functional limitations and disability; and (3) secondary conditions resulting from the primary disability. The system should also monitor causal phenomena, risk factors, functional status, and quality of life, and provide state-specific data for program planning and evaluation of interventions" (IOM, 1991, p. 275). The report suggested that the National Health Interview Survey should be revised to include more items relevant to understanding disability. For example, it proposed that core survey questions on mental disorders and other potentially disabling conditions should be added to the survey to estimate the magnitude of these conditions in the general population and the extent to which they contribute to disability. The report also called for more data on the personal and social effects and the economic consequences of disability in the United States, for longitudinal surveys to collect data on the incidence and prevalence of functional limitations and disease, for additional questions to be developed for the year 2000 decennial census, and for consideration of panel studies that monitor individuals over time.

On the basis of its review of existing national surveys and related activities, the committee concluded that, although the monitoring system has improved since 1991, the situation is, in many respects, much as it was then.[10] The number of surveys that collect disability data has increased,

---

[9]Although not a form of population surveillance or monitoring, another initiative that should be noted is the National Institutes of Health's PROMIS (Patient-Reported Outcomes Measurement Information System) project. As discussed further in Chapter 10, the project aims to improve measures of patient-reported symptoms and other health outcomes and make them more easily and widely used in clinical research and practice. In the resources consulted by the committee, the domains of outcomes and measures are not explicitly mapped to ICF concepts, which would be desirable as part of the initiative's further development.

[10]The committee notes the important contributions of other surveys that have been more limited in scope (e.g., the 1993 to 1995 Women's Health and Aging Study, which focused on women ages 65 and over in Baltimore [Guralnik et al., 1995]), that have examined a single topic in depth (e.g., the 2001 National Survey on Assistive Technology and Information Technology [Carlson and Berland, 2002]), or that have focused on health care providers (e.g., the National Nursing Home Survey conducted by the National Center for Health Statistics).

but analysts and policy makers continue to be limited in making straight-forward comparisons across surveys and across time. For example, several surveys include questions about limitations in activities of daily living (ADL) and instrumental activities of daily living (IADL), but the specific questions vary.[11]

Notwithstanding the limitations of the data, one area of progress involves the greater availability of existing data for use by researchers and policy analysts. For example, the National Institute on Disability and Rehabilitation Research (NIDRR) has funded centers on disability statistics that generate policy-relevant analyses using existing data and that also explain the available data sets and their strengths and limitations. The current NIDRR-designated center is based at Cornell University.

Important gaps in survey content also remain that impede the tracking of progress in federal goals related to the removal of barriers to participation and the equalization of opportunities for people with disabilities. This is, in part, because the traditional "medical model" of disability—in which disability is attributed primarily to chronic health conditions without recognition of environmental contributions—still underlies many of the items embedded in contemporary federal surveys. Overall, despite the advances that have been made since 1991, a national, ongoing, coherent, and adequately informative disability monitoring system remains a partly realized goal rather than a reality.

Since 1991, the CDC's National Center for Health Statistics launched one major survey that focused on disability—the 1994–1995 Disability Supplement to the yearly National Health Interview Survey. In many ways, this supplemental survey was an important starting point for the kind of detailed surveillance recommended in 1991 (see NCHS [2006a] for survey details and Altman et al. [2003] and Hendershot [2005] for summaries of the significant research findings). The survey covered many of the key components of a disability monitoring system for children and adults living in the community. Although it was fielded in two parts (a core questionnaire as part of the main interviews for 1994 and 1995 and then an in-depth follow-up interview 7 to 17 months later), the Disability Supplement provided essentially cross-sectional data, meaning that it did not provide true panel data that measures changes involving the survey respondents. The survey data are now 10 years old, and the committee is not aware of plans for another similar effort.

Another important milestone in disability monitoring was the redesign

---

[11]ADLs include personal care activities such as bathing, dressing, eating, transferring, walking across a room, and toileting. IADLs include activities essential to living independently, such as shopping, household chores, managing medications, using the telephone, and managing money.

of the National Health Interview Survey in 1997 (see NCHS [2006b] for details and Box 2-3 for a brief overview of disability-related items). Although the redesign has complicated comparisons with data from earlier time periods, the revised questions are likely to lead to an improved future assessment of trends in functioning for both adults and children. (See Chapter 3 for a discussion of the special challenges in defining and measuring disability for children.) Nonetheless, the survey continues to include few measures that are relevant to participation restrictions or the role of the environment. The cross-sectional nature of the National Health Interview Survey precludes an in-depth exploration of the onset and recovery of disability.

The U.S. census is an important source of information for the distribution of federal dollars and planning at the local level. For the 2000 census,

---

BOX 2-3
Disability-Related Content in the Redesigned
National Health Interview Survey

For each family member:
• The need for help with personal care needs (such as eating, bathing, dressing, or getting around)
• The need for help with routine needs (such as everyday household chores or doing necessary business, shopping, or getting around for other purposes)
• Limitations because of difficulty remembering or confusion
• Difficulty waking without special equipment
• If a limitation, difficulty, or need for help is noted, the respondents were asked to select from a list of 18 health conditions the condition(s) that caused the limitation

For one randomly sampled adult:
• Difficulty with physical functioning in a context that is not activity specific (e.g., the degree of difficulty experienced doing activities such as walking three city blocks, standing for 2 hours, or lifting or carrying something as heavy as 10 pounds, such as a bag of groceries)
• Difficulty engaging in social activities and recreation
• Mental distress

For children:
• Receipt of special education or early intervention services
• Limitation in movement (such as walking, running, or playing)
• Whether the child has a health problem that requires prescription medicine
• Ever been told by a school official or health care provider that the child has a learning disability
• Mental disorders

the agency redesigned questions to provide information on limitations in the ability to perform major life activities. The census long form (administered to one in six households) contained new questions about long-lasting health conditions that limit vision or hearing, physical activities (such as walking, climbing stairs, reaching, lifting, or carrying), cognitive tasks (such as learning, remembering, or concentrating), taking care of personal needs (such as bathing, dressing, or getting around inside the home), going outside the home, or working at a job. These items were subsequently incorporated into the ongoing annual American Community Survey, administered by the U.S. Census Bureau (and highlighted in Chapter 3). Studies evaluating the quality of these items have produced mixed results (Andresen et al., 2000; Stern, 2003; Stern and Brault, 2005). Some have called for the questions to be redesigned for the 2010 census (NCD, 2004b).

Recently, the U.S. Census Bureau tested a revised set of items recommended by the American Community Survey Disability Work Group (Miller and DeMaio, 2006). Based on this testing, the agency then tested the questions again to assess whether the new question set (Box 2-4) improved reliability, validity, and item response.

BOX 2-4
Disability Items in the American Community
Survey 2006 Content Test

16a. Is this person deaf or does he/she have serious difficulty hearing?
  b. Is this person blind or does he/she have serious difficulty seeing even when wearing glasses?

Answer question 17a if this person is 5 years old or over. Otherwise skip to the questions for Person 2 on page 12.

17a. Because of a physical, mental, or emotional condition, does this person have serious difficulty concentrating, remembering, or making decisions?
  b. Does this person have serious difficulty walking or climbing stairs?
  c. Does this person have difficulty dressing or bathing?

Answer question 18 if this person is 15 years old or over. Otherwise skip to the questions for Person 2 on page 12.

18. Because of a physical, mental, or emotional condition, does this person have difficulty doing errands alone such as visiting a doctor's office or shopping?

SOURCE: Stern (2006).

Although it was not explicitly mentioned in the 1991 recommendations, the CDC's Behavioral Risk Factor Surveillance System, which was established in 1984, is another component of disability monitoring. Beginning in 1993, the survey included one core item related to limitations in activities (see BRFSS [2006] for questionnaires by year). Optional disability items were available and were used by a number of states (CDC, 2000b). In 2001 and from 2003 forward, the CDC added two items related to disability to the core questionnaire. Now, all states administer two questions: "Are you limited in any way in any activities because of physical, mental, or emotional problems?" and "Do you now have any health problem that requires you to use special equipment, such as a cane, a wheelchair, a special bed, or a special telephone?" Still, the content relevant to disability remains quite limited. For example, the questions do not ask about the severity of activity limitations. In addition to the limited scope of the questions themselves, another weakness of this telephone survey is that response rates have generally been lower (in the 40 to 70 percent range by state) than for national surveys using face-to-face interviews (NCCDPHP, 2006).

Through its Child Health Assessment and Monitoring Program, the Behavioral Risk Factor Surveillance System has also been used occasionally to provide uniform data on the health conditions and behavioral risks of children and adolescents, but the topic of disability per se has not been a focus.[12] Items related to secondary conditions, which are also relevant for studying issues related to aging with a disability, have been fielded by Washington State but are not part of the core survey.[13]

Since 1991, the number of surveys focused on older adults has expanded. The National Institute on Aging, for example, has provided support for the Health and Retirement Study (covering people age 50 or older), the National Long-Term Care Survey (covering people age 65 or older), and the second Longitudinal Survey on Aging (covering people age 70 or older), the last of which was conducted in collaboration with the National Cen-

---

[12]For example, in 2004 the survey was used to collect information on child vaccination rates across all states; and in 2005 optional random child selection, childhood asthma prevalence, and child immunization modules became official optional modules. More extensive follow-up surveys (for example, the 2005 Behavioral Risk Factor Surveillance System Asthma Follow-up Survey) have also been implemented.

[13]In 1991, Washington State included in its disability supplement questions about 16 secondary conditions (whether respondents had experienced the condition in the past 12 months as a result of their primary impairment and, if so, how big a problem the condition had been). Secondary conditions, which were broadly defined to cover certain social circumstances as well as health conditions (see Chapter 5 for the definition used in this report), included chronic pain, sleep problems, fatigue, weight or eating problems, periods of depression, skin problems, muscle spasms, respiratory infections, falls or other injuries, bowel or bladder problems, serious episodes of anxiety, lack of romantic relationships, problems getting out or getting around, problems making or seeing friends, feelings of isolation, and asthma (Kinne et al., 2004).

ter for Health Statistics. Together with the Medicare Current Beneficiary Survey (which also includes beneficiaries under age 65), these surveys have provided important information on aging, disability, and long-term care, including information about trends in disability among older adults (see Chapter 3 for more discussion of trends). These surveys, however, offer few opportunities for studying participation by older individuals in activities beyond those considered in traditional ADL and IADL measures.

As noted above, many key national surveys do not include individuals living in institutional settings. For the purposes of profiling and monitoring disability, the exclusion of people living in residential care settings, such as nursing homes and group homes, is a shortcoming because these individuals often are—by virtue of their qualification for this type of care—significantly limited physically or cognitively, or both. Many of the surveys that focus on older adults include those living in group residential care settings, such as assisted living facilities, but there currently is no standard approach for identifying them (Spillman and Black, 2006).

Improving Disability Monitoring

Expanding the Goals of Monitoring

Disability monitoring serves multiple functions. Altman and colleagues (2006a,b) have highlighted three distinct purposes:

- To aid in the development and evaluation of service provision programs and policies for people with disabilities, for example, by identifying individuals who need or use housing, long-term care, transportation, assistive technology, or rehabilitation services
- To monitor functioning, for example, by tracking population-level trends in work limitations or self-care limitations
- To assess the equalization of opportunities, for example, by comparing employment levels among individuals with and without mobility limitations[14]

In the past, federal surveys efforts in the United States have emphasized the first two goals. For example, the Survey of Income and Program Participation includes items on the receipt of federal disability and cash assistance from Social Security Disability Insurance and Supplemental Security Income programs. Measures of functioning in the survey have allowed projec-

---

[14]This discussion draws upon materials developed for a meeting of the Washington Group, a city group formed under the auspices of the United Nations to develop internationally comparable measures. For more details, see Altman et al. (2006b).

tions of the future sizes of these programs (Lahiri et al. 1995; Toder et al., 2002). The aim of tracking health (and, to some degree, functioning) in the population has been a primary aim of the National Health Interview Survey, whereas the Behavioral Risk Factor Surveillance System tracks health conditions and risk behaviors. The Current Population Survey, the nation's primary data source on employment statistics, includes a measure of work limitations, which can be tracked over time (Burkhauser et al. 2002).

In recent years, the removal of barriers to participation by people with disabilities is increasingly being recognized by federal agencies as an important policy goal. For example, as described in Chapter 1, *Healthy People 2010* (DHHS, 2000b) includes a chapter on promoting the health of people with disabilities, preventing secondary conditions, and eliminating disparities between people with and without disabilities. Similarly, the *Surgeon General's Call to Action to Improve the Health and Wellness of Persons with Disabilities* sets forth the goals of promoting accessible health care and support services for people with disabilities (U.S. Public Health Service, 2005). In addition, the latest strategic plan from the U.S. Department of Health and Human Services calls for increasing the independence and quality of life of people with disabilities (DHHS, 2006c).

Unfortunately, despite the advances that have been made since 1991, current survey efforts remain inadequate to assess progress in these stated goals and, likewise, to assess progress in the equalization of opportunity since the passage of the Americans with Disabilities Act and other legislation intended to remove barriers to participation in community life. Information on barriers in public transportation, public accommodations, and telecommunications is not widely or systematically available. The identification of appropriate questions to add to surveys has been challenging. For example, despite a 1998 Executive Order (now expired) to develop an accurate and reliable measure of the employment rate for people with disabilities, the most recent Current Population Survey still includes only a measure of work limitation (McMenamin et al., 2005, 2006). The Bureau of Labor Statistics has undertaken efforts to develop and test measures of disability for the survey, but it has not yet adopted any new measures and is, instead, considering further testing.

The approach used to improve the items in the American Community Survey may be useful in this regard (see earlier discussion). Rather than focusing on health conditions or impairments in body systems and structures (i.e., the factors emphasized in the medical model) or introducing circularity of thinking by measuring work disability or limitations in other major life activities, the items relate to limitations in more basic activities such as hearing, seeing, remembering, making decisions, walking, personal care, and doing errands. Although items focusing on an inherent capacity to do an activity rather than actual performance of the activity are preferable for assessing unequal opportunities, in practice it is difficult to assess capacity in a brief survey instrument. Consequently, the revised disability items for the American Community Survey (if they are shown to be reliable and valid) may be useful for adoption by surveys for the purpose of identifying individuals at risk for inequality in employment, income, poverty, and health care.

Expanding Measures of the Environment

The 1997 IOM report recommended that measures of disability reflect a model in which disability (as more narrowly defined in that report) is jointly determined by the characteristics of individuals and their environment. It further recommended that these survey items should be incorporated into ongoing surveys, including the National Health Interview Survey, the Current Population Survey, and the Survey of Income and Program Participation.

Several new measures of the environmental components of disability have recently been developed (for a review, see Keysor [2006]), but few have been incorporated into ongoing national surveys. Some surveys include a broad range of demographic, medical, socioeconomic, and behavioral items by which individuals with disabilities can be cross-classified, but they do not measure aspects of the environment that may contribute to activity limitations or participation restrictions. Although certain surveys have adopted a few measures of the use of assistive technologies and others include measures of the family context, measures of the environment otherwise continue to be quite limited. For example, questions about the accessibility of public spaces, barriers in the home or workplace, or insurance coverage for assistive technologies are not routinely included.[15] Because these items are missing from national health surveys, investigations into the causes of disability inevitably emphasize only those characteristics that are covered in the surveys, such as chronic health conditions or demographic characteristics (e.g., education).

Developing and Implementing Panel Surveys

The 1991 IOM report also suggested that a comprehensive longitudinal survey of disability be developed and implemented (Recommendation 9). Such a survey would include specific conditions and a variety of measures

---

[15]In some cases, separate data collection efforts have been mounted to fill these gaps. See, for example, the work of Carlson and Berland (2002), who report highlights from a 2001 U.S. survey of assistive technology and information technology use and need by individuals with disabilities.

reflecting the personal and social impacts and the economic burden of disability in the United States. Panel studies—those that monitor the same individuals over several years or even decades—are particularly useful in understanding the dynamic nature and natural course of disability, including risk factors for the onset of a disability and recovery from the disability.

In 1991, few national panel studies that could be used to study disability trajectories existed. The National Long-Term Care Survey, which began in 1982, and the first Longitudinal Study of Aging (1984 to 1990) provided some national longitudinal data. Both of those studies focused on older adults. In the last 15 years, a number of new panel surveys that include repeated measurement of disability have been undertaken. The Health and Retirement Study, for example, focuses on adults age 50 or over, and the Medicare Current Beneficiary Survey monitors beneficiaries (including adults under age 65 who qualify for Medicare because of a disability) for several years. A second Longitudinal Study of Aging (1994 to 2000) provided a panel survey of health and disability among older adults that was comparable to the one undertaken in the 1980s. These surveys and several smaller panel studies (e.g., the Women's Health and Aging Study) have provided important insights into the dynamics of disability and risk factors related to disability onset and recovery in late life. As discussed earlier in this chapter, these surveys most often include measures of basic activity limitations (usually ADLs and IADLs) and functional deficits, but little else to understand the nature of the gap between underlying functional abilities and the demands of the physical environment. Moreover, opportunities to study young adults who are aging with disabilities remain limited.

Because it has included the full age spectrum, the Survey of Income and Program Participation has served as an important panel resource in the past. In addition to core information on participation in disability-related programs, the survey collects more detailed information about impairments, work limitations, and other activity limitations in topical modules. The "functional limitation and disability" module, for example, which includes questions for adults, young adults, and children, has in the past been administered multiple times to the same panel. The current 2004 panel participants have, however, received this module only once.

The proposed reengineering of the Survey of Income and Program Participation by the U.S. Census Bureau (the new Dynamics of Economic Well-Being System; see U.S. Census Bureau [2006a,b]) raises some concerns. If changes in the survey eliminate the topical modules or reduce the collection of data on people with disabilities, the nation's ability to track gaps in economic well-being for those at risk for disability could be jeopardized. Like the Current Population Survey, it is important that the Survey of Income and Program Participation identify the populations with limitations in basic activities who are at risk for unequal economic well-being.

Although some recent cross-sectional survey efforts have been geared to understanding children with special health care needs (DHHS, 2004),[16] panel studies have not historically been aimed at identifying and monitoring the progress of children with disabilities.[17] As part of the assessment of the 1997 Individuals with Disabilities Education Act (IDEA 97), the U.S. Department of Education has launched a series of panel studies to monitor children using special education services: the National Early Intervention Longitudinal Study (focusing on infants and toddlers), the Pre-Elementary Education Longitudinal Study (for children ages 3 to 5), the Special Education Elementary Longitudinal Study (for elementary and middle school youth), and the National Longitudinal Transition Study-2 (the second multiyear study of high school-age children who are moving into young adulthood) (see descriptions of these studies at http://www.ed.gov/about/offices/list/osers/osep/studies.html). (Chapter 4 presents data from the last of these studies.) These panel studies monitor children over several years, including their development; functional status; and participation in social, academic, and family activities. In addition, although they are not an explicit focus, children with disabilities have been included in the department's Early Childhood Longitudinal Study, which includes two large and overlapping cohorts, one monitored from birth through the first grade and another monitored from kindergarten through the eighth grade (see descriptions of these studies at http://nces.ed.gov/ecls/).

Another useful source of information on children with disabilities has been the National Longitudinal Survey of Labor Market Experience, Youth Cohort (BLS, 2005). This Bureau of Labor Statistics survey has monitored a nationally representative sample of 12,686 young men and women who were 14 to 22 years old when they were first surveyed in 1979. Since 1986, detailed information has been collected about the health, functioning, and

---

[16]As defined by the U.S. Maternal and Child Health Bureau, children with special health care needs are "those who have or are at increased risk for a chronic physical, developmental, behavioral, or emotional condition and who also require health and related services of a type or amount beyond that required by children generally" (McPherson et al., 1998, p. 137). This broad definition was developed to help in implementing amendments to the Social Security Act that provided for the development of community-based services to serve children with special needs and their families.

[17]In the 1920s and 1930s, three cohort studies in California monitored children's physical and mental development, and one study (Hauser, 2002) included periodic follow-up data collection into the early 1980s. In the United Kingdom, longitudinal cohort studies include two studies of all children born within brief time frames in 1946 or 1958 as well as later studies of a 1970 birth cohort, a 1991–1992 cohort, and a 2001–2003 group (see, e.g., Wadsworth and Kuh [1997], Plewis et al. [2004], Reilly et al. [2005], and Wright et al. [2006]). These studies have provided substantial information about the interaction of biological phenomena with family, developmental, educational, and other environmental variables that may affect the prevention and management of disease and disability.

home environment of the children of the women in this sample. For example, 3,315 mothers along with 7,467 children were interviewed in 2002.

The state of knowledge about children with disabilities could potentially be enhanced by the National Children's Study (see http://www.nationalchildrensstudy.gov/). That study, if it is funded to full implementation, would enroll more than 100,000 newborns and monitor them to age 21 (Branum et al., 2003). Beginning even before a child's birth, the study is designed to collect information on a variety of environmental and genetic variables and assess their effects on children's birth outcomes and their longer-term health and development. Environment is broadly defined to include natural, human-made, social, and cultural factors. The sample is large enough to allow the study of a number of specific disabilities among children over time.

RECOMMENDATIONS

Since the publication of the 1991 IOM report *Disability in America*, many agencies and individuals have taken significant steps to advance the conceptual understanding of disability and to improve aspects of disability assessment and monitoring. At the same time, continued improvements are needed to prepare the country for the future and the challenges that it entails. This section presents the committee's specific recommendations.

The committee recognizes that improvements in the country's system for measuring and monitoring disability will involve costs, both financial costs and comparability costs as some previously used questions are dropped and new or revised questions are added. Agency budgets will need to be adjusted (at least temporarily) to reflect new costs, trade-offs will have to be made between continuity and improved measures, and areas of policy and other dispute will need to be resolved. For example, some argue that the inclusion of the same questions in different national surveys represents unnecessary duplication and costs (GAO, 2006). In the case of disability measures at least, this committee disagrees with this viewpoint. It is important for surveys not only of health but also of employment, housing, transportation, and other areas to include a core group of disability-related questions, just as they include core questions on race and gender. Otherwise, disparities in key areas of activity and participation will be difficult or impossible to identify and monitor for people with disabilities.

Adopting and Improving the ICF

Achieving universally accepted and understood terminology, language, and concepts with which to describe and discuss the concept of disability will remove one barrier to progress in disability research and public policy.

This will not happen immediately but, rather, will involve a long-term process of further movement toward the adoption and application of the ICF conceptual framework combined with continued efforts to refine and improve that framework and to develop tools and methods for applying it. The adoption of the ICF framework and the use of validated measures based on the framework in disability monitoring will support the use of the framework in disability research. This will, in turn, help improve the comparability of research findings over time and across studies, cultures, and nations, which will help build the knowledge base needed to better meet existing needs and prepare the country for the future challenges identified in Chapter 1.

The committee recommends that federal agencies involved in disability monitoring explicitly adopt the ICF conceptual framework *and* support efforts to strengthen it. It further recommends that these agencies cooperate, under the auspices of the Interagency Subcommittee on Disability Statistics of the Interagency Committee on Disability Research (ICDR), to develop and test new measures of disability that correspond to the major elements of the ICF and that fit the specific objectives and needs of each agency. The subcommittee should apply state-of-the-art measurement and research methodologies to evaluate these new measures for their reliability, validity, and relevance to different policy objectives. (Chapter 10 discusses the ICDR in more detail and proposes ways to strengthen it.)

> Recommendation 2.1: The National Center for Health Statistics, the U.S. Census Bureau, the Bureau of Labor Statistics, and other relevant government units involved in disability monitoring should adopt the *International Classification of Functioning, Health and Disability* (ICF) as their conceptual framework and should actively promote continued refinements to improve the framework's scope and utility for disability monitoring and research. The Interagency Subcommittee on Disability Statistics of the Interagency Committee on Disability Research should coordinate the work of these agencies to develop, test, validate, and implement new measures of disability that correspond to the components of the ICF, consistent with public policy priorities.

Although it recommends adoption of the ICF concepts, the committee recognizes that the ICF is still a framework under development and that it needs to be refined and strengthened in various areas, as described earlier in this chapter. Box 2-5 summarizes the directions that the committee identified for further work on the ICF. These refinements—combined with a program of further research to evaluate the application of the framework—should help to correct some shortcomings in the classification scheme and respond to concerns that have been discussed by the disability research community

---

BOX 2-5
Directions for Further Work on the *International Classification of Functioning, Health and Disability*

As the World Health Organization and others work to improve and refine the ICF, priority areas for attention include

- clarifying or otherwise resolving the lack of operational differentiation between the concepts of activity and participation;
- explicitly incorporating quality of life in the framework of key concepts for understanding health and disability and conducting research;
- developing classifications for personal factors affecting functioning and disability;
- further developing the classification of environmental factors;
- incorporating secondary health conditions as an ICF concept; and
- supplementing the ICF with a dynamic model of factors that influence the movement of individuals among states of functioning or disability.

---

and by ICF users across the world. Although some steps, such as the refinement of the coding or classification of environmental factors and the development of codes for personal factors require the formal modification of the ICF by WHO, the consideration of quality-of-life and secondary conditions in monitoring and research activities can still proceed, as can the development of core measures of ICF concepts as discussed below.

The committee recognizes that different disability measures serve different purposes. It therefore does not recommend that a single measure of disability be used in all national disability monitoring programs or that every component of the ICF be equally emphasized in all activities. Specific steps can, however, be taken to move toward greater consistency in disability assessment and monitoring, for example, developing, testing, and then adopting a set of core survey questions.

First, for surveys that aim to provide information on the removal of barriers to participation for individuals at risk for unequal opportunity by virtue of their physical, cognitive, mental, or sensory impairments, one priority is the adoption of a uniform set of measures of such impairments of body structure and function. Again, the ICDR can coordinate work to identify a set of core measures of impairment that can be used to measure progress in removing barriers to independent living and participation in community life. The classification scheme of the ICF will be helpful in guiding these efforts, but it does not by itself provide these core measures. For activity limitations, the measures proposed for the American Community Survey (as discussed earlier) may be a useful starting point.

Second, in addition to refining the classification of environmental factors, further work is needed to measure various environmental contributors to disability, particularly those that contribute to activity limitations and participation restrictions. Important steps include the review of existing measures for their reliability and validity and the development and testing of new items, if necessary. Those measures found to be valid and reliable can then be incorporated into appropriate national surveys.

Third, continued refinement is needed of age- or developmentally appropriate measures of disability for children that correspond to the ICF concepts of impairment, activity limitation, and participation restriction (see, e.g., Ogonowski et al. [2004], McConachie et al. [2006], and Simeonsson [2006]). In addition, instruments that identify children with special needs related to their disabilities (e.g., higher than typical rates of use of health care or social services) are valuable, although surveys should continue to identify chronic health conditions that may contribute to disability.

Fourth, to the extent that new measures replace old ones in a particular survey, the committee encourages the use of both measures in the years surrounding the transition. This will allow analysts to assess the influence of the wording changes on the survey results.

Finally, in addition to the adoption of the new measures by the agencies that are most identified with disability monitoring, the committee encourages other agencies leading or funding relevant national surveys (as listed earlier in Table 2-1) to update their measures to reflect the concepts in the ICF as such measures become available. These agencies include the National Institute on Aging, the Centers for Medicare and Medicaid Services (CMS), and the Agency for Healthcare Research and Quality.

Improving the Scope and Quality of National Disability Monitoring Data

In addition to adopting the ICF framework, which itself would help harmonize the country's disability monitoring efforts, the federal government should move in other ways toward a more coherent disability monitoring program. Disability statistics must now be taken piecemeal from multiple surveys to obtain disability-related information on people of all ages and in all living situations. Federal agencies have not harmonized measures across surveys, and surveys pay scant attention to the environmental components of disability. Adopting a common conceptual framework does not in itself correct these shortcomings or fill gaps in existing data.

Recommendation 2.2: The National Center for Health Statistics, in collaboration with other relevant federal agencies, should continue to

improve the scope and quality of data—including longitudinal or panel data—on disability, its causes, and its consequences. These improved data sources should serve as the cornerstone of a new national disability monitoring system.

As new measures of the ICF become available, agency coordination through the Disability Statistics Subcommittee of the ICDR will help achieve consistency across surveys. Agencies can collaborate now to develop and test a set of core measures for incorporation into key national surveys, including surveys on housing, employment, income, and other topics that do not now include questions on disability.

Action by the CDC, in particular, the National Center for Health Statistics, is critical to an improved disability monitoring system. Priorities include the development of a new panel survey of disability as a supplement to the National Health Interview Survey and enhancements to the Behavioral Risk Factor Surveillance System to provide more comprehensive state-specific estimates of disability. A primary purpose of the panel study on disability would be to track changes in barriers to activity and participation by monitoring the surveyed individuals over time, including as they enter or leave supportive living environments and institutional settings. To secure sufficient representation, the survey would need to oversample children. By monitoring people of all ages over time, a new panel study would also permit investigation of issues related to aging with a disability. In addition, CDC should also consider ways to supplement the National Health Interview Survey framework by surveying individuals living in institutional settings so that the full spectrum of living arrangements can be represented. In developing the panel study, CDC will need to balance the need to reflect new language, concerns, and understandings of disability with the desirability of making some comparisons with the 1994–1995 Disability Supplement.

Priorities for enhancements to the Behavioral Risk Factor and Surveillance System include expansion of core disability measures, assessments of disability among children, and measures to track changes in the accessibility of public and private spaces, including schools, health care facilities, and offices. Such measures can be developed first as optional modules and then eventually incorporated into core survey modules.

Because employment and economic security are such central issues for the independence and the community integration of people with disabilities, better data on the employment status of and economic opportunities for people with various kinds of limitations are also high priorities. Thus it is important for the Bureau of Labor Statistics to include core disability measures in the Current Population Survey and for the U.S. Census Bureau to include such measures in the reengineered survey in the Dynamics of

Economic Well-Being System that will replace the Survey of Income and Program Participation.

Remedying gaps in knowledge about disability among children is another important direction for a national disability monitoring program. As this chapter and the next make clear, the data on children with disabilities are limited. Moreover, as described in Chapters 4 and 5, policy makers, clinicians, educators, and families lack key longitudinal data on the relationship between childhood conditions, physical and social environments, medical treatments, and other events and the long-term functioning and well-being of children as they move into and through adult life. The inclusion of children in a new CDC panel study of disability and the incorporation of measures of disability among children into the Behavioral Risk Factor Surveillance System would help remedy some of these gaps.

The committee's recommendations to this point focus on the "data production" side of the disability monitoring system. The use of the data for monitoring and other purposes is also important. Although agencies generally make their data available for use by others, it would be helpful for users to have access to some kind of data or information intermediary that would simplify and support user access to the resources of multiple agencies. The NIDRR-supported disability statistics center at Cornell University has taken steps in this direction by preparing guides to disability statistics sources (e.g., the American Community Survey) and data summaries (e.g., annual disability status reports). The center will also develop options for activities to bridge the divide between users and sources of disability data. One possible prototype for such an activity is the Research Data Assistance Center at the University of Minnesota (www.resdac.umn.edu), which is supported by CMS to encourage researchers' use of the agency's data by supplying free technical assistance in obtaining and using the data.

This chapter has argued for the development of a common conceptual framework based on the ICF framework and a set of actions to strengthen the quality and usefulness of this country's data on disability and to move toward the development of a coherent, coordinated, ongoing disability monitoring system. Good data are essential to understanding the current situation of people with disabilities, identifying problems, and creating the conditions for the independence and fuller participation of people with disabilities in all aspects of national life. Using data currently available from monitoring programs, the next chapter summarizes trends in disability among Americans in early, middle, and late life.

3

Disability Trends

Disability is an ambiguous demographic, but one that is unambiguously increasing.

Glenn T. Fujiura (2001)

As described in Chapter 1, demographic trends—notably, the aging of the American population—promise to increase substantially the numbers of people at risk for disability. Whether such trends will translate in the future into increasing numbers of people with limits on their activities and participation in community life is less clear. Avoiding such increases will depend in part on the nation's will to promote equalization of opportunity for all Americans, irrespective of age or ability.

The good news is that for many people the chances of experiencing activity limitations or participation restrictions can be reduced through a variety of means. These include making effective assistive technologies and accessible general-use technologies more widely available (see Chapter 7) and promoting broader acceptance and stronger enforcement of policies to remove environmental barriers to access and participation in areas such as health care, employment, transportation, and telecommunications (see Chapter 6 and Appendixes D, E, F, and G). In addition, public health and clinical interventions can help prevent the onset of illness or injury and associated physical or mental impairments, as well as minimize the development of secondary health conditions and limit the effects of atypical or premature aging among young adults with disabilities (see Chapter 5).

To provide insight into the future of disability, this chapter reviews recent trends in the amount, type, and health-related causes of disability—primarily in the form of activity limitations—for people in early, middle, and late life. It considers projections of future levels of disability. The analysis here should be read in the context of the review in Chapter 2 of the inadequacies in the nation's current disability surveillance system. As in 1991, when the Institute of Medicine (IOM) report *Disability in America* was published, data sources that can be used to guide the future of disability in America, particularly efforts to identify and remove environmental barriers to participation for people with disabilities, are inadequate.

Current statistics, discussed further below, indicate that the number of people with disability (broadly defined as impairments, activity limitations, or participation restrictions) now exceeds 40 million—and that number could be more than 50 million. Data on trends in disability during early, middle, and late life present a mixed picture of the changes that have taken place during the last two decades and more. Among children, evidence points to increases in some health conditions—including asthma, prematurity, autism, and obesity—that contribute to disability. These increases have been accompanied by increases in certain activity limitations that are not entirely explained by increased health and educational screening of children. The percentage of adults under the age of 65 who had activity limitations, including work limitations, grew during the 1990s, although this increase appears to have leveled off recently. In contrast, among older adults, declines in the prevalence of personal care and domestic activity limitations have been reported, although not all groups appear to have benefited equally, and the reasons for these declines remain unclear.

As described in Chapter 2, data on participation restrictions, in particular, remain relatively limited. Thus a full portrait of trends in disability is not possible. Moreover, although the equalization of opportunities for people with disabilities is an increasing focus of researchers, they cannot yet track the broad range of environmental factors that contribute to activity limitations and participation restrictions. This chapter focuses on trends during the past two decades in a relatively narrow set of activity limitations, the health conditions that contribute to those limitations, and, where relevant, possible explanations for these trends.

CURRENT ESTIMATES OF DISABILITY AND RELATED CONDITIONS

As discussed in Chapter 2, the omission of key groups from national population surveys has important implications for the development of basic

BOX 3-1
Selected Recent Chartbooks and Other
Profiles of Statistical Data on Disability

Federal Resources

Centers for Disease Control and Prevention
   Disability and Health State Chartbook 2006: Profiles of Health for Adults with Disabilities

U.S. Census Bureau
   Americans with Disabilities, 2002 (Steinmetz, 2006)
   Disability and American Families, 2000 (Wang, 2005)

Health Resources and Services Administration, Maternal and Child Health Bureau.
   National Survey of Children with Special Health Care Needs Chartbook, 2001 (HRSA, 2004)

National Institute on Disability and Rehabilitation Research
   Chartbook on Mental Health and Disability in the United States (Jans et al., 2004)

Other Resources

Cornell Center on Disability Demographics and Statistics
   2004 Disability Status Reports: United States Summary (Houtenville, 2005)

Disability Statistics Center, University of California at San Francisco
   Improved Employment Opportunities for People with Disabilities (Kaye, 2003)

Population Reference Bureau
   Disability in America (Freedman et al., 2004b)

estimates of the population with disabilities. Such estimates must be pieced together from various sources, and the figures vary depending on the choice of survey and definition.

Box 3-1 lists several chartbooks and other profiles of disability data in the United States. The U.S. Census Bureau and most other agencies supply public use data sets so that researchers and others can obtain data more recent than those available in such profiles, and a few agency resources also allow some online analysis of the data.[1]

One challenge in using information from different surveys is that different surveys rely upon different conceptual notions of disability, which in

---

[1]As indicated in the source citations for most of the figures in this chapter, the committee contracted with H. Stephen Kaye of the University of California at San Francisco to supply information from the public use data sets for the National Health Interview Survey.

turn lead to different population estimates. For example, Stein and Silver (2002) found estimates of the rates of disability among children to be in the range of 14 to 17 percent, depending on whether children were identified through chronic conditions, special health care needs, or reports of disability. Moreover, even seemingly minor differences in the phrasing of questions or response options or in the ways of summarizing the data may yield different or even inconsistent pictures of a particular aspect of disability. For example, for older adults, some surveys ask whether they "have difficulty" with an activity, whereas others ask if they "need help" and others ask if they "get help or use special equipment" to perform the activity. Such differences can lead to different estimates of disability levels and trends. Hence, the use of these measures outside of a coherent conceptual framework and the lack of sufficient attention by users to the implications of differences in measures contribute to inconsistency and confusion.

Recognizing these caveats, the committee reviewed recent disability statistics and concluded that the total number of people in the United States with disabilities (defined to include individuals with impairments in body structure or function, activity limitations, or participation restrictions) currently exceeds 40 million. Depending on the survey from which statistics are drawn, the figure could exceed 50 million. No single data source yields estimates for all age groups living in the community and in institutional settings, so the estimate of the population with disabilities must be drawn from several different surveys.

The committee began with data from the U.S. Census Bureau's 2004 American Community Survey. As summarized in Table 3-1, an estimated 38 million people (4.1 million people between the ages of 5 and 20, 20.2 million people between the ages of 21 and 64, and 13.5 million people ages 65 and older) who live in the community report a disability.[2] This estimate does not include people living in nursing homes and other institutional settings or children under age 5. The Medicare Current Beneficiary Survey estimates that approximately 2.2 million Medicare beneficiaries live in long-term care facilities and that about 350,000 of this population are adults under age 65 (CMS, 2005a). In addition, other surveys suggest that approximately 16,000 children with intellectual or developmental disabilities are living in out-of-home residential settings, about half which have four or more residents (Prouty et al., 2005). Data from the 2004 National Health Interview Survey indicate that perhaps 700,000 children under age 5 have a limitation in one or more activities because of a chronic condition, which

---

[2]In the American Community Survey, "disability" is defined as a long-lasting sensory, physical, mental, or emotional condition that can make it difficult for a person to walk, climb stairs, dress, bathe, learn, remember, go outside the home alone, or work at a job or business. The term also covers vision or hearing impairments.

TABLE 3-1 Disability Rates by Sex and Age (Excluding Ages 0 to 4), Civilian Population (Excluding Residents of Nursing Homes, Dormitories, and Other Group Housing), 2004

Population	With a Disability		By Type of Disability (number, in millions)[a]					
	Number (millions)	Percent	Sensory	Physical Activity[b]	Cognitive[c]	Self-Care	Go Outside Home	Employment
5 years and over								
Male	17.8	13.8	5.0	10.2	6.8	2.8	NR	NR
Female	20.1	14.8	4.6	13.6	6.9	4.2	NR	NR
Both	37.9	14.3	9.5	23.8	13.8	7.1	NR	NR
5 to 15 years								
Male	1.8	8.0	0.3	0.3	1.5	0.2	NA	NA
Female	1.0	4.5	0.2	0.2	0.8	0.1	NA	NA
Both	2.8	6.3	0.5	0.5	2.3	0.4	NA	NA
16 to 20 years								
Male	0.7	7.8	0.1	0.1	0.5	0.1	0.1	0.2
Female	0.5	5.9	0.1	0.1	0.3	0.1	0.1	0.2
Both	1.3	6.9	0.3	0.3	0.9	0.1	0.3	0.4
21 to 64 years								
Male	9.8	11.9	2.6	5.8	3.4	1.6	2.1	5.6
Female	10.4	12.2	2.0	6.8	3.6	1.9	2.9	6.2
Both	20.2	12.1	4.7	12.7	7.0	3.3	5.0	11.7
65 years and over								
Male	5.4	37.1	2.5	3.9	1.5	1.1	1.7	NA
Female	8.1	41.4	2.9	6.4	2.3	2.1	3.8	NA
Both	13.5	39.6	5.5	10.3	3.7	3.2	5.6	NA

[a]One person may have more than one type of disability, so the overall figure may be smaller than the sum of the types. NA = not asked; NR = not reported.

[b]The U.S. Census Bureau refers to "physical" rather than "physical activity" disabilities or limitations.

[c]The U.S. Census Bureau uses the term "mental" rather than "cognitive" to refer to difficulties remembering, learning, or concentrating.

SOURCE: U.S. Census Bureau (2005a, Tables S1801and B18002 to B18008).

brings the total of children ages 0 to 17 with disabilities to approximately 4.8 million. With these additional groups added to the American Community Survey estimate, the total estimate of people with disabilities exceeds 40 million.

Surveys that use a broader conception of disability than that adopted by this committee yield higher estimates. For example, based on the 2002 Survey of Income and Program Participation, which includes numerous questions to identify individuals of all ages with disabilities living in the community, the U.S. Census Bureau estimated that 51 million people have disabilities, including 32 million who have a severe disability (Steinmetz, 2006).[3] The Behavioral Risk Factor Surveillance System, which includes two broad items to identify the adult community-based population with disabilities, also places the figure for all states close to 50 million (CDC, 2006a).[4] Based on its review, the committee concluded that the number of people in the United States with disabilities exceeds 40 million and may exceed 50 million. Although these figures are not directly comparable to the 35 million estimate from the 1991 IOM report (because the survey questions differ), the number of people with disabilities has almost certainly increased since 1988, when most of the data used in that report were collected.

Table 3-2 lists the most common health conditions reported by respondents in the National Health Interview Survey as "causing" or contributing to limitations among people of different ages residing in the community. The survey questions reflect a largely medical model of disability. The committee could identify no national data on the extent to which features of the physical and social environments contribute to disability (see also Chapter 6).

For children, the primary health conditions contributing to a limitation are cognitive, emotional, or developmental problems, although speech prob-

---

[3]For adults, questions in the Survey of Income and Program Participation ask about mobility-related assistive technology use; activity limitations; learning disabilities; the presence of a mental or emotional condition, or both; mental retardation; developmental disabilities; Alzheimer's disease; and conditions limiting employment or work around the house. For children, the questions involve specified conditions (autism, cerebral palsy, mental retardation, developmental disabilities); activity limitations (seeing, hearing, speaking, walking, running, taking part in sports); developmental delays; difficulty walking, running, or playing; or difficulty moving the arms or legs (Steinmetz, 2006). Not all the questions in the survey involve disability as defined in this report.

[4]Widely cited estimates from the 2000 decennial census also put the estimate of the civilian, noninstitutional population with disabilities near 50 million. However, U.S. Census Bureau analysts attributed this estimate to a formatting problem with the census questionnaire that may have incorrectly increased positive responses to questions about disabilities with going-outside-the-home and work limitations (Stern and Brault, 2005). Subsequent estimates from the American Community Survey of the U.S. Census Bureau put the figure closer to 40 million.

TABLE 3-2 Leading Chronic Health Conditions Reported as Causing Limitations of Activities, by Age, Civilian, Noninstitutional Population, 2002 and 2003

Chronic Condition	Number of People with Activity Limitations Caused by Selected Chronic Health Conditions per 1,000 Population		
	Under 5 years	*5–11 years*	*12–17 years*
Speech problem	10.7	18.5	4.6
Asthma or breathing problem	8.2	8.4	8.3
Mental retardation or other development problem	7.0	10.2	9.6
Other mental, emotional, or behavioral problem	2.7	12.0	14.2
Attention deficit or hyperactivity disorder	2.1	17.6	21.8
Learning disability	2.9	23.3	33.9
	18–44 years	*45–54 years*	*55–64 years*
Mental illness	12.9	23.1	24.1
Fractures or joint injury	7.0	15.5	20.6
Lung	5.0	12.6	25.6
Diabetes	2.5	13.4	33.4
Heart or other circulatory	5.9	28.4	74.3
Arthritis or other musculoskeletal	22.2	61.9	100.7
	65–74 years	*75–84 years*	*85 years or over*
Senility (dementia)	6.8	30.5	96.1
Lung	34.7	41.4	44.4
Diabetes	41.1	49.4	38.4
Vision	18.2	44.3	96.6
Hearing	10.0	27.8	84.9
Heart or other circulatory	101.9	162.6	223.5
Arthritis or other musculoskeletal	125.8	171.0	267.6

NOTE: The table shows the numbers per 1,000 population. The respondents could mention more than one condition.
SOURCE: NCHS (2005a, spreadsheet data for Figures 18, 19, and 20, based on the 2002 and 2003 National Health Interview Surveys).

lems figure prominently for children under the age of 12 and asthma contributes to activity limitations among children in all age groups. For the 0.7 percent of children who had limitations so severe that they could not attend school, Msall and colleagues (2003), using data from the 1994–1995 disability supplement to the National Health Interview Survey, found that the most common reported reasons for nonattendance were life-threatening or other physical disorders, neurodevelopmental disorders, learning-behavior disorders, and asthma.

Among adults under age 65, musculoskeletal problems (including arthritis) and heart problems become increasingly important as people grow older. Mental illness is the second leading chronic condition mentioned as a cause of activity limitation for individuals ages 18 to 44 and is the fifth most frequently mentioned cause for individuals ages 55 to 64. For some people in this age group who are aging with disabilities, their primary health condition (e.g., cerebral palsy or spinal cord injury) is a risk factor for the development of secondary health conditions that have the potential to contribute to additional impairments, activity limitations, or participation restrictions. In general, survey questions have limited ability to distinguish such secondary disabling conditions from primary disabling conditions. (See Chapter 5 for further discussion.) For people ages 65 and over, musculoskeletal and heart problems continue to be leading contributors to limitations. Among people age 75 and over, senility (the term used by the National Center for Health Statistics but now more commonly referred to as dementia) is a major contributor to limitations.

MONITORING TRENDS IN DISABILITY

Monitoring trends in disability is important for several reasons. First, trend data provide a barometer of the nation's achievements in terms of disability prevention. Second, when such data include measures of social, medical, and environmental risk factors, they can point policy makers to effective strategies for future interventions that will prevent or limit disabilities. Third, by including individuals of all ages, trend data can provide important insights into the future and serve as a basis for making assumptions that can be incorporated into projections.

Studies that track and attempt to explain changes over time in the population require a high degree of consistency in survey design. Changes in the wording of questions, the type and coverage of the sample frame, the use of proxy respondents, and the frequency and timing of interviews, among other factors, can all influence the conclusions drawn from such studies (Freedman et al., 2002). Unfortunately, despite the growing number of data sources and the repetition of certain major surveys, the available data—on the whole—permit few direct comparisons with data from the 1980s and earlier. Notably, although several surveys that focused on older adults have allowed analysis of late-life trends since the 1980s, discontinuities in the surveys make comparisons of present survey data with data from previous surveys difficult for those in early and middle life. This difficulty will be particularly evident in discussions of data from the National Health Interview Survey before and after the major revisions made to that survey in

1997 (see Chapter 2 for further discussion of the revisions). The 1991 IOM report used data from the 1988 National Health Interview Survey.

With these limitations noted, the next three sections of this chapter review trends in disability in early, middle, and late life. These divisions of the human life span are necessarily artificial to some degree. They are based on a mix of social conventions, statistical convenience, and public policy considerations; but they reflect important distinctions. Thus age 18, when people become legal adults in nearly all states, is used as the endpoint for early life (childhood and adolescence), even though important physical and psychological development continues past that age and well into the third decade of life (see the discussion of the transition into adult life in Chapter 4). Midlife, ages 18 to 64, encompasses a particularly broad period of life, almost five decades. As discussed in Chapter 5, many people in this group have conditions that in years past commonly led to early death, and many are experiencing premature or atypical aging that neither they nor their physicians have anticipated. The late-life period is defined as beginning at age 65, although some studies focus on an older group (age 70 and older or age 85 and older) that is at a considerably higher risk of disability than younger groups within the older population.

TRENDS IN EARLY LIFE

In a background paper prepared for an IOM workshop held in August 2005, Stein observed that "over a 40-year period, the proportion of children reported to have major limitations in their activities related to play and school has gone from less than 2 percent to close to 7 percent" (Stein, 2006, p. 146). The reasons for this trend are complex and varied. In part, the trend reflects changes in the epidemiology of childhood illness and functioning. For example, data show disturbing increases in recent years in the number of children who are reported to have potentially disabling chronic conditions, such as asthma and autism, as well as increases in the prevalence of preterm births (Stein, 2006). In addition, longer-term trends likely reflect increases in the recognition and treatment of learning-related disabilities and other conditions. The next section reviews these trends in more detail, and the subsequent section describes two public health successes: declines in the rates of spina bifida and lead poisoning.

Activity Limitations

Examining disability trends among children presents special challenges. Especially in the first few years of life, children's developmental changes make it difficult or inappropriate to identify certain kinds of behaviors as impairments or activity limitations. Furthermore, "the functioning of children is always a moving target, as children mature at different rates, live in different cultures with different expectations of independence and self-sufficiency, and grow up in environments that vary markedly in the demands that they place on the performance of activities by children" (Stein, 2006, p. 145). Estimates of disability also vary depending on whether children are identified as having disabilities because of chronic conditions, special health care needs, or reports of activity limitations (Stein and Silver, 2002).[5] In addition, as it is true for all age groups, revisions in national surveys complicate comparisons of disability trends for children. Despite these challenges and complexities, the data suggest increases in the proportion of children with activity limitations and conditions that put them at risk of disabilities.

The earliest data from the National Health Interview Survey (Newacheck et al., 1984, 1986) reported activity limitations for only 1.8 percent of children under age 18 in 1960. The rate group increased to 3.8 percent for 1979 to 1981. For the period from 1984 to 1996, reports of the rates of activity limitations for this group increased from 5.1 to 6.1 percent (Table 3-3).

More recent data, based on new National Health Interview Survey questions that asked about the receipt of special education services, the need for assistance with personal care, and limitations in walking and cognition, suggest that increases in the numbers of children with activity limitations also occurred between 1997 and 2004 (Table 3-4). In this more recent period, the increase in activity limitations was particularly affected by the increasing receipt of special education services, especially for boys. Boys are almost twice as likely as girls to be reported to be receiving such services. In addition, pooled data from the 2000 to 2002 National Health Interview Survey show that boys have higher rates of mental retardation, learning disabilities (including attention deficit or hyperactivity disorder), asthma, and vision or hearing problems (Xiang et al., 2005). Although special education services may be aimed, in particular, at children with conditions that primarily affect cognition (e.g., mental retardation), they also serve children with medical conditions that may secondarily affect the ability to learn.

---

[5]As defined by the U.S. Maternal and Child Health Bureau, children with special health care needs are "those who have or are at increased risk for a chronic physical, developmental, behavioral, or emotional condition and who also require health and related services of a type or amount beyond that required by children generally" (McPherson et al., 1998, p. 137). This broad definition was developed to help in implementing amendments to the Social Security Act that provided for the development of community-based services for children with special health care needs and their families.

TABLE 3-3 Percentage of Children (Under Age 18) with Activity Limitations, by Type of Limitation and Age, 1984 to 1996

Activity Limitation	1984	1986	1988	1990	1992	1994	1996
Limited in activity (ages 0–17)	5.1	5.0	5.3	4.9	6.1	6.7	6.1
Limited in activity (ages 0–4)	2.5	2.5	2.2	2.2	2.8	3.1	2.6
Limited in activity (ages 5–17)	6.1	6.0	6.6	6.1	7.5	8.2	7.5
Needs ADL help (ages 5–17)	0.3	0.3	0.3	0.3	0.4	0.5	0.4

NOTE: Only limitations in activity caused by chronic conditions or impairments are included. Data for children residing in group settings are not included. Respondents are classified as having no activity limitation if they report a limitation due to a condition that is not known to be chronic. An activity limitation is defined as follows: children are classified in terms of the major activity usually associated with their particular age group. The major activities for the age groups are (1) ordinary play for children under 5 years of age and (2) attending school for those 5 to 17 years of age. A child is classified as having an activity limitation if he or she is (1) unable to perform the major activity, (2) able to perform the major activity but limited in the kind or amount of this activity, and (3) not limited in the major activity but limited in the kinds or amounts of other activities. ADL = activities of daily living.
SOURCE: H. Stephen Kaye, Disability Statistics Center, University of California at San Francisco, unpublished tabulations from the National Health Interview Survey, as requested by the committee.

(For the activity limitations and major activity limitations reported before 1997, boys also showed a higher prevalence of disability.)[6]

Potential Explanations of Trends

As suggested above, the tripling of activity limitations among children over four decades likely reflects a confluence of forces. In part, there have been real changes in the epidemiology of illnesses and related disabilities among children. In addition, the trend may be capturing in part the increasing awareness by parents, health professionals, and other agencies

---

[6]Other surveys besides the National Health Interview Survey suggest significant increases in the rates of certain potentially disabling chronic conditions among children and youth, especially in recent years. For example, the National Longitudinal Survey of Labor Market Experience, Youth Cohort, provides information on the health-related conditions of children born to women who were ages 14 to 21 in 1979. These data show an increase in the prevalence of chronic conditions from 11 percent in 1994 to 24 percent in 2000 among children who were ages 8 to14 in those years (unpublished tabulations from James Perrin, committee member).

TABLE 3-4 Percentage of Children (Under Age 18) with Activity Limitations, by Type of Limitation, Age Group, and Gender, 1997 to 2004

Limitation	1997	1998	1999	2000	2001	2002	2003	2004
Limited in activity								
All (ages 0–17)	6.6	6.2	5.9	5.9	6.7	7.0	6.8	7.0
Male (ages 0–4)	4.2	4.4	3.8	4.0	4.2	4.0	4.2	4.2
Male (ages 5–17)	9.9	9.3	8.7	8.8	10.3	10.6	10.0	10.5
Female (ages 0–4)	2.7	2.3	2.4	2.4	2.4	2.5	2.9	2.7
Female (ages 5–17)	5.5	5.2	5.1	5.0	5.5	6.1	6.0	6.1
Needs help with ADL								
All (ages 5–17)	0.55	0.45	0.50	0.51	0.44	0.66	0.46	0.65
Male (ages 5–17)	0.64	0.51	0.60	0.64	0.53	0.76	0.52	0.79
Female (ages 5–17)	0.46	0.38	0.39	0.38	0.34	0.55	0.41	0.50
Has difficulty walking								
All (ages 5–17)	0.25	0.29	0.30	0.29	0.23	0.33	0.23	0.29
Male (ages 5–17)	0.27	0.27	0.33	0.35	0.27	0.31	0.18	0.34
Female (ages 5–17)	0.23	0.31	0.26	0.22	0.19	0.34	0.28	0.25
Uses special education								
All (ages 5–17)	6.2	6.1	5.9	5.8	6.7	7.1	6.8	7.1
Male (ages 5–17)	8.1	7.8	7.5	7.5	8.9	9.2	8.7	9.0
Female (ages 5–17)	4.1	4.3	4.2	3.9	4.4	5.0	4.9	5.1

NOTE: Only limitations in activity caused by chronic conditions or impairments are included. The respondents are reclassified as having no activity limitation if they report a limitation due to a condition that is not known to be chronic. A child is considered to have an activity limitation if the parent responded positively to at least one of the following questions: (1) "Does [child's name] receive Special Education Services?" (2) "Because of a physical, mental, or emotional problem, does [child's name] need the help of other persons with personal care needs, such as eating, bathing, dressing, or getting around inside the home?" (3) "Because of a health problem does [child's name] have difficulty walking without using any special equipment?" (4) "Is [child's name] limited in any way because of difficulty remembering or because of periods of confusion?" (5) "Is [child's name] limited in any activities because of physical, mental, or emotional problems?"
SOURCE: H. Stephen Kaye, Disability Statistics Center, University of California at San Francisco, unpublished tabulations from the National Health Interview Survey, as requested by the committee.

(especially schools) of conditions that merit attention and intervention, particularly through educational programs.[7]

---

[7]Increased awareness may affect the estimation of disability rates for other age groups besides children; see, for example, the work of Waidmann and Liu (2000) for the influence of changes in Social Security Disability Insurance policies and criteria on self-reports of disability by adults.

Shifts in Conditions Potentially Contributing to Disability

Over the last few decades, the rise in the rates of potentially disabling childhood conditions—in particular, asthma—along with increases in the rates of preterm births, deserves special consideration in the analysis of activity limitation trends in children. During the early 1970s, when the rates of severe limitations grew from 2.7 to 3.7 percent, Newacheck and colleagues (1984, 1986) found increasing rates of several health conditions, especially mental health conditions, asthma, orthopedic conditions, and hearing loss. Unfortunately, changes in the questions as part of the redesign of the National Health Interview Survey in 1997 make comparisons over the entire time period inappropriate.[8] Instead, the committee focused its review on the role of changes in the prevalence of a few potentially disabling health conditions.

Approximately 12 percent of children have at some time been diagnosed with asthma—the single most prevalent condition associated with childhood disability—and 8 percent currently have asthma (Federal Interagency Forum on Child and Family Statistics, 2005). In 2000, an analysis by the Centers for Disease Control and Prevention (CDC) reported that the prevalence of asthma among children increased by approximately 5 percent per year during the period from 1980 to 1995 but dropped by 17 percent in 1996 (CDC, 2000a). For the period from 1969–1970 to 1994–1995, Newacheck and Halfon (2000) documented the contribution of asthma to the rise in the overall prevalence of disabilities among children. They reported that the prevalence of disability related to asthma (based on data from the National Health Interview Survey) increased 232 percent over this time span, whereas the prevalence of disability related to all other chronic childhood conditions increased by 113 percent over the same period.

Changes in the questions about asthma in the National Health Interview Survey in 1997 preclude a comparison of recent data with earlier data. The prevalence of asthma did not, however, change much between 1997 and 2004. During this more recent time period, the percentage of children with asthma or breathing problems that caused limitations declined from 0.9 percent in 1997 to 0.6 percent in 2004 (unpublished tabulations of the National Health Interview Survey prepared by this committee).

---

[8]In addition, because of further changes in questions in the National Health Interview Survey *after* 1997, of the six leading conditions (speech problems; asthma or breathing problems; mental retardation or other development problems; other mental, emotional, or behavioral problems; attention deficit or hyperactivity disorder; and learning disabilities), only the survey questions related to speech problems and asthma are comparable over the 1997 to 2004 time period. For example, before 2000, parents were asked only if they had been told that their child had attention deficit disorder; after that they were also asked about attention deficit or hyperactivity disorder (Pastor and Reuben, 2005).

Why the rate of asthma has increased and whether the rates have truly leveled off remain unclear. A recent review of evidence to explain the increase in the prevalence and severity of asthma in the United States and a number of other countries since the 1960s suggested that "the combination of the control of infectious diseases, prolonged indoor exposure, and a sedentary lifestyle . . . is the key to the asthma epidemic and, in particular, the key to the rise in severity" (Platts-Mills, 2005, p. 1026).

Another condition potentially contributing to disability is preterm birth. For a variety of reasons, including the increased rates of survival of high-risk infants and the growth in the number of multiple births associated with certain fertility treatments, the numbers of infants born prematurely and with low birth weights have increased (IOM, 2006a). For example, the rate of premature births (as a percentage of all births) increased from 10.6 percent in 1990 to 12.5 percent in 2004. Prematurity (birth before 37 weeks of completed gestation) and low birth weight (birth weight less than 2,500 grams) are risk factors for a number of short-term and long-term neurodevelopmental and other health problems and disabilities related to cerebral palsy, mental retardation, and sensory impairments, as well as more subtle disorders, such as attention deficit or hyperactivity disorder.

The reported prevalence of autism and related disorders has also grown significantly (Newschaffer et al., 2005; CDC, 2007). These conditions are characterized by impairments in social interactions and communication patterns and restricted, stereotyped, repetitive sets of activities and interests (WHO, 2006). CDC recently reported data from 14 sites showing an average rate of autism of 6.5 per 1,000 children aged 8 years in 2002 or approximately one child in 150 (CDC, 2007), a figure that is considerably higher than those suggested in earlier studies and reviews (see, e.g., Gillberg and Wing [1999] and Fombonne [2002]). The range reported in the CDC study was 3.3 to 10.6 per 1,000 children. An IOM study that examined the relationship between autism and childhood vaccines concluded that the published literature was generally uninformative in helping assess trends in the condition (IOM, 2004c). The growth in the reported rates of autism undoubtedly reflects a variety of factors, including the broader range of conditions currently encompassed in the spectrum of autism disorders (e.g., Asperger's syndrome, other childhood disintegrative disorder, and pervasive developmental disorder, unspecified) and the addition of a substantial number of young people on the milder edge of the autism spectrum (APA, 2000; Shattuck, 2006). A substantial growth in the levels of awareness of autism and related disorders by both parents and clinicians has also led to the better identification of children who have autism spectrum disorders. In years past, these children might have been given another diagnosis (e.g., unspecified mental retardation) (Gurney et al., 2003; Barbaresi et al., 2005;

Newschaffer, 2006). Some of the growth in autism rates likely reflects a true growth in the prevalence of autism.

Although the connection of obesity to disability warrants more investigation, another IOM committee has described the increasing prevalence of childhood obesity as a "startling setback" for child health (IOM, 2005a, p. 21). Obesity is a risk factor for a number of serious health conditions, such as diabetes, that are, in turn, risk factors for disabilities. Figure 3-1 shows trend data for children 6 to 11 and 12 to 19 years of age. Based in part on concerns about the stigmatization of children and in part on concerns about the reliability of the body mass index (BMI) as a measure of fatness for children, CDC has used the term "overweight" for children who would count as overweight or obese on the basis of BMI criteria (Wechsler, 2004). The earlier IOM committee, however, concluded that the term "obesity"

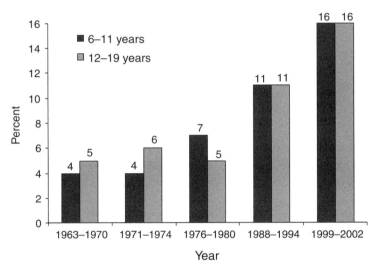

FIGURE 3-1 Trends in overweight (obesity) for children ages 6 to 11 and adolescents ages 12 to 19, civilian noninstitional population, 1963 to 2002. Overweight (the term used by CDC) is defined as a BMI value at or above the 95th percentile cutoff points in the sex- and gender-specific BMI growth charts developed by CDC in 2000, based on BMI data from earlier surveys (see IOM [2005a]). Data exclude those for pregnant women starting with the period from 1971 to 1974. Pregnancy status was not available for the periods from 1963 to 1965 and 1966 to 1970. Data for 1963 to 1965 are for children 6 to 11 years of age; data for 1966 to 1970 are for adolescents 12 to 17 years of age, not 12 to 19 years.
SOURCE: CDC National Health and Nutrition Examination Surveys (CDC, 2005b).

was appropriate for children 2 years of age and older who have a BMI at or above the 95th percentile for their age and sex groups (IOM, 2005a).

Explanations for the increases in the rates of childhood obesity, which occurred primarily in the 1980s and 1990s, were cited in a 2001 report from the U.S. Surgeon General (U.S. Public Health Service, 2001). Factors include inactive lifestyles (e.g., watching television and playing computer and video games) and unhealthy eating patterns exacerbated by media exposure.

The Role of Increased Identification

Although the data of Newacheck and colleagues (1984, 1986) did not allow an estimate of how much of the growth in the activity limitations among children in the 1970s might reflect an increased awareness and identification of these limitations, their data raised the possibility that these factors might have played a role. For example, after noting that the marginal increase in activity limitations in the late 1970s (from 3.7 to 3.8 percent) was primarily accounted for by an increase in educationally related impairments, the authors proposed that the increase might have been associated with the implementation of the Education for All Handicapped Children Act of 1975 (which was renamed Individuals with Disabilities Education Act in 1990) and associated efforts to identify and provide mainstream education to children with disabilities (see additional discussion in Chapter 4).

In addition, other policies that have promoted screening of children for health and learning problems may have contributed to increases in the measured prevalence of disabilities. For example, the Social Security Amendments of 1967 created the Early and Periodic Screening, Diagnostic, and Treatment (EPSDT) benefit for children eligible for Medicaid. The objective was the early identification and management of problems that can impede children's normal development. (Screening for the EPSDT benefit includes a comprehensive health and developmental history and a physical examination.) The implementation of the EPDST benefit has been far from universal, but millions of children in low-income families have been evaluated for disabling or potentially disabling conditions and were identified to have conditions that might otherwise have gone undiagnosed (Herz et al., 1998; GAO, 2001a).

Changes in eligibility criteria for the Supplemental Security Income (SSI) program in the early 1990s could also have influenced the rates of diagnosis or identification of functional limitations in children, especially among children with more severe disabilities (Ettner et al., 2000; Perrin et al., 1999). One change (resulting from the 1990 U.S. Supreme Court decision in *Sullivan v. Zebley* [493 U.S. 521]) required that disability determinations for children include individual functional assessments, and the implementing regulations allowed the enrollment of children who had multiple health problems that, taken together (if not singly), were disabling.[9] Also in 1990, the Social Security Administration expanded from 4 to 11 the number of qualifying mental impairments for children, one of which was attention deficit or hyperactivity disorder. Moreover, both the U.S. Congress (in 1989) and the U.S. Supreme Court provided for increased efforts to inform families of the SSI program and the eligibility criteria for the program, with an emphasis on active outreach to hard-to-find populations. Between 1989 and 1996, the number of children receiving SSI benefits grew from approximately 265,000 to 955,000 (or from 5.8 to 14.4 percent of all SSI beneficiaries) (SSA, 2006a). A study by Perrin and colleagues (1999) suggests, however, that the SSI changes had some impact but that the impact on the rates of reported potentially disabling conditions was fairly minimal. That study examined Medicaid claims for the period from 1989 to 1992 and found similar increases in the rates of asthma and mental health conditions among children insured by Medicaid, whether they received SSI benefits or not. A tightening of eligibility criteria in 1996 cut the number of children's receiving SSI benefits to 847,000 by 2000, after which the number grew again to almost 960,000 at the end of 2003 and to more than 1,035,000 by the end of 2005 (Schmidt, 2004; SSA, 2006a).

Declines in Selected Health Conditions That Contribute to Disability in Childhood

For a number of health conditions that contribute to disability, such as spina bifida and exposure to lead paint, the trends have been encouraging (Stein, 2006). These two conditions illustrate the success of public health interventions aimed at women of childbearing age and their children.

Decreases in the rates of spina bifida reflect the successes of a major public health strategy, specifically, the implementation of campaigns to promote folic acid supplementation for women of childbearing age. During the period from 1991 to 2003, the incidence of spina bifida dropped from 24.9 to 18.9 per 100,000 live births (Mathews, 2006). All of the decrease came after the U.S. Food and Drug Administration authorized the enrichment of cereals with folic acid in 1996 and then made it mandatory in 1998. The decrease in the incidence of spina bifida was larger and the economic benefit was greater than had been projected before adoption of the policy (Grosse et al., 2005). To reduce further the rates of spina bifida and other

---

[9]The *Zebley* decision was based on a notion of equity. Until that decision, the Social Security Administration provided functional assessments for adults who might not otherwise qualify for SSI benefits on the basis of their clinical symptoms alone.

neural tube defects, CDC is actively promoting the greater consumption of folic acid by women of childbearing age (the agency estimates that 50 to 70 percent of these conditions are related to folic acid deficiency [NCBDDD, 2005]).

Another public health success involves lead exposure. In years past, lead exposure was an important risk factor for neurodevelopmental problems and the associated functional limitations for many children, especially children who live in low-income areas. As measured by the periodic National Health and Nutrition Examination Surveys, in the roughly 10-year period from 1976–1980 to 1988–1991, the percentage of children with elevated lead levels dropped from 88 to 9 percent after federal and state government regulations sharply reduced the use of lead in gasoline, paints, and a range of consumer products (NCEH, 2004). For the period from 1999 to 2002, the figure dropped below 2 percent after efforts to eliminate continuing sources of lead exposure, such as contaminated soil and deteriorating house paint applied before the presence of lead in paint became regulated (Schwemberger et al., 2005). Children in low-income families remain particularly at risk in many communities with stocks of old, deteriorated housing that have not been renovated or that have been subjected to unsafe renovation practices (CDC, 2004).

TRENDS IN DISABILITY IN MIDDLE LIFE

Trends in impairments, activity limitations, and disability in middle life are important not only in themselves but also for what they may suggest about the future of disability in America when people now in the middle decades of life enter late life. Analyses of trends involving these adults have mostly focused on work limitations and employment issues, as discussed below, rather than on other kinds of activity limitations. Few systematic analyses have tracked trends in the health and environmental factors that contribute to disability in this age group. On balance, such studies that do exist suggest that the rates of disability are rising among America's non-elderly adults, at least in part because of increases in the rates of obesity.

Personal Care or Routine Care Limitations

Figure 3-2 presents National Health Interview Survey data on personal care limitations (referred to as activities of daily living [ADLs]) and routine care limitations (referred to as instrumental activities of daily living [IADL]) over the period from 1984 to 2004 for individuals ages 18 to 44 and individuals ages 45 to 64. Although the numbers are generally low, Figure 3-2 shows that the prevalence of ADL limitations for both age groups rose through the early 1990s, followed by a slight decrease. The ADL trend

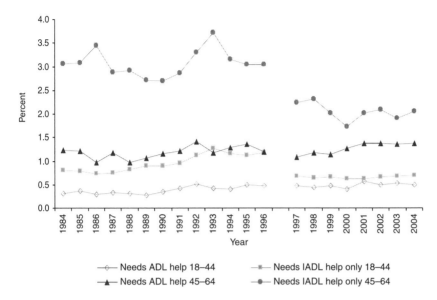

FIGURE 3-2 Trends in the proportion of the civilian, noninstitutional population ages 18 to 44 and 45 to 64 needing help with ADLs or IADLs only, 1984 to 2004. ADL = needs help with personal care activities, such as eating, bathing, dressing, or getting around the home; IADL only = needs help only with routine needs, such as everyday household chores, doing necessary business, shopping, or getting around for other purposes.
SOURCE: H. Stephen Kaye, Disability Statistics Center, University of California at San Francisco, unpublished tabulations from the National Health Interview Survey, as requested by the committee.

line was essentially flat both before and after the 1997 survey redesign. Between 1997 and 2004, the percentage of those in the group ages 45 to 64 needing assistance with ADLs rose but only from 1.09 to 1.37 percent. For IADL limitations, Figure 3-2 shows considerable fluctuation, with a rise in prevalence during the early 1990s, followed by some decline. Since 1997, the rates have been flat.

In a study that used National Health Interview Survey data for the population ages 18 to 69, Lakdawalla and colleagues analyzed trends in personal care (ADL) and routine care (IADL) needs among the working-age population between 1984 and 1996 and between 1997 and 2000 (Lakdawalla et al., 2005). During the period from 1984 to 1996, when the percentages of both kinds of disabilities increased among those ages 18 to 59 overall, the largest percent change occurred among those ages 30 to 39. In contrast, the prevalence of both kinds of disability decreased for people 60 to 69 years of age.

Limitations in Work

The last decade has seen considerable analysis of work limitations. It has also seen considerable controversy about the concept of work disability, the data used for analyses of disability and work, the analytic techniques used, and the interpretation of the data, particularly with respect to the effects of public policies on the employment of people with disabilities (Acemoglu and Angrist, 2001; Burkhauser et al., 2002; Autor and Duggan, 2003; Stapleton and Burkhauser, 2003; Burkhauser and Houtenville, 2004; Kaye, 2005). Several of these analyses are reviewed in Appendix E.

In contrast to the questions about personal care and routine care needs, the National Health Interview Survey does not ask people whether they need assistance to work. Rather, it asks whether they have a health problem or disability that (1) prevents them from working or (2) limits the amount or the kind of work that they can do. The Current Population Survey asks the same question, although the context is different, in that that survey does not focus primarily on health status. The American Community Survey asks whether a person has any difficulty working at a job or business because of a physical, mental, or emotional condition that has lasted for 6 months or more, although that question would be eliminated in proposed revisions to the survey (see the discussion in Chapter 2).

Figure 3-3 shows data for 1984 to 2003 from the National Health Interview Survey for people ages 18 to 44 and ages 45 to 64 who were reported to be unable to work. Among those ages 18 to 44, the percentage of people unable to work rose from the 1980s through the 1990s, before the survey redesign. The prevalence of people ages 45 to 64 reporting an inability to work (which was much higher overall than that for the younger age group) decreased in the 1980s but rose in the early 1990s. After 1997, the figures for both groups showed slight decreases, before increasing after 2000, especially for the older age group. The trends in reported work limitations (as opposed to an inability to work) were substantially similar, although the levels of work limitation are lower than the levels of inability to work among those ages 45 to 64.[10]

---

[10]Burkhauser and colleagues (2002) point out that many people with impairments that would seem to be work limiting are not actually reporting such work limitations in the National Health Interview Survey. One explanation is that many people who report no work limitations make such a report on the basis of their experience of having found a job that they can do without ongoing difficulty either because of the nature of the job or because of the accommodations in work conditions that employers or workers have made, or both.

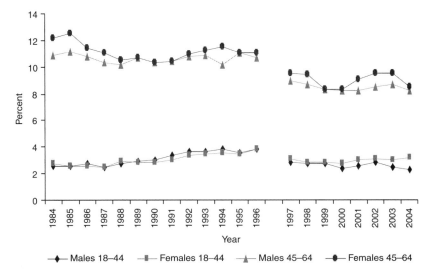

FIGURE 3-3 Trends in the proportion of the civilian, noninstitutional population who are unable to work, by gender, ages 18 to 44 and 45 to 64, 1984 to 2004. SOURCE: H. Stephen Kaye, Disability Statistics Center, University of California at San Francisco, unpublished tabulations from the National Health Interview Survey, as requested by the committee.

Employment Trends Among Adults with Disabilities

Most studies of disability and employment have found some reductions in the rates of employment among adults with disabilities over time (DeLeire, 2000; Acemoglu and Angrist, 2001; Bound and Waidmann, 2002; Houtenville and Burkhauser, 2004; Jolls and Prescott, 2004; Moon and Shin, 2006), but some analyses have reported increases in the rates of employment among individuals with severe functional limitations who report the ability and desire to work (Kruse and Schur, 2003). Consistent with the controversies over measurement, the interpretation of data on employment trends among adults with disabilities has generated considerable disagreement (see Appendix E). For example, some suggest that declines in employment reflect employer anxiety about the requirements of Title I of the Americans with Disabilities Act, which was passed in 1990 (DeLeire, 2000; Acemoglu and Angrist, 2001). Others attribute the declines to changes in the Social Security Disability Insurance (SSDI) and SSI programs during the 1980s that liberalized eligibility criteria (Houtenville and Burkhauser, 2004).

Figure 3-4 shows the trends in employment rates for people with and people without activity limitations. Overall, the graph suggests an increas-

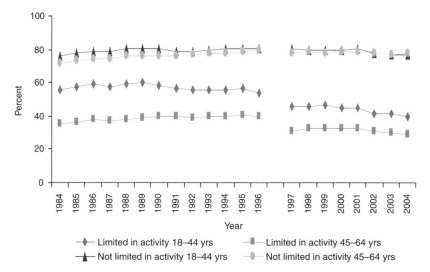

FIGURE 3-4 Trends in employment rates for people with any type of activity limitation and for people without such limitations, ages 18 to 44 and 45 to 64, civilian, noninstitutional population, 1984 to 2004. Any type of activity limitation is indicated by a positive answer to any question about limitation in activities because of a chronic condition.
SOURCE: H. Stephen Kaye, Disability Statistics Center, University of California at San Francisco, unpublished tabulations from the National Health Interview Survey, as requested by the committee.

ing gap between the level of employment for people without activity limitations and the level for people with activity limitations. The recessions of the early 1990s and 2000s appear to have affected all groups, but people with activity limitations have not experienced the more recent recovery in employment levels shown for people without such limitations. In addition, as employment rates among those with limitations have fallen faster than the rates among those without such limitations, the gap in employment between the two groups has grown.

Conditions Contributing to Disability in Middle Life

Few systematic analyses have investigated the health conditions that contribute to disability among nonelderly adults. In a recent review, Bhattacharya and colleagues (2006) report that adults under age 65 are increasingly likely to have chronic bronchitis (ALA, 2002), congestive heart failure (NHLBI, 1996), and diabetes (Mokdad et al., 2000). At the same time, other data suggest that the rates of heart disease (Reynolds et al., 1999), stroke (Carandang et al., 2006), and arthritis (CDC, 1997) have been declining in this age group. The National Health Interview Survey also allows a glimpse into trends since 1997 in the rates of selected conditions identified by respondents as causing activity limitations. Again, note that the survey questions reflect a largely medical model of disability, without regard to the contribution of environmental factors. For the most common conditions that were listed earlier in this chapter (Table 3-2) as contributors to activity limitations, Table 3-5 suggests very recent declines in fractures and joint injuries, lung disease, heart or other circulatory diseases, and arthritis as "causes" of or contributors to activity limitations. Diabetes, in contrast, increased in importance in 2003 and 2004. Further analysis is needed to sort out whether these changes are statistically significant, whether they are maintained after controlling for demographic shifts during the period, and whether all groups have been equally affected.

The Medicare Current Beneficiary Survey offers additional insights into the chronic conditions that exist among a subgroup of people between the ages of 18 and 65: those who have qualified for Medicare benefits not by age but by virtue of having qualified for SSDI. About 4 percent of Medicare beneficiaries are under age 45, and 11 percent are between the ages of 45 and 64. Perhaps the most striking trend revealed in Table 3-6 is the increase in the numbers of beneficiaries with a mental disorder, which is consistent with significant increases in SSDI awards because of mental disorders (Loftis and Salinsky, 2006).

Finally, much has been written about the obesity epidemic in the United States (and elsewhere) and its implications. On the basis of data from the

TABLE 3-5 Trends in Chronic Health Conditions Causing Limitations of Activity as Reported for Civilian, Noninstitutional Population, Ages 18 to 64, 1997 to 2004

Type of Chronic Health Condition	Number of People with Activity Limitations Caused by Selected Chronic Health Conditions per 1,000 Population							
	1997	1998	1999	2000	2001	2002	2003	2004
Mental illness	14.2	13.2	13.2	13.1	15.3	17.3	16.0	14.5
Fractures and joint injuries	12.1	10.6	11.0	10.2	11.3	11.4	11.2	9.5
Lung	10.6	9.3	9.3	8.6	9.4	10.1	9.5	9.0
Diabetes	9.7	8.1	9.2	9.3	9.7	9.6	11.1	10.5
Heart, other circulatory	20.7	19.3	19.3	18.9	19.9	20.0	20.6	18.8
Arthritis, other musculoskeletal	42.5	38.9	37.7	33.8	37.5	38.0	37.7	35.5

SOURCE: Committee's analysis of National Health Interview Survey data, 1997 to 2004.

TABLE 3-6 Trends in Self-Reported Health Conditions and Mobility Limitations, Community-Dwelling Medicare Beneficiaries Under Age 65, 1992 to 2002

Self-Reported Health Condition[a]	Percentage of Total Medicare Beneficiaries Under Age 65					
	1992	1994	1996	1998	2000	2002
Chronic conditions[b]						
None	20.9	16.8	17.8	18.1	17.4	15.3
Two or more	56.6	64.4	64.6	60.3	64.3	65.9
Disease or condition[b]						
Heart disease	33.2	32.9	33.0	32.0	33.3	35.7
Hypertension	42.9	47.5	47.8	45.6	48.3	52.1
Diabetes	17.3	18.2	19.5	18.8	20.3	22.0
Arthritis	46.6	49.6	49.3	49.1	50.3	52.7
Mental disorder	32.5	35.4	34.4	41.2	49.4	55.8
Mobility limitation						
No limitation	36.9	38.0	38.1	35.9	33.7	31.4

[a]Beneficiaries who were administered a community-based interview answered health status and functioning questions themselves, unless they were unable to do so. A proxy, such as a nurse, always answered questions about the beneficiary's health status and functioning for long-term care facility-based interviews.

[b]In 1997, the facility instrument was changed from a paper-and-pencil interview to a computer-assisted personal interview, and questions about certain diseases or conditions were asked differently. Consequently, there are significant fluctuations in the prevalence of certain diseases or conditions before and after 1997.

SOURCE: Compiled from Medicare Current Beneficiary Survey, Health and Health Care Sourcebooks, 1992 to 2002.

National Health and Nutrition Examination Surveys beginning in 1960, Figure 3-5 presents trend data on the rates of obesity among adults ages 20 to 39 and ages 40 to 59. The figure shows substantial increases in the rates of obesity among individuals in both age groups. In a paper prepared for the August 2005 IOM workshop on disability, Bhattacharya and colleagues (2006) linked these increases to increases in ADL and IADL limitations in middle life. Sturm and colleagues (2004) project increases in the prevalence of disability of 1 percent per year in the group ages 50 to 69, if current trends in obesity continue unabated. The link between obesity and disability needs further investigation because not only can obesity be a risk factor for disability but disability can likewise be a risk factor for obesity (see the discussion of secondary conditions in Chapter 5).

TRENDS IN DISABILITY IN LATE LIFE

Reflecting the high prevalence of disability in late life and concerns about the implications of an aging population on the economy, the health

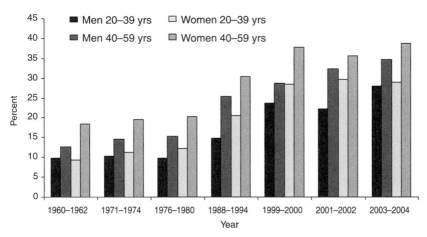

FIGURE 3-5 Trends in the prevalence of obesity for men and women ages 20 to 39 and 40 to 59, civilian, noninstitutional population, 1960 to 2004.
SOURCE: Compiled from the work of Flegal et al. (2002) and Ogden et al. (2006) on the basis of data from the National Health Examination Survey (1960 to 1962) and the National Health and Nutrition Examination Survey (other years).

care system, and other areas of life, trends in disability have best been mapped and analyzed for older age groups. Generally, studies of disability trends in late life have focused on measures of activity limitations: ADLs and IADLs. Variations in the wording of questions across surveys, time periods, and other survey features have led to seemingly conflicting results in some cases. On balance, however, as first noted by Manton and colleagues (1993), trends in the prevalence of disability in late life are largely positive, with the evidence suggesting a substantial decline in the rates of IADL-related disabilities and smaller declines for ADL-related disabilities.

This discussion relies primarily on data from the 1982 to 2004 National Health Interview Surveys. For older individuals, comparison of pre-1997 survey data with data from the revised survey suggested only minor discontinuities in the data on personal care and routine care limitations.[11] Therefore, the data are presented without discontinuity by year.

Personal Care and Routine Care Limitations

Figure 3-6 shows the ADL and IADL trend data for 1982 through 2004. These data show a clear overall pattern of decline during the 1980s and 1990s in the percentage of the community-based population who need

---

[11]This discussion draws on a background paper prepared for the August 2005 IOM workshop organized during the first phase of this study (Freedman, 2006).

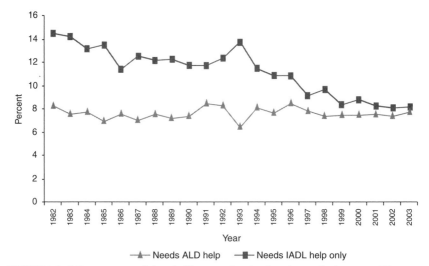

FIGURE 3-6 Percentage of the civilian, noninstitutional population ages 70 years and older reporting need for help with personal care or help with routine care activities only, 1982 to 2003. ADL = needs help with personal care activities, such as eating, bathing, dressing, or getting around the home; IADL only = needs help only with routine needs, such as everyday household chores, doing necessary business, shopping, or getting around for other purposes.
SOURCE: Analysis by Freedman (2006) of the 1982 to 2003 National Health Interview Survey data.

assistance with limitations in routine care activities, such as shopping or preparing meals, but who do not need help with personal care. The decline has continued in the current decade but at a slower pace.

Other data also point to declines in the percentage of the older people with limitations in routine care activities. For example, analyses based on data from the National Long-Term Care Survey suggested particularly large declines in three IADL measures from 1984 to 1999: doing laundry, managing money, and shopping for groceries (Spillman, 2004). A review of 16 relevant studies that used data from eight different surveys found substantial agreement that declines in IADL-related disabilities occurred through the 1980s and early 1990s (Freedman et al., 2002). A few more recent studies (Schoeni et al., 2005; Manton et al., 2006) suggest that such declines have continued into the current decade.

Changes in trends for limitations with personal care activities, such as dressing or bathing, are not as large. As presented in Figure 3-6, data from the National Health Interview Survey showed a small decline in the prevalence of personal care limitations during the entire period, from 8.2 percent in 1982 to 7.8 percent in 2003. The Medicare Current Beneficiary

Survey also collects data on ADLs, although it asks about difficulty in performing an activity without help or special equipment. On the basis of data from that survey, Figure 3-7 shows decreases in limitations for community-dwelling beneficiaries in each category for the period from 1992 to 2003. A technical working group explored the inconsistencies in ADL trends across surveys and concluded that during the 1990s there were declines in difficulty with daily activities and the use of help with daily activities and increases in the percentage of individuals who used equipment to assist them with some activities (Freedman et al., 2004a).

Despite the percent declines in IADL-related disabilities and the relative steady state of ADL-related disabilities, the total number of people with ADL or IADL limitations increased from approximately 4 million in 1982 to 4.2 million in 2003. (The numbers were calculated by using U.S. Census Bureau data on population by age group, available at http://www.census.

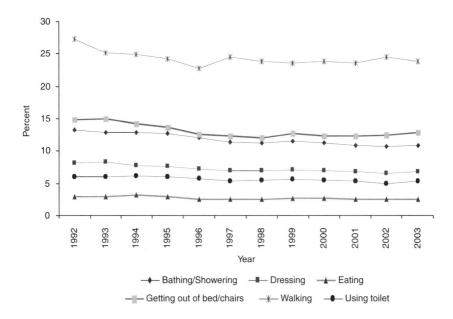

FIGURE 3-7 Percentage of community-dwelling Medicare beneficiaries ages 65 and over who have difficulty in performing selected personal care activities without help or special equipment, 1992 to 2003.
SOURCE: NCHS, 2007 (data from the Medicare Current Beneficiary survey obtained from tables compiled by CDC, available at http://209.217.72.34/aging/TableViewer/tableView.aspx?ReportId=362).

gov/cgi-bin/ipc/idbagg.) Without the declines in IADL limitations, the 2003 number would be much larger.

The concern that not all groups may be benefiting equally from the declining rates of disability has led some researchers to investigate disparities in trends by race and socioeconomic status. Findings by race have been inconsistent thus far. On the one hand, data from the National Long-Term Care Survey suggest that racial disparities in chronic ADL- or IADL-related disabilities increased during the 1980s and decreased during the 1990s (Clark, 1997; Manton and Gu, 2001). On the other hand, three studies that used data from the National Health Interview Survey found no statistically significant changes in relative disparities in disabilities between racial minorities and whites, although the absolute size of the gaps may have narrowed (see, for example, the work of Schoeni et al. [2005]).

A review of analyses of disparities in the rates of disabilities by level of education again found inconsistent results (Freedman et al., 2002). One study based on the National Long-Term Care Survey reported no clear pattern for the period from 1982 to 1999 (Manton and Gu, 2001). Another study that was also based on data from the National Health Interview Survey reported a decline in the prevalence of disabilities only among those with 13 or more years of education (Schoeni et al., 2001). More recently, using data from the National Health Interview Survey for the period 1982 through 2002, Schoeni and colleagues (2005) demonstrated widening gaps in the prevalence of disabilities by socioeconomic status.

Disabilities Within Group Residential Care Settings

Because of data limitations, many trend analyses have omitted data for the 2 million older individuals living in nursing homes and other group residential care settings. Data from the 1977 to 2004 National Nursing Home Surveys indicate that the proportion of older individuals living in nursing homes may have declined in recent years (Alecxih, 2006). Other analyses suggest that the short-stay population (those with stays of less than 3 months) has increased sharply, primarily as a result of Medicare's adoption of hospital prospective payment, which gave hospitals strong incentives to discharge people more quickly, whether it was to home or to a post-acute care facility (Decker, 2005).

Further insight into trends in disability among the population living in long-term care facilities is provided in Figure 3-8, which is based on data from the Medicare Current Beneficiary Survey. Figure 3-8 shows ADL-related data from 1992 to 2003 for beneficiaries age 65 and over living in long-term care facilities. (Note that the y-axis for Figure 3-6 extends from 0 to 16 percent, whereas it extends from 0 to 100 percent for Figure 3-8). Figure 3-8 shows increases in ADL disabilities for this group and, as ex-

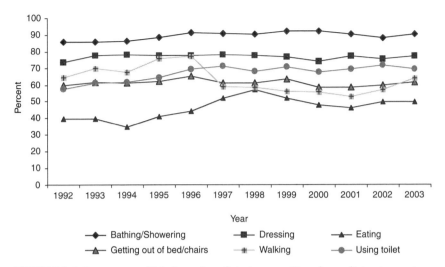

FIGURE 3-8 Percentage of Medicare beneficiaries ages 65 and over living in nursing homes and other facilities who have any difficulty in performing selected personal care activities because of a health or physical problem, 1992 to 2003.
SOURCE: NCHS, 2007 (data from Medicare Current Beneficiary Survey obtained from tables compiled by CDC, available at http://209.217.72.34/aging/TableViewer/tableView.aspx?ReportId=362).

pected, very high levels of limitations. Data from the National Nursing Home Survey cited above show that the percentage of nursing home residents ages 85 and over increased from 35 to 47 percent between 1977 and 1999 (Decker, 2005).

Other evidence also suggests that older adults living in nursing homes are frailer and have higher levels of disability now than older adults did a decade ago, perhaps because alternative care arrangements are more available for people with lesser but still significant levels of impairment (Spillman and Black, 2005b). For example, assisted living facilities, which offer supported living arrangements for those who need assistance but who do not require 24-hour skilled nursing care, grew from being almost nonexistent in the 1970s to serving about 750,000 older adults in 2000 (Spillman and Black, 2006).[12] As described in Chapter 9, state Medicaid programs are paying for an increasing proportion of long-term care in home rather than institutional settings.

---

[12] At a minimum, these facilities offer 24-hour supervision and assistance, as well as meals in a common dining area. Other services may include housekeeping and laundry services, medication reminders or help with medications, help with personal care activities, transportation, security, health monitoring, care management, and activities.

Health Conditions Associated with Disability in Late Life

The extent to which some chronic conditions develop into disability may have been ameliorated in recent decades, in particular for arthritis (Freedman and Martin, 2000) and cardiovascular diseases (Cutler, 2003), even as the prevalence of many of the conditions in the older population has increased (Crimmins and Saito, 2000; Freedman and Martin, 2000; Crimmins, 2004). With respect to sensory functioning, the findings are mixed. Data from the Survey of Income and Program Participation suggest substantial declines in the percentage of older Americans with difficulty seeing from 1984 to 1993 (Freedman and Martin, 1998) and in the percentage with difficulty seeing or hearing from 1984 through 1999 (Cutler, 2001). Data from the Supplements on Aging to the National Health Interview Survey, however, show that the rates of blindness, deafness, and hearing impairment remained constant between 1984 and 1995 (Desai et al., 2001). Like the review for the nonelderly adult population, this summary of trends in health conditions and certain kinds of disabilities draws upon many data sources, data from different time periods, and different measures.[13]

The committee also reviewed trends in conditions that contribute to disability using data from the 1997 to 2004 National Health Interview Survey. The most common conditions linked to activity limitations among the population age 65 and older (Table 3-7) include arthritis and other musculoskeletal conditions, heart and other circulatory conditions, hearing and vision problems, diabetes, lung disease, and senility (dementia). The prevalence of these conditions as contributors to activity limitations declined for all conditions except diabetes and senility.

Potential Explanations for Late-Life Trends

Researchers are still trying to explain the declines in certain aspects of late-life disability and are debating whether past patterns are likely to continue (Cutler and Wise, in press). Several different factors have probably played roles in the recent declines. Increasing levels of education have likely played a role in decreasing disability; but the exact nature of this link remains unclear, and it appears that increases in educational attainment in the future will not match those of the past two decades (Freedman and Martin, 1999). Also, as noted previously, certain common chronic conditions appear to be less debilitating today than they were in the past (Crimmins and Saito, 2000; Cutler, 2003; Freedman and Martin, 2000).

Moreover, as discussed in Chapters 1 and 7, assistive technologies may be replacing some kinds of personal caregiving (Spillman, 2004; Freedman

---

[13]See IOM workshop paper prepared by Freedman (2006) for more details.

TABLE 3-7 Trends in Chronic Health Conditions Related to Activity Limitations, Civilian, Noninstitutional Population, Ages 65 and Over, 1997 to 2004

Type of Chronic Health Condition	Number of People with Activity Limitations Caused by Selected Chronic Health Conditions per 1,000 Population							
	1997	1998	1999	2000	2001	2002	2003	2004
Senility (dementia)	22.8	22.9	23.8	25.3	24.5	24.6	27.5	25.6
Lung	39.5	39.8	39.4	38.6	38.0	38.0	38.7	35.0
Diabetes	44.2	44.0	41.8	46.4	50.6	45.3	49.4	49.2
Vision	49.3	41.1	42.9	42.9	45.7	42.0	35.7	34.9
Hearing	29.1	27.2	24.5	23.9	27.2	28.2	22.9	21.6
Heart, other circulatory	149.4	141.3	131.4	134.8	137.2	131.4	130.9	128.4
Arthritis, other musculoskeletal	161.9	146.1	146.6	139.5	143.4	139.2	149.1	145.5

SOURCE: Committee's analysis of National Health Interview Surveys, 1997 to 2004.

et al., 2006). This development could affect how people respond to questions about disability, particularly questions about the use of personal assistance (Wolf et al., 2005). Uncertainty remains, however, about the possible changes in people's perceptions of disability at all stages of life and the relative contributions of changes in medical care, health behaviors, and living and working environments to declines in disability.

PROJECTING THE FUTURE OF DISABILITY IN AMERICA

The number of people with impairments in body structures or functions is likely to grow substantially in the coming years. Unless substantial progress is made in reducing the chances of such impairments developing into activity limitations and participation restrictions, particularly at older ages, the number of people in the United States facing barriers to work, health care, and independent living will no doubt escalate. The number of individuals needing personal assistance, whether it is from family members or from paid caregivers, will also increase. Designing and implementing strategies and policies to promote the health and well-being of people with existing disabilities and to prevent the development or progression of potentially disabling conditions should, therefore, be national priorities.

In preparing this report, the committee reviewed the few existing studies that project the size of the population with disabilities. The review included, for example, projections related to the SSDI and SSI programs, the demand for long-term care services, and the rates of disability among the elderly population (see Bhattacharya et al. [2004] and Waidmann and Liu

[2000]).[14] Although a comprehensive review of different methodologies is beyond the scope of this report, a few key issues can be cited. In projections of the future size of the older population, assumptions about life expectancy (that is, how long people can be expected to live) are key, whereas projections of the size of younger populations rely more heavily on assumptions about future birth rates. Also, projection methodologies generally make some assumptions about whether disability rates will increase, decline, or remain unchanged in the future. Some projection models have built elaborate assumptions about such rates (allowing variation, for example, in the timing of disease onset and progression), whereas others simply project forward the existing rates onto the numbers of people in each age group. Methods also vary in whether changes in other factors linked to disability (e.g., years of completed education) are incorporated into projections or are held constant. Finally, projections of program enrollment (in, e.g., the SSDI program) rather than disability per se may involve assumptions about additional variables, such as labor force participation rates.

No source for projections of the number of children with disabilities could be identified. However, in the last half century and more, advances in biomedicine have saved many children who once would have died from conditions such as prematurity, traumatic injury, and a variety of genetic conditions or fetal developmental problems. Some of these children have gone onto experience slight to substantial physical or cognitive impairments. Other children have experienced impairments related to exposures to toxic substances. Furthermore, because disabling or potentially disabling conditions that are present at birth or that arise during childhood can have long-term consequences (Forrest and Riley, 2004; IOM, 2003a, 2005a, 2006a), the increases in the numbers of children with conditions such as childhood obesity and diabetes could eventually add to the numbers of adults and older adults with disabilities. The lack of projections based on these developments represents an important gap in present knowledge.

The number of working-age adults eligible for SSDI (meaning that they have a qualifying disability and have worked long enough in Social Security-covered jobs to qualify for benefits) is projected to increase. For example, the Congressional Budget Office projects that caseloads will increase from 6.7 million in 2000 to 10.4 million in 2015 (CBO, 2005b). The number of beneficiaries per covered worker is also projected to increase, as described in Chapter 1. However, the consequences of premature aging or atypical aging for people with disabilities—including individuals with conditions that once were incompatible with long-term survival—have been

---

[14]Projections of SSDI caseloads are available from CBO (2005b) and the work of Toder et al. (2002). Long-term care projections are available from CBO (1999). Social Security projections of SSI and SSDI are available from SSA (2006c).

little discussed with respect to their potential impact on the SSDI program. More generally, analysts have predicted that ADL disabilities and work limitations among adults will increase (irrespective of program eligibility), in part as a consequence of the growing prevalence of obesity and related disorders (Sturm et al., 2004).

Focusing on older adults, if the rate of activity and other limitations for those ages 65 or over were to remain what it is today (roughly 40 percent from Table 3-1), the number of older people with impairments or limitations would increase from approximately 14 million today to more than 28 million in 2030. Using different definitions and a more complex methodology, Waidmann and Liu (2000) have projected that the numbers of older adults with activity limitations would grow from 22 million in 2005 to 38 million by 2030. They also projected that the number of people with limitations in ADLs or IADLs would increase from 12 million to 22 million over this period, if the rates of people with limitations in ADLs and IADLs remained constant but the numbers of people classified by age, sex, and education change according to U.S. Census Bureau projections. Importantly, Waidmann and Liu also project that if rates of activity limitations did not hold constant in the future but, instead, declined at the same rate observed during the 1990s, the number of people with such limitations would still grow to about 38 million by 2030. In contrast, the number of older people with limitations in ADLs or IADLs would stay steady at about 12 million. Another analysis, which assumes that disability rates remain constant, estimates that the number of Americans of all ages with limitations in ADLs only will increase from 5.2 million in 2000 to 9.3 million in 2030 (Friedland, 2004).

Taken together, these projections suggest that the number of people with disabilities is likely to increase in the coming years, unless steps are taken to reduce the environmental barriers that contribute to avoidable activity limitations and participation restrictions. The good news is that the rates of limitations for some activities have already been declining for older individuals. As discussed earlier in this chapter, it is not completely clear why this is the case. As discussed in later chapters of this report and as recommended in Chapter 10, further research is needed to identify and disseminate practices and programs that minimize activity limitations and participation restrictions.

4

Health Care Transitions
for Young People

When our son was 3 months old, he was diagnosed with cystic fibrosis (CF), a progressive, genetic condition that primarily affects breathing and digestion. Soon after his diagnosis, his physician, in his typically family-centered approach, asked me where I wanted my son to be in 20 years. I can remember being a little confused by his question. I was still very focused on getting through each day and really did not have much energy to think beyond taking 1 day at a time. He persisted. Where did I want my son to be in 20 years? What had I wanted for him before he was diagnosed? Forced to think about it, I finally said that we were hoping that all of our children would be able to go to college. His response was very positive and explained that because CF would mean physical limitations, it would be wise to think of ways that our son could make a living using his mind. He said that planning for college was one way to begin thinking about the future. For him to go away to school, we would also need to begin to think of ways to help him gradually assume more responsibility for his own health care.

Donna Olsen (Olsen and Swigonski, 2004 [used with permission])

For children with cystic fibrosis, congenital heart disease, spina bifida, and other conditions that once were often or always fatal in infancy or childhood, what might earlier have seemed a fantasy of the future—planning for college and work life—is now a reality for many families. Depending on an individual child's physical and mental condition, that planning may have some special dimensions, such as particular attentiveness to the presence of physical barriers or hazards in the home or to the capacity of schools to provide a safe and positive environment. When it is done sensitively, as described in the account above, an early focus on long-term planning for the child's transition to adult life can help enlarge a family's range of concerns to include not only their child's immediate medical situation but also the child's future—even when a shortened life expectancy is still likely, given current therapies.

The story of Donna Olsen and her son also illustrates that health and disability—like most of life—are dynamic and not static for both individuals and societies. With advances in biomedical science and technology, many people with early-onset health conditions are living years, even decades, longer than they did in the past, although often with some degree of physical or mental impairment. In addition, advances in early diagnosis and treatment for heart disease, stroke, and other serious chronic diseases associated with aging have meant longer survival—also with various degrees of impairment—for many people in middle and late life.

Disability and health are dynamic in other respects. Over time, some health conditions, such as certain forms of multiple sclerosis and arthritis, exhibit a significant course of waxing and waning that affects the ease or difficulty that people with these conditions have performing daily activities and underscores the significance of environmental characteristics, such as the accessibility of transportation systems. People with other conditions, such as Down syndrome, tend to exhibit periods of long-term stability, although changes in their environment may enlarge or reduce the scope of their activities and participation. Yet other health conditions are characterized by a fairly steady course of increasing impairment (which happens with amyotrophic lateral sclerosis) or improvement (which is typical for certain types of serious injuries). The promotion of health and well-being and the creation of supportive environments play a part in the dynamics of disability in all these pathways.

Research on risk factors for disability has highlighted the interaction between individual characteristics and physical and social environments as a critical dynamic in the development of disability. This interaction was a theme in the Institute of Medicine (IOM) reports *Disability in America* (1991) and *Enabling America* (1997). In addition, the latter report identified the study of change over time and transitions to different states of physical and social functioning as essential dimensions of disability and rehabilitation research. Indeed, the report defined rehabilitation research as "the study of movement among states [that is, pathology, impairment, functional limitation, and disability] in the enabling-disabling process" (IOM, 1997, p. 25).

Anyone can experience an injury or illness that unexpectedly and dramatically alters his or her life. Moreover, as described in Chapter 3, people who live long enough are very likely to develop disabilities, although the pathways of disabilities in late life may still be quite variable. Using data from the Women's Health and Aging Study, Guralnik and colleagues (see, e.g., Ferrucci et al. [1996] and Guralnik et al. [2001]) have identified two distinct types of disability onset in later life: the sudden, catastrophic onset of multiple limitations (which often happens with a stroke or a traumatic injury) and the slow, steadily progressive decline in functioning (which often occurs with osteoarthritis or congestive heart failure). Other studies are revealing the diverse, recurrent, and episodic nature of many of the disabilities that occur in late life (see, e.g., Fried et al. [2001], Gill and Kurland [2003], Hardy et al. [2005], and Gill et al. [2006]). This variability underscores the importance of continued research on the biological and environmental risk factors for disability.

In addition to experiencing function-related transitions, people with disabilities experience a range of other transitions, many of which mark common social milestones, such as starting school or work or moving out of the family home. This chapter examines one especially dynamic period of transition: that experienced by children and youth with disabilities as they become adults and move from the pediatric to the adult health care system. For young people with disabilities, a poor transition in this arena of life can threaten their health and undermine other transitions, for example, in education, work, social relationships, and independent living.

The chapter begins by placing the transition from child to adult in the broader context of changes and risk factors for disability that can be studied throughout the life span. It then discusses the population of young people at particular risk for problems with health care transitions and examines goals for successful transition planning. The remaining sections examine child and family characteristics that may affect transitions, relevant public policies and other environmental factors that may ease or complicate those transitions, models of care for children and adults with chronic health conditions and disabilities, and approaches to health care transitions for young people with disabilities. The chapter concludes with the committee's recommendations. Chapter 5 follows with an examination of related but different dynamics: aging with disability and the development and prevention of secondary conditions.

TRANSITIONS TO ADULT CARE IN A LIFE SPAN PERSPECTIVE

As used here, a *transition* involves a significant change or set of changes in a person's life circumstances during a relatively limited time period rather than over the life span. Transitions may involve changes in social roles (e.g., from a minor to a legal adult), changes in living arrangements (e.g., from the family home to an independent living arrangement or from the family home to an institutional setting), or changes in functioning related to events such as traumatic injuries. Over a life span, a person will typically experience many transitions, with the transition to adult life being one of the most momentous.

Adopting a *life span* or *life course* perspective on health, disability, and transitions reinforces the understanding that disability is dynamic and that a physical or social transition is a process rather than a point in a person's life. It also involves the seemingly simple recognition that what happens earlier in life affects what happens later (Meaney and Szyf, 2005; Champagne and Meaney, 2006). Research has focused particularly on the health and other consequences for adolescents and adults of what happens

in childhood in such areas as family relationships, peer interactions, education, nutrition, health care, and exposures to such obvious hazards as air pollution or violence (see, e.g., Kuh and Ben-Schlomo [1997], Thyen et al. [1998], Dell and To [2001], Sears et al. [2002], and Forrest and Riley [2004]). A number of conditions that commonly affect adults—including heart disease, diabetes, certain cancers, asthma, and obesity—are associated with childhood environments that can affect a child's physiology or shape personal behaviors that persist into adulthood (see, e.g., Seidman et al. [1991], Rona et al. [1993], Barker [1997], and Shaheen [1997]).

In addition, physicians and families are also becoming more aware that some unwanted effects associated with the improved survival rates for premature infants and the successful treatment of cancer and other childhood illnesses may not be evident for years (Perrin, 2002; Brandt et al., 2003; IOM, 2003a, 2006a; Castro et al., 2004). For example, a recent large, retrospective study that compared the survivors of childhood cancer with their siblings reported that 62 percent of survivors but only 37 percent of their siblings had at least one chronic condition; 28 percent of the survivors but only 5 percent of the siblings had a severe or life-threatening condition (Oeffinger et al., 2006). If accurate information about these childhood experiences, conditions, and treatments does not accompany a young person as he or she makes the transition to health care as an adult, the primary care or specialist physicians treating that person may fail to adopt or recommend appropriate monitoring and preventive measures.

At a general level, taking a long view of disability across the life span requires a significant, sustained investment in longitudinal research. Chapter 2 stressed this point as it applies to epidemiological research. It applies equally to clinical and social intervention research, including research related to transitions for young people, aging with disability, and secondary conditions. Unfortunately, in both health care and policy research, very long-term studies, which tend to be costly and complicated to administer, are the exception rather than the rule, particularly for younger populations. One such exception is the National Children's Study, which was described in Chapter 2. As important as this study will be to the identification of risk factors, it will not include the range of data needed to track transitions and identify variables associated with successful transitions for young people.

A CRITICAL TRANSITION: FROM CHILD TO ADULT

Systematic attention to health care transitions for young people dates back more than two decades. In 1989, the U.S. Surgeon General convened a conference on the topic that built on a smaller 1984 conference with the same theme (Magrab and Miller, 1989). Currently, the U.S. Maternal and Child Health Bureau (MCHB; which is part of the Health Resources and

Services Administration of the U.S. Department of Health and Human Services) has made the following one of its six primary goals: "[a]ll youth with special health care needs will receive the services necessary to make appropriate transitions to adult life, including adult health care, work, and independence" (McPherson et al., 2004, p. 1538).[1] MCHB funds the development and evaluation of model programs on transitions and also funds the Healthy & Ready to Work Center to promote successful transition planning and outcomes (see www.hrtw.org). The National Institute on Disability and Rehabilitation Research has supported projects that conduct research on health care transitions, prepare informational materials for young people and their families, and develop guidance for health care professionals. To cite a few other examples, the American Academy of Pediatrics (AAP) (see below), a number of states, and several medical centers and children's hospitals have developed transition resources or programs. In the United Kingdom, the National Health Service also supports research on transitions (NCCSDO, 2002).

Adolescent Population "At Risk" for Transition

Statistical data underscore the importance of planning for the transition to adulthood for young people with disabilities. Data from the 2004 National Health Interview Survey indicate that approximately 1.4 million children with some kind of activity limitation were in the 14- to 17-year-old age group, a critical period for transition planning (data supplied by committee consultant H. Steven Kaye, September 5, 2006). More than half of these young people were reported to have a learning disability or attention deficit hyperactivity disorder (or both). Another quarter had a mental health condition or a developmental disability (other than mental retardation). Approximately 70,000 had a limitation in activities of daily living. Data from the U.S. Department of Education (2006c) indicate that over 1.8 million children in this age group received special education services in 2002 and that over 375,000 were age 17 and, thus, soon to turn 18. Data from a 2001 survey of children with special health care needs suggest that perhaps a half a million or more children with such needs turn age 18 each year (Lotstein et al., 2005). As described below, reaching age 18 can trigger critical changes in a young person's legal, financial, and health care status.

Well before they turn age 18 and for various periods of time thereaf-

---

[1]As defined by MCHB, children with special health care needs are "those who have or are at increased risk for a chronic physical, developmental, behavioral, or emotional condition and who also require health and related services of a type or amount beyond that required by children generally" (McPherson et al., 1998, p. 137).

ter, many young people with disabilities will be involved in an active and complex process of transition planning that reaches beyond their families and health care professionals to include individuals from multiple service sectors, especially the public schools. School transition planning services are discussed later in this chapter.

Goals of Health Care Transition Planning for Young People

For a young person with a disability or serious chronic health condition, the ultimate goal for the transition from pediatric to adult health care services is to maximize "lifelong functioning and potential through the provision of high-quality, developmentally appropriate [and technically sophisticated] health care services that continue uninterrupted as the individual moves from adolescence to adulthood" (AAP et al., 2002, p. 1304). More specific individual goals include helping young people (consistent with their medical condition) achieve the skills in self-care, health care decision making, and self-advocacy that will prepare them to take more responsibility for their health and health care. For young people with disabilities as a population, the goals for health care transitions include the capacity of relevant health care and social agencies to identify and respond appropriately to different health and personal characteristics, family situations, and physical and social environments.

The discussion here emphasizes health care transitions. Successful health care transitions, however, usually require attention to other dimensions of a young person's life, including living arrangements, transportation, postsecondary education, work, family and other social relationships, and financial self-sufficiency. For example, housing and transportation conditions can affect the ease of self-care and physical access to supportive health care services. Although clinicians do not manage these aspects of a young person's life, they should be alert to how such factors might support or interfere with a successful health care transition.

For many young people with serious disabilities, successful health care transitions will also depend on public policies that support access to health insurance, assistive technologies, personal care services, housing, vocational training or postsecondary education, and income support, as well as public policies that support nondiscrimination in employment and the physical accessibility of transportation and public spaces. Several policies that include specific provisions for transition planning or assistance for young people are discussed below as environmental factors that affect health care transitions.

INDIVIDUAL AND FAMILY FACTORS AFFECTING HEALTH CARE TRANSITIONS

Becoming an adult involves many steps and stages in a complex process. Some steps are fairly abrupt, in particular, reaching legal adulthood. Other aspects of the transition to adult life occur much more gradually and unevenly across different dimensions of a young person's life. Major domains of transition include transitions from pediatric to adult health care, from school to work, and from living with parents to living independently.

The nature of the transitions, including health care transitions, necessarily varies according to the specific situation and the characteristics of the individual young person. Family characteristics and resources will also influence the transitions. The next sections discuss these factors as they affect health care transitions.

Individual Factors

Box 4-1 summarizes several broad characteristics of health that will affect health care transitions for children. In general, the more complex the young person's health situation is, the more complex the transition process will be. Children with conditions that are chronic but mild and not dis-

---

BOX 4-1
Characteristics of Child and Adolescent Health That May Affect the Complexity of Health Care Transitions

$\longleftarrow\!\!\!\!\longrightarrow$

Simpler Transition	More Complex Transition
Single health condition	Multiple health conditions
Low risk of future health problems	High risk of future health problems
No dependence on medical equipment	Reliance on life-sustaining medical equipment
Rare acute illness, medically stable	Frequent acute episodes, medically unstable
Few medications	Multiple medications, medication problems
No cognitive impairments	Profound mental retardation
No physical impairments	Serious physical impairments
Mentally healthy	Mentally ill
No behavioral concerns	Serious behavioral concerns

SOURCE: Adapted from Kelly et al. (2002).

---

abling (e.g., eczema) or that only slightly impair activities (e.g., mild talipes equinovarus, or clubfoot) may need little if any transition planning, other than that appropriate for most young people. Certain other conditions, such as early-onset schizophrenia, will almost always present major challenges for the transition from pediatric to adult health care. The transitions for young people with many health conditions, such as cerebral palsy or asthma, are much more variable, however. For example, some young people with cerebral palsy have severe physical or mental disabilities that require considerable transition planning, whereas others experience barely noticeable effects of the disorder and therefore do not require the same intensity of attention to their transition to adult care.

A small but important group of children and adolescents survive with major assistance from certain technologies, especially respiratory, nutritional, and mobility assistance. With appropriate educational, recreational, and workplace accommodations, these technologies typically allow young people to participate in many kinds of social and other activities. Careful monitoring is, however, important to ensure that equipment (including software) is performing correctly and is adjusted as needed to accommodate developmental, medical, or environmental changes. Planning for transitions in health care and living arrangements and other transitions can be particularly complex for this group of young people. Planning for transitions in health care requires very knowledgeable clinicians who have experience working with this population and their devices in diverse settings.

Placing individual or condition-specific differences aside, considerable evidence suggests that young people in general are still developing neurologically, emotionally, and intellectually well into their 20s. They will therefore differ in some respects from older individuals, who comprise the majority of patients seen by most physicians and other health care professionals who care for adults. The creation of adolescent medicine as a specialty was a response to the particular challenges of caring for teenagers and young adults and, in itself, represents a transition strategy particularly attuned to the developmental stage of adolescence, although it does involve an additional health care transition that must be managed. In any case, adult care professionals will be better prepared to manage the health care needs of young people if they have the education and experience that allow them to understand how continuing development may affect risk taking and other decision making by their young adult patients with disabilities. As discussed later, the amount of education that professionals receive in these and other dimensions of health care transitions for young people is minimal.

In addition to a young person's health condition, planning for health care transitions must also consider what the *International Classification of Functioning, Disability and Health* (ICF) terms "personal factors" (WHO, 2001). These factors include maturity and readiness for self-care, coping styles, and personality characteristics. As noted in Chapter 2, the identification and study of these factors are sometimes controversial and may raise charges of blaming the victim and ignoring environmental influences on behavior. Nonetheless, transition planning that does not consider a young person's behavioral, psychological, and other personal characteristics runs the risk of failure. For example, research on children with asthma has found that adolescents are less likely to adhere to preventive drug regimens than their younger counterparts and, as a result, have poorer control over their condition (Jonasson et al., 1999; McQuaid et al., 2003). Decreasing oversight by parents likely accounts for some of the relationship between increasing age and decreasing adherence to drug or other treatment regimens.

In general, as Rosen and colleagues (2003) have observed, "[m]any adolescents with chronic conditions are at higher risk than peers for unnecessary dependency, developmental difficulties, and psychosocial delay" (p. 309). One objective for a successful transition process is to counter these risks by helping young people with disabilities become—and see themselves as—more independent and self-reliant.

No clear milestone heralds the readiness of a particular young person to transfer his or her health care from a pediatrician to a health care provider for adults or for other dimensions of the transition to adult life, such as living independently. Several guidelines for transition planning have suggested personal factors that health care professionals, parents, and even young people themselves may consider in assessing readiness (see, e.g., McDonagh and Kelly [2003], Ardoin and Schanburg [2005], Adolescent Transition Project [undated], and Children's Hospital Boston [undated]). They include

- maturity of judgment and reasoning skills and a maturity of response to anticipatory guidance and transition preparation;
- understanding of the medical condition and treatment and the ability to participate in medical visits;
- self-care skills, including the ability to fill prescriptions, follow prevention and treatment regimens, and seek assistance in an emergency;
- self-advocacy skills; and
- medical status and stability.

Family and Guardian Factors

For most young people with disabilities, families play a critical role in successful health care transition planning and implementation. Health care and social service professionals recognize that various family characteristics, such as education, income, marital status, living arrangements, health insurance coverage, and the availability of support from the extended family, can influence health care transitions.

Family dynamics are also important. McDonagh (2006), for example, cites research indicating that family support (without overprotectiveness) is associated with emotional resilience and independence in young people with a chronic illness or disability. Other factors, such as differences in child and parent perceptions of the child's situation, parental discord, and parents' difficulty in accepting a young person's increasing maturity, can complicate transition planning, youth readiness for independence, and other outcomes (see, e.g., Resnick et al. [1997], Werner [1997], McDonagh [2006], and Shaw et al. [2006]).

Even when young adults have assumed legal responsibility for making decisions about their care, parents often provide practical, emotional, and financial support with the transition process and beyond. When young adults cannot assume such responsibility, parents usually continue as the legal decision makers. For many young people with cognitive impairments, reliance on parental financial, caregiving, and other resources may be much more important than it is for young people with other disabilities (Thorin et al., 1996).

For some children with disabilities, state agencies assume the role of guardian and act in lieu of the parents. An analysis of 1998 data found that 14 percent of children in foster care had a disability, usually one involving a cognitive or psychological condition (Smith, 2002). It also found that 20 percent of foster children had not received a clinical evaluation. Although young people with more severe disabilities may receive ongoing support from social service agencies, critics have noted deficiencies in how state foster care programs plan and support the transition from child to legal adult (see, e.g., English et al. [2003, 2006] and Reilly [2003]).[2] Some have recommended the extension of Medicaid coverage to age 21 to assist young people leaving the foster care system (CPPP, 2001).

ADOLESCENT TRANSITIONS, PUBLIC POLICY, AND OTHER ENVIRONMENTAL FACTORS

One milestone in becoming an adult is marked by a distinct and abrupt role shift—that from legal minor to legal adult, usually at age 18. Still, the parents of young people with complex health challenges often remain deeply involved in making decisions about the young person's health care

---

[2]Of the approximately 280,000 children of all ages who left foster care in 2004, 8 percent were described as emancipated (by virtue of reaching age 18 or meeting other state criteria, such as living independently and being financially self-supporting), 2 percent were runaways, and 2 percent transferred to another state agency (ACF/DHHS, 2006).

and other matters, although they may no longer be legally responsible. At the same time, before an adolescent has the legal authority to make decisions about his or her own health care, pediatricians, parents, and others tend to give increasing weight to the young person's views, preferences, and perceptions (AAP, 1995; IOM, 2004b).[3]

Turning age 18—or age 20 or 22, for that matter—may bring other age-triggered transitions. Among the potentially more consequential of these is the transition from being covered by a parent's employer-sponsored health insurance or by Medicaid (or other public insurance for children) to being uninsured. In addition, poor children with disabilities who have qualified for Supplemental Security Income (SSI) must, when they turn 18, undergo a new assessment to determine whether they meet the eligibility criteria applied to adults (Loprest and Wittenburg, 2005). Various federal-state programs for children with special heath care needs have upper age limits of 18 to 21. Planning for age-related transitions for these programs is particularly important for children who have complex chronic conditions or disabilities and who are poor.

In addition, child health care professionals and organizational providers may have their own age-based policies for transferring young patients to professionals or providers providing adult services, although they will usually work with young people with serious chronic problems or disabilities and their families to plan the transfers of care and smooth the transition (Reiss and Gibson, 2006). The involvement of multiple providers and service agencies with different policies will, in some respects, add to the complexity of the transition.

For young people with disabilities, a number of federal and state policies may directly or indirectly support or complicate transition planning. The rest of this section briefly describes policies related to health insurance and other health programs, income support, and public education. The focus is on their possible relevance to the health care transition process.

Medicaid and Other Public Health Programs

As described in Chapter 8, children with special health care needs or disabilities are slightly more likely than their peers to have health insurance and are particularly more likely to have public health insurance, primarily through Medicaid. Approximately 29 percent of children with special health care needs but only 17 percent of other children have Medicaid (For

---

[3]Under certain circumstances, young people under the age of majority may acquire the authority to make their own decisions about health care and other matters. State policies vary; but these circumstances typically include living independently of one's parents by virtue of marriage, military service, or financial independence (Campbell, 2004).

the State Children's Health Insurance Program [SCHIP], the figures are 3 and 2 percent, respectively.)

The rules for the federal-state Medicaid program are complex and difficult to summarize. Children may qualify for Medicaid in different ways. Depending on the category under which they qualify, their school status, and, in some cases, state discretion, Medicaid may cover children through age 17, 18, 19, or 20 (CMS, 2005d). After that, young people must meet the criteria for coverage applied to adults. For children with disabilities who would qualify for SSI benefits except that their family income is too high, the Family Opportunity Act (passed and signed as part of the Deficit Reduction Act of 2005) allows states to create a "buy-in" option that provides access to Medicaid for families with incomes up to 300 percent of the federal poverty level (Kaiser Commission, 2006a). (States are permitted to charge premiums based on family income.)

Children who are covered by Medicaid by virtue of receiving SSI benefits may lose both SSI benefits and Medicaid coverage at age 18 if they do not meet the SSI eligibility criteria for adults. These and other age-related aspects of both public and private insurance complicate health care transition planning and implementation.

As described in more detail in Chapters 8 and 9, federal regulations require that Medicaid programs must cover Early and Periodic Screening, Diagnostic, and Treatment (EPSDT) services for children.[4] Transition planning is not specifically cited as an EPSDT-covered service, and, in any case, implementation of EPSDT requirements has been uneven across the states (see, e.g., Foltz [1982], Sardell and Johnson [1998], Rosenbaum et al. [2005], and Peters [2006]). Nonetheless, the EPSDT benefit should, in theory, cover various assessments and services in preparation for the transition of a young person with disabilities to adult health care services. In addition, the basic Medicaid benefit package covers a number of long-term care services, including specialized therapies and some home care services that are often not available through private plans but that can ease the transition to adult health care for some young people with disabilities.

The federal rules for SCHIP do not require states to include EPSDT benefits, but SCHIP is still an important resource for children with special needs who would otherwise be uninsured. As recommended at the end of

---

[4]As discussed in Chapter 9, the Deficit Reduction of Act of 2005 made complex changes in federal Medicaid policies. EPSDT benefits are still required for children, but in some cases, the benefits could be structured as a wraparound to an otherwise less comprehensive benchmark benefit plan (Kaiser Commission, 2006a). By adding another complexity to EPDST coverage, this policy change could have unintended consequences. West Virginia is said to have recently approved an alternative Medicaid basic benefit plan that excludes the follow-up EPSDT diagnostic and treatment services that are prescribed on the basis of the findings of screening examinations (Peters, 2006).

this chapter, extending Medicaid and SCHIP benefits through age 21 for all young people with disabilities would help them through a vulnerable period as they transition to adult life.

A variety of other health-related public programs may help children with disabilities obtain services and prepare for the transition to adult health care. For example, Title V of the Social Security Act authorizes MCHB to administer a major program of state block grants that offer support services for mothers, infants, and children and a series of specialized national programs, many of them related to children with special health care needs or disabilities. By law, 30 percent of funds for these grants are reserved for "family-centered, community-based programs for children with special health needs," although the states may spend more (Peters, 2005, p. 16; see also Gitler [1998]).

One review of Title V programs for children with special needs noted that they "have traditionally focused on short-term goals and medical needs and have not focused on long-term issues such as transfer to adult care systems, employment, and independent living" (HRTW National Resource Center, undated, unpaged). In recent years, however, MCHB and state programs have expanded their focus beyond specialty services and have directed more attention to transition and longer-term issues, as evidenced by the transition goal and programs cited earlier.

Transition Support and Public Schools

For children who are eligible, federal education policy requires, at least in principle, the provision of extensive support for transition planning and implementation in several, mostly nonmedical aspects of a young person's life and environment, including independent living arrangements, work, and postsecondary education. Problems in these nonmedical areas of life can have negative consequences for health and health care transitions.

The transition support requirements were included in 1990 amendments to the Individuals with Disabilities Education Act (IDEA), which requires free appropriate public education for children with disabilities who need special education and related services.[5] The requirements apply until an eligible young person completes school or, in most cases, reaches age 22. In 2002, IDEA covered approximately 1.8 million young people in the 14- to 17-year-old age group, 200,000 18-year-olds, and 87,000 people

---

[5]Other laws also apply to the education of children with disabilities, including the Rehabilitation Act of 1973 (as amended) and the Americans with Disabilities Act. Section 504 of the Rehabilitation Act states that "[n]o qualified handicapped individual shall, solely by reason of his handicap, be excluded from participation in, be denied benefits of, or otherwise be subjected to discrimination under any program or activity which receives or benefits from Federal financial assistance."

in the 19- to-21-year-old age group (U.S Department of Education, 2006c, Table 1.7). The U.S. Department of Education funds the National Center on Secondary Education and Transitions to provide technical assistance and information on transition planning and resources for young people with disabilities.

Since 1990, further amendments to IDEA have changed some transition planning requirements. Currently, a student's individual education plan must include a description of the transition services that he or she requires (Apling and Jones, 2005). These services are now defined as a coordinated set of activities that is designed to be "results oriented" and "focused on improving the academic and functional achievement of the child with a disability to facilitate the child's movement from school to post-school activities, including post-secondary education, vocational education, integrated employment (including supported employment), continuing and adult education, adult services, independent living, or community participation" (21 U.S.C. 1401). The 2004 amendments to IDEA changed the required start date for transition planning to age 16, which many view as too late (Cortiella, 2005; SSAB, 2006). Other provisions specified that every state is to develop a transition monitoring and improvement plan (U.S. Department of Education, 2006a).

Although health care transitions are not an explicit focus of IDEA, when a young person has a health condition that interferes with his or her academic achievement, the transition plan may directly address that problem and the services needed to address that problem. Some attention to health-related issues is implicit in aspects of transition planning, for example, guidance or education related to risk taking and safety skills (see, e.g., Blessing [2003] and Wood et al. [2004]). Although contacts with health care organizations are generally not tracked, the U.S. Department of Education does report on contacts with mental health agencies. For an estimated 11 percent of covered students in 2002, schools contacted mental health agencies as part of the transition planning process (U.S. Department of Education, 2006c, Figure 1-48).

An evaluation of IDEA and its transition planning requirements was beyond the scope of this study, but the committee did find reason for concern that the program was not living up to expectations. In 2000, a report from the National Council on Disability based on data from the U.S. Department of Education concluded that nearly 45 percent of states were not in compliance with requirements for individualized education plans and that nearly 90 percent were not in compliance with transition planning requirements (NCD, 2000a). In 2002, the U.S. Commission on Civil Rights noted a lack of full federal funding for IDEA and inadequate resources for program monitoring (USCCR, 2002).

In a 2005 interim report from a 10-year longitudinal study funded by the U.S. Department of Education, researchers described the transition experiences and other circumstances of a national sample of young people ages 15 to 19 who were out of school in 2003 and who had also been the subject of interviews in 2001, when they were still receiving special education services (Wagner et al., 2005). (The researchers also questioned their parents and teachers.) The study, which began in 2000 and which will continue until 2009, includes 12,000 young people who were 13 through 16 years of age when the study began. Researchers reported that the average age at which transition planning began was 14.7 years (at the time, the legal requirement was that it was to begin at age 14) and that 95 percent of young people had a transition plan. The researchers reported that, overall, about 83 percent of teachers described the transition planning program as being well suited or fairly well suited to preparing youth for transition, although only 73 percent of the youth received instruction that focused specifically on transition planning.

Box 4-2 lists several of the study's initial findings about the postschool experiences of the young people with disabilities evaluated in the study. The researchers emphasized the great diversity among the young people, noting that "some youth are struggling because of their disability, poverty, the absence of a high school education, or other factors" (Wagner et al., 2005, p. ES10). They also reported that, compared with the other young people studied, young people with emotional disabilities, mental retardation, or multiple disabilities experienced more limitations related to work, postsecondary education, and other factors related to community participation. The researchers urged caution at this early point in the study in describing the outcomes as successes or failures,

Income Support and Work

In 2005, approximately 1 million children qualified for SSI because they met the law's definition of disability for children and their and (usually) their family's incomes and resources fell within the eligibility limits (SSA, 2006a). For about two-thirds of these children, the disability involved a mental disorder, including mental retardation. When children receiving SSI benefits reach age 18, their medical condition is reviewed by using the disability rules for adults to determine their continued eligibility. At that point, their family's income and resources no longer count for financial eligibility determinations. Some young people lose benefits on the basis of the application of adult disability criteria, but others become eligible for SSI

BOX 4-2
Selected Survey Findings About the Postschool
Experiences of Young People with Disabilities

• Overall, 72 percent completed high school, including over 85 percent of those with hearing, vision, or orthopedic impairments or autism. School completion rates were 56 percent for young people with emotional disturbances, 65 percent for those with multiple disabilities, and 75 percent for those with learning disabilities.

• Overall, 96 percent had no reported problems with self-care, 78 percent had high reported functional abilities scores, and 78 percent had medium or high reported social skills. Seventy-two percent had health described as excellent or very good.

• Approximately 80 percent were attending school, working, or preparing to work.

• Approximately 20 percent were attending postsecondary school, which is about half the rate for other young people. About half of this group said they did not consider themselves to have a disability.

• Over 40 percent were employed, whereas the rate was over 60 percent for other young people. During the initial interviews, for all categories of disability except multiple disabilities, over 90 percent of parents expected that their children would definitely or probably work.

• About 75 percent were living with their parents up to 2 years after leaving school, a rate similar to that for other young people.

SOURCE: Wagner et al. (2005).

---

because their family's resources are no longer considered in their eligibility determination.[6]

To support independence and community participation, the U.S. Congress and the Social Security Administration have developed various dem-

---

[6]Beginning at age 18, young people with disabilities also may become eligible for SSDI benefits on the basis of a parent's Social Security earnings record, even if they have no such earnings record of their own. Under one SSDI provision, the program may cover adult children who have a disability that began before they reached age 22. Under another provision, the program may cover adult children who received dependents' benefits under their parent's Social Security before age 18 if they are disabled at age 18 (based on disability determination criteria for adults) (SSA, 2007a). Young people who qualify for SSDI become eligible for Medicare after 24 months after they begin receiving benefits. (Chapter 9 recommends that this waiting period for Medicare coverage be phased out.)

onstration and other programs to help adult SSDI and SSI recipients begin or return to work by providing vocational and other assistance, including a continuation of Medicare or Medicaid benefits. In addition, one program, Ticket to Work, has a component for young people ages 18 to 21 that is intended "to ensure the successful transition of youth with disabilities from school to work and adulthood through the provision of employability services, supports, and incentives" (SSA, 2006b, unpaged; see also U.S. Department of Labor [2004b]). This program does not extend to young people under age 18 who receive SSI benefits, although these young people may be eligible for vocational and other transition services through IDEA. In a report to Congress, the federal Ticket to Work and Work Incentives Panel (SSA, 2003b) recommended that 16- and 17-year-olds be allowed to participate in the Ticket to Work program, and the committee reinforces this recommendation at the end of this chapter.

A recent report on the reform of Social Security disability programs also recommended several changes related to children (SSAB, 2006). Among other directions, it proposed an integrated system for children with disabilities that would include (1) comprehensive, functional assessments early in childhood; (2) expectations of independence, self-support, and participation; and (3) continuing guidance and management to plan for these goals and secure the supports necessary to achieve them. It did not describe how this integrated system would be financed, for example, what local school districts would be expected to fund. With respect to reform directions overall, the report acknowledged that "no substantial body of evidence-based research" provides clear direction about what programs to encourage work are effective and with what populations (SSAB, 2006, p. 8).

Other Environmental Factors

For young people, the nature of health care transitions and transition outcomes—including their participation in community life—may be influenced by many environmental factors in addition to those cited above. For example, among the environmental domains identified in the ICF (listed earlier in Box 2-2), *support and relationships* involving family and friends can affect how well prepared young people are to manage health care and other transitions and how much assistance is available to help them when problems arise. *Attitudes*, including cultural biases and anxieties, may lead primary care professionals to avoid accepting adults with disabilities as patients. Assistive *products* and accessible home *technologies* can help young people with disabilities achieve and sustain independent living. Accessible *built environments* can affect the ease with which young people are able to find a combination of physically manageable (and affordable) housing, transportation, and employment arrangements that allows them to live independently.

In most of the domains just cited, *services, systems,* and *policies* beyond those discussed in this chapter can impose or remove barriers to young people's transition to an adult life of independence and community participation. For instance, a wide range of social service and advocacy programs and organizations—both public and private—seek to help people with disabilities achieve fulfilling lives and manage or overcome the physical, cultural, economic, and other environmental barriers that they encounter. Examples of such programs include the state Assistive Technology Programs, other technology-access programs described in Chapter 7 and 9, and the Centers for Independent Living.[7] Such organizations may fill gaps in public services, provide alternative styles or types of services, assist people in dealing with bureaucratic and legal obstacles to obtaining needed services, provide information about options that public officials may not mention without explicit inquiries, and engage in more general advocacy for people with disabilities. Even when such organizations do not exist in a given community, many groups have websites that offer extensive information and advice, for example, about how to qualify for and then manage consumer-directed personal care services.

The next section considers health services and system factors that may affect the transition from pediatric to adult health care. It also discusses the "disability competence" of health plans more generally.

HEALTH CARE SERVICES AND SYSTEMS

Efforts to plan and manage health care transitions for children with chronic medical problems and disabilities are inevitably complicated by the diversity of this country's health care delivery and financing arrangements. One feature of this diversity is persistent disparities in access to care among different populations. Moreover, even for young people with mild conditions, differences in pediatric and adult health care services can be a challenge—particularly as they relate to the expectations for primary care practice and routine preventive and health promotion services.

Survey data clearly show a shift in the health care experiences of young people as they enter adult life. For young people ages 12 to 17, in com-

---

[7]As described by the U.S. Department of Education, which administers the Centers for Independent Living grant program under the Rehabilitation Act, these centers are "consumer-controlled, community-based, cross-disability, nonresidential, private nonprofit agencies that are designed and operated within a local community by individuals with disabilities and provide an array of independent living services" (U.S. Department of Education, 2006b, unpaged).

TABLE 4-1 Usual Sources of Health Care for Young People With and Without Activity Limitations, Ages 12 to 17 and 18 to 24, 2005

| | Percentage of Young People | | | |
| | Ages 12–17 | | Ages 18–24 | |
Source of Health Care	With Limitation	Without Limitation	With Limitation	Without Limitation
Clinic or health center	19.6	18.6	18.0	16.3
Doctor's office or HMO	71.5	72.1	57.8	47.7
Hospital emergency room	1.4	0.4	2.1	1.7
Hospital outpatient department	1.4	0.9	0.2	0.8
Other/unspecified	0.3	0.7	3.4	2.9
Totals for:				
Those with a usual source of care	94.2	92.7	81.5	69.4
Those with no usual source of care	5.8	7.3	18.5	30.7

SOURCE: H. Stephen Kaye, Disability Statistics Center, University of California at San Francisco, unpublished tabulations from the National Health Interview Survey, as requested by the committee. The questions used to identify limitations that differ by age group are described in Chapter 3.

parison with young people ages 18 to 24, the transition to adulthood is accompanied by a reduction in the percentage of individuals with a usual source of care (Table 4-1).[8] The drop is, however, larger for the group without disabilities. For both groups, most of the decline is accounted for by a drop in the use of a doctor's office or a health maintenance organization (HMO) as the usual source of care. Additional data from the same survey show that young adults ages 18 to 24 are the least likely among all age groups to have a usual source of care.

Several factors undoubtedly contribute to the differences in the sources of health care by age and disability status. Young adults without disabilities, particularly males, often have no pressing need to see a physician. They typically will have "aged out" of their pediatrician's practice and may not have thought to ask for a referral. Young adults also may lose insurance coverage because they are no longer covered by their parent's health insurance or Medicaid and may have moved out of the family home and the sphere of family oversight.

In 2005, approximately 26 percent of young people with disabilities

---

[8]The respondent for individuals under age 18 is usually a parent, whereas individuals age 18 and over usually report for themselves. The sample sizes for young people with specific kinds of limitations are too small to allow reliable subgroup estimates.

and 28 percent of other young people lacked insurance, a figure substantially higher than that for working-age adults overall (see Chapter 8). The combination of a lack of insurance and a lack of a usual source of health care can be significant for young people with disabilities. A recent analysis of 1999 to 2002 National Health Interview Survey data reported that 45 percent of young people ages 19 to 29 who had a disability and who were uninsured had no usual source of health care and two-thirds said that they had unmet health needs (Callahan and Cooper, 2006).

Organization of Pediatric and Adult Care for Individuals with Chronic Health Conditions or Disabilities

A comprehensive review of the diverse and complicated organization of health care children, adolescents, and adults with chronic health conditions or disabilities is beyond the scope of this report. As briefly described below, however, desirable models of such care have been identified for both children and adults. To the extent that the features of these models become more widely adopted, young people should experience better planning for health care transitions.

Medical Home Model of Pediatric Care

For children with disabilities or special health care needs, efforts to improve the provision of health care have proceeded along many fronts. Some initiatives focus on advances in specialty medical care, whereas others focus on primary care, in particular, the development and implementation of the medical home model of care. The medical home model, which is endorsed and supported by the AAP, promotes health care that is accessible, family centered, continuous, comprehensive, coordinated, and compassionate (AAP, 2002; see also AAP [1999a, 2005a]).[9] For MCHB, one of its six goals for children with special health care needs (which includes children with disabilities) is that all such children "receive coordinated, ongoing comprehensive care within a medical home" (McPherson et al., 2004, p. 1538).

The medical home is intended to provide ongoing primary care for children with special health care needs, help educate children and families about the child's condition and its treatment, coordinate health services

---

[9]With funding from MCHB and others, the AAP administers the National Center of Medical Home Initiatives for Children with Special Health Care Needs, which develops educational materials, training, guidelines, and other resources to help physicians, families, and others provide children with access to medical homes (AAP, 2005b). MCHB also helped fund two medical home "learning collaboratives" that had as one focus extending state Title V agency relationships with pediatric primary care under Title V of the Social Security Act (NICHQ, 2005).

(especially subspecialty, surgical, and specialized therapies) with the family, facilitate the integration of the child into community services, and address the child's psychological and social needs. In addition, it should aid children and families through critical health care and community transitions, including the transition to adult life and adult health care services. As noted above, planning for health care transitions may involve attention to educational, developmental, psychosocial, and other service needs and the coordination of health care plans with educational and other community organizations as well as adult care providers.

A 2001 survey of families of children with special health care needs suggested that although most of these children had access to some features of the medical home model, the full model was not available for a significant proportion of them (Strickland et al., 2004).[10] A North Carolina study reported that 56 percent of children with special health care needs had a medical home (Nageswaran et al., 2006). Surprisingly, the researchers found that children with some or severe functional limitations were less likely to have a medical home than children with no functional limitations. This is unfortunate, because early reports suggest that the medical home approach may particularly benefit children who have the most severe conditions (Broyles et al., 2000; Palfrey et al., 2004).

Adult Care Models

Proponents of the medical home model for children with special health care needs are increasingly linking it to a model for chronic care management that has focused primarily on adults (see, e.g., NICHQ [2005]).[11] At the same time, the medical home is increasingly being invoked in discussions of the chronic care model. For example, in a position statement endorsing the chronic care model, the American College of Physicians (ACP) noted its support for "a patient-centered, physician-guided model of chronic care management that gives the patient a 'medical home' from which all care needs are coordinated" (ACP, 2004, p. 2). In 2006, the ACP endorsed the "advanced" medical home as the basic model for all primary care (ACP, 2006).

---

[10]The study assessed five components of the model: the child and family had a usual place to receive health care, a personal physician or nurse, no problems in obtaining appropriate referrals to specialists or other appropriate services, appropriate coordination of care, and family-centered care.

[11]The model, which was developed by Edward Wagner with support from the Robert Wood Johnson Foundation, differs from disease management programs in several respects. The latter tend to be focused on single medical conditions, to involve little or no use of nonmedical services, and to rely more heavily on standardized care management protocols (see, e.g., ACP [2004] and MedPAC [2004]).

The chronic care model is widely cited and endorsed (see, e.g., IOM [2003b], Eichner and Blumenthal [2003], and ACP [2004]). Although both models emphasize the importance of coordinated care and active patient involvement, the pediatric medical home model is more explicit in defining the roles of the parent and the child in education and participation in decision making. Most descriptions of the chronic care model are more explicit in emphasizing the crucial roles of system-level elements. These elements include overall delivery system design, evidence-based decision making, clinical decision support systems, and clinical information systems that can track the performance of the care team and provide feedback.

Palsbo and Kailes (2006) recently analyzed the chronic care model to identify features that would make applications of the model "disability competent" (see also the work of DeJong et al. [2002]). Although these features do not take the specific needs of young people into account, they are broadly relevant to this group (Box 4-3).

As discussed in Chapter 8, federal policy makers have been promoting Medicare special needs plans for beneficiaries who live in institutional settings, who are dually eligible for Medicare and Medicaid, or who have severe or disabling chronic conditions (Section 231 of the Medicare Modernization Act of 2003). The great majority of the existing plans (226 of 276 as of 2006) serve dually eligible individuals; only 13 focus on individuals with severe or disabling chronic conditions (Verdier and Au, 2006). Most plans have contracts only with Medicare. Although these plans have not been aimed at young people in transition, experience with them may contribute to the dissemination of the chronic care model to this younger group.

If the pediatric medical home and chronic care models were in place, transitions from pediatric to adult health care would undoubtedly become easier and more predictable for young people with disabilities. Such ease and predictability are not at hand, however. The widespread implementation of both the chronic care model and the medical home model depends on extensive changes in the organization, delivery, and financing of health care in the United States; but such changes have been slow to materialize (see, e.g., Berenson [2006]). For example, despite the heavy promotion of electronic medical records, their implementation in physicians' offices has proved slow (see, e.g., Jha et al. [2006]). Evidence-based guidelines are becoming more available, but acceptance of the guidelines is uneven and decision support tools to promote adherence are not in widespread use (see, e.g., Cabana et al. [1999], Solberg et al. [2000], and Shekelle et al. [2003]). Financing barriers to transition planning and implementation are discussed further below.

BOX 4-3
Features of Disability-Competent Chronic Care Systems

• "Gate-opener" mechanisms, for example, standard protocols for specific health situations that allow the bypassing of "gatekeeper" procedures that control specialty referrals and access to other expensive specialized services

• Extended appointment times, for example, for individuals who use augmented communications tools or technologies or who need assistance in getting ready for an examination

• Benefit management mechanisms that facilitate waivers of benefit restrictions when the provision of additional services would likely reduce a health plan's overall costs for a person's care

• Care that considers the whole person and his or her environment, including needs for social services or home modifications

• Specialized health education and behavior modification programs, for example, programs suitable for individuals with bipolar disorder

• Accessible websites and other communications tools

• Information systems that support the integration of clinical and social services as well as quality monitoring and improvement activities appropriate to this array of services

• Providers with accessible facilities and equipment

• Clinicians and other personnel who have the appropriate knowledge, skills, attitudes, and organizational support (e.g., communications training and access to specialized expertise) to serve people with disabilities, including expertise in assessing the needs and options for assistive technology, general-use technologies, and home modifications

---

SOURCE: Palsbo and Kailes (2006).

Approaches to Health Care Transitions for Young People

This period of late adolescence and young adulthood too often is at risk of becoming a twilight zone with young people falling out of [pediatrics] but not yet falling into adult medicine.

McDonagh (2006, p. 4)

Most discussions of health care transitions for young people reflect the perspectives of pediatric and adolescent medicine, with relatively little contribution from adult-oriented medicine (but see the work of Barbero [1982] and Schidlow and Fiel [1990]). In 2002, however, the AAP, the ACP, and the American Academy of Family Physicians collaborated on a statement on health care transitions for young adults (AAP et al., 2002).[12] In 2003 the Medicine-Pediatrics Program Directors Association created a Committee on Transition Care (Melgar et al., 2005). Today, about 15 percent of pediatrics graduates come from combined medicine-pediatrics residencies.

A good model of transition for young people with disabilities would combine the features emphasized in the medical home and chronic care models with the disability-competent features described above in Box 4-3. Even then, the specific approaches to transition and the transfer of care will vary depending on the complexity of the person's health condition; the availability of relevant medical and other services in the community; and other individual, family, and environmental factors, as described earlier.

Several options exist for transferring responsibilities for a young person's health care. For example, the transfer might be from a general pediatrician to an adult internist or family practitioner, from a pediatric subspecialist to an adult subspecialist, from a pediatric subspecialist to an internist or family practitioner with specialized experience, or from a pediatric medical home to a coordinated adult chronic care team. Today, the fourth option—with a coordinated team on both sides of a planned transition—is uncommon. In addition, although many young people with disabilities will experience a transfer of health care from a pediatrician (or adolescent medicine specialist) to an adult care physician, some who have been under the care of a family practitioner may continue with that individual as their primary care physician.

A survey of 126 interdisciplinary adolescent transition programs reported that a primary care transition approach was uncommon (Scal et al., 1999). (These programs were developed before the intense promotion of the medical home model of care.) The majority of programs (62 percent) were organized around a specific condition, such as cystic fibrosis; the rest provided services for a range of conditions. Nonetheless, the actual services provided differed little among the different approaches. Program respondents cited multiple difficulties in achieving successful transitions, including a lack of institutional support, a lack of time, and inadequate education in the areas of behavioral change and sexuality and reproduction. Several reports have called for transition service education for physicians but have not proposed specific educational strategies (Leslie et al., 2000).

---

[12]The AAP has also issued statements on the physician's role in the development and implementation of the individualized education plans that are required under IDEA and, more generally, the transition of young people with disabilities from school to work or college (AAP, 1999b, 2000). These statements stress that the physician role includes promoting self-advocacy and self-determination and providing anticipatory guidance to help prepare young people for health, health care, and other challenges or issues that may lie ahead.

An analysis commissioned by the National Health Service in the United Kingdom used four problem-oriented models of health care transition as a means of describing different arrangements (NCCSDO, 2002). The *direct transition model* involves a handoff from pediatric to adult health care providers that includes strong attention to communication and information sharing but minimal attention to developmental issues (e.g., maturity for self-care). The analysis suggests that this approach is best suited to young people with mild impairments and few personal, family, or environmental risk factors. The *sequential transition model* entails considerably more support (e.g., support from an adolescent transition clinic) for a young person whose circumstances are more complex and who still needs to develop the skills and maturity required to negotiate the health care system and to manage his or her own care independently. The *developmental transition approach* puts even more emphasis on psychosocial and other developmental issues and support for young people identified as medically or socially vulnerable. Finally, the *professional transition model* shifts the focus to the professional infrastructure needed to support health care transitions for young people with complex medical conditions, such as cystic fibrosis or advanced sickle cell disease. This might include a stepwise process of (1) physician visits that include some time with the parents present, (2) introductions to adult care physicians, (3) assessments of readiness for health care transfer, and (4) transfer to adult health care with continuing access to counseling and peer support groups.

Although physicians in organized health care systems will have more support and resources to manage the transitions outlined in the professional transition model, all physicians—regardless of the setting—will, ideally, have basic competencies and characteristics that reproduce certain elements of the chronic care model at the individual level of the clinician and the patient. These elements include

- a comprehensive approach to assessment and planning;
- a willingness to acquire expertise when needed to manage the individual's health care and transition to adult health care;
- a readiness to work collaboratively;
- a patient-centered philosophy of care;
- good skills in communicating with patients, families, other health care professionals, and social service professionals, when necessary; and
- an ability to negotiate and resolve differences when professional and patient or family preferences differ.

The elements of a professional health care transition infrastructure have been examined in a number of articles that focused on particular health conditions, such as asthma (Couriel, 2003), sickle cell disease (Anie and Telfair, 2005), inflammatory bowel disease (NASPGHAN, 2002), diabetes (Kipps et al., 2002), and cystic fibrosis (Anderson et al., 2002). For example, in one study higher rates of clinic attendance were seen among adolescents with diabetes who had had the opportunity to meet the adult diabetes consultant before their transfer to adult health care (Kipps et al., 2002). Although some of these articles summarize the findings for only a small series of patients, who were often evaluated by the use of surveys, their common themes provide some opportunity to identify frequent characteristics of transition. This is relevant, because research on health care services for children's chronic conditions suggests that what works is often not disease specific but, rather, is applicable across a broad range of conditions (Hobbs et al., 1985; Perrin et al., 1993).

Box 4-4 outlines the steps in transition planning that will be particularly important for a young person with a serious chronic condition or disability. Most of these steps involve the collaboration of the physician with the young person (to the extent that his or her condition permits) and the young person's family beginning well before the time that a transfer in care is anticipated. They also involve considerable attention to detail so that important needs are not overlooked and the practical aspects of a successful transition are identified well in advance of the actual transfer of care. These practical aspects include the identification of every service that a young person is receiving, the determination of what transfer options are available for each service (including self-care), the assessment of the financial resources required to support the transfer, the evaluation of patient and family understanding of the care plan and their needs for education and counseling, and the evaluation of the psychosocial and practical as well as the medical aspects of the transition. The description in Box 4-4 assumes that the young person has been cared for by a pediatric specialist or generalist. For family practitioners who continue to care for a young person, some of these assessments may still be needed if a transition from pediatric to adult subspecialist care must be arranged and if the effects of changes in a young person's living arrangements need to be considered.

The importance of the last element listed in Box 4-4—counseling and the preparation of young people for the health care transition—is illustrated by the findings of Hauser and Dorn (1999) about adolescents with sickle cell disease who were undergoing transitions in care. They found that about half of the small group of adolescents they studied (n = 22) did not know such basic information as their hemoglobin type or their insurance status or that their condition is hereditary.

Barriers to Successful Transition Planning and Outcomes

A 1999 analysis of barriers to care coordination for children with special health care needs is also relevant to the transition of young people to the adult health care system (AAP, 1999a). Box 4-5 expands upon that

BOX 4-4
Care Coordination and Transition Planning

• The young person's physician or care team begins working with the patient (as appropriate) and the patient's family to discuss the process and timing for the shift to adult health care and the steps needed to prepare for that shift. The process should begin by age 14 for patients with more complex conditions.

• In collaboration with the family and all providers involved in the young person's care, the physician or care team prepares a detailed description of the patient's diagnoses with supporting diagnostic data and a plan of care that documents all aspects of care, including hospital care, specialty care, home care (formal and informal), medications, medical devices, and other relevant information. It includes a roster of patient diagnoses with dates and status, therapeutic plans with medication management, and other interventions.

• On the basis of the care plan and an assessment of the patient's or family's understanding of the child's condition and needed care, the health care plan is amended to include steps to address known and anticipated gaps.

• In light of the assessment described above, the physician or care team works with the patient and the patient's family to assess the young person's readiness for the transfer of care and evaluate the adequacy of his or her environmental supports, including health insurance, living arrangements, work arrangements or plans, and transportation needs.

• The physician or care team works with the patient (as appropriate) and family to identify and contact adult care providers consistent with the care plan and to identify other appropriate resources (e.g., social service agencies, support groups).

• The physician or care team develops a medical summary that provides a common information resource for adult health care providers and facilitates the transfer of relevant records and other information to adult health care providers with the patient's written permission.

• The patient and the patient's family receive a notebook or file with documentation of the patient's diagnoses, essential medical history, treatments, and self-care needs; questions for the patient's new health care providers; and information about community resources and supports.

• The physician or care team provides counseling and education about new roles and responsibilities of the patient for components of the health care plan. Anticipatory planning covers both disease-specific and developmental aspects of care and includes special attention to sexual development, family planning, and risk taking as part of the developmentally appropriate patient care plan.

BOX 4-5
Examples of Barriers to Care Coordination and
Transition for Young People with Disabilities

• Involvement of multiple service delivery systems and, possibly, multiple care coordinators with no organized system overall for care coordination

• Lack of clearly defined or agreed-upon roles for each member of the primary health care practice team and the specialty team, the family, and educational and social services agencies

• Inadequate communication among health care professionals and the other organizations involved in the young person's care

• Inadequate knowledge about community resources and the process of coordinating care and transitions

• Insufficient reimbursement for the knowledge, time, and administrative work required to effectively coordinate care and care transitions

• Language and cultural barriers

SOURCES: AAP (1999a) and McDonagh (2006).

---

analysis, which focuses on the challenges facing the primary care pediatrician. Given that different providers, funding programs, and social services agencies may need to be involved as a young person moves from pediatric to adult health care, the potential for care coordination difficulties is likely to multiply during that transition.

A small survey of primary care physicians ($n = 13$) with experience in transitions reported that the most significant barriers to the process were difficulty finding an adult health care provider, youth resistance to the transition, family resistance to the transition, and a lack of institutional support for the process (Scal, 2002). The physicians generally reported success in dealing with youth and family resistance, however.

Others have described similar transition barriers. For example, Tuffrey and Pearce (2003) identified the following barriers to the transition placed by the patient, the family, and the health care provider (see also the work of Koop cited in Magrab and Millar [1989]).

•   *Young person.* Young people, particularly young people with complex conditions who have spent years with the same pediatric care team, may see the transition process as abandonment and may feel uncomfortable or threatened by the style of practice of physicians who care for adults.

• *Family.* Parents, too, may see the transition from the pediatric care team as abandonment. They can also feel threatened by the loss of authority over care for an adult child, especially if the adult health care provider is not sensitive to parental anxieties and to parental involvement in their child's ongoing process of achieving independence.

• *Pediatrician.* Pediatricians may be reluctant to initiate a transition. They may also see physicians who care for adults as less prepared to provide comprehensive, developmentally appropriate patient- and family-centered care.

• *Adult health care providers.* Physicians who care for adults may have had little training for many conditions that were once fatal in childhood and may have little experience working with young adults with disabilities or potentially disabling conditions and with their parents. Many will be subspecialists with a less comprehensive, less interdisciplinary approach to care than is characteristic of providers in pediatric or family practice.

Health care financing issues loom large in discussions of barriers to successful health care transitions and, more generally, to effective implementation of the medical home and chronic care models. One set of financial barriers involves coverage, in particular, the potential for young people (1) to lose coverage altogether when they turn 18 or (2) to experience a disruption in their source care and covered services during a switch from one health plan to another or from Medicaid coverage for children to Medicaid coverage for adults. As noted earlier, the relatively high rates of uninsurance for young adults with disabilities compared with rates for children with disabilities create access problems that can undermine the transition to appropriate health care as an adult. In addition, the avoidable interruptions in children's enrollment in public insurance programs, as discussed in Chapter 8, can disrupt health care coordination generally and transition planning specifically. A recommendation in Chapter 8 calls for the states to limit recertification for and reenrollment in SCHIP to no more than once a year.

A second set of financial issues involves provider payment methods. These issues are often intertwined with coverage issues. Several studies have described shortfalls in the financing of health care for children with special needs and noted that payment for care coordination is typically limited with respect to both payment levels and the coverage of nonmedical services or services provided by nonmedical personnel (see, e.g., Fox and Newacheck [1990], Fox et al. [2002], and Markus et al. [2004]). Although it is not specific to young adults or health care transitions, a recent literature review by Jeffrey and Newacheck (2006) found strong evidence that health insurance coverage had positive effects on access to care for children with special health care needs and on their use of services. The studies reviewed did not assess the effects of coverage on health outcomes.

Pediatricians and internists, among others, have long argued that coordination-of-care activities and other nonprocedural services are poorly reimbursed compared with the payments provided for services that involve surgical, imaging, or other procedures.[13] The website for the AAP medical home initiative devotes one section to the provision of advice on coding and reimbursement to help pediatricians secure the maximum appropriate payment for their services and time (AAP, 2006; see also the work of McManus et al. [2003] and Sophocles [2003]). For example, the AAP website recently provided advice about revisions in the Current Procedural Terminology coding scheme for physician services. The revisions added a code for 15 to 30 minutes per month of care plan oversight for patients who are not enrolled in home health or hospice and who are not in a nursing facility. Given the extensive demands that care coordination makes on physician time and the time of nursing, office, and other personnel, as well as the documentation required for meticulous coding of services, some pediatric practices limit the number of children with special health care needs or disabilities that they will accept as patients (see, e.g., Mitchell et al. [2001] and Valet et al. [2004]).[14]

Another concern for pediatricians is that if they choose to participate in Medicaid managed care contracts, they may be required to accept full-risk capitated payment (i.e., payment per managed care member rather than payment per service provided). Despite progress in developing health-based risk adjustment methods that more fairly compensate health plans that care for patients with serious chronic conditions or disabilities (see Chapter 8 and Appendix C), limited information and analyses are available for use in developing reliable and equitable risk adjustments for capitated payments for the care of children or young adults with special health care needs (White, 2002).

Notwithstanding the risks of capitated payment for health plans or in-

---

[13]Medicaid reimbursements are a particular point of contention, as is the application to pediatric practice of payment models (e.g., resource-based relative value scale) that were originally developed for Medicare (AAP, 1997, 1999a, 2004; see also GAO [2001a]). Nonetheless, a 2003 study reported that pediatricians' caseload of Medicaid patients increased significantly between 1993 and 2000 (Tang et al., 2003). The study did not focus on children with special health care needs.

[14]Recognizing the limits on financing of coordinated care for children with special health care needs, researchers examined the extent and costs of care coordination activities in one four-physician pediatric practice organized around the medical home model (Antonelli and Antonelli, 2004). Considering only nonbillable encounters, they found that about half of the encounters involved activities that are not typically considered medical, for example, managed care referrals and consultations involving educational programs. Physicians were involved in about half of the coordination activities. Using Bureau of Labor Statistics (BLS) data, the researchers estimated the annualized cost of the unreimbursed coordination activities for the practice to be $28,500 (setting staff labor costs at the BLS median). They did not discuss this figure in the context of overall practice expenses or revenues.

dividual providers and concerns about restrictions on patients' timely access to needed services and providers, capitated payment theoretically allows more flexibility in how professionals manage care, including how they delegate services to nonphysicians. It also offers the potential for providers to benefit from the savings achieved through more effective care management. One recent examination of alternatives to the full-fledged model of chronic care endorsed by the ACP and others concluded that it is more difficult to support the management of patients with complex chronic conditions in a fee-for-service setting than in a capitated setting (Berenson, 2006).

As noted earlier in this chapter, federal policy makers have been promoting Medicare special needs plans for beneficiaries who live in institutional settings, who are dually eligible for Medicare and Medicaid, or who have severe or disabling chronic conditions. In addition, the U.S. Congress has increased payments for capitated Medicare Advantage plans (not just plans participating in the special needs program and not just traditional managed care plans), such that payments to health care plans are projected to be higher than historic costs, particularly for dually eligible beneficiaries who are relatively healthy (Peters, 2005; Gorman Health Group, 2006). (See the work of Peters [2005] for a discussion of the complexities associated with various initiatives to coordinate and integrate care for Medicare and Medicaid beneficiaries with significant chronic care needs.)

As described earlier, Title V of the Social Security Act provides for a program of state block grants for services to aid mothers, infants, and children and also supports programs for children with special health care needs or disabilities. Although they make needed services available to people who might otherwise go without them, the range of specialized Title V programs creates transition challenges in at least two dimensions. One dimension relates to the complexities of collecting the required information and planning and coordinating the appropriate transfers of care for a particular young person or for the group of young people served by a pediatric practitioner. The other dimension is financing. Multiple eligibility criteria may need to be tracked, and eligibility for some services may end when a young person "ages out" of the program (Szilaygi et al., 2003). As transfers of care occur for young people, the tracking and tapping of financing sources for care coordination and other transition activities can be a major challenge, particularly for the nonmedical dimensions of care and for young adults who are eligible for benefits from multiple sources (e.g., Medicaid, Medicare, and providers of vocational rehabilitation and assistive technologies).

A 2000 review of state care coordination programs under Title V of the Social Security Act reported that although 41 (of 46 responding) programs assisted families with obtaining early intervention services and specialty medical services, only 33 offered assistance with transition planning (Zimmerman et al., 2000). That study also reported that only 18 state programs sought reimbursement for care coordination services through their state's Medicaid program (e.g., under EPSDT case management benefits, among other options). Nine of the 30 states that provided services to children enrolled in SCHIP obtained reimbursement through that program.

Research on Health Care Transition Planning

Notwithstanding the attention focused on health care transitions by the 1989 U.S. Surgeon General's conference and various initiatives to promote organized transitions programs, research on the health care transition experiences of young people is limited (see, e.g., McDonagh [2000, 2006] and Bennett et al. [2005]). As a Canadian group put it, "[t]ransition is discussed frequently . . . but studied rarely" (Reid et al., 2004, p. 198). The investigators involved in one 1993 study reported that most young people with chronic conditions made the transition to adult life without serious problems, although those individuals with more complex conditions were more likely to experience difficulties (Gortmaker et al., 1993).

A more recent and much larger study that used data from the 2001 national survey of parents of children with special health care needs reported low rates of discussion with a child's physician about transition issues, including the identification of adult health care providers (Scal and Ireland, 2005; see also the work of Lotstein et al. [2005]). Positive responses in all the areas covered in the survey were reported for only 16 percent of the children; those children were more likely to have more extensive health care needs. These two studies found that the type of insurance was not significantly associated with the adequacy of transition planning (Scal and Ireland, 2005; see also Lotstein et al. [2005]).

Using attendance at a congenital heart disease center as a measure of successful transfer, a Canadian study of young people ages 18 to 21 who had been treated as children at a children's hospital found that not quite half had successfully transferred (Reid et al., 2004). Successful transfer was more likely for young people who were older at the time of their last children's hospital appointment, who had undergone more surgeries, and who had a recommendation for follow-up documented in their medical chart.

In an extensive review of the literature on transitions, McDonagh (2006) reported that studies of formal transition activities generally showed positive results. In studies of populations with cystic fibrosis or human immunodeficiency virus infection, one strategy that both young people and their parents viewed as successful was interaction with the designated adult care clinician during the transition period (Westwood et al., 1999; Miles, 2004). During such interactions, the patient and family can gain confidence in that clinician's knowledge and capabilities. A study of young people with rheumatologic conditions (Shaw et al., 2005) and two studies involving young people with diabetes (Salmi et al., 1986; Vanelli et al., 2004) also found positive results by use of this transition strategy.

Most of the studies reviewed by McDonagh focused on process, satisfaction, and knowledge measures, but some of the studies reported improved health outcomes related to organized transition processes. Most studies involved small populations, often at a single center. Some focused on a single aspect of transition, for example, the role of a care coordinator. Few of the studies monitored the children over time.

DIRECTIONS FOR RESEARCH

Although the committee's review identified useful research, many unanswered questions exist about the transition of young people with disabilities to adult health care and the circumstances that support successful transitions. The committee did not attempt to rank priorities for a program of research but identified several broad areas for further investigation (Box 4-6). It encourages researchers and research agencies to involve young people and their families, advocacy and support groups, pediatric and adult health care providers, and representatives of educational and social service agencies and health plans in planning a program of further research. The development of such a program of research should be part of the expanded support for disability and rehabilitation research called for in Chapter 10.

EDUCATION OF PEDIATRICIANS AND ADULT CARE PHYSICIANS

Despite the growth in the numbers of young people with chronic conditions and disabilities, professional education to prepare pediatricians and adult care physicians to guide the health care transitions for their young patients with serious chronic conditions and disabilities appears to be minimal or less in medical school and residency training (Reiss and Gibson, 2006). This lack reflects a broader problem with the preparation of health care professionals to care for people with chronic conditions and disabilities across the life span, as discussed also in Chapter 5 (Holman, 2004). Well-functioning health care systems can create an environment that supports good care for people with disabilities, but such care still requires appropriately educated physicians.

Survey data suggest that today's physicians may be poorly prepared to meet the complex medical and psychosocial needs of people with disabilities. For example, a national survey of physicians ($n = 1,236$) reported that nearly two-thirds regarded their training as inadequate in 10 chronic care skill areas: geriatric syndromes, chronic pain, nutrition, developmental milestones, end-of-life care, psychosocial issues, patient education, assessment of caregiver needs, coordination of services, and interdisciplinary teamwork (Darer et al., 2004). Another study of 70 clerkship directors for 16 medical schools reported that the directors varied considerably in

BOX 4-6
Directions for Research on Health Care
Transitions for Young People

Child Development and Personal Factors

• What are critical periods in child development that affect the transition process? Does planning for transition from the onset of a disability make a difference?

• How do stages in adolescent development, including risk-taking behaviors in earlier adolescence and maturation in later adolescence, affect the characteristics of transition planning and implementation? How may a young person's physical and mental condition interact with development to affect the transition?

• What are developmentally appropriate ways and times for increasing an adolescent's self-care and self-management responsibilities and involving adolescents with disabilities in decision making? To what extent should the process vary depending on the characteristics of the child?

Family Factors

• What family characteristics influence transition and in what ways? How should transition programs account for and respond to these characteristics?

• What education and other types of support are most effective in helping parents prepare for their child's transition to adult health care?

Health Care Services Organization and Financing

• What are the most critical components of a model of health care transition for young people with disabilities?

• What does each component contribute to the effectiveness of transition care? For example, what characteristics of electronic health records and record systems best support the gathering and timely sharing of relevant medical, social, and other information among the parties involved in transition planning (e.g., young people, family members, the referring and the accepting physicians, and other health care providers). How does the effectiveness of different aspects of the model vary depending on the characteristics of the young person, the family, and their environment?

• How can transition care best be planned and implemented when the features of the medical home and chronic care models are not in place?

• What roles do assistive technologies, including those for cognitive disabilities, play in easing the transition?

• What specific changes in coverage of services, payment to providers, or other characteristics of health care financing would be most useful in improving the transition of care for young people with disabilities?

• Does training in teamwork in planning and coordinating the transitions for young people with disabilities improve the process and outcomes?

the importance that they assigned to an array of skills or competencies in chronic care management (Pham et al., 2004). Such skills or competencies are also relevant to care for many people with disabilities. Of concern to the committee is the relatively low ratings assigned to the need for physicians to know strategies to maximize their patients' potentials, to be able to discuss alternative information sources, and to have the ability to assess equipment needs, which may involve identifying the need for a referral to an expert in this area.

In addition to shortfalls in education on the care of chronic illnesses generally, another concern is an inconsistency between recognition of the importance of transition planning by providers and their personal involvement with the transitioning of their own patients. For example, Telfair and colleagues (2004) reported that although the majority of providers agreed on the importance of a formal transition program for young people with sickle cell disease, few actually facilitated the transition process with their patients. A survey of parents and physicians found differences of opinions about the extent to which they believed that it was the provider's responsibility to assist in various transition activities and the extent to which providers actually did provide such assistance (Geenen et al., 2003).

An encouraging sign of increasing attention to the requisites of chronic care management is the recent identification by the Accreditation Council on Graduate Medical Education (ACGME) of the need to make competency in systems-based care a priority in residency program curricula (ACGME, 2006a). As described earlier, systems-based care is a key element of the chronic care model. The ACGME discussion stresses the importance of working with other health care professionals, helping patients negotiate the health care system, and understanding coding and other dimensions of health plan operations. Other competencies involve medical knowledge, patient care, interpersonal and communication skills, professionalism, and practice-based learning and improvement. All of these competencies are relevant to physicians caring for young people with disabilities, either as aspects of direct patient care or in managing interactions with health plans so that payment and other procedures are followed to minimize coverage denials and other problems.

In another initiative, the Institute for Improving Medical Education of the Association of American Medical Colleges has created the Enhancing Education for Chronic Illness Care initiative (AAMC, 2006). The institute has awarded grants to 10 medical schools to redesign their curricula and residency programs to improve graduates' understanding and knowledge of treatments for chronic conditions.[15] Although it cannot be expected to cover the many specific dimensions of health care for young people with mobility, speech, cognitive, and other types of impairments, many aspects of general training in chronic care management will be relevant for the care of children with disabilities related to chronic health conditions.

With respect to pediatric professionals specifically, pediatric residency programs require only a month of adolescent medicine experience (ACGME, 2006b). In addition, adolescents are underrepresented in continuity-of-care clinics, constituting less than 10 percent of clinic patients identified in a 1995 survey (Marilyn Dumont-Driscoll, professor of pediatrics, University of Florida College of Medicine, personal communication, December 11, 2006). Continuity-of-care clinics offer pediatric residents experience in providing longitudinal and continuous care for well children and children with chronic conditions or disabilities. The committee found no data on formal education for pediatricians about the transition to adult care for young people with disabilities.

RECOMMENDATIONS

The transition to adult health care is a complex process that is influenced by the characteristics of the young person, his or her family, and the larger environment of policies and organizational arrangements that affect the availability and coordination of health care services, the sharing of health care information, and the support provided by schools and social services available in the community. As outlined in this chapter, many barriers to successful health care transitions for young people with disabilities are basic features of health care in this country. These include the fragmented organization of health care services, dysfunctional provider reimbursement methods, the high levels of uninsurance or incomplete insurance (e.g., a lack of coverage for nonmedical consultations and services), and the limited availability of sophisticated information technology to support information sharing among generalists and specialists who care for children with complex health conditions. The limited education of health care professionals in chronic care management is another barrier. In addition, most physicians who treat adults have little exposure to pediatric medicine and thus to the conditions and patterns of care that their young adult patients with disabilities have experienced.

---

[15]Other initiatives can also be cited. For example, more than a decade ago, the U.S. Department of Veterans Affairs began a 3-year realignment of its graduate medical education program by reducing specialty training positions and increasing primary care positions (Stevens et al., 2001). The shift came in response to a restructuring of patient care to improve services for the system's large population of seriously and chronically ill veterans.

The committee was impressed by the potential and promise found in the medical home and chronic care models. If these models were widely adopted and sustained, young people would be much more likely to receive the comprehensive and multifaceted care that would help them to make a successful transition from pediatric to adult health care.

Although further development of these models is needed, as is more research on the circumstances that contribute to their effectiveness, several elements appear to be critical if health care consistent with that offered through these models is to expand and reach more young people. These elements include reforms in the organization and financing of health care and better preparation of health care professionals for the provision of co-ordinated care for people with serious chronic conditions and disabilities.

> **Recommendation 4.1: To improve the transition of young people with disabilities from pediatric to adult health care, policy makers, pro-fessional societies, public and private payers, and educators should work to**
>   • **align and strengthen incentives in public and private health care programs to support coordinated care and transition planning;**
>   • **expand the use of integrated electronic medical records for chronic disease management and during the transition of young people with disabilities from pediatric to adult health care; and**
>   • **expand chronic care education in pediatric and internal medi-cine residency programs and add skills in the management of individu-als with chronic health care needs to specialty board requirements.**

This chapter makes clear that young people face major changes in their eligibility for public or private health coverage and are at risk for the loss of benefits just as they are in the process of making the transition from pediatric to adult health care. As described earlier, Medicaid, SCHIP, IDEA, and SSI all change eligibility or coverage policies at age 18 or by the time a young person reaches age 21. MCHB, despite its emphasis on planning for transition, has neither the jurisdiction nor the resources to support transition programs for individuals beyond age 21. Thus the com-mittee recommends several changes in public programs to support young people with making a successful transition to adult health care services and independent living.

> **Recommendation 4.2: To support the successful transition of young people with disabilities from pediatric to adult health care and indepen-dent living, the U.S. Congress should**
>   • **extend Medicaid and State Children's Health Insurance Program (SCHIP) coverage through age 21 for young people with disabilities**

and specify that Medicaid and SCHIP benefits cover transition assessment, coordination, and management services for these young people;

• fund the Maternal and Child Health Bureau so that it may expand its work to develop and implement medical home and other services for young people with special health care needs who are over age 21 and who need continued transition support;

• revise the Ticket to Work program by lowering the eligibility age to 16 years and directing the U.S. Department of Education and the Social Security Administration to develop guidance for the coordination of Ticket to Work services with the transition services and supports provided under the Individuals with Disabilities Education Act; and

• direct the Centers for Disease Control and Prevention to work with other relevant agencies to examine opportunities for the monitoring of transitions through additions to state and national youth surveys or other cross-sectional and longitudinal data collection efforts.

In addition, as discussed in Chapter 9, it important that policy makers monitor the effects of changes in Medicaid program requirements that were made in the Deficit Reduction Act of 2005. Some of these changes may threaten the provision of services to children with special needs. It will also be important to monitor the implementation of the act's provisions for states to expand enrollment of low-income children and youth with disabilities.

Although not a formal recommendation, the committee encourages the Centers for Disease Control and Prevention, in conjunction with the Social Security Administration, the Maternal and Child Health Bureau, the Centers for Medicare and Medicaid Services, and the Department of Education to convene a conference on transition planning for young people with disabilities. The topics for such a conference could include discussions of best practices in transition services, transition monitoring, continued research to strengthen the evidence base for transition planning, health professions education, and issues in coordinating the transition services provided by different public programs.

This chapter has focused on young people with disabilities who are in the process of moving into the world of adult health care and adult life generally. The next chapter focuses on the continuing experiences of people with early-onset disability as they grow older. It also considers the risk of secondary health conditions for people with disabilities—regardless of age.

5

Secondary Conditions and Aging with Disability

I was about 35 years old when I started to feel the signs of aging that I later learned were being brought on prematurely by my disability (cerebral palsy). The timing was ironic, because it coincided with my involvement as the principal investigator of one of the country's first studies of how disability affects the [process of aging]. . . . I became aware that I wasn't alone with these symptoms, that they weren't 'all in my head.' . . . But I was frightened because aging with a disability was an uncharted course.

Kathleen Lankasky (2004 [used with permission])

One surprising and sometimes frightening feature of life with certain potentially disabling conditions acquired at birth or in early life is that people who have managed their lives successfully for years may find, as they reach their 30s or 40s, that they are experiencing the effects of aging earlier than others or are developing secondary health conditions.[1] This is not what they had expected. For clinicians, researchers, policy makers, and others, the challenge is, on the one hand, to prevent or delay secondary conditions and premature aging and, on the other hand, to prepare for and mitigate their effects, once they develop. Meeting this challenge will involve progress on several fronts, including improving professional and consumer awareness and responses based on existing knowledge, strengthening further that base of knowledge, developing supportive public policies, and identifying and removing environmental barriers such as inaccessible transportation systems.

---

[1]As discussed later in this chapter, secondary health conditions are additional physical or mental health conditions—such as pressure ulcers or urinary tract infections—that can result from a primary health condition but that are not a diagnostic feature of that condition.

136

Secondary conditions related to a primary health condition and atypical or premature aging with disabilities are important because they can affect physical and psychosocial functioning, independence, and participation in community life, including work. They can diminish a person's quality of life, add to the demands on family members or others as caregivers, expose previously unnoticed environmental barriers that limit activity and participation, and challenge health care professionals whose education has not prepared them to care knowledgeably for people aging with early-onset or long-standing disabilities.

As noted in Chapters 3 and 4, more and more children and young adults with once fatal conditions that contribute to disability are surviving into middle and late life, thus increasing the number of individuals at risk for secondary conditions and premature or atypical aging. Some individuals are also at risk of long-term complications of treatment, including treatments (e.g., chemotherapy, radiation, and surgery) that were undertaken to cure or mitigate their condition. On the basis of data from the 1994–1995 Disability Supplement to the National Health Interview Survey, Verbrugge and Yang (2002) estimated that approximately 7 to 9 percent of adults had a disability that began before age 20 (Table 5-1). Approximately 20 to 30 percent of adults experienced the onset of their disability between ages 20 to 44. An analysis of Canadian data reported that approximately two-thirds of people ages 65 to 74 who had a disability had acquired that disability before age 65, whereas for people age 75 and older, the figure was less than 30 percent (HRSDC, 2005).

Focused interest in secondary conditions and aging with disability is relatively recent and reflects, in part, the survival and life expectancy trends for children and adults noted above. Citing the attention-directing observations of Michael Marge (1988), the Institute of Medicine (IOM) report *Dis-*

TABLE 5-1 Age of Disability Onset for Individuals with Disabilities by Category of Disability, 1994

Type of Disability	Percentage of Individuals with Disability Onset at Age:						
	At birth	>0–19	20–24	25–44	45–65	65–74	75+
ADL	4.1	4.5	2.7	18.3	25.2	18.9	26.3
IADL	3.9	4.9	3.2	22.3	29.4	18.8	17.5
PLIM	2.3	5.1	4.1	27.0	31.7	16.7	13.1

NOTE: ADL = limitation in activities of daily living; IADL = limitation in instrumental activities of daily living; PLIM = limitation in physical tasks. Data are from the National Health Interview Survey Disability Supplement, Phase 1 (1994), and are weighted to be representative of the U.S. civilian noninstitutional populations ages 18 and older. Row distributions add to 100 percent.
SOURCE: Verbrugge and Yang (2002 [used with permission]).

ability in America (1991) devoted a chapter to secondary conditions. Both the 1991 report and the report *Enabling America* (IOM, 1997) recognized aging as a risk factor for secondary conditions and noted that interventions that prevent secondary conditions will promote health and well-being as people with disabilities grow older. A number of other reports, articles, and conferences have explored these topics, including the 2005 workshop and associated publication sponsored as part of the activities used to develop this report (Treischmann, 1987; Simeonsson and McDevitt, 2002; Kemp and Mosqueda, 2004; IOM, 2006b). In addition, the National Institute on Disability and Rehabilitation Research has funded three relevant research centers, one focusing on aging with a disability, a second one focusing on aging with developmental disability, and a third one focusing on secondary conditions. Longitudinal research that can guide consumer health practices and clinical care is still in short supply, but at least the rationale for such research is better understood.

The significance of secondary conditions as a legitimate target for public health strategies is also evident in *Healthy People 2010*, which includes a chapter on disability and secondary conditions (CDC, 2001). An overarching goal stated in that report is to "promote the health of people with disabilities, prevent secondary conditions, and eliminate disparities between people with and without disabilities in the U.S. population" (p. 6-8). The goals do not explicitly mention aging with disability, but discussions of secondary conditions and aging with disability (including those reviewed in this chapter) often overlap and cite the same health issues and literature.

Efforts to prevent secondary conditions or to delay and slow the progression of conditions linked to aging with certain kinds of disability are a form of tertiary prevention (IOM, 1991). In a public health or clinical context, *primary prevention* aims to avert the creation or onset of illnesses, injuries, or other conditions (e.g., through vaccination programs to prevent polio and other contagious diseases and through the promotion of folic acid use during pregnancy to prevent spina bifida). For health conditions that are already present but that are either not recognized or not symptomatic, *secondary prevention* emphasizes early detection and intervention to halt or delay the progression of the condition (e.g., through screening for breast cancer and through infant testing and the use of early dietary interventions to prevent symptoms of phenylketonuria). *Tertiary prevention* seeks to reduce or stabilize the consequences of a primary health condition and prevent or mitigate secondary health conditions associated with a primary condition. Examples of tertiary prevention include evaluating the bone density of young people with mobility impairments such as cerebral palsy to prevent fractures from secondary osteoporosis, monitoring individuals who have had a stroke for shoulder pain, and educating individuals with sensory impairments on the selection and safe use of assistive technologies.

In addition to clinical care, tertiary prevention may involve environmental modifications, such as changes in household technologies or arrangements that reduce the risk of falls or that help a person remain independent in self-care. Tertiary prevention also extends to the policy arena, for example, through the removal of barriers and hazards in public spaces and the adoption of policies that help people pay for home modifications or assistive technologies. These outcomes may also benefit family members and society generally.

Although scientific and clinical knowledge about secondary conditions and aging with disability has advanced and strategies for preventing additional disabilities have improved, much remains to be learned—and to be applied consistently where knowledge does exist. Before selected segments of the research literature on secondary conditions and aging with a disability are reviewed, the next section puts these aspects of living with disability in a broader framework.

A LIFE SPAN PERSPECTIVE ON SECONDARY CONDITIONS AND AGING WITH A DISABILITY

In discussions of disability across the life span, one frequent goal is to draw attention to the long-term aspects of living with a disability. As people with many kinds of chronic health conditions acquired in early, middle, or late life live longer and as the impact on later life of what happens earlier in life is more fully appreciated, clinicians, families, and people with disabilities are recognizing how important it is to consider and plan for the long-term future.

Experience and research have prompted reconsideration of some traditional ways of managing and living with certain conditions to reduce unwanted long-term effects. For example, as Kemp and Mosqueda (2004) have written, "instead of encouraging everyone [with conditions such as polio or cerebral palsy] to work as hard as possible . . . 'the use it or lose it attitude' . . . a philosophy akin to 'conserve it to preserve it' may be more appropriate" (p. 4). This shift reflects one theory behind postpolio syndrome, which holds that after the initial assault of the polio virus, the remaining motor neurons are overworked, particularly during intensive and prolonged exercise. Unfortunately, clinicians and consumers with postpolio syndrome still lack solid scientific evidence about the role of exercise, including how to strike a balance between sufficient exercise for the prevention of illnesses such as cardiovascular disease and sufficient rest for the prevention of severe fatigue and weakness.

This example underscores points made in earlier chapters. First, longitudinal studies are vital, and second, consideration of the long-term future should start soon after the onset of a potentially disabling condition. In addition, given the impact on later life of what happens earlier in life, evaluations of adults with long-standing disabilities should also consider the long-term past (Verbrugge and Yang, 2002). That is, it is important for clinicians to obtain thorough medical and personal histories from these adults, even though it may be difficult to document some elements of the past. People with childhood-onset conditions may not know key details about the onset of their condition, its initial treatment, and potentially relevant environmental circumstances, such as exposure to toxic substances. Their parents likewise may not remember or may not be alive, and childhood medical records may not be available.

The implications of aging with a disability and the potential for acquiring a secondary condition vary by the nature of an individual's primary health condition. Later sections of this chapter review several conditions for which data on secondary conditions and aging are comparatively good.

Although the discussion in this chapter focuses on the medical and cognitive aspects of aging with disability, the committee recognizes the need to better understand the role of environmental and personal factors in premature or atypical aging. Lankasky (2004) has, for example, stressed such psychosocial issues as helping children with disabilities to develop a strong sense of self-worth that will prepare them for sometimes negative attitudes from peers, health care professionals, and others. Others have also pointed to the influence of personal factors, in particular, styles of coping with adversity (see, e.g., Hansen et al. [1998]) and family circumstances (see, e.g., Kemp et al. [1997] and Kemp [2006]) in shaping an individual's responses to declines in health or functioning.

Secondary Conditions

In 1988, Michael Marge observed that people with disabilities are at significant risk for "additional or secondary disabilities" (Marge, 1988). The 1991 IOM report (p. 35) defined *secondary condition* as "any additional physical or mental health condition that occurs as a result of having a primary disabling condition."[2] (A "disabling condition" is any mental

---

[2]Others have defined the term far more broadly to include many additional possible consequence of a primary disabling condition, such as social isolation or a lack of romantic relationships (see, e.g., DHHS [2000a]). Nonetheless, just as this report distinguishes primary physical or mental health conditions from poverty, pollution, discrimination, and other environmental conditions that may contribute to illness, injury, impairment, activity limitations, or participation restrictions, so, too, does it distinguish secondary physical or mental health conditions from the social and economic consequences that may follow the onset of a primary health condition. Excluding unwanted social and economic outcomes from the definition of secondary conditions does not, in any sense, diminish their significance or the importance of taking steps to help people lead rewarding social lives.

or physical health condition that can lead to disability.) Some secondary conditions, for example, depression, arthritis, and cardiovascular disease, are also common primary health conditions (see, e.g., Kemp [2006]).

In the clinical and research literature, frequently mentioned secondary conditions include arthritis, pain, pressure ulcers, fatigue, depression, contractures, and urinary tract infections. The risk of developing a particular secondary condition, however, depends in part on a person's primary condition. For example, people who have vision or hearing impairments are generally not at higher-than-average risk of pressure ulcers or urinary tract infections.

As is the case with a primary disability, the interaction of biology, lifestyle and behavior, and environmental factors affect whether a secondary condition contributes to the development of additional impairments, activity limitations, or participation restrictions. Some secondary conditions, such as an infected pressure ulcer, can become life-threatening, and some can be more disabling than the primary condition, for example, when intractable pain causes someone to cut back on work or social activities. One challenge for researchers, who are still building a descriptive base of knowledge on secondary conditions, is sorting out the contributions of different health, personal, and environmental factors to these conditions.

People with a given primary health condition will not necessarily experience all the secondary conditions for which they are at increased risk, especially if good preventive strategies exist and are used. For those who do develop them, severity may vary. For example, not all children with cerebral palsy will have contractures, and among those who do, some children will have more severe contractures than others. Again, individuals' experiences may reflect the specific features of their primary condition, the quality of their medical and rehabilitative services, their ability to adhere to treatment or prevention regimens, their access to personal care assistance, and other personal and environmental factors.

Many secondary conditions appear to be linked through common physiological processes or functional characteristics across several different primary health conditions. For example, as discussed later in this chapter, people with significant mobility limitations—which might be related to spinal cord or brain injury, multiple sclerosis, or a number of other conditions—are at risk of pressure ulcers or contractures. As more longitudinal research is undertaken, more linkages and common risk factors may be identified. Likewise, long-term clinical or well-designed observational studies may identify the extent to which common interventions (e.g., prescribed exercises) can reduce the probability or severity of secondary conditions that are common to different primary health conditions (see, e.g., Rimmer and Shenoy [2006]).

Discussions of secondary conditions are complicated by confusion with several other types of health conditions. According to the definitions offered by Turk (2006), *associated conditions* are aspects or features of the primary condition; that is, they are expected elements of its pathology, although their expression may be variable. Thus, for people with cerebral palsy, spasticity is an aspect of upper motor neuron impairment and, therefore, an associated rather than a secondary condition. Although many people with cerebral palsy do not experience them, seizures and mental retardation are also considered features of the disorder's pathology and not secondary conditions. To cite other examples, limited skin sensation is an associated condition with spinal cord injury. Dysphagia is an associated condition of Parkinson's disease and other disorders that affect the muscles or nerves used in swallowing, such as amyotrophic lateral sclerosis. Muscle weakness is a defining feature of post-polio syndrome. Clinically, an inability to make distinctions between features of the primary health condition and secondary conditions may not affect individual patient care.

Another distinction is between secondary conditions and *comorbidities*. Comorbidities are health conditions that develop independently of the primary condition. They are neither a feature of the condition nor a secondary condition. A person with a traumatic brain injury may develop skin cancer. An individual with hearing loss may develop heart disease. Sometimes, however, researchers identify links between conditions formerly thought to be independent of each other. One example is the link between spinal cord injury and the development of insulin-resistant diabetes, as discussed later in this chapter.

Treatment complications are caused by treatment for a condition rather than by the condition itself. Like secondary conditions, they may sometimes be preventable. Also like secondary conditions, they can contribute to additional disability. In practice and especially over the long term, it can be difficult to distinguish treatment effects, secondary conditions, and age-related phenomena.

Age may affect the development and treatment of secondary conditions. For example, although secondary conditions such as pressure ulcers or recurrent urinary tract infections can occur at a very young age, prevention or management may be more difficult with older people who have less physiological reserve capacity, more comorbid chronic conditions, and other age-related changes, such as thinning of the skin. In addition, age may make a person more susceptible to the side effects of treatment, such as gastrointestinal bleeding in association with the use of nonsteroidal anti-inflammatory drugs for treatment of pain (see e.g., Laine et al. [2002] and Pilotto et al. [2003]).

Aging and Disability

I write . . . [as] someone who is a living, aging-with-disability 'labora-tory.'. . . When I talk with older people without disabilities about their aging experiences, I often identify with what they describe and think to myself, 'I'm already there!'

June Isaacson Kailes (2006)

Although genetics, environment, and behavior contribute to significant variations in individual patterns of aging, aging as a biological process begins at a relatively young age. For example, declines in muscle mass, hormone levels, organ function, and other biological structures or processes begin well before people reach their 50s (see, e.g., Masoro [1999] and Schulz et al. [2006]). Over a normal life span, such natural physiological declines are not preventable, although they may be accelerated or slowed by a variety of individual genetic factors, personal behaviors (e.g., diet and exercise), health care practices (e.g., screening and treatment for heart disease), and other environmental circumstances (e.g., working conditions).

In most discussions about disability and in most disability-related research, a focus on aging typically means a focus on the increasing level of chronic illness and disability in late life. That is, the emphasis is on people *aging into disability.*

In contrast, the emphasis in this chapter is on *aging with a disability*, which typically refers to the experience of people who were born with physical or mental impairments or who acquired them in early to middle life. A Canadian government report limits the description to people under the age of 65 (HRSDC, 2005).

Understanding and studying the nature of aging with disabilities requires an appreciation of the different dimensions of time that may be at work (see, e.g., Campbell [1993] and Krause and Adkins [2004]). These dimensions include

- the usual process of development and aging through childhood, middle life, and late life;
- the number of years spent with a particular disability, for example, having lived with multiple sclerosis for 10 years, whether its onset occurred at age 25 or age 35;
- in some cases, the years of exposure to a particular medication (e.g., corticosteroids) or other therapy or environmental factor with cumulative adverse side effects;
- the individual's cohort or era of disability onset and initial medical treatment, which may be associated with different treatment experiences,

attitudes, and opportunities, depending, for example, on whether the individual experienced a traumatic brain injury in 1985, 1995, or 2005; and

- the age at onset of a disability in relation to the individual's developmental maturity.

The last factor—the age of onset in relation to developmental maturity—may be important for some conditions, such as a spinal cord injury, that typically involve prolonged periods of hospitalization for acute treatment and rehabilitation. A 5-year-old, for example, is dealing with different developmental tasks than a 15-year-old, which means that younger and older children may experience different long-term psychosocial or physical effects from an extended hospitalization. In addition, the severity of a condition sometimes varies with the age at onset.

As the list above suggests, a variety of mechanisms likely explain the aspects of aging with a disability considered in this chapter. For example, for disabilities that typically lead people to compensate for impairments in one aspect of the body with additional demands on other aspects of the body (e.g., people with impairments in lower limb mobility compensate with greater reliance on their arms and shoulders), the existence of a disability for a longer period of time may accelerate use-related musculoskeletal pain or other problems. The time that a person lives with a disability may also interact with the metabolic or other biological processes and changes triggered by a primary health condition, leading eventually to the earlier-than-usual development of, for example, cardiac or orthopedic problems.

SELECTIVE REVIEW OF THE LITERATURE

Despite the many complexities and questions surrounding the definition of secondary conditions, consumers, practitioners, and researchers have adopted the concept as a useful way of understanding certain potentially preventable health conditions that can contribute to additional disability. Researchers are generating an increasing amount of information about secondary conditions, usually in studies of specific primary health conditions, such as spinal cord injury. Likewise, researchers are investigating the experiences of people aging with different kinds of primary health conditions. In addition, researchers are recognizing that a number of primary conditions, particularly those involving musculoskeletal impairments, show certain common patterns of secondary conditions or aging, although the underlying pathophysiologies may vary. In some cases, better understanding of these kinds of common patterns may lead to interventions that are effective for people with a range of primary health conditions.

The research reviewed in this section focuses on secondary conditions, but much, if not most, of this research has also been considered in presentations or papers about aging with disability. The research largely involves disabilities and impairments that have relatively high prevalence rates (e.g., cerebral palsy), are easy to associate with a disability group (e.g., polio survivors), benefit from organized and dedicated service programs (e.g., spinal cord injury), and—reflecting these characteristics—have attracted research funding sufficient to generate a significant body of knowledge about the condition.

Most studies focus on biological and clinical processes and health outcomes. Some consider or acknowledge the contribution of environmental or personal factors, such as a lack of health insurance coverage for relevant services or equipment (e.g., a proper wheelchair), inaccessible fitness equipment and facilities, or the failure of individuals or their caregivers to follow preventive or treatment regimens (e.g., recommended exercises and proper positioning in a bed or a chair). They may emphasize a particular secondary condition, such as pain, or they may consider multiple conditions. Few consider activity and participation outcomes or effects on family members.

The research reviewed here suffers from various other limitations. The literature includes a combination of scientifically observed and anecdotal information. Secondary conditions are sometimes the central focus of research; but they may also be noted in descriptive studies, reports on the health status or life course of people with disabilities, and health promotion studies.

For the most part, studies are cross-sectional rather than longitudinal, although a few have focused on aging and the life course for specific chronic conditions. They often involve convenience samples or case series that may not be representative of the larger population of individuals with a particular disability. Studies that include more than one primary condition may have a higher representation of people with certain conditions and may not report data for each condition group, so it may be difficult or inappropriate to generalize about each group. Still, methodologically sound cross-condition studies in areas such as exercise interventions may be useful to the extent that the biological processes of the response to the intervention are similar.

Another limitation of much research is that conclusions are drawn from patient reports and clinical observations without the use of standardized measures of individual characteristics or outcomes. A few studies use a very broad definition of secondary conditions and include disability-related social conditions, such as unemployment or social isolation. Embedded in these studies, however, may be useful descriptive information about secondary health conditions. Further complicating the picture, some research describes as secondary conditions what this report describes as associated conditions (e.g., poor urinary control and incontinence in individuals with spinal cord injuries) or direct residuals of the primary impairment (e.g., behavior dysregulation in individuals with brain injuries). Again, a critical review may sort out such labeling differences to glean useful descriptive information about secondary conditions from these reports.

The review in the following sections is illustrative rather than comprehensive. It covers research on secondary conditions associated with four specific primary conditions that have been the focus of considerable research and other attention: spinal cord injury, cerebral palsy, postpolio syndrome, and Down syndrome. The review also considers some cross-condition studies.

Spinal Cord Injury

The typical person experiencing a spinal cord injury is a young male (National Spinal Cord Injury Statistical Center, 2006). Better early treatment of spinal cord injuries has led to improved survival, although often with severe long-term impairments. In addition, better treatment of certain associated and secondary conditions, including urinary tract complications, has increased survival beyond the initial treatment stage. Young survivors can typically expect decades of living—and aging—with the disability.

The secondary conditions and aging experiences of individuals with spinal cord injuries are probably the best defined of all disability groups. Many medical centers have organized spinal cord injury centers or programs, and both institutions and professionals may be certified or credentialed to provide these services. These organized and focused care settings can support systematic data collection, surveillance, and ongoing research, including research on secondary conditions. Research on spinal cord injury has been consistently funded through the model systems programs of the National Institute on Disability and Rehabilitation Research and the National Center for Medical Rehabilitation Research and through the Veterans Health Administration with support from the Paralyzed Veterans of America. (Chapter 10 discusses the desirability of better coordination of the model systems programs supported by the National Institute on Disability and Rehabilitation Research and National Center for Medical Rehabilitation Research model.)

Because a spinal cord injury involves multiple organ systems, many of the associated health conditions (as defined earlier) are often erroneously identified as secondary conditions. For example, neurogenic bladder and bowel can be expected in people with spinal cord injuries and may involve either over- or underactive functioning. Autonomic dysreflexia (overactivity of the autonomic nervous system, leading to dangerously high blood pressure), is possible in injuries at and above the sixth thoracic vertebra (approximately waist level), and spasticity can be anticipated in 70 percent of people with spinal cord injuries (Levi et al., 1995). Each of these medical conditions is a residual of the injury, that is, an associated condition.

Each condition, of course, warrants management and preventive strategies in its own right.

In his paper for the 2005 IOM workshop on disability, Bauman (2006) reviewed pulmonary and cardiovascular diseases, metabolic syndrome,[3] osteoporosis, vitamin D deficiency, and pressure ulcers as common secondary conditions and health concerns for people with spinal cord injuries. He noted that cardiovascular disease has replaced urinary complications as the leading cause of death among those with spinal cord injuries and thus has become a major focus of research to identify preventive interventions. Most of the secondary conditions discussed (e.g., cardiovascular disease and metabolic syndrome) are also concerns for people with other conditions that limit the regular use of large muscle groups.

Many case series report on the occurrence of pain in people with spinal cord injuries, with approximately 30 to 50 percent of individuals complaining of shoulder pain that is severe enough to interfere with function (Bayley et al., 1987; Gellman et al., 1988; Sie et al., 1992; Curtis et al., 1999a). Pain prevalence increases with time from injury. This pain may have multiple musculoskeletal etiologies, but the most common is chronic shoulder (or rotator cuff) impingement syndrome, which affects about half of case series populations (Bayley et al., 1987; Curtis et al., 1995; Campbell and Koris, 1996; Escobedo et al., 1997, Lal, 1998). These case series have led to recommendations for prevention and treatment strategies. In addition, some research has evaluated the effectiveness of exercise protocols that can be used to prevent further shoulder problems, finding that regular strengthening and flexibility programs decrease their recurrence (Olenik et al., 1995; Curtis et al., 1999b).

As discussed below, a consortium of professionals, payers, and consumers has developed clinical practice guidelines for the preservation of upper limb functioning in people with spinal cord injuries. For many people, shoulder problems are linked to long-term wheelchair use or other actions that place great physical demands on the upper extremities. Thus advances in wheelchair design and systematic evaluations of an individual's wheelchair use have the potential to reduce shoulder damage in the short and the long term. Individuals may not, however, be able to take advantage of improved equipment and proper evaluations if their health plans have outdated coverage policies and criteria (see Chapter 9 for a discussion of coverage for assistive technologies and services).

Neuropathic pain, often severe enough to limit activities and participation and decrease quality of life, is reported in 47 to 96 percent of people

---

[3]Metabolic syndrome refers to a group of risk factors for heart disease, including, among other elements, elevated blood pressure, obesity (especially around the abdomen), high levels of triglycerides and low levels of high-density lipoprotein, and insulin resistance.

with spinal cord injuries (Yezierski, 1996). Researchers have studied many interventions for this kind of pain, although most involve case series and surveys (often involving small numbers of participants) rather than controlled research. Disappointingly, the research does not clearly point to a particular intervention that provides significant relief or control of pain related to damage to the peripheral or central nervous system (Davis and Lentini, 1975; Cole et al., 1991; Tai et al., 2002; To et al., 2002; Warms et al., 2002).

The Paralyzed Veterans of America (PVA) has been particularly active in promoting the development of evidence-based clinical practice guidelines on the prevention and management of secondary conditions through the Consortium on Spinal Cord Medicine (CSCM). The consortium, which the PVA has funded and managed, involves more than 20 health professional, consumer, and payer groups and has developed guidelines in several areas, for example, the prevention of pressure ulcers (CSCM, 2000), respiratory management (CSCM, 2005b), the preservation of upper limb function (CSCM, 2005a), and bladder management (CSCM, 2006). The group has also developed companion guides for consumers on pressure ulcers (CSCM, 2002), neurogenic bowel (CSCM, 1999), and other topics.

Cerebral Palsy

Cerebral palsy is a significant contributor to lifelong disability. The term *cerebral palsy* covers several neurological disorders involving brain abnormalities that affect muscle control. It is usually identified early in life. The rate of early mortality is higher than average for children born with severe impairments, such as profound mental retardation, significant motor impairments, and the pulmonary complications associated with cerebral palsy (Kudrjavcev et al., 1985; Eyman et al., 1990; Evans and Alberman, 1991; Hemming et al., 2005). Overall, however, more than 90 percent of children born with the condition survive into adulthood (Murphy and Bliss, 2004). Encouraged by individuals with cerebral palsy, their families, and the United Cerebral Palsy Association, all federal research funding agencies have named cerebral palsy as a condition of interest.

Adults with cerebral palsy report that they enjoy generally good health, with their self-rated health being comparable to that of a community at large in one study (Murphy et al., 1995; Turk et al., 1995, 1997a). People with this condition have health care needs specific to the condition but also benefit from common health promotion and disease prevention services (e.g., routine childhood vaccinations, screening for breast cancer, and counseling about tobacco use). Many communities support specialized health care programs for children with cerebral palsy but not for adults with the condition.

Adults with cerebral palsy have reported worries and concerns about their long-term health and functional status as they age (Turk et al., 1997a). These concerns are well-founded. Published reports of studies with adults with cerebral palsy (involving cross-sectional or convenience samples) show that about one-third of study participants report declines in walking ability beginning in early adulthood (Murphy et al., 1995; Schwartz et al., 1999; Ando and Ueda, 2000; Andersson and Mattsson, 2001; Bottos et al., 2001; Turk et al., 2001; Strauss et al., 2004). Case series have also reported on cervical myelopathy (spinal cord pathology) in adults with cerebral palsy (Fuji et al., 1987; Kidron et al., 1987; Sakai et al., 2006), but these reports do not explain the decline in walking ability or its prevalence.

Pain is a typical secondary condition among adults with cerebral palsy (Murphy et al., 1995; Turk et al., 2001; Engel et al., 2002; Jensen et al., 2004), with reports of back and leg pain being the most common (Murphy et al., 1995; Turk et al., 1996, 1997b; Schwartz et al., 1999; Jahnsen et al., 2004). Pain is reported at relatively young adult ages among adults with cerebral palsy (Schwartz et al., 1999; Turk et al., 2001; Jahnsen et al., 2004) and may influence individuals' performance at these young ages and in the future. Studies have also documented pain complaints among children and adolescents with cerebral palsy (Houlihan et al., 2004; Engel et al., 2005; Tervo et al., 2006). Chronic pain is often increased with inactivity and fatigue and decreased with higher levels of activity (Schwartz et al., 1999; Engel et al., 2002; Jensen et al., 2004). Fatigue is another common secondary condition in people with cerebral palsy (Jahnsen et al., 2003), and it is often associated with reports of pain (Schwartz et al., 1999; Jahnsen et al., 2003).

Given the predominance of cross-sectional and case series reports in the literature reviewed here, longitudinal controlled studies are needed to confirm the prevalence of pain in people with cerebral palsy, map the types and the sites of pain, identify the etiology, and evaluate prevention and intervention strategies. In addition, the information and best clinical judgments accumulated to date need to become more widely and systematically included in graduate, postgraduate, and continuing medical education for physicians who care for children and adults with cerebral palsy.

Poliomyelitis

Survivors of childhood poliomyelitis are a vocal group who began to note unexpected changes in their functional and health status as they moved into their adult years (see, e.g., Halstead and Rossi [1985], Aston [1992], and Farbu et al. [2006]). People who had walked with only minor difficulty found themselves needing canes. Many experienced pain and fatigue with no apparent cause. Familiar exercises became difficult or impossible. Vigorous self-advocacy and organized lobbying combined with an intriguing medical puzzle attracted the attention of health care professionals and researchers. This was the first group to be evaluated for aging and secondary conditions through a focused clinical cross-sectional study (Halstead and Rossi, 1985; Maynard et al., 1991).

The term *postpolio syndrome* was coined to describe the phenomenon of new weakness after a prolonged stable period in individuals who had had poliomyelitis. It has been studied under the rubric of aging with a disability as well as secondary conditions. Secondary conditions associated with the syndrome include fatigue, temperature sensitivity, and joint pain (see, e.g., Halstead and Rossi [1987], Jubelt and Cashman [1987], Ramlow et al. [1992], and Perry [2004]). On the basis of concerns that exercise might be a risk factor rather than a protective factor, a number of studies have investigated the effectiveness and safety of exercise to improve strength, endurance, and function for polio survivors, generating recommendations for graded and monitored exercise (Dean and Ross, 1988; Jones et al., 1989; Einarsson, 1991; Grimby and Einarsson, 1991; Birk, 1993; Ernstoff et al., 1996; Spector et al., 1996). The link between exercise and the manifestations of postpolio syndrome remain an important area for research.

A 2001 study of 30 adult polio survivors noted fatigue, sleep problems, temperature sensitivity, and chronic pain as the most commonly reported secondary conditions (Harrison and Stuifbergen, 2001). Conditions noted to occur at frequencies greater than 50 percent were hypertension, depression, and scoliosis and related back conditions. Osteoporosis was reported at a frequency more than 35 percent. Some of these conditions, such as osteoporosis, are likely due to a mix of factors; that is, they have components of secondary health conditions, comorbid conditions, and associated conditions.

Klein and colleagues (2000) have reported that shoulder pain in polio survivors is related to lower-extremity weakness and body weight. These findings point to the problems created when people whose legs are weak and who are also heavy pull themselves up and around with their arms—problems that may arise for others with similar characteristics but different primary health conditions. The researchers are comparing the outcomes of programs of exercise for the upper extremities with those of programs of exercise for the lower extremities.

Down Syndrome

Down syndrome is the most common mental retardation syndrome and the most common autosomal chromosome abnormality in humans. The condition occurs in about 1 in 800 infants. Individuals with Down syndrome have facial and limb features that are not morphologically abnormal, but the specific constellation is distinctive. Common associated conditions include cardiac and gastrointestinal anomalies and abnormalities. Children with Down syndrome have a 15-fold increased risk for leukemia and hematological aberrations (Lange, 2000; see also Kivivuori et al. [1996] and Roizen and Patterson [2003]). Molecular studies have not yet provided an explanation for this predisposition to leukemias for children with Down syndrome. Older individuals with Down syndrome are often more obese, are of shorter stature, and have more medical problems than older individuals with other cognitive conditions (Carmeli et al., 2004).

According to an analysis of mortality data conducted by the Centers for Disease Control and Prevention, life expectancy for people with Down syndrome increased at a rate of almost 2 years per year from 1968 to 1997 (Friedman, 2001). The analysis also identified a very large gap in the median life expectancies of whites and blacks with the condition: 57 years for whites and only 25 years for blacks. The data did not help in identifying the source of this disparity, except to suggest that it did not appear that it was associated with differences in life-threatening malformations or congenital heart conditions and likely was associated with poor access to health care and other environmental factors.

As their life expectancy has increased, people with Down syndrome are experiencing an array of new physical and mental conditions in middle and late life. In clinical terms, these conditions probably include a mix of associated conditions (i.e., conditions that are aspects of the primary condition but that were not commonly seen until life expectancy increased) and secondary conditions related to aging or environmental factors (e.g., low levels of physical activity). People with Down syndrome experience higher rates or the earlier onset of hearing loss, cataracts, and endocrine disorders (e.g., diabetes mellitus). Thyroid function requires monitoring into adulthood, since the signs of hypothyroidism can be confused with dementia (Smith, 2001). Although cardiac abnormalities are usually diagnosed in infancy and childhood, adults with Down syndrome without known cardiac disease can develop valve dysfunction (Cohen and Patterson, 1999). Obstructive sleep apnea occurs in up to 50 percent of individuals with Down syndrome (Southall et al., 1987; Stebbens et al., 1991) and is related to obesity, decreased muscle tone, and structural abnormalities (Smith, 2001).

A recent review of the literature reported that individuals aging with Down syndrome are more likely than the rest of the population to develop Alzheimer's disease in middle age (Connolly, 2006). Furthermore, some research suggests that postmenopausal women with Down syndrome and low serum estrogen levels are four times more likely to develop Alzheimer's disease than women with Down syndrome and higher hormone levels (Schupf et al., 2006). Because of this increased risk for Alzheimer's disease, physicians may jump to the conclusion that the symptoms of people with Down syndrome are related to Alzheimer's disease and fail to evaluate other potential causes (e.g., depression, bladder incontinence because of narrowing of the spinal canal, and memory problems related to medications). Other medical or health conditions may also be overlooked. These include hypothyroidism, drug effects, delirium, and myelopathy.

Obesity is common in people with Down syndrome, and people with the condition are known to have reduced resting metabolic rates (Luke et al., 1994; Allison et al., 1995). Although research has not confirmed their effectiveness, suggested prevention strategies include the monitoring of growth, the adjustment of food selections, the promotion of exercise, and the use of behavioral techniques (Roizen and Patterson, 2003). Also well known are the low muscle tone and joint laxity associated with Down syndrome. If joint instability is detected clinically or radiographically, individuals with Down syndrome may be placed under activity restrictions, especially those related to sports activities. Several follow-up studies of children with asymptomatic instability have, however, shown no development of subluxation or spinal cord compression with and without sports activity restrictions (Pueschel et al., 1992; Cremers et al., 1993a,b). Research also suggests that cervical myelopathy has an earlier onset in adults with Down syndrome (Bosma et al., 1999) and that outcomes from surgical stabilization vary (Doyle et al., 1996; Bosma et al., 1999; Taggard et al., 2000).

To encourage the early identification and management of various conditions associated with Down syndrome, the American Academy of Pediatrics (AAP, 2001) and the Down Syndrome Medical Interest Group (Cohen and Patterson, 1999) have developed guidelines for pediatricians and family practitioners. Specific recommendations include routine immunizations; cardiac evaluation with echocardiogram before 6 months of age; audiologic evaluation, including a tympanogram, by 6 months of age; screening of newborn infants with Down syndrome for hypothyroidism and periodic testing for hypothyroidism throughout childhood and into adulthood; and ophthalmological evaluations beginning in infancy and routinely thereafter, given that ophthalmological disorders increase in frequency with age in individuals with Down syndrome (Roizen et al., 1994; Cohen and Patterson, 1999).

Cross-Condition Studies

The discussion earlier in this chapter noted a number of secondary conditions that appear to be related not to a specific disease but to functional impairments, such as muscle weakness and limited use of muscles. Some studies have directly investigated secondary conditions among people with different primary health conditions. The objectives of such research include the identification and understanding of the association of these primary conditions with common secondary conditions and the extent to which the latter might be responsive to common preventive or therapeutic interventions (see, e.g., Ravesloot et al. [2006], Rimmer and Shenoy [2006], and Seekins et al. [2006]). Most studies have involved people with physical mobility disabilities, with little representation of individuals with sensory-related conditions (e.g., vision impairment and hearing impairment) or cognitive disabilities. Some studies use a broad definition of secondary conditions that covers social participation (see, e.g., Ravesloot et al. [2006] and Seekins et al. [2006]). Most studies employ survey or questionnaire methods of data collection.

Several cross-condition studies (Seekins et al., 1994; Ravesloot et al., 1997; Wilber et al., 2002; Kinne et al., 2004; Nosek et al., 2006) have identified three common secondary conditions: fatigue, chronic pain, and depression. Other conditions listed in these studies—such as spasticity or spasms, weakness, and mobility impairments—may represent associated conditions. Sleep problems and eating or weight control issues are also named, but with various rates of prevalence or identification, depending on the study. Nevertheless, each study offers insights into the associations between these conditions and health status, activities, and participation. Individuals with a larger number of secondary conditions tend to have poorer health outcomes and poorer general health status (Wilber et al., 2002). Individuals with spinal cord injuries report more secondary conditions than other groups (Wilber et al., 2002), and women reported more interference in activities from secondary conditions (Nosek et al., 2006).

Using a different approach, Chan and colleagues (2005) investigated the secondary conditions occurring in a large sample of Medicare beneficiaries with motor performance disabilities. That study showed a high prevalence of secondary conditions, although, again, the conditions examined included both secondary conditions and impairments from the primary disability (e.g., dysphagia, spasms, and weakness). Musculoskeletal system-related conditions were more common than other conditions. Higher levels of mobility and limitations in activities of daily living were associated with a higher number of secondary conditions and an increased need for the medical management of those secondary conditions.

DIRECTIONS FOR RESEARCH AND EDUCATION

The research reviewed above focused on a few primary health conditions for which considerable data on secondary conditions and aging are available. The review reveals an increasing knowledge base as well as knowledge gaps. Gaps also exist in the education of health care professionals in caring for people with serious chronic conditions and disabilities.

Research Challenges, Knowledge Gaps, and Research Directions

The identification of secondary conditions or atypical aging with a disability depends on the understanding of the etiology and pathophysiology of particular primary conditions and the expected trajectory (or range of trajectories) of health and function typically associated with such conditions. Thus many studies are disability specific.

The ability to generalize about aging and secondary conditions for multiple disability groups is difficult without an in-depth understanding of the linkages among common physiological processes, functional characteristics, or the underlying pathophysiology to a set of primary health conditions. For example, people with a variety of chronic health conditions experience similar associated and secondary conditions in the musculoskeletal and neuromuscular realms. Spasticity, contractures, and pain are common among people with spinal cord injuries, multiple sclerosis, cerebral palsy, brain injuries, and stroke. In the realm of function, problems such as fatigue, falls, and a decline in one's ability to handle daily activities, such as dressing or bathing, are common among people with these and several other primary conditions. In contrast, with a number of more traditional medical problems, such as bladder dysfunction, it may be difficult to make generalizations across impairment groups. People with damage at the spinal cord level have difficulty with bladder function arising from a physiological mechanism different from that in people with bladder dysfunction caused by brain pathology (e.g., cerebral palsy, stroke, or a brain injury). Thus a common functional characteristic may have different pathophysiological sources. This complexity requires research that identifies such differences in ways that are relevant to clinical practice.

Some challenges relate to data collection and measurement. Large databases often rely on patient reports of medical conditions, which may result in the misclassification of conditions. For example, people may report that they have arthritis as an additional medical problem, when a problem with pain or stiffness may actually stem from soft tissue musculoskeletal conditions rather than joint abnormalities. Such reporting errors may result both from a patient's assumptions and from health professionals' misunderstanding of the patient's signs and symptoms.

A different challenge and need is the involvement of people with disabilities in establishing priorities for research; developing research questions and emphases; and, when they are qualified, participating as investigators, contributors, collaborators, and managers (Kailes, 2006). To the extent that clinical or other researchers focus primarily on medical aspects, they may overlook the basic issues of functioning and social participation that matter the most to people aging with a disability or grappling with secondary conditions. The involvement of family members and caregivers may likewise be valuable both in identifying outcomes relevant to those close to an individual with disabilities and in developing a fuller understanding of secondary conditions; aging issues; and potentially constructive clinical, environmental, and other interventions.

As discussed earlier in this chapter, pain is a common secondary condition for adults with many chronic conditions, and recent studies note that pain is also present in children with cerebral palsy (Tervo et al., 2006). Given that shoulder pain is a common complaint of those who propel wheelchairs over a long period of time and that pain and osteoarthritis are noted in the intact knees of those with lower limb amputation over time (Hungerford and Cockin, 1975; Norvell et al., 2005), a theoretical basis exists for a rehabilitation focus on prevention as well as performance-enhancing strategies. To date, however, there has been no direct study of the effect of rehabilitation and therapeutic strategies focused on the conservation of physiological capacity and function.

Also in need of further development more generally are evaluations of prevention and intervention programs. In general, health and function monitoring is inconsistent clinically. Unless an index of suspicion exists, clinicians may not routinely question individuals to identify changes in health and performance. Moreover, the interventions typically prescribed are those strategies used for the treatment of similar conditions in individuals without disabilities. That is, the principles of treatment for shoulder derangement syndromes for people without disabilities are used for the treatment of shoulder dysfunction in people who propel wheelchairs, with some modifications (e.g., advice to use a power wheelchair instead of a manually propelled wheelchair). These interventions have been seen to be effective on the basis of anecdotal evidence or case reports but have not been systematically evaluated. Other interventions are even less well supported. Use of medications that are commonly prescribed for menopausal osteoporosis to reduce bone resorption or increase bone formation have shown some promise for the treatment of secondary osteoporosis in children with osteogenesis imperfecta (a genetic disorder associated with weak, easily broken bones) and in women with spinal cord injuries, but the long-term benefits and effectiveness of these medications in preventing bone mineral loss are unclear.

Research directions therefore involve several fronts. These include

- further study and classification of secondary and aging conditions related to specific primary health conditions;
- classification of secondary conditions and conditions associated with aging with a disability that are common across primary health conditions, with the identification of the similar and the different physiological origins of the secondary problems;

•   clarification of the extent to which different kinds of levels of functioning and performance in earlier life are associated with the development of secondary and aging conditions;
•   evaluation of prevention and intervention strategies, including the use of assistive technologies, exercise, medications, and environmental modifications;
•   assessment of the effects of secondary conditions and aging with a disability on family members and caregivers; and
•   systematic reviews of the literature, with the consolidation, development, and dissemination of practice guidelines.

The second direction cited above has implications for the design and conduct of research. To the extent that certain secondary conditions are strongly linked to functional characteristics, such as limitations in mobility, this implies the need for more cross-condition research.

As noted earlier in this chapter, groups have developed evidence-based practice guidelines for specific conditions related to individuals with spinal cord injuries. In general, however, these guidelines apply to an adult population with spinal cord dysfunction and are specific to the identified condition (e.g., autonomic dysreflexia, urinary tract infections, and neurogenic bladder). They are not intended to broadly guide the monitoring and promotion of general health and functioning. For childhood-onset conditions and disabilities, it is particularly important that guidelines describe anticipatory care to identify and prevent common secondary health and aging conditions that may develop in the decades after the onset of the primary condition. Some examples of monitoring and anticipatory care guides for children with disabilities can be cited (see, e.g., Ohio Department of Health [1995a,b,c,d] and the Down syndrome guidelines noted earlier [Cohen and Patterson, 1999; AAP, 2001]). Overall, despite the increasing amount of information available, only a limited number of standards and quality markers now exist to help physicians, especially primary care physicians, monitor their patients with disabilities for common preventable or manageable aging and secondary conditions.

Education of Health Care Professionals

Although a critical review of the similarities and differences in secondary conditions and aging conditions among categories of disability was beyond the resources of this committee, it is clear that clinical care for some groups has undergone a paradigm shift as longer life spans have brought new questions and new research. In general, as people with early-onset disabilities grow older, the conservation of function and the prevention of secondary conditions become high priorities.

In the committee's experience, despite the availability of increased amounts of information about secondary conditions and aging with disability and changes in care for some conditions, primary care and other clinicians outside the field of rehabilitation continue to display a limited appreciation of both concepts. This limitation is subsidiary to broader deficiencies in clinical education about chronic care management, as discussed in Chapter 4. These deficiencies extend to education about both general and specialized health promotion and preventive care needs of people with disabilities. Today, the basic medical curriculum generally includes little meaningful content specific to disability, as it is defined in this report. Most medical school graduates have minimal experience providing care to people with long-term disabilities. Among the medical and other health care professions, few beyond physical medicine and rehabilitation, physical therapy, and occupational therapy have comprehensive clinical requirements relating directly to the provision of health care for people with disabilities.

Education theory identifies attitudes, knowledge, and skills as requirements for competent patient care; and undergraduate, graduate, and continuing education for health care professionals is important in each of these three areas. Research on the provision of care for people with disabilities has noted negative attitudes among health care providers, but has also documented that education about disability and experience with people with disabilities creates more positive attitudes (Estes et al., 1991; Gething, 1992; Lindgren and Oermann, 1993; Oermann and Lindgren, 1995; Rainville et al., 1995; Ralston et al., 1996; White and Olson; 1998; Packer et al., 2000; Chan et al., 2002; Tervo et al., 2002). Such attitudes are important for the establishment of unbiased approaches to history taking, the performance of physical examinations, and the consideration of nonmedical issues and supports, such as home and family environments. The committee recognizes the intense competition for space in an already crowded medical curriculum but believes that it is important for clinicians to have a basic grounding in disability concepts and issues common to the care of people with disabilities, including routine primary care, the prevention and management of secondary conditions and premature aging, the provision of timely referrals, and respectful attention.

The better dissemination of existing knowledge is also important. Currently, publications about secondary conditions and issues related to aging with a disability appear in a variety of journals or search formats but often without these terms appearing as key words. The consolidation of existing information and the design of more usable electronic and other formats could increase the dissemination of information to clinicians and the use of that information by clinicians. In addition, tools or systems that could be used to monitor changes in an individual's health and functioning over time would be of significant assistance to clinicians and people with disabilities.

Systematic reviews of the research in this area would provide a credible evidence base for practice guidelines, monitoring systems, best practices, and quality markers.

RECOMMENDATIONS

Since the publication of the 1991 IOM report on disability, clinicians, consumers, researchers, and the public health community have—to various degrees—become more aware of and knowledgeable about secondary health conditions and aging with disability. Nonetheless, clinicians need better preparation, awareness, and evidence-based guidance to manage the care for their patients with disabilities and advise their patients about these conditions and processes. The guidance developed for clinicians will often not be directly useful to consumers but can provide a foundation for the development of additional resources for individuals with disabilities and their families. The committee's recommendations focus on organizing the knowledge base and improving professional education.

Organizing the Knowledge Base

In addition to continuing research to expand the knowledge base about secondary conditions and aging with disability, it is important to organize that knowledge in ways that are useful to both professionals and consumers. As exemplified in the PVA-sponsored guidelines for the prevention of secondary conditions related to spinal cord injuries, this will likely involve different information products and different dissemination strategies for these two groups.

Organized knowledge in the form of evidence-based reviews is an important starting point. Such reviews will likely need to be framed in two different ways. One way will be with a focus on a particular primary health condition and what is known about related secondary conditions and aging. The other will be with a focus on secondary conditions and aging issues that are common to several primary conditions. In some cases, separate reviews may be needed for children or other groups if comprehensive documents would be unwieldy or unlikely to reach key audiences.

The committee believes that people with disabilities and clinicians, including rehabilitation specialists, would benefit from additional systematic assessments of the evidence as a basis for developing practice guidelines or critical pathways for the prevention and management of secondary conditions or the care of people aging with disabilities. One feature of such reviews should be the identification of practices for which evidence is lacking. Given its experience in managing evidence-based reviews to support the development of clinical practice guidelines, the Agency for Healthcare Research and Quality in the U.S. Department of Health and Human Services is well situated to oversee this activity and to involve other government agencies, professional societies, advocates, and researchers in identifying priorities for systematic reviews. The Agency for Healthcare Research and Quality also sponsors a clinical practice guidelines clearinghouse that is a useful vehicle for disseminating guidelines (see http://www.guideline.gov). The agency has identified people with disabilities as a priority population for its health services research agenda (Clancy and Andresen, 2002). New work focused on secondary conditions and aging with a disability would require additional resources.

> **Recommendation 5.1: The U.S. Congress should direct and fund the Agency for Healthcare Research and Quality so that it may take the lead in**
> • evaluating the evidence base to support the development of clinical practice guidelines, quality goals, and monitoring standards for the prevention and management of secondary health conditions among people with disabilities and for the monitoring and management of people aging with a disability;
> • evaluating the evidence base about environmental contributors to secondary health conditions; and
> • identifying research gaps and directions for further research on secondary health conditions and aging with a disability.

Improving the Education of Health Care Professionals

As noted in the 1991 IOM report, "[m]ost schools of medicine, nursing, and allied health have not properly prepared health care professionals to address problems and issues related to disability and chronic disease" (p. 231). In the committee's experience and judgment, too little progress has occurred since then. The committee recognizes that health care professions programs face challenges in better preparing professionals in these areas, especially generalists and others who do not specialize in rehabilitation or the provision of health care for individuals with specific chronic health conditions. Those designing curricula face the challenge, not only of including basic medical and health knowledge, but also covering leading-edge information regarding the multiplying medical advances in areas such as genomics, pharmacology, and materials science that may be applicable to people with disabilities. Even with a fairly long period of physician training, competition is fierce for space in didactic educational modules or coverage during clinical rotations. In this competition, education and experience involving care for people with disabilities have fared poorly. Recent graduates tend to be better versed in management of acute medical conditions, and seasoned clinicians often become focused on limited practice areas that direct their self-study. The available information on disabilities thus tends to be disseminated to a restricted audience.

Given the expected growth in the numbers of people aging with disability or aging into disability and the increasingly understood opportunities for clinical care and guidance to prevent or mitigate secondary conditions, health care professions education has a critical role to play. The building of a knowledge base about disability should begin early in a clinician's education and training and be reinforced through direct clinical experience with people with disabilities. Physicians who do not routinely care for patients with disabilities still need core knowledge and skills and appropriate support systems (see Chapter 4), for example, to guide the provision of timely and accessible preventive care services, the prevention of secondary conditions, and the referral of patients with disabilities to experts with more specific knowledge, when appropriate.

The committee recognizes that the increased knowledge required of health care professionals can be daunting and that they often welcome evidence-based reviews and well-crafted, evidence-based guidelines for practice that help them maintain and update their knowledge and skills. In addition, accreditation, certification, and licensing boards and agencies have required documentation of self-assessment and lifelong learning to promote excellence in health care, and guidelines and evidence-based reviews may also be useful for that purpose. Health plans have also developed or adopted guidelines or similar tools to monitor services and to promote cost-effective care, and they are increasingly seeking to couple provider payment to performance using such tools, which may or may not be based on systematic reviews of the relevant evidence and well-designed consensus development methods. Given the discussion of cross-condition interventions earlier in this chapter, screening and other prevention or treatment approaches and guidelines may increasingly be focused on functional limitations (e.g., lower extremity weakness) as well as on primary conditions.

Recommendation 5.1 calls for the evaluation of evidence to support the development of guidelines and pathways to improve the health care of people with disabilities. Recommendation 5.2 calls for the development of such guidelines and for the formulation of disability-related educational modules and competency standards for health care professionals. The principles for the development of evidence-based practice guidelines have been articulated elsewhere, including in three IOM reports (IOM, 1990a, 1992, 1995). Involvement by professional societies, researchers, and advocates in the process should be useful in developing guidance that will be helpful to different categories of clinicians, health care organizations, and health care professions educators. Different formats and contents may be appropriate for different purposes and audiences, for example, clinical generalists versus rehabilitation specialists. Once guidelines are developed for professionals, the development of additional documents for people with disabilities and their family members should be considered.

> **Recommendation 5.2: As part of broader efforts to improve the quality of care provided to people with disabilities, health care professionals, educators, people with disabilities, and their family members should work together to**
> • **develop, disseminate, and apply guidelines for the prevention and management of secondary conditions and for the monitoring and care of people aging with disability;**
> • **design educational modules and other curriculum tools for all relevant types of health care professionals and all levels of education; and**
> • **develop competency standards for these educational programs.**

Even with improved guidance and information, well-informed clinicians, and knowledgeable consumers, the maintenance of health and functioning can be difficult in the face of the environmental barriers that people with disabilities often encounter in daily life and in health care environments. These barriers include inaccessible transportation that can make health care appointments difficult, hazards in the home, information technologies that are unfriendly to people with sensory and other impairments, insurance plans that limit access to technologies that increase safety and functioning, and inaccessible health care equipment and facilities. The next several chapters (and Appendixes D through G) discuss aspects of these environmental barriers.

6

The Environmental Context of Disability: The Case of Health Care Facilities

My primary physician and several specialists I respect all practice at a major university medical center fairly close to my home. Recently, though, when I requested a gynecology referral there, I was told that I would not be seen unless I could bring my own assistants to help me get on the examining table. This is a huge world-renowned hospital. This is the era of ADA [Americans with Disabilities Act]. Still I am treated as though I don't belong with the other women who seek services in OB/GYN unless I can make my disability issues go away. This news makes me weary. I know it means once again that I can't simply pursue what I need as an ordinary citizen. I can't be just a woman who needs a pelvic exam; I must be a trailblazer. I must make the many bits of legal information and persuasive arguments it will take to get me into that clinic.

Female power-wheelchair user with postpolio syndrome
Carol J. Gill (1993 [used with permission])

This story illustrates how physical and social environments can affect a person's opportunities to participate in everyday life—in this case, by getting routine preventive health services—without making a disproportionate effort. The woman recounting this experience of discrimination had the knowledge, skills, and determination to get what she needed, despite equipment inadequacies and administrative obstacles. Others with less education, savvy, and resilience, however, may be discouraged and may abandon their efforts to obtain appropriate preventive, diagnostic, and treatment services.

The creation of accessible environments that promote independence and community participation has been and remains a focal point of advocacy by and for people with disabilities. The conceptual framework in the 1991 Institute of Medicine (IOM) report *Disability in America* particularly stressed the role of environmental barriers in contributing to disability. Indeed, the report defined disability as reflecting "a gap between a person's capacities and the demands of relevant, socially defined roles and tasks in a particular physical and social environment" (IOM, 1991, p. 81). Thus defined, disability is not an inherent attribute of the individual but, rather, is the result of the interaction of the individual with the environment, including social norms. Also, as described in Chapter 2, the *International Classification of Functioning, Health and Disability* (ICF) (WHO, 2001) stresses this interaction.

Over several decades, legislative and regulatory changes as well as technological innovations, advances in biomedicine, and shifts in attitudes about disability have helped to reduce or mitigate some kinds of environmental barriers. To cite a few examples of the environmental progress that has been made since the 1991 IOM report was published, technological advances and telecommunications regulations have made it easier for people with vision, hearing, and other impairments to communicate electronically with clients, coworkers, friends, family, and others, although keeping pace with product innovation and building in access from the outset are significant policy challenges (see Appendix F). Getting around the community and traveling beyond it are becoming easier for many people with disabilities because of the barrier removal and accessibility requirements of the Americans with Disabilities Act (ADA) and other policies—notwithstanding continuing problems with compliance, enforcement, and financing and the need for more research to evaluate the effectiveness of policies (GAO, 1993, 1994a; NCD, 2000c, 2001; Harrison, 2002; see also Appendix G).

In addition to the removal of barriers, interest is growing in strategies of universal and accessible design. The goal for these strategies is to create—from the outset—physical environments and products that are easily used and accessible to as wide a range of potential users as practicable. The aging of the baby boom generation is one force driving greater attention to transgenerational design, including the design of attractive, broadly accessible housing and public spaces (see, e.g., Pirkl [1994], Luscombe [2003], and the AARP web page at http://www.aarp.org/families/home_design/). In general, the more that universal design principles are applied to products, services, and environments, the less the need for assistive or adaptive technologies will be, although the latter will continue to be necessary for many tasks and environments.

Despite progress in barrier removal and advancements in universal design-based practices, significant environmental barriers remain, sometimes in places where one would not expect them, for example, hospitals and physicians' offices that lack buildings, equipment, and services suitable for people with physical mobility, sensory, and other impairments. The persistence of such environmental barriers will only become more serious as the number of people at the highest risk of disability grows substantially in coming decades. Still, growing numbers should mean a larger market for accessible products and an increasing demand for accessible environments.

Part of the charge to the IOM included examination of the role of assistive technologies and physical environments in increasing the participation in society of people with disabilities. The next section of this chapter briefly reviews the state of research on the link between environmental factors and disability. The chapter then examines accessibility in health care facilities as important in itself and also as illustrative of the dimensions of the physical environment and of public policies that can impede or support independence and participation. The concluding section of the chapter presents the committee's recommendations. The next chapter discusses assistive technologies and universal or accessible design, which extend to the design of buildings and other physical spaces. Other chapters of this report (as well as Appendixes D to G) also consider the physical and social environments in which people conduct their lives. The committee initially planned to examine accessibility in several areas, including housing, transportation, and work, but it determined that such an examination would exceed its resources and would require another report (or several reports).

Given the sparseness of well-designed studies on the relationship between environmental factors and disability outcomes, the discussion in this chapter is informed by the committee's experience and observations as well as available research. Furthermore, the discussion reflects value judgments, particularly the judgment that certain types of environmental barriers should be reduced or eliminated as a matter of fundamental equity, even if many people with chronic health conditions and impairments have demonstrated resiliency, persistence, and creativity in finding ways around such barriers and living full lives despite them.

RESEARCH ON THE ROLE OF THE ENVIRONMENT IN DISABILITY

As described in Chapter 2, the ICF systematically categorizes and codes features of the environment that may support or impede health and functioning (WHO, 2001). The major categories of the environment in the ICF are (1) products and technology (e.g., personal assistive technologies and communications products); (2) the natural environment and human-made changes to the environment (e.g., physical geography and air quality); (3) support and relationships (e.g., immediate family and health professionals); (4) attitudes (e.g., the individual attitudes of strangers and social norms); and (5) services, systems, and policies (e.g., transportation or economic policies).

The ICF states that the environment interacts with "all components of functioning and disability" (WHO, 2001, p. 8). That interaction tends, however, to be more evident for activity limitations and participation restrictions (e.g., traveling or working) than for impairments in body functions or structure (e.g., restricted motion of a joint or the absence of a limb). The small research literature on disability and environmental factors reflects this.

For the 2005 IOM workshop on disability in America, Keysor (2006) summarized the ICF and other taxonomies of the environment, described instruments for measuring the relationship between the environment and disability, and reviewed research on how the environment influences disability. She found a limited amount of research, especially prospective, controlled studies, that directly evaluated people's functioning and participation in the community. Of the studies that she identified, most involved mobility limitations and the built environment (e.g., buildings and pedestrian spaces).

In her review, Keysor pointed to evidence suggesting "that some environments that are more facilitative are associated with less disability, whereas other environments that are facilitative are associated with more disability" (Keysor, 2006, p. 98). This seeming paradox may reflect a complex and dynamic process of human adaptation to or modification of the environment. For example, people with greater levels of physical impairment and more difficulty getting around may modify their environments to reduce barriers and make life easier; they may also choose their home or work environment, or both, to minimize barriers. Studies that can untangle such causal relationships are important but difficult.

In general, research has tended to examine how or whether people perceive environmental features as barriers and has less often attempted to observe directly the effects of environmental features on such outcomes as functioning, social participation, and costs. Assessments of interventions to modify the environment are uncommon. A few controlled studies have evaluated home modifications (see e.g., Mann et al. [1999], Gitlin [1995], and Gitlin et al. [2006]). Each of these types of research is important, although some strategies are more difficult to design and implement than others. Assessing people's perceptions of the effects of environmental barriers on activities and participation is usually easier and less expensive than directly measuring the effects of environmental features on these outcomes and, especially, undertaking controlled studies of interventions to modify these features. The final section of this chapter includes recommendations about directions for further research on environmental factors.

ACCESSIBLE HEALTH CARE FACILITIES

[A] commonplace but counterintuitive aspect of our health care delivery system [is] the failure to provide safe and accessible care to those who have most frequent need of it—people with disabilities.

Reis et al. (2004, p. 2)

Discussions of disability and health care access often focus on financial access, in particular, access by people with disabilities to public or private health insurance plans that cover needed services and technologies.[1] The following discussion examines physical access to health care facilities and equipment and access to information in appropriate forms for people with vision, hearing, cognitive, or other impairments affecting communication. Many accessibility problems in health care facilities are representative of problems with poorly designed buildings, inaccessible equipment, and inattention to alternative modes of communication that can impede or support independence and participation in schools, stores, government offices, workplaces, and other physical settings. Deficient access to health care facilities and equipment can, however, be particularly shocking, as the following quotations from focus group participants reveal:

We can't treat you here; this is an ambulatory clinic, which means you have to be able to walk. You are wheelchair bound.

Told to a woman about to start chemotherapy

I literally chose my doctors because of those [adjustable examination] tables, so that it would be easier for them to examine me.

Female power-wheelchair user with cerebral palsy

I've not been on a wheelchair scale since rehab, over 22 years [ago]. . . . My HMO has one, but apparently it's in a storage room down by emergency somewhere, and nobody has ever seen it.

Male manual-wheelchair user with spinal cord injury
All cited in Kailes (2006)

As used here, *physical access* refers to features of individual facilities rather than to the geographic distribution of facilities, which is also an important issue for people with and without chronic health conditions or impairments. For convenience, the term *physical access* will sometimes encompass information or communications access.

Physical and communications access to health care facilities and other public spaces may be improved through a universal or "access-for-all" design strategy that, as described above, attempts to create environments or products usable by people with as wide a range of abilities as practical. Special equipment or accommodations may still be necessary for certain purposes and users, but even then, an accessible design strategy will consider how an environment or product can facilitate the use of such equipment or

---

[1]Chapters 8 and 9 of this report examine certain financial dimensions of health care access. Appendix D discusses the application of the Americans with Disabilities Act to health care, including the U.S. Supreme Court decision in *Olmstead v. L.C.*

modifications. As described in Chapter 4, a "disability-competent" health care system will include appropriate features for people with disabilities (see, e.g., DeJong et al. [2002] and Palsbo and Kailes [2006]).

Box 6-1 includes selected universal design features for health care facilities that were identified by the North Carolina Office on Disability and Health. Some of the cited features are not physical but, rather, refer to the knowledge, training, and sensitivity of the people who work in these facilities. Additional recommendations, not listed in the box, cover the space outside buildings, including entryways, sidewalks, and parking areas.

BOX 6-1
Selected Universal Design and Other
Features for Health Care Facilities

- Protection from the weather at entrance doors
- Power door mechanisms at interior and exterior entrances
- Spaces in waiting areas where wheelchair users can sit out of traffic lanes but with other people
- Chairs for use by people who cannot stand while transacting business
- Chairs that can be set at different heights for use by children, adults, and older people, some equipped with armrests for those who need assistance rising to their feet
- Weight scales that allow people with difficulty standing to hold on, and weight scales that allow people to be weighed while they are sitting in a wheelchair
- Motorized, adjustable-height treatment and physical examination tables and chairs
- Mammography machines that can be used for a woman in a seated position
- A portable, amplified communications system or device with volume control at service desks and treatment spaces for people who are hard of hearing
- More than one accessible toilet and dressing room, with some left-handed and some right-handed
- A TTY for use by people who are deaf to make phone calls from health care facilities*
- Staff awareness and training in using the telephone relay systems*
- Awareness and sensitivity training for all staff and professional personnel on interacting with people with disabilities

---

*Originally, TTY stood for "text teletypewriter," but today the abbreviation is more often explained as "text telephone," a device that allows those with hearing or speech impairments to type and read messages sent over telephone lines. These devices are also called TDDs (as in the Americans with Disabilities Act) for "telecommunications device for the deaf." A telephone relay system usually involves an operator who reads typed messages to and types voice messages from telephone users who do not have hearing impairments. For further discussion, see Appendix F of this report.

SOURCE: Center for Universal Design and North Carolina Office on Disability and Health (undated).

Data on Difficulties with Physical and Communications Access in Health Care Facilities

Many people have vivid memories of medical procedures and the instructions they received, such as, "Just hop up, look here, read this, listen up, don't breathe, and stay still!"

June Isaacson Kailes (2006)

Although the committee encountered many personal accounts of access barriers in health care facilities, it located very few consumer or patient survey data on these problems. In their recent examination of the financial, physical, and other barriers to accessible health care, Iezzoni and O'Day (2006) reported no findings on such barriers from data from the disability supplement to the National Health Interview Survey or other surveys. The authors relied primarily on interviews, focus groups, and their own observations and experiences to describe access problems and their consequences.

DeJong and colleagues (2002) have observed that health services researchers have tended to overlook people with disabilities, and to the extent that that is true, it may contribute to the limited research on environmental barriers. Moreover, occupational therapists and others knowledgeable about rehabilitation and the barriers that people encounter in health care facilities may not gravitate to health services research (see, e.g., Andresen et al. [2006]).

Two recent surveys suggest the scope of the accessibility problem in health care facilities. One survey, which involved approximately 400 Californians with mobility limitations, found that nearly one in five people surveyed had problems with the main entrance to their physician's office and one-third had problems entering examination rooms (Markwalder, 2005). Among those using wheelchairs, 45 percent reported difficulty using mammography and other imaging equipment, 69 percent reported difficulty using physical examination tables, and 60 percent reported problems with inaccessible weight scales. More than 90 percent of people with vision problems did not receive medical information in alternative formats.

A second survey of approximately 400 people nationwide, which was conducted by the Rehabilitation Engineering Research Center on Accessible Instrumentation, found that respondents identified physical examination tables, radiology equipment, exercise and rehabilitation equipment, and weight scales as the most difficult-to-use equipment in health care settings (Winters et al., 2007). Safety was a primary concern, as were comfort, ease or possibility of transferring, and poor visual displays.

These survey findings are consistent with those from a small study by Mele and colleagues (2005). In extended face-to-face interviews with 20 women with different kinds of disabilities, the interviewers reported that not one woman could recall having encountered an accessible examination table or weight scale. The women also said that they often found that toilet facilities and entryways were inaccessible.

A few studies have examined the views of facility administrators about access. For example, Sanchez and colleagues (2000) compared perceptions of accessibility by clinic managers with the investigators' direct evaluations of physical accessibility in 40 clinics in a midwestern city. The focus was access for people with spinal cord injuries. Although all the managers reported that their clinics were accessible, direct evaluation showed otherwise. Less than 18 percent of the clinics had an examination table that could be lowered to a standard manual wheelchair-seat height, yet nearly 40 percent of managers reported that their clinics did have such tables. Most clinics did, however, have buildings, examination rooms, and bathrooms that were wheelchair accessible.

Another small survey (62 general practitioners, family practitioners, internists, and obstetricians-gynecologists of 220 contacted) asked practitioners about their policies and practices, including physical, communications, and other aspects of accessibility and compliance with the requirements of the Americans with Disabilities Act (ADA) (Grabois et al., 1999). Almost one-fifth of the physicians said that they could not serve some patients with disabilities. Among other reasons, they cited a lack of accessible equipment, which is not an excuse under the ADA, unless accommodation would not be "readily achievable" as described below. With respect to accessible communications, the most common technology reported to be available was audio recordings, which were mentioned by only 15 percent of practitioners. Other researchers found generally similar results in a survey involving chiropractic clinics; moreover, the survey respondents reported that they had few patients with disabilities and saw no need for the clinics to become more accessible (Rose, 1999).

These small studies are consistent with the interviews, observations, and experiences reported by Iezzoni and O'Day (2006). In their chapter on health care settings, several headings highlight areas in which people encounter difficulties: getting in the door, getting around inside facilities, and getting on and off examination tables. Another chapter focuses on communications issues, some of which relate to access to information but others of which relate to the knowledge, sensitivity, and respectfulness of health care professionals and support staff and to their ability to see situations "through a patient's eyes."

Studies of the use and underuse of health care services by people with disabilities generally do not directly assess the effects of physical access problems. Underuse of services may be due to a number of environmental factors in addition to physical access, including a lack of adequate health insurance, transportation barriers, and problems with clinician attitudes and competence in caring for people with disabilities.

Some studies of the use of health care services by people with disabilities hint at possible physical access effects. For example, an analysis based on the Medicare Current Beneficiary Survey found that disability, especially severe disability, was a significant risk factor for not receiving mammograms and Pap smears but not influenza and pneumococcal vaccinations, which do not require major equipment or equipment modifications (Chan et al., 1999). An analysis of data from the California Health Interview Survey reported that people with a probable disability were statistically significantly less likely than others to have received screenings for breast, cervical, or prostate cancer; the differences for colon cancer screening were not statistically significant (Ramirez et al., 2005). People with a probable disability were, however, more likely than others to report a usual source of care and health insurance coverage, characteristics that usually predict increased use of preventive services. Another study that used data from the Behavioral Risk Factor Surveillance System in 2000 reported that "people with mild and moderate disability received influenza and pneumonia vaccinations somewhat more frequently than people without disabilities, but people with the most severe disabilities least frequently received vaccinations" (Diab and Johnston, 2004, p. 749). A recent review of studies of screening for breast and cervical cancer and osteoporosis concluded that women with more severe disabilities were less likely to be screened than women with mild or moderate disabilities (Smeltzer, 2006). An earlier study with data from the National Study of Women with Physical Disabilities found similar results for pelvic examinations but no differences for mammograms for women with or without disabilities (Nosek and Howland, 1997). Again, these various survey findings could reflect a number of factors other than or in addition to the physical accessibility of facilities and equipment.

Public Policies to Improve Health Care Facility and Equipment Accessibility

The federal government has taken a number of steps over several decades to make public spaces and buildings more accessible to people with disabilities, first in federal facilities and then in many private facilities that are used by the public. (State policies are not reviewed here.) These policies have had positive effects, although as described below, changes in both the content and the implementation of federal policies would allow more progress.

In 1968, the Architectural Barriers Act (ABA) established requirements for accessibility in buildings designed, built, altered, or leased with federal funds. As discussed in more detail below, the Rehabilitation Act of 1973 created the Architectural and Transportation Barriers Compliance Board (known as the Access Board) to develop and enforce minimum accessibility guidelines (sometimes referred to as ABA guidelines) for federal agencies.

Then, in 1990, in a major expansion in the scope of accessibility requirements, Title III of the ADA defined private health care providers as public accommodations (without regard to the receipt of federal funds). Title II of the ADA covers health care facilities and services provided by state and local governments. Health care providers include acute and long-term care hospitals, nursing homes, medical and dental offices and clinics, diagnostic and rehabilitation facilities, and similar providers. For health care providers, the U.S. Department of Justice has enforcement responsibilities related to Title III, and the U.S. Department of Health and Human Services (DHHS) has enforcement responsibilities related to Title II. The U.S. Department of Justice cannot, however, investigate complaints involving state or local government facilities without a referral from DHHS. (See Appendix D for an additional discussion of the ADA in a health care context.)

Some general requirements of the ADA (e.g., that services be provided in the most integrated setting appropriate to the needs of an individual with disabilities) apply to all covered entities. Additional requirements apply only to certain service providers, including medical care facilities. In some cases, exemptions from requirements (e.g., for elevators in buildings less than three stories tall) that apply to other facilities do not apply to health care facilities.

Some physical access requirements apply only to new construction and remodeling. Others apply to removal of barriers in existing structures when—in the words of the statute—compliance is "readily achievable," which means "easily accomplishable and able to be carried out without too much difficulty or expense," taking into account the characteristics of the organization (including its resources) and the nature and cost of the changes in question (U.S. Department of Justice, 1995).[2] As might be expected, interpretation of what is readily achievable can be a contentious issue.

As noted in Chapter 1, enforcement of the ADA is, to a considerable extent, reactive (NCD, 2000c). It depends substantially on federal agency responses to complaints by or on behalf of individuals who have encountered violations of the law. Complaints can be communicated to enforcement agencies such as the U.S. Department of Justice, or they can take the form of lawsuits. (Complaints to federal agencies may follow unsuccessful

---

[2]In addition to federal ADA accessibility guidelines, the American Institute of Architects publishes broad guidelines in *Guidelines for Design and Construction of Health Care Facilities* (AIA, 2006). Architects, engineers, and health care professionals use that document in the planning or renovation of health care facilities; and state and federal agencies and the Joint Commission for the Accreditation of Healthcare Organizations use the document as a guide or standard for the review of construction plans or completed facilities.

complaints to offending institutions.) Many individuals are, however, unaware of their rights under the law, or they lack the financial and other resources to pursue a complaint administratively or through the courts. Also, remedies for violations of ADA requirements may be limited. For example, individuals who successfully sue for violations of Title III public accommodations requirements are entitled only to injunctive relief and not monetary damages (although such a provision was included in draft legislation) (Colker, 2000). Injunctive relief specifies or directs some action by the offending party, such as providing wheelchair access to a restroom or agreeing to provide medical care to a person with human immunodeficiency virus (HIV) infection. If the government brings suit in cases involving a pattern of discriminatory practice in public accommodations, however, it can seek monetary damages or fines (Colker, 2000). In suits involving Titles I and II of the ADA, individuals can seek monetary relief under certain circumstances, although the U.S. Supreme Court has ruled that the Constitution bars monetary damages for state employees (EEOC, 2002; Jones, 2003; see also ILRU [undated]). Also, individuals may be able to seek monetary damages under state law. The argument for allowing monetary damages is that such penalties create stronger incentives for compliance with the law than allowing only injunctive relief.

As noted above, the Rehabilitation Act of 1973 created the Access Board, which develops and enforces the ABA minimum accessibility guidelines for federal agencies. It also develops design and accessibility guidelines to help implement the ADA. The Access Board is thus responsible for two broad sets of guidelines, the latest of which were issued in 2004, with some amendments made in 2005 (Access Board, 2005).

The original ABA guidelines form the basis for the Uniform Federal Accessibility Standards (issued in 1984). These standards, which apply to federal and federally funded facilities, were developed to minimize differences among earlier standards used by the General Services Administration, the U.S. Departments of Housing and Urban Development and Defense, and the United States Postal Service, each of which has the authority to issue standards for federal agencies under the ABA (Access Board, undated).

Another goal of the Access Board and the other agencies involved is to achieve consistency between federal standards and standards set by the American National Standards Institute (ANSI) as far as possible (Access Board, undated). ANSI is a private organization that oversees the development of voluntary standards that affect thousands of products, processes, and services, including medical equipment.[3] Also among ANSI products

---

[3]Before the passage of ABA in 1968, ANSI worked with the President's Committee on Employment of the Physically Handicapped and the National Society for Crippled Children to develop the first national accessibility standards (Beneficial Designs, Inc., 1999). The vol-

are human factors standards (developed in collaboration with the Association for the Advancement of Medical Instrumentation) for medical device engineering and design. These standards are intended to promote the easy and safe use of devices based on knowledge of how humans interact with devices and the environment in which the devices are used.

A recent review suggested that attention to human factors had increased the accessibility of medical devices for people with disabilities, although that was not the initial intent (Wiklund, 2007; see generally Winters and Story [2007a]). The review cited examples of what it called "user interface design affordances" (accessibility features) (p. 273), including open magnetic resonance imaging scanners that allow access by very large individuals and glucose meters designed with minimal buttons to reduce problems with their use for people with arthritis or other conditions that affect an individual's dexterity. The review also noted that the medical industry was generally regarded by human factors experts as a "laggard" in adopting both human factors practices and accessibility objectives and that a "disturbing proportion of new [medical] devices still have significant shortcomings" (pp. 273, 278). The development of accessibility standards for medical equipment (as recommended at the end of this chapter) would provide an important supplement to the health care facility standards issued by the Access Board.

After passage of the ADA, the Access Board published the first ADA Accessibility Guidelines in 1991. These guidelines cover two broad areas: facility construction and alteration and transportation facilities and transportation vehicles.[4] The U.S. Department of Justice has adopted the facility guidelines as standards that it enforces (28 CFR Part 36),[5] and the U.S. Department of Transportation likewise has adopted the transportation

---

untary ANSI standards were first issued in 1961 as a six-page document and were updated and substantially expanded in 1980.

[4]In 2004, the Access Board adopted revised ADA Accessibility Guidelines that included additions in several areas, including building elements designed for use by children (Access Board, 2005). Subsequently, the U.S. Department of Justice (2005a) published an advance notice of proposed rulemaking announcing its intention to publish a regulation that would adopt all Access Board amendments to the guidelines issued since 1998, but it had not yet done so by the end of 2006.

[5]A 1995 U.S. Department of Justice checklist of "readily achievable barrier removal" for existing facilities lists four priority areas with questions for users and suggested solutions for identified problems (Adaptive Environments, 1995). The priority areas are (1) accessible approaches and entrances (e.g., a route of access that does not include stairs, adequate accessible parking, curb cuts to sidewalks, and an accessible entrance that can be used without assistance); (2) accessible goods and services (e.g., all public spaces and levels are accessible, doors can be opened without too much force, all obstacles in circulation paths are detectable with a cane, elevator controls are properly located, and signs have raised characters and braille text); (3) accessible restrooms (e.g., at least one fully accessible restroom if public restrooms are provided, adequate maneuvering space for wheelchairs inside and outside stalls, and

guidelines as enforceable standards (49 CFR Part 37). In 2004, after the U.S. Supreme Court decision on the ADA's application to physical access to state and local courts, the Access Board created a 35-member Courthouse Access Advisory Committee (2006) that recently produced a report with recommendations that covered both courthouse design and the design of courtrooms, jury deliberation rooms, and other spaces.

The ADA does not explicitly mention medical equipment, nor do the accessibility guidelines or standards, although they do cover certain equipment (e.g., drinking fountains and toilets) that is found in many types of facilities. Instead, the general nondiscrimination provisions of the statute, which prohibit exclusion, segregation, and unequal treatment, offer an avenue for claims related to inaccessible medical equipment. Several high-profile settlements negotiated by the U.S. Department of Justice have included provisions related to equipment, usually examination tables and lift devices (see the discussion below of the case involving the Washington Hospital Center and other settlements). Nonetheless, neither the general provisions nor the individual settlements provide detailed, authoritative guidance for equipment or facility access.

The U.S. Department of Justice has been more visible in the area of communications access, undertaking (in the agency's words) "an ambitious, nationwide campaign to improve communications access in our nation's hospitals for people who are deaf, are hard of hearing, or have speech disabilities" and using a consent decree with 10 Connecticut hospitals as a "model for enforcement in other states" (U.S. Department of Justice, 2002b, unpaged). It has also issued a business brief on communicating in hospitals with people who are deaf or hard of hearing (U.S. Department of Justice, 2006a). The committee's recommendations call on the U.S. Department of Justice to issue explicit guidance for health care providers based on the broader settlements involving the Washington Hospital Center and other organizations.

The federal accessibility guidelines and standards have only a few provisions directly related to medical facilities. Dimensional and similar specifications for ramps, doorways, shower stalls, and other architectural features do not differ for hospitals and nursing homes.

The U.S. Department of Veterans Affairs (VA) examined provisions of the Uniform Federal Accessibility Standards relevant to the agency's medical facilities and concluded that they were not adequate for the population served in its medical facilities. It then created a set of supplementary guidelines for barrier-free design that differ in a number of areas from the federal accessibility standards (VA, 2006a). The VA document notes that

---

faucets operable with one closed fist); and (4) other (e.g., accessible drinking fountains and telephones, if they are provided for public use).

some government accessibility standards for the design, construction, and alteration of buildings (e.g., for acceptable ramp slopes) have been set by using individuals who were younger and stronger than the people served by VA facilities.[6] The standards do not specially consider user populations who may be ill, elderly, or new users of wheelchairs or other assistive technologies. For example, as described in the VA document, the standards for showers barely allow the entry of a person in a wheelchair and do not allow maneuvering of the wheelchair or room for other people to provide assistance to the user. For that reason, many of the VA's guidelines for its own facilities differ from those prepared by the Access Board. Another general study of standards for ramps (which was commissioned by the Access Board) suggested the need for further assessment of standards appropriate for facilities with high proportions of older users (Sanford, 1996).

The VA guidelines advise that "100% accessibility makes nursing simpler, puts less strain on staff, gives patients more independence, and requires less patient supervision by a limited staff" (VA, 2006a, p. 5). These observations appear to be applicable to many if not most other health care facilities.

Administrative and Judicial Responses to Continuing Problems with ADA Compliance

The committee located no formal, systematic nationwide survey or evaluation of compliance with or enforcement of ADA provisions related to medical facility accessibility.[7] Reis and colleagues (2004) reviewed U.S. Department of Justice quarterly status reports from 1994 to 2003 and found 114 cases related either to the accessibility of health care facilities (including equipment and communications) or to the denial of service. Almost half (65 cases) involved access to effective communications services by people with hearing limitations. Physical access to facilities or equipment (primarily in medical or dental office settings) was the next most common problem (38 cases).

The continued lack of common accessibility features in places where

---

[6]Also, VA hospitals serve a population that is a different and a considerably older population than the population in community acute care hospitals, in which, for example, 11 percent of the admissions are accounted for by childbirth (AHRQ, 2005). These and other characteristics of the population served are reflected in shorter lengths of stay in community hospitals, about 5 days in 2002 (AHRQ, 2005), in comparison with 12.5 days in VA hospitals (Pfizer Pharmaceutical Company, 2003).

[7]In a U.S. Department of Justice status report marking the tenth anniversary of the passage of the ADA, the discussion of health care accessibility mentioned services for people with HIV infection or hearing impairments but did not cite any cases related to the physical accessibility of facilities or equipment (U.S. Department of Justice, 2000a).

people might expect them—notably, hospitals—was spotlighted during the course of this study by the settlement in 2005 of an ADA case involving the Washington Hospital Center, the U.S. Department of Justice, and the plaintiffs (the Equal Rights Center and four individuals) (U.S. Department of Justice, 2005b,e). The scope of the accessibility problem at this major medical center is suggested by features of the complaint and the settlement, as summarized in Box 6-2. The settlement included provisions involving architectural features, equipment, and institutional policies and procedures.

On the same day that the Washington Hospital Center settlement was announced, the U.S. Department of Justice announced two other agreements with health care providers. One involved another Washington hospital that agreed to provide appropriate auxiliary aids and services for deaf patients (U.S. Department of Justice, 2005c). In the second case, which involved a group of California radiologists, the department announced that the radiology group had agreed (1) to purchase mechanical lift devices and transfer boards to assist wheelchair-to-examination table transfers; (2) to establish appointment scheduling procedures that include asking people if they need assistance or special equipment or practices and discussing ways to meet their needs; (3) to provide appropriate assistance during the appointment; and (4) to train staff to meet their responsibilities (U.S. Department of Justice, 2005d).

The details of a 2001 settlement involving Kaiser Permanente (*Meltzer v. Kaiser Permanente*) also reveal significant shortfalls in accessibility for people with disabilities in a large, well-respected health care system. In that settlement, the organization agreed to provide accessible medical equipment in its facilities (37 medical centers and 282 medical offices in California), survey its facilities and policies for barriers and remove such barriers or review policies, and provide appropriate staff training (Levine, 2005). Since then, the plaintiff organization has tracked implementation. It recently announced plans (using funds from a foundation grant) to conduct site visits at Kaiser Permanente facilities and offices to review progress and provide consumer feedback (DRA, 2006). The group is also collecting information from consumers on access problems at other California health care facilities.

Cases such as those summarized here underscore the fact that health care providers have legal—as well as ethical and professional—responsibilities to provide accessible facilities, equipment, and services. Nonetheless, achieving accessibility remains a long-term vision that will require clear guidance for providers, continuing education and enforcement, and examination of the appropriateness of existing standards.

BOX 6-2
Highlights of ADA Settlement Involving
Washington Hospital Center (U.S. Department
of Justice Complaint Number 202-16-120)

Allegations

Among the problems cited by plaintiffs were "not being placed in an accessible inpatient room; being examined on inaccessible equipment which required them to be lifted onto an examination table; having such lifting performed in an improper manner; having to wait significantly longer than other patients for an outpatient exam because the examination room with an accessible table was occupied; not receiving adequate inpatient services required as a result of a disability, such as assistance with eating, drinking, and having bowel movements; and [a lack of timely receipt of] accessible equipment needed as an inpatient, such as an accessible call button and telephone."

Selected Elements of Hospital Responsibilities Under the Settlement

• Adopt goal of making 10 percent of inpatient rooms (other than those in the intensive care unit) meet ADA accessibility standards (including having an accessible toilet room); 35 of 600 rooms to be made accessible within 5 years
• Purchase adjustable-height beds for the accessible inpatient rooms
• Hold the accessible rooms for patients with disabilities, unless hospital is operating at full capacity
• Provide each department with at least one accessible examination table
• Survey all equipment and purchase equipment needed for accessibility (e.g., examination tables and chairs, lifts, wheelchair-accessible weight scales, and radiology equipment)
• Survey public areas to identify barriers to access and then remove those barriers
• Review and, if necessary, revise hospital policies related to accessibility (e.g., communications methods for individuals with vision and hearing impairments or cognitive limitations, lifting techniques, service animals, and shuttle bus accessibility)
• Post information in reception and common areas on ADA rights and remedies for hospital patients and prepare a brochure on ADA for inpatients and outpatients
• Provide training on equal access for all employees who assist patients, including doctors, nurses, receptionists, orderlies, and admissions staff
• Establish an advisory group of people with disabilities and appoint consultants to assist with facility and policy reviews, policy development, and training
• Appoint an ADA equipment expert
• Appoint an ADA officer and establish a formal, timely complaint process

---

SOURCE: U.S. Department of Justice (2005e).

RECOMMENDATIONS

Expanding Research on Environmental Factors

The 1997 IOM report on disability recommended further research on the impact of environmental factors on disability. Some helpful studies have been conducted since then, but the amount of research is still quite limited as discussed earlier in this chapter. Chapter 2 discussed the further work that needs to be undertaken to develop the environmental component of the ICF framework so that the framework can better support research on environmental contributors to disability. It also recommended improving the country's disability surveillance system by adding measures that will help researchers identify environmental influences on activity and participation and monitor changes over time. Chapter 7 includes recommendations on assistive and accessible technologies as features of the environment, and Chapter 10 presents a recommendation for additional research on interventions to reduce environmental and other factors that contribute to activity limitations and participation restrictions.

Policies related to research and science and technology generally are not mentioned in the ICF classification scheme, but they, too, are part of the environmental domain of services, systems, and policies. The conceptual and policy emphasis on the interaction between person and environment that has been endorsed by the IOM, the World Health Organization, and others should be supported by research that evaluates this interaction. Although the federal government, particularly through the National Institute on Disability and Rehabilitation Research, has supported some research on environmental contributors to disability, the committee believes that such research should become a higher priority in all agencies engaged in disability research. General directions for such research include evaluations of population-level data, studies of people's perceptions of barriers, and observational and interventional assessments of the effects of environmental features and modifications on disability outcomes. In view of the enormous range of environmental factors across the physical, interpersonal, attitudinal, economic, and service and policy domains, an organized process to assess research priorities would be useful.

Recommendation 6.1: Given the limited research on the effects of environmental factors on disability, the National Institute on Disability and Rehabilitation Research, the National Institutes of Health, the Veterans Health Administration, the Centers for Disease Control and Prevention, and other relevant agencies should collaborate to develop a program of research in this area. As part of developing such a program, these agencies should

- organize a symposium to engage people with disabilities, relevant governmental agencies, researchers, methodologists, and other interested parties in a collaborative process to recommend priorities for research on environmental factors, as defined in the *International Classification of Functioning, Disability and Health*;
- apply these priorities in a plan for outcomes research to investigate the relative effects of different aspects of the environment on disability; and
- intensify current efforts to improve epidemiological, observational, and experimental measures and methods to assess the effects of specific environmental features on independence, participation, and quality of life over the short term and long term for people with disabilities.

A number of criteria may be taken into account in setting priorities for research on the effects of environmental factors on disability (see, e.g., IOM [2003b]). Although few data may be available to guide such assessments, which means judgments may be largely subjective, examples of possible criteria include

1. the importance of an environmental feature as a potential barrier for people with disabilities;

2. the number of people with chronic health conditions or disabilities potentially affected by a particular environmental barrier or set of features;

3. the ethics and feasibility of research, especially interventional research, involving a barrier or feature;

4. the potential of research findings to influence public or private actions to reduce a barrier and improve outcomes for people with disabilities; and

5. the likelihood that such actions might have specific additional positive outcomes or spillover effects (e.g., reducing disparities among people with disabilities; improving accessibility for other individuals; and reducing costs to families, firms, or governments).

Improving the Accessibility of Health Care Facilities

On the basis of available literature and the committee member's collective experience as health care professionals and health care consumers, the committee concludes that inaccessible equipment, deficits in communication, and burdensome and inaccessible health care physical plants remain commonplace and create significant barriers to the receipt of timely, high-quality health care by people with disabilities. The enforcement of federal accessibility standards in the health care sector is critical, as are education of providers, the implementation of guidelines, and the use of other steps that promote voluntary adherence to the ADA, the ABA, and other laws. The right to access applies to both public and private health care settings, regardless of whether providers participate in federal programs such as Medicare. The committee developed two recommendations that involve actions by both federal agencies and private organizations to make health care facilities more accessible to people with disabilities.

> **Recommendation 6.2: To improve the accessibility of health care facilities and equipment and to strengthen the awareness of and compliance with the provisions of the Americans with Disabilities Act related to accessible health care facilities,**
>   • **the U.S. Department of Justice should continue to vigorously pursue and publicize effective settlements and litigation (if necessary) of complaints of accessibility violations in major health care institutions;**
>   • **the U.S. Department of Justice should issue and widely disseminate guidelines for health care providers that describe expectations for compliance with the accessibility provisions of the act; and**
>   • **the Joint Commission and other organizations that accredit or set federal program participation conditions for health care organizations should explicitly consider compliance with federal accessibility standards and guidelines in making their accreditation and participation decisions.**

> **Recommendation 6.3: The U.S. Congress should direct the Architectural and Transportation Barriers Compliance Board (the Access Board)**
>   • **to develop standards for accessible medical equipment to be supported with technical assistance and with dissemination and enforcement efforts by the appropriate federal agencies and**
>   • **to collaborate with the U.S. Department of Veterans Affairs, groups representing people with disabilities, and other relevant experts to assess whether the accessibility standards developed by the Access Board are appropriate for health care facilities serving people with disabilities and an aging population.**

The first recommendation above calls for the U.S. Department of Justice to pursue a vigorous course of enforcement. Its strategy should include attention to high-profile cases that have a particular potential to underscore the responsibilities of health care institutions to make their facilities accessible to people with disabilities. In addition, it is important that the department do more to make its expectations known. Although it has investigated ADA-related access barriers in health care facilities and has reached individual settlements with noncompliant providers, it has not issued comprehensive compliance guidelines or specific technical assistance. Such guidelines or technical assistance would supplement case-by-case enforcement efforts and promote a better understanding by health care professionals and providers of their responsibilities under the law. The guidelines on the provision of services to patients with limited English proficiency are an example of this approach (U.S. Department of Justice, 2002a, see also U.S. Department of Justice [2001]). The committee understands that work on efforts to provide guidance or technical assistance is under way, but it is not clear when such guidance might be issued or when assistance might provided. Once the guidance is published, it should be widely disseminated as part of departmental activities to educate providers on their responsibilities.

Beyond the U.S. Department of Justice, many other public and private organizations have roles to play in promoting adherence to accessibility standards in health care facilities as critical elements of the quality and safety of patient care and the rights of patients. For example, the Joint Commission (formerly the Joint Commission on the Accreditation of Healthcare Organizations), which evaluates and accredits hospitals and other health care organizations, states that hospitals should comply with the ADA (JCAHO, undated). Unfortunately, the commission has established specific requirements (under standard RI 1.7) only in the area of communication for people who have hearing and speech impairments. The commission's description of its "environment-of-care" standards mentions the promotion of a safe, functional, and effective environment for patients, staff, and visitors; but access for people with disabilities is not explicitly cited. In contrast, the Commission on Accreditation of Rehabilitation Facilities (CARF) more directly recognizes barriers to access. Its standards require a written accessibility plan that must address environmental and other barriers identified by stakeholders (Reis et al., 2004). In 2004, the organization published the *CARF Guide to Accessibility* for use by the facilities that it accredits (CARF, 2004). The Joint Commission and other accrediting groups should move in this direction as well.

In general, accrediting organizations and organizations that set criteria for facility participation in Medicare and other federal programs should explicitly consider compliance with federal accessibility standards and guidelines in making accreditation decisions. This might require the development of educational materials, guidance, and standards for facility accessibility that clearly and specifically identify requirements for compliance. Potentially, the Disability and Business Technical Assistance Centers, funded by the National Institute on Disability and Rehabilitation Research to facilitate compliance with the ADA, could also help focus the attention of health care facilities on their responsibilities under the statute and associated regulations.

Recommendation 6.3 proposes that the Access Board be charged with developing accessibility standards for medical equipment to supplement existing facility standards. As is the case with facility standards, it will be important for other agencies to participate in the dissemination of information about equipment standards, the provision of technical assistance, and the formulation of enforcement policies. Further, the committee is concerned about the conclusion by the U.S. Department of Veterans Affairs that the Uniform Federal Accessibility Standards fall short of ensuring accessibility in the department's health care facilities. It encourages the Access Board to join with the U.S. Department of Veterans Affairs and others to examine this question and to determine whether certain ADA accessibility guidelines and standards should be revised as they apply to health care facilities.

The next chapter goes beyond the consideration of health care facilities and considers more generally the design of accessible technologies, the principles of universal design, and the importance of accessibility in "mainstream" technology that is not intended specifically for people with disabilities. It also examines assistive technologies that are specifically intended to support functioning, independence, and participation by people with various kinds of physical and cognitive impairments. One major challenge for both assistive technologies and broadly accessible general use technologies is securing resources for new product development and commercial distribution. Another is creating health care consumer and health care professional awareness of useful existing technologies.

7

Assistive and Mainstream Technologies for People with Disabilities

As she nears her 70th birthday, Ms. G has increasingly severe arthritis in her hands. She is feeling more and more restricted in her everyday life as daily tasks have become difficult or painful and many products—from the kitchen blender to the little pencils for filling out election ballots—have become hard or impossible for her to use. Recently, during an urgent visit to her physician's office after she sliced her hand with a kitchen knife, she had to see the practice's new partner. She explained that the knife had slipped because it was hard for her to grasp it firmly. The doctor asked whether she had heard of the knives and other ordinary household tools that are designed to be easier—and sometimes safer—for everyone to use. Did she have a computer so she could find out more from groups that had practical advice about technologies and other strategies for people with arthritis? Ms. G said she did. The doctor jotted down a note for her and added "You should check out these two web sites for information about equipment and other Internet resources for people with arthritis and other conditions. Unfortunately, though, you can't buy your own voting equipment."

As this story illustrates, people with conditions such as arthritis may encounter the myriad technologies of modern life in somewhat different ways than people without disabilities. Doorknobs, kitchen tools, or shirt buttons that do not produce a second thought for most people can become obstacles for someone with arthritis. In turn, a lever door handle substituted for a doorknob may be a significant aid to that individual—and also be welcomed by many others, such as parents juggling packages and children. A simple buttonhook device, although not useful to most people, can assist someone who finds it difficult to manipulate buttons. Thus, although certain technologies create obstacles to independence for people with disabilities, other technologies—some of which are designed to accommodate impairments and some of which are designed for general use—provide the means to eliminate or overcome environmental barriers. These helpful technologies may work by augmenting individual abilities (e.g., with glasses or hearing aids), by changing the general environment (e.g., with lever door handles or "talking" elevators), or by some combination of these two types of changes (e.g., with computer screen readers).

Given the projected large increase over the next 30 years in the numbers Americans at the highest risk for disability, as discussed in Chapter 1, designing technologies today for an accessible tomorrow should be a national priority. Otherwise, people who want to minimize the need for personal assistance from family members or others, who want to avoid institutional care, who want or need to work up to and beyond traditional retirement age, or who have talents to volunteer in society will face avoidable barriers that will diminish their independence and role in community life. Accessible technologies are also a matter of equity for people with disabilities, regardless of age. One of the goals of *Healthy People 2010* is a reduction in the proportion of people with disabilities who report that they do not have the assistive devices and technologies that they need (DHHS, 2001; see also DHHS [undated]).

Since the publication of the 1991 Institute of Medicine (IOM) report *Disability in America*, the world of assistive technologies has changed significantly in a number of areas. Perhaps the most dramatic advances involve the expanded communication options that have accompanied the improvement and widespread adoption of personal computers for use in homes, schools, and workplaces. Spurred in part by federal policy incentives and requirements, industry has developed a range of software and hardware options that make it easier for people with vision, hearing, speech, and other impairments to communicate and, more generally, take advantage of electronic and information technologies. In many cases, these options have moved into the realm of general use and availability. For example, people who do not have vision or hearing loss may find technologies like voice recognition software valuable for business or personal applications. Prosthetics technology is another area of remarkable innovation, with research on the neurological control of devices resulting in, for example, prosthetic arms that people can move by thinking about what they want to do (Murugappan, 2006).

Research suggests that assistive technologies are playing important and increasing roles in the lives of people with disabilities (see, e.g., Russell et al. [1997], Carlson and Ehrlich [2005], Spillman and Black [2005a], and Freedman et al. [2006]). For example, using data from the 1980, 1990, and 1994 National Health Interview Surveys, Russell and colleagues (1997) concluded that the rate of use of mobility assistive technology increased between 1980 and 1994 and that the rate of increase was greater than would have been expected on the basis of the growth in the size of the population and changes in the age composition of the population. A more recent analysis by Spillman (2004), which examined data from the National Long-Term Care Survey (for the years 1984, 1989, 1994, and 1999), found that the steadily increasing use of technology was associated with downward trends in the reported rates of disability among people age 65 and over. Other research, discussed later in this chapter, suggests that assistive technologies may substitute for or supplement personal care. Surveys also report considerable unmet needs for assistive technologies, often related to funding problems (Carlson and Ehrlich, 2005).

Findings such as those just cited suggest that the greater availability and use of assistive technologies could help the nation prepare for a future characterized by a growing older population and a shrinking proportion of younger people available to provide personal care. The increased availability of accessible general use technologies is also important.

Chapter 6 pointed out that people with disabilities encounter technology barriers in many environments, including health care. As surprising as it may seem, individuals with mobility limitations and other impairments may find that examination tables, hospital beds, weight scales, imaging devices, and other mainstream medical products are, to various degrees, inaccessible (see, e.g., Iezzoni and O'Day [2006] and Kailes [2006]). Chapter 6 urged the stronger implementation of federal antidiscrimination policies and the provision of better guidance to health care providers about what is expected of them in providing accessible environments.

Many kinds of technologies, such as medical equipment, voting machines, and buses, cannot be purchased or selected individually by consumers and are, in a certain sense, public goods even when they are privately owned. Their development and accessibility often depend on policies that require or encourage public and private organizations to make environments, services, and products more accessible. Other public policies tackle environmental barriers by encouraging consumer awareness of assistive and accessible products or by helping people purchase or otherwise obtain such products. Yet other policies promote research and development to make all sorts of technologies more usable and accessible to people with different abilities.

This chapter examines the role of assistive and mainstream technologies in increasing independence and extending the participation in society of people with disabilities. It also considers how technologies may act as barriers. Many of the topics discussed are themselves worthy of evaluation in separate reports, so the committee's review has necessarily been limited in scope and depth. The chapter begins with definitions of assistive technology, mainstream technology, and universal design. It then briefly reviews public policies affecting the availability of assistive and accessible technologies, summarizes information on the use of assistive technologies, discusses obstacles to the development of better products and the effective use of existing products, and highlights how mainstream technologies can limit or promote independence and community participation. The chapter concludes with recommendations.

TYPES OF TECHNOLOGIES USED OR ENCOUNTERED
BY PEOPLE WITH DISABILITIES

*Though coming from quite different histories, the purpose of universal
design and assistive technology is the same: to reduce the physical and attitudinal barriers between people with and without disabilities.*

Story et al. (1998, p. 11)

The intersection between technology and disability is a complex topic
for a number of reasons. As noted earlier, technology can be a barrier or
a means to independence and participation in the community. For some
people, technologies, such as mechanical ventilators, allow life itself—as
long as systems are in place to protect the users when natural disasters or
other events disrupt electrical power, caregiving arrangements, and other
essential services.

As the term is used in this chapter, *technology* generally refers to equipment, devices, and software rather than to medications (e.g., drugs to control the potentially disabling effects of epilepsy), procedures (e.g., physical
therapy techniques to restore function), administrative systems (e.g., rules
and implementing mechanisms for determining eligibility for disability income benefits), or a body of knowledge (e.g., rehabilitation medicine). In
other contexts, the term may be used much more comprehensively to refer
to some or all these additional areas.

Assistive technologies and general use or mainstream technologies, as
defined below, may serve similar or quite different purposes in people's
lives. Whether a technology is assistive or mainstream may affect how
people acquire the technology. For example, certain assistive technologies,
such as prostheses, require a physician's prescription and expert training in
safe and effective use. The distinction may also affect what health plans pay
for, as discussed in Chapter 9. In addition, for any given product category,
a mainstream or general use technology is likely to have larger prospective
markets and thus may be more likely than an assistive technology to attract
private-sector innovation and investment without government incentives
or rules.

Assistive Technology Defined

The Technology-Related Assistance for Individuals with Disabilities
Act of 1988 and the Assistive Technology Act of 1998, which replaced the
1988 legislation, define an *assistive technology device* as "[a]ny item, piece
of equipment, or product system, whether acquired commercially, modified,

or customized, that is used to increase, maintain, or improve the functional capabilities of individuals with disabilities" (29 U.S.C. 3002).[1] This policy definition is extremely broad and can be interpreted to cover a very large range of products—such as Velcro and microwave ovens—that are useful to people with disabilities but that are not specifically designed or adapted to assist them.

The broad legislative language intentionally permitted the information and funding programs created by the legislation to cover general use or mainstream products if, for a given individual, such a product worked as well as or better than a specially designed product. Nonetheless, as noted in a report developed for the American Academy of Physical Medicine and Rehabilitation and the Foundation for Physical Medicine and Rehabilitation, "a health plan or program could never include coverage [for assistive technology as defined in the Act] . . . because the benefit would be completely open-ended" (AAPM&R/The Foundation for PM&R, 2003, p. 9). For similar reasons, most discussions of assistive technology, at least implicitly, focus more specifically on items "*designed for* and used by individuals with the *intent* of eliminating, ameliorating, or compensating for" individual functional limitations (OTA, 1982, p. 51, emphasis added).[2]

Environmental modifications, for example, the widening of a bathroom doorway, are not explicitly covered by the Assistive Technology Act, although equipment (e.g., grab bars) installed during modifications is included. Building modifications are sometimes referred to as "fixed assistive technology," not all of which involves equipment installations (see, e.g., Tinker et al. [2004]).

Assistive technologies can be subdivided to distinguish many kinds of products. For example, *personal assistive devices*—such as canes, scooters, hearing aids, and magnifying glasses—act, essentially, as extensions of a person's physical capacities. They often move with the person from place to place. *Adaptive assistive devices* make an inaccessible mainstream or general use device usable by a person with a disability, although usually at additional cost. One example is the computer screen reader, which allows people with low vision to hear what is shown on a computer screen, for

---

[1]The committee recognizes that all technologies—scissors, wheelchairs, or computers—are assistive in some sense, that is, are tools to serve some human purpose.

[2]The statutory definition of *assistive technology* could be interpreted to include medications (as an "item"), as well as an array of implanted medical devices, such as cardiac pacemakers, orthopedic rods and plates, electronic neurostimulators, artificial joints, and catheters. Although some implanted devices and certain medications may improve functional capabilities, such as the ability to walk, bend, or reach, this report—consistent with most reports consulted by the committee—generally excludes both implanted devices and medications from the definition of assistive technology.

example, text documents. To operate effectively, computer screen readers require appropriate design of what appears on the screen (e.g., text labels for graphics or photos) (Tedeschi, 2006; see also Vascellaro [2006] and http://www.w3.org). Other examples of adaptive assistive technologies are the hand controls that operate braking and acceleration systems for automobiles.

Certain assistive technologies qualify as *durable medical equipment* under the Medicare statute and regulations. That is, they can withstand repeated use, are primarily and customarily used to serve medical purposes, are generally not useful to individuals in the absence of an illness or injury, and are appropriate for use in the home (42 CFR 414.202). The Medicare statute also mentions certain other categories of assistive products, such as prosthetics and orthotics. In general, insurance plans do not cover assistive technologies, as broadly defined by the Assistive Technology Act. (See Chapter 9 for a discussion of financing for assistive technologies under Medicare, Medicaid, private health plans, and other programs.) In some situations, health plans may pay for a more expensive assistive technology when a less expensive mainstream technology would serve as well.[3]

For children, assistive devices include adapted or specially designed toys that not only are entertaining and usable but that also make a contribution to their physical and emotional development (see, e.g., Robitaille [2001]). Continued implementation of the Individuals with Disabilities Education Act has focused attention on a range of educational assistive technologies for children with learning and other disabilities (see Chapters 4 and 9). Some of these technologies may also benefit adults with learning or cognitive limitations, increasing their ability to live independently, work, and otherwise participate more fully in community life.

Examples of cognitive assistive technologies include visual or auditory prompting devices that provide simple cues to help people perform a task (e.g., prepare food) or remember things that they need to do (e.g., take medications). Other examples include alarm devices that help warn caregivers that someone with dementia or some other cognitive condition may be in danger, tracking devices that use Global Positioning System technology to determine the location of an individual, and simplified versions of e-mail.

In addition, although they may be financially out of reach for many potential beneficiaries, a range of new assistive technologies are being developed to take advantage of advances in electronics and computing power

---

[3]Health plans with case management or similar programs or policies will sometimes waive usual policy limitations and pay for a mainstream product for an individual when it is clear that the product will perform at least as well as a specialized assistive product and will be less costly. See NHATP (2001) for an extensive discussion of how consumers can use cost-effectiveness arguments to persuade health plans to pay for technologies that are not normally covered; see also RESNA (2002).

that have stimulated innovation throughout the economy. Examples of these technologies include communications devices based on the tracking of individual eye movement (e.g., for people with severe speech and movement impairments because of a stroke), complex prosthetic devices that respond to neural impulses, and stair-climbing wheelchairs. As with all technologies, individual and environmental circumstances will influence the usefulness and the availability of specific technologies.

Mainstream Technology and Universal Design Defined

The term *mainstream technology* has no statutory definition or precise technical meaning. As the term is used here, it refers to any technology that is intended for general use rather than for use entirely or primarily by people with disabilities. The setting in which a technology is used may determine the classification of a technology. For example, a handrail in a place where one is normally found (e.g., beside steps in a school building) would be mainstream device, whereas a handrail installed along the hallway in the home of someone with mobility limitations would be an assistive device and an environmental modification.

Mainstream technologies include such disparate items as pens and pencils, personal computers, kitchen gadgets and appliances, cash machines, automobiles, cell phones, alarm clocks, trains, microwave ovens, and elevators. Some mainstream products, for example, Velcro, were not developed for people with disabilities but have come to have a variety of assistive uses. In some cases, the inclusion of accessibility features in general use products is required under Section 508 of the Rehabilitation Act or other legislation, as described below.

Universal design is the process of designing environments, services, and products to be usable, insofar as possible and practical, by people with a wide range of abilities without the need for special adaptation.[4] Other common terms for this process are "design for all," "inclusive design," and "accessible design."[5] Although "accessible design" might be considered a more inclusive term that encompasses mainstream products or environments with certain adaptations (e.g., wheelchair ramps), the term is often used interchangeably with universal design.

Among the most widely known examples of accessible mainstream products cited by proponents of universal or accessible design is a popular brand of kitchen tools and other gadgets that were designed from the start

---

[4]The term "universal design" was coined by the late Ron Mace, The Center for Universal Design, North Carolina State University College of Design.

[5]Some suggest reserving the term "accessible design" for design features or processes that meet legal requirements (Erlandson et al., 2007).

both to be attractive and generally useful and to be easily used by people with limited hand strength or dexterity (Mueller, 2000). In some cases, accessible design may mean the creation of a product or a building that is compatible with assistive technologies (e.g., wide doorways or ramps that accommodate wheelchairs) or that can be easily adjusted for different user characteristics. (See Box 6-1 in the preceding chapter for a list of selected universal design features for health care facilities.)

Another path to safer and more useful products is human factors engineering, which considers how people use products and how human capacities and expectations interact with the characteristics of products in different environments. As is also true of universal design, one focus of human factors engineering is the design of products and processes to reduce the opportunity for human error.

Human factors engineering often does not consider the capacities of people with visual, hearing, mobility, or other impairments. Nonetheless, its principles and methods can be applied to the design of mainstream and assistive technologies to take into account how people with different kinds of impairments interact with such technologies. Unfortunately, Wiklund (2007) concludes that although the application of human factors standards appears to have made some medical equipment more accessible, "a disturbing proportion of new devices still have significant shortcomings" (p. 273).

A recent edited work on accessible medical instrumentation proposed a number of design principles to improve accessibility and safety for a wide range of equipment users, including health care professionals as well as consumers and informal caregivers (Winters and Story, 2007a).[6] Desirable product features include easily located device controls with "on" and "stop" buttons that have common, distinctive designs and colors.

It must be kept in mind, however, that universal design is a *process* and not an outcome. In practice, a product or environment that can be used without adaptation by people with every possible kind of physical or mental impairment will rarely if ever be possible. Nevertheless, the process of universal design can significantly extend the range of users for many products and environments. It can also make the use of adaptive assistive

---

[6]In one definition, medical instrumentation is broadly defined to include "any furniture, measuring device, device that comes in contact with or is designed to be manipulated, monitored or read by health care professionals, lay person caregivers or end-user patients themselves as part of the provision or receipt of medical services, interventions or care, and any user-controlled software designed or required to be installed and used in connection with such technology, or any process or control system with which such patients or caregivers must interact in order for medical services, medical information, or treatment results to be achieved, measured or communicated" (Mendelsohn, 2007, p. 65).

technologies much simpler and less obtrusive. A web page designed so that it can easily be used with computer screen readers is an example.

Box 7-1 lists widely cited principles of universal design that may be applied to the planning of products, services, buildings, and environments such as parks and pedestrian spaces. (Story et al. [2003] have prepared a set of performance measures that can be used to assess how well products meet these principles.) Most of these principles are also useful reference points for those designing an assistive device, for example, to make its use simple and intuitive, to limit the physical effort required to use it, and to minimize the opportunity for error or unsafe use. Another principle that appears to guide much accessible design relates to style or attractiveness, that is, giving products pleasing designs that do not invite stigma.

In general, the broader the application of universal design principles to products, services, and environments is, the less the need for assistive or adaptive technologies will be. For public technologies, such as voting machines or buses, accessible design is the only method that works, because individuals cannot purchase or choose accessible versions of these kinds of devices on their own.

BOX 7-1
Principles of Universal Design

Equitable use. The design is useful and marketable to people with diverse abilities.

Flexibility in use. The design accommodates a wide range of individual preferences and abilities.

Simple and intuitive. Use of the design is easy to understand, regardless of the user's experience, knowledge, language skills, or current concentration level.

Perceptible information. The design communicates necessary information effectively to the user, regardless of ambient conditions or the user's sensory abilities.

Tolerance for error. The design minimizes hazards and the adverse consequences of accidental or unintended actions.

Low physical effort. The design can be used efficiently and comfortably and with a minimum of fatigue.

Size and space for approach and use. Appropriate size and space are provided for approach, reach, manipulation, and use, regardless of the user's body size, posture, or mobility.

SOURCE: Center for Universal Design (1997 [copyrighted but available for use without permission; guidelines on file]).

KEY POLICIES THAT PROMOTE ASSISTIVE TECHNOLOGY AND UNIVERSAL DESIGN OF MAINSTREAM TECHNOLOGIES

Both before and since the publication of the 1991 and 1997 IOM reports, the U.S. Congress has taken steps to promote assistive and accessible technologies for people with disabilities. Some policies—notably, the Assistive Technology Act—aim to make different kinds of technologies more available, more useful, and more affordable. Other policies, such as coverage provisions of health insurance programs such as Medicare and Medicaid, do not focus on assistive technology as such but significantly affect access to it (see Chapter 9).

Section 508 of the Rehabilitation Act

In 1986, responding to the proliferation of copiers, computers, and other electronic and information technologies, the U.S. Congress added the Electronic Equipment Accessibility amendment to the Rehabilitation Act of 1973 (U.S. Department of Justice, 2000b). The amendment directed the General Services Administration and the National Institute on Disability and Rehabilitation Research (NIDRR) to develop guidelines for federal agency procurement of accessible electronic equipment. As described in Appendix F, the Congress responded to lax enforcement of the 1986 provisions with the Workforce Investment Act of 1998.

The 1998 legislation requires the electronic and information technologies acquired by federal agencies to be accessible to federal workers and members of the public with disabilities and to do so on the basis of standards developed by the Architectural and Transportation Barriers Compliance Board (known as the Access Board; see the description of the board in Chapter 6). The standards, which were issued in December 2001, establish technical criteria for making electronic technology accessible to people with sensory and mobility limitations. They cover telephones and other telecommunications, computers, software applications, video and multimedia products and applications, World Wide Web-based intranet and Internet information and applications, information kiosks, and office equipment such as copiers and fax machines.[7]

As described by the U.S. Department of Justice, the standards "cannot—and do not pretend to—ensure that all [electronic and information technology] will be universally accessible to all people with disabilities" (U.S. Department of Justice, 2000b, unpaged). Reasonable accommoda-

---

[7]The law does not require accessibility for equipment that has embedded information technology, such as heating and ventilation system controls, as long as the principal function of the equipment is not information management, storage, manipulation, or similar activities.

tions will still be necessary in some situations, but more attentiveness to accessibility will limit the need for accommodations.

Under Section 508, the U.S. Department of Justice is supposed to oversee federal agencies in conducting evaluations of their activities to assess the extent to which their electronic and information technologies are accessible to people with disabilities. The agency published its last such evaluation in 2000 (U.S. Department of Justice, 2000b). That report noted that Section 508 is "technology centered" and focuses on whether mainstream products meet regulations, whereas other provisions of the Rehabilitation Act (Sections 501 and 504) are "person centered" and focus on accommodations related to individual needs.

The National Council on Disability has recommended extending the provisions of Section 508 so that organizations receiving federal funds would be "prohibited from utilizing federal dollars to develop or procure technology that is inaccessible" (NCD, 2000b, unpaged). The council criticizes, in particular, the One-Stop employment centers (funded under the Workforce Investment Act) for not reliably providing or employing accessible information and telecommunications services. In addition, the council suggests that federal and state officials involved in acquiring electronic and information technology need more training in the evaluation of products for accessibility. This committee agrees that these enhancements to Section 508 would contribute to the expansion of accessible electronic and information technologies.

Assistive Technology Act of 1998

The Assistive Technology Act of 1998, which replaced a 1988 law and which was reauthorized in 2004 to continue through 2010, is the legislation most directly supportive of assistive technology. It authorizes federal support to states to promote access to assistive technology for individuals with disabilities. For fiscal year (FY) 2006, the U.S. Congress appropriated $26 million for the program. At this level of federal spending, most state programs are funded at levels below the $410,000 minimum grant award specified in the law (ATAP, 2006). Overall, the level of funding is quite low.

The 2004 reauthorization shifted the focus of the policy from infrastructure development to direct support for technology access by people with disabilities through financing assistance (loans), device exchange or reuse, and device loan programs. Funds can also be used for training, public awareness, and other programs. Programs cannot pay directly for devices for individuals.

Other Policies

In addition to the Rehabilitation Act and the Assistive Technology Act, a number of other policies affect the availability of assistive and accessible technologies. As described in more detail in Appendix F, these include policies on the compatibility of telecommunications equipment with hearing aids and the captioning of television programs. For example, the Telecommunications Act of 1996 requires that new video programming, including cable as well as broadcast television, provide closed captions that make programs accessible to people with hearing loss.

Although it does not fund the development of assistive technologies and implementation has been disappointing in many areas (see Appendixes D and E), the ADA potentially creates demand for certain assistive and accessible technologies as public and private organizations remove environmental barriers, as required by the law. For example, workplace accommodations may involve the purchase or rental of a variety of aids that allow the use of computers and other electronic equipment.

As mentioned earlier in this chapter, education policies and health care financing programs—notably, the Individuals with Disabilities Education Act, Medicare, and Medicaid—also affect access to assistive technology. In addition, the New Freedom Initiative, which was announced in a 2001 Executive Order proposed a number of steps to remove barriers to equal participation in society by people with disabilities (Executive Order 13217).[8]

EXTENT OF ASSISTIVE TECHNOLOGY USE

Assistive technologies have been developed to meet a wide range of needs. A database (ABLEDATA) developed by NIDRR includes information on more than 21,000 currently available assistive devices, up from about 6,000 devices listed in the early 1980s (OTA, 1985; ABLEDATA, 2006).[9] The database also includes some useful items that were not designed as assistive devices.[10] In addition, the database provides links to organizations

---

[8]How much has been accomplished under this initiative is difficult to gauge. A New Freedom Initiative website created by the U.S. Department of Health and Human Services does not provide much information specific to the initiative, and most of the specific information dates back to 2003 or earlier (http://www.hhs.gov/newfreedom/links.html).

[9]Beyond supporting research, as discussed in Chapter 10, NIDRR is also charged with providing practical information to professionals, consumers, and others; disseminating the knowledge generated by research; and promoting technology transfer.

[10]For example, some items, including a convection oven, are convenient for people with disabilities but appear to have been neither intended for their specific use nor deliberately designed to be accessible to as wide a range of users as possible. Items designed by applying universal design principles include a vegetable peeler aimed at the mass market but intentionally designed to be easy to use by people with limited hand strength or dexterity. Examples

that offer services or assistance, companies, publications, conferences, and consumer reviews of products. (The database service does not itself sell products.) According to a report by the U.S. Commerce Department, world-wide sales of American assistive technology products and services exceeded $2.85 billion in 1999 (Baker et al., 2003).

In a review of data from six national population surveys, Cornman and colleagues (2005) estimated that 14 to 18 percent of people age 65 and over used assistive technology. The authors noted that such surveys may underes-timate assistive device use if they restrict questions about such use to people who have already reported that they have difficulty with daily activities and, thereby, exclude respondents who report device use but no difficulty. People may, for example, use a device but report no difficulty because the device is so successful and so familiar to them that they do not think of their underlying impairment when responding to survey questions.

Not surprisingly, when questions are limited to people with disabilities rather than the general population, surveys show much higher levels of as-sistive device use. A Kaiser Family Foundation survey found that 45 percent of nonelderly adults who reported having a physical disability said that they relied on equipment to help them with basic needs at home or work (Hanson et al., 2003).

A 2001 University of Michigan survey sponsored by NIDRR also focused on people with disabilities (Carlson and Ehrlich, 2005). On the basis of the survey responses, the researchers coded 75 different types of assistive devices. The four most commonly used technologies were canes or walking sticks, wheelchairs, hearing aids, and walkers. Other commonly used devices were scooters (often those provided at grocery and other stores rather than personally owned equipment), back braces, oxygen tanks, and crutches. Other surveys also find that mobility devices are the most com-mon type of assistive equipment reported to be used (see, e.g., Russell et al. [1997] and Cornman et al. [2005]).

The University of Michigan survey found that 64 percent of the respon-dents used some form of assistive technology (Carlson and Berland, 2002; Carlson and Ehrlich, 2005). More than 85 percent reported the need for equipment or personal assistance, or both. Respondents under age 40 were more likely than older respondents to report that they have unmet needs for assistive technology. People with unmet needs were also more likely to be nonwhite, to have low levels of education and personal and family income, and to not be working. The majority of respondents reported that they had received little or no information about assistive technologies or

---

of listed items that are intended primarily for use by people with specific impairments include a vegetable peeler with a clamp that allows use with only one hand and a carbon monoxide detector for use by people with hearing limitations.

about where to obtain them. They also thought that public awareness of the need for these technologies had increased in the preceding decade. The great majority (approximately 90 percent) agreed that changes in laws or program policies in the previous decade had helped people with disabilities get access to assistive technologies. As reported below, the survey asked respondents some questions about their use of other technologies and environmental access features.

Other surveys have also identified unmet needs for assistive technologies. For example, in a national survey of people with a spinal cord injury, multiple sclerosis, or cerebral palsy, Bingham and Beatty (2003) found that half of those surveyed reported that they needed assistive technology during the preceding year and that one-third of this group did not receive it every time that it was needed.

OUTCOMES OF ASSISTIVE TECHNOLOGY USE

Today, AT [assistive technology] provides alternate ways of providing transportation for those who cannot walk, communicating for those who cannot speak, reading for those who cannot see or read print, using the telephone for those who cannot hear and remembering for those who forget.

NTFTD (2004)

Assistive technologies may meet the needs of users in different ways. They may allow people to do something that they could not do before (e.g., use a computer or drive a car) or to do it more safely, more easily, or more independently. The ability to perform a discrete task, such as using an appliance, driving a car, or putting on socks, may translate directly or indirectly into better general functioning in daily life (e.g., getting dressed and preparing meals); more independence (e.g., traveling outside the home); or improved abilities to perform social roles, such as attending school, working, or taking care of one's children. These outcomes may, in turn, translate into a better quality of life. They may also reduce demands on family or paid caregivers.

In general, the usefulness of an assistive technology will depend on interactions involving several factors (see, e.g., Batavia and Hammer [1990], Thorkildsen [1994], and Scherer [2005]). These factors include

- characteristics of the individual user, such as a person's particular impairment, income, education level, and adherence to therapy regimens, as well as his or her preferences and goals;
- characteristics of the technology itself, including ease of use (with

respect to both physical and cognitive demands), ease of maintenance, need for training in use, reliability, safety, durability, portability, cost, and obtrusiveness; and

- environmental circumstances, including characteristics of an individual's home or workplace, family relationships, social attitudes, the knowledge and attentiveness of health care professionals, and supportive public policies.

In various ways that reflect their personal characteristics and environments, users (and those who advise them) balance the various pluses and minuses of specific devices or categories of devices. This balance helps determine what devices they will seek to use, what they will actually use (once a device is obtained), and when they will consider using a new device.

Despite the increasing use of assistive technologies and the creation of a number of federal programs to promote the development and availability of these technologies, the amount of information on the effectiveness of these technologies in improving function and, in particular, increasing independence and community participation appears to be relatively sparse across the range of available technologies and users (AAPM&R/The Foundation for PM&R, 2003; Carlson and Ehrlich, 2005).[11] As discussed in Chapter 10, government funding for disability-related research is, in general, very small in relation to the personal and societal impact of disability. More research to assess the effectiveness of existing and emerging technologies is important to guide consumer, clinician, and health plan decision making. The development of health outcomes measures as part of the National Institutes of Health's Patient-Reported Outcomes Measurement Information System (PROMIS) initiative (see Chapter 10) should improve the use of such measures in clinical studies, including studies that evaluate assistive technologies.

Some privately funded research is undertaken to support approval by the U.S. Food and Drug Administration (FDA) for certain complex devices. FDA makes the submission of clinical data demonstrating safety or efficacy in humans a condition of approval for only a small percentage of medical devices (FDA, 1999; IOM, 2005b).[12] Manufacturers must supply FDA with

---

[11]Consistent with the definitions used in much clinical and health services research, *effectiveness* refers to the extent to which an assistive (or mainstream) technology meets the needs of users in everyday life. (It may also refer to the extent to which the technology performs as intended.) *Efficacy*, in contrast, refers to outcomes in clinical trials or other controlled research settings.

[12]For example, in 2003, the FDA approved the iBOT, a battery-powered wheelchair that can rise to eye level, climb stairs and curbs, and traverse uneven surfaces by using a computer-controlled system of sensors, gyroscopes, and electric motors (FDA, 2003). The agency reviewed test data on the device's mechanical, electrical, and software systems and also

nonclinical safety and other technical data for a larger group of devices; and they must register a very much larger group of relatively simple devices, such as manual wheelchairs, canes, and braces. FDA also regulates the claims that manufacturers may make about devices. For example, in 1993, the agency warned hearing aid manufacturers to stop making misleading claims and to supply clinical data to justify certain claims (FDA, 1993).

Since publication of the 1991 IOM report, researchers have continued to work on outcome assessment tools that are suitable for testing the effects of technology use on different dimensions of functioning and disability.[13] NIDRR has funded research centers and projects to improve the measurement of outcomes from the use of assistive technologies and to promote the use of valid measures (NARIC, 2006a). It has also supported assessments of specific assistive technologies and funded several engineering research centers that focus on various types of technologies or technology needs (see Box 7-2 later in this chapter). Many of these activities involve other agencies, including the U.S. Department of Veterans Affairs and the National Center for Medical Rehabilitation Research. These agencies and a number of others also independently fund evaluations of technologies.

The committee identified a few controlled studies that compared assistive technologies or that compared the use of an assistive technology with no use. For example, several studies have compared hearing aids and other devices used to enhance hearing (see, e.g., Cohen et al. [2004], Mo et al. [2004], and Morera et al. [2005]). A number of studies have also focused on different features of wheelchairs or other aspects of wheelchair use (see, e.g., Cooper et al. [2002], Fitzgerald et al. [2003], Levy et al. [2004], Trefler

---

evaluated information from a prospective, nonrandomized study with 18 individuals (of 29 who were initially enrolled). These research participants were trained to use the device and were then observed for 2 weeks in the test device and 2 weeks in their regular wheelchair or scooter. As described in the agency's approval notice, 12 of the participants could climb up and down stairs alone with the device, whereas 6 required an assistant; but none could climb a single step with their regular device. (The only injuries that occurred involved minor bruising related to a fall out of the chair.) On a test of independence in functioning for a range of tasks (e.g., stair climbing), the participants showed more independent functioning when the task involved the device's special features but equal functioning when the device offered no advantage over the person's regular equipment. The device was, however, rated as difficult to maneuver compared with the maneuvering difficulty of the participant's regular device in the home. As a condition for approval, the device manufacturer agreed to provide data on device failures and adverse events for 2 years following its approval. In 2006, the Centers for Medicare and Medicaid Services concluded that several of the device's advanced features (e.g., its stair-climbing capacity) did not provide a clinically significant benefit (CMS, 2006d), as discussed later in this chapter.

[13] A recent review of instruments for measuring the outcomes of assistive technology use reported that most published reports about instruments or their use date to the mid-1990s or later (Smith et al., 2005).

et al. [2004], and Holliday et al. [2005]; see also Consortium for Spinal Cord Medicine [2005a]).[14]

Most controlled studies appear to involve technologies related to mobility or sensory impairments, although a number of studies have investigated the use of computer-based and other assistive technologies for children and adults with learning or cognitive disabilities. Controlled studies of equipment typically cannot use "blinding" strategies that limit researcher or participant awareness of which group is receiving a test product. For equipment essential to basic functioning (e.g., mobility equipment), the use of a no-treatment or placebo control group might be unethical.

Studies of outcomes may include functional assessments, but most research relies on self-reports of satisfaction or usefulness rather than direct assessments of functional outcomes. In the University of Michigan survey cited earlier, more than 90 percent of respondents reported being satisfied or very satisfied with their assistive technology (Carlson and Ehrlich, 2005). Approximately half reported that assistive technology reduced their need for personal assistance somewhat or a lot; less than 30 percent said that it had no effect. In addition, the majority of respondents reported that universally designed products, better-designed products, or environmental access features reduced their need for assistive technology and services a lot or some. Only about one-quarter reported no effect. Other mostly small, mostly European studies of several kinds of assistive technologies have also found that the majority of users report positive experiences (see, e.g., Sonn et al. [1996], Hammel et al. [2002], Roelands et al. [2002], Thyberg et al. [2004], and Veehof et al. [2006]).

Several population-based studies suggest that assistive technologies may substitute for or supplement personal care (Manton et al., 1993; Agree, 1999; Agree and Freedman, 2000; Allen, 2001; Hoenig et al., 2003; Agree et al., 2005). Some of this research suggests more specifically that the use of simple devices may substitute for informal care, whereas the use of complex devices may supplement the use of formal or paid care (Agree and Freedman, 2000; Allen, 2001; Agree et al., 2005). As might be expected, those whose difficulties are not resolved by the use of a technology are more likely than others to use personal assistance (Taylor and Hoenig, 2004). Using responses from the 1994–1995 National Health Interview Survey, Verbrugge and Sevak (2002) concluded that "controlling for factors that route people to different types of assistance, equipment is more efficacious

---

[14]For example, one pilot study in a nursing home setting examined functional outcomes and quality of life before and after the provision of individually prescribed seating and mobility systems for 60 users of wheelchairs (Trefler et al., 2004). The investigators concluded that after the new system was provided, the participants "had less difficulty independently propelling their systems and increased forward reach, quality of life for social function and physical role, and satisfaction with the new wheelchair technology" (p. 18).

than personal assistance" (p. S366). They also noted that their conclusions needed to be tested with longitudinal studies.

At least one controlled trial (Mann et al., 1999) found cost savings with the substitution of assistive technology for some personal care.[15] Using a variety of outcome measurement tools, the investigators also found that the group that used the technology experienced slower rates of functional decline and less pain than the control group.[16]

As is evident from this discussion, the availability of assistive and accessible mainstream technologies may have consequences that reach beyond individual users to affect formal and informal caregivers, including family members. Family member caregivers may, for example, find that a new assistive technology reduces physical and emotional stress. In some cases, it may reduce the caregiving requirements sufficiently that family members can work outside the home or be more productive in their paid work. Assistive technologies that allow children to perform better at school and adults to work or to work more productively will also likely benefit others, including teachers, employers, and coworkers. Overall, then, the effective use of assistive technologies may benefit society as a whole to the extent that such use reduces dependency and increases productivity (per worker and per member of society). The committee found little empirical research on these kinds of outcomes (however, see, e.g., Pettersson et al. [2005]). Evaluations of outcomes involving family members and others would permit a fuller understanding of the effects of an assistive or accessible technology.

ENHANCING ACCESSIBILITY THROUGH UNIVERSAL DESIGN OF MAINSTREAM TECHNOLOGIES: PROMISES AND PROBLEMS

When technology and disability are discussed, assistive technologies are usually the first things that come to mind. As emphasized earlier in this chapter, however, people with disabilities encounter and must use—or be disadvantaged by an inability to use—a very wide range of mainstream technologies in their daily lives. Standard alarm clocks, microwaves, ovens, washing machines, thermostats, computers, and a host of other products

---

[15]Another controlled study with older adults with chronic conditions evaluated a package of interventions (e.g., exercise, instruction in problem-solving strategies, home modifications, and related training), most of which did not involve equipment (Gitlin et al., 2006). The investigators reported that participants in the intervention group had fewer difficulties with activities of daily living and instrumental activities of daily living, a greater sense of self-efficacy, and greater use of adaptive strategies.

[16]Assessment instruments included the Functional Independence Measure (motor and cognitive sections), the Older Americans Research and Services Center Instrument, and the Craig Handicap Assessment and Reporting Technique (physical independence, mobility, occupation, and social integration sections).

may not be accessible (either directly or with adaptive technologies). In that case, then, people must do without, accept products with significant shortcomings, or buy special products, often at a higher cost. The nation's aging population should spur the growth of a market to support—and demand—the development and availability of more accessible mainstream products, although the larger part of this market will be people with milder impairments. Table 7-1 summarizes some key mainstream technologies and the barriers that they can present to people who have various kinds of physical or cognitive impairments.

With electronic technology being integrated into products and services in education, employment, health care, and many other aspects of daily life, the inability to use these electronic features can itself be disabling. For example, a person with vision loss who could work a traditional stove

TABLE 7-1 Examples of Barriers Created by Mainstream Technologies

Mainstream Use	Example of Barrier
Medical diagnosis	Magnetic resonance imaging devices that do not allow use by people with spinal deformities or morbid obesity Mammography machines do not accommodate women in wheelchairs or scooters
Medical therapy or monitoring	Home blood pressure monitoring devices that are difficult for people with low vision to read Alarm systems on glucose monitoring devices that have no visual indicator for people with hearing loss
General built environment	Buildings with doors, hallways, seating areas, and other features that are awkward or impossible for people with mobility limitations to use
Activities of daily living	Ovens, washing machines, and other appliances in rental apartments that have touch screens or other features that limit their use by people with vision or other impairments New products that require complex sequences of commands that exceed the capacities of people with cognitive impairments or that require intensive training
Information technology	Displays on fax and other machines that are positioned so that they are not visible to people in wheelchairs Commercial firms that operate only through the Internet and that have websites that are not compatible with computer screen readers used by people with vision impairments
Transportation	Buses that have access features that are not functioning because of a lack of timely maintenance and repair Fare machines that are difficult to use by people with cognitive limitations or that assume a person's familiarity with operating procedures

with knobs that click through the heat settings may not be able to use a replacement that relies entirely on touchpad controls with no audible or tactile cues.

In addition, electronic devices are increasingly replacing human agents for transacting business—whether the business is getting cash, checking out groceries, or purchasing tickets. Often, these devices and their specific features are designed without attention to people with vision, hearing, manual dexterity, or other impairments.

Progress, albeit slow, is being made in some areas to counter some of these barrier-creating developments. For example, in 2004, the Access Board published final guidelines advising that automated teller machine (ATM) instructions and other user information be accessible to people with vision impairments (Access Board, 2004). In the preamble to the guidelines, the Access Board noted that it was not extending the guidelines to other types of interactive transaction machines and that it would monitor application of the existing standards under Section 508 of the Rehabilitation Act for federal agencies purchasing such machines. (These guidelines have not yet been formally adopted as regulations by the U.S. Department of Justice, although a notice of proposed rule making was published in 2005 [Department of Justice, 2005a].)

Although ATMs were mentioned explicitly in the ADA, the Internet was a thing of the future in 1990, when the ADA legislation was passed. Now, the Internet is becoming the primary or least expensive place to obtain certain types of goods, particularly specialty items that may not be available in many smaller communities. If computer technologies in general and websites in particular are not accessible, people with disabilities may face serious limits in their ability to find and purchase these less common products, including certain assistive technologies.

The accessibility of computers generally and the Internet specifically is a particular concern of many policy makers, consumer advocates, researchers, and software and hardware producers (see, e.g., Novak [2001], Kirkpatrick et al. [2006], and W3C [2006]; see also Appendix F to this report). A report from the U.S. Department of Commerce, which used data from the September 2001 supplement to the Current Population Survey, reported that "with the exception of those individuals with severe hearing impairment, those who have [one of several categories of] disabilities are less likely than those without a disability to live in a home with a personal computer. And even in homes with a computer, people who have at least one of these disabilities are less likely to use the computer or the Internet" (NTIA/ESA, 2002, unpaged). Some access problems may relate to the economic disadvantages of people with disabilities and their lack of financial resources to buy a computer or Internet access. Inadequate design remains a factor, particularly for people with visual impairments who may find, for example, that web pages are not compatible with computer screen readers.

Sometimes designing mainstream devices so that they are compatible with an assistive technology—as is done by designing computer screen readers—is the only practical strategy for achieving access. Often, however, the most economical and effective approach is to have the mainstream device designed so that no additional adaptive equipment is needed, as happens when buildings are designed without steps or when elevators "announce" their arrival and their stop status.

Although the desirability of having mainstream products accessible to a wide range of individuals is clear, product research and development incentives in this area follow the same principles identified below for assistive technologies. Unless there is the prospect of a market and significant additional revenues, companies have little motivation—other than the need to comply with regulations—to include any particular accessibility features in a product. Regulatory approaches do not, however, work well if enforcement is lax or if the perceived real or opportunity costs of complying are higher than the costs (e.g., fines) of not complying.

Even accessibility features that are known or expected to increase revenues must compete with other features for engineering and marketing time. If another feature appears to have a significantly greater profit potential, then the accessibility feature is likely to get a lower priority (Tobias and Vanderheiden, 1998; Vanderheiden and Tobias, 2000). As a result, access features may sit fairly near the top of a list of proposed features for a product and yet never make it into new releases of the product.

As discussed earlier, the U.S. Congress has adopted policies to require accessibility for certain services or products, primarily in the area of telecommunications. One significant challenge to policy makers and regulators is keeping up with technological advances. An example is the development of wireless and Internet-based telephone services (see Appendix F).

CHALLENGES TO DEVELOPMENT AND EFFECTIVE PROVISION AND USE OF ASSISTIVE TECHNOLOGIES

As illustrated in the discussion to this point, assistive technologies constitute a quite broad and varied array of products that are directed toward a very diverse population of device users. Encouraging private firms and individuals to imagine, develop, and produce useful technologies presents many challenges and obstacles. Even when a good product is available, a number of barriers—such as a lack of consumer awareness of technologies and a lack of financial access—may lie in the path that leads to its successful, continued use by people with disabilities.

Viewed broadly, the process of creating, providing, and supporting technologies for use by people with disabilities has several stages. They stretch from the earliest glimmerings of a product or process idea through the end of a product's useful life or its replacement by an improved product. These stages, which also characterize many—if not most—mainstream consumer products, include

- product research and development;
- commercial application and production;
- consumer and professional awareness;
- guidance and product selection;
- financial access to equipment and related services;
- personal adaptation, training, and use; and
- product maintenance, repair, and replacement.

The characteristics of these stages vary considerably for different kinds of products and companies. Some products, such as advanced prosthetic limbs, may be characterized by complexity at every stage, requiring substantial investment in applied research and commercial development as well as major financial, technical, and other support for users. After their initial conceptualization and development, other products, such as the shower chair or the button hook, may see little continued innovation, minimal user training (even when advice about the product's safe use might be advisable), and a limited risk of obsolescence, even though competitive products may emerge (e.g., Velcro and other fastening options for clothing). Lack of consumer awareness may be the biggest challenge for such established products.

Nonetheless, even for relatively simple devices, human factors engineers and others may see ways to improve the safety and functionality of the devices, for example, by changing the dimensions or the shape so that a device is more easily gripped or manipulated. As the next section describes, that a device can be improved does not necessarily mean that a manufacturer will be motivated to invest in bringing the improved device to market, particularly if the likelihood of a reasonable return on its investment appears to be low.

Many of the challenges or problems reviewed below relate to weaknesses in the market for assistive technologies, including prescribed medical devices of various sorts. On the demand side of the market, sales may be limited by the small numbers of prospective purchasers for many products, the lower-than-average incomes of many people with disabilities (see Chapter 3), and health plan coverage of assistive technologies that is more restrictive than coverage of medical and surgical services (see Chapter 9). In addition, consumers, their families, and the health care professionals who advise them may not even be aware of relevant product options or may find them difficult to evaluate. On the supply side, innovators and entrepreneurs may, depending on the product, face high capitalization costs for manufacturing facilities and distribution networks, as well as significant research and development costs, particularly if the product requires the submission of data on safety and efficacy to the FDA. In comparison to the pharmaceutical industry, the medical device industry is characterized by a greater presence of small firms, a lesser reliance on patents as a source of competitive advantage, and a more continuous process of product refinement and innovation (Gelijns et al., 2005).

The following discussion first examines the stages of research, development, and commercial application for assistive technologies. It then considers the use of technologies by consumers.

Product Research and Development

It's mind boggling when you think of the things [assistive technologies] they're coming up with. What higher-level quads like me couldn't do before, we can do now. What a big incentive to keep going. There are so many advantages . . . I mean I'm glad I broke my neck in this century.

Brian, as quoted by Scherer (2005)

This enthusiastic, if somewhat startling, view of what technology can do to increase functioning and independence for people with disabilities was offered not in 2005 but in 1986. By that time, innovations in materials and in electronic and computer technologies had brought significant improvements in technologies for people with spinal cord injuries and other mobility-limiting conditions. The next two decades have seen many further technological advances and benefits, including lighter and more effectively controlled wheelchairs and prosthetic limbs and better knowledge of how to fit and maintain such devices to minimize the development of pressure ulcers and other secondary health conditions.

A number of analyses have, however, identified an array of obstacles to technological development and innovation in assistive technologies (see, e.g., IOM [1997], NCD [2000b, 2004a, 2006] and Baker et al. [2003]). Most relate to the relatively small market for many products, but product affordability is also an issue. Obstacles may also include a continuing legacy of discrimination and inattention to people with disabilities in medical research and engineering (Seelman, 2007).

Role of the Private Sector in Research and Development

In the private sector, the development and production of assistive technologies involve a diverse population of organizations (Baker et al., 2003). These organizations range from relatively large companies that produce wheelchairs or hearing devices to niche firms that produce products for small and dispersed populations (e.g., adults and children who are both blind and deaf).[17] In addition, the assistive technology industry includes individual professionals who custom produce items such as adapted vans, braces, and orthotics. In general, small firms play a much bigger role in the medical device and assistive technology sector than they do in the pharmaceutical sector.

For products for which the potential for profit is good, private companies will typically take the lead in product research and development and continuing improvement. For many assistive products, however, the potential for sales and profits will appear low. For example, among people who could potentially benefit from electronic augmented communications devices, the range of abilities and communications needs is quite varied. Thus actual core technologies may likewise be quite varied. For example, several device control options are available (keyboard, infrared head pointer, hand gestures) (see, e.g., Bauer [2003]). As a result, the market for the general product category is quite fragmented, which tends to increase costs and limit profit potential.

Restrictive insurance coverage exacerbates the disincentive for product development for these and other product categories (see Chapter 9). For example, in a controversial and disappointing decision, the Centers for Medicare and Medicaid Services has determined that the iBOT (described earlier in footnote 12) meets the definition of durable medical equipment and qualifies as reasonable and necessary for people with certain mobility limitations; but it further determined that several integrated functions of the device, such as those that allow it to climb stairs, do not offer clinically significant benefits (CMS, 2006d). The agency also declined to create a new coverage category for the device, which critics argue effectively denies coverage since Medicare covers only the least costly device in a category, which in this case is the category for a standard power wheelchair (see the critique from the ITEM Coalition [2006]). (The iBOT sells for more than $25,000, and the company sold approximately 1,000 of the devices in its first 3 years on the market [Young, 2006].)

A 2003 report by the U.S. Department of Commerce cited a number of difficulties facing the assistive technology industry. They include "the prevalence of small firms [who lack resources for sophisticated product de-

---

[17]People with low-incidence disabilities and children with certain disabilities are two examples of populations that may require public-sector support for product development. Even when the number of children with a condition is sizeable, children's growth and development mean that many different sizes of a product may be required. Unlike a medication, which often can be provided in different doses to people of different ages, many medical devices and assistive technologies cannot be manufactured in one form and then easily "sized" at the time of delivery or use (IOM, 2005b).

velopment] . . . ; problems in hiring and retaining a trained workforce; . . . and the disconnect between . . . industry and the resources of the federal laboratory system" (Baker et al., 2003, unpaged). The report cited survey data indicating that research and development was a significant activity for less than half of the firms surveyed, and only 15 percent of the firms surveyed cited activity in basic research.

The 1997 IOM report *Enabling America* suggested that the situation for assistive technologies is similar to that for so-called orphan drugs for people with rare medical conditions.[18] Unfortunately, it has proved difficult for the U.S. Congress to identify incentives for the development of medical equipment for small user populations similar to those identified for the development of orphan drugs (IOM, 2005b). In language accompanying the 2002 appropriation for the U.S. Department of Education and other agencies, the Senate Committee on Appropriations stated that "priority for grants [under the Assistive Technology Development Fund] should be given to the development of technology that has a limited number of users, or orphan technology" (U.S. Senate, Committee on Appropriations, 2001).

Role of Government in Research and Development

If private industry finds investment in product development activity in a particular area unattractive, the primary alternative is government-supported research and development or, occasionally, research supported by private foundations. As described in Chapter 10, government investment in disability and rehabilitation research of all kinds—including most kinds of product innovation and development—is limited relative to the population that could benefit. One exception is investment in prosthetic research, which has received substantial support from the U.S. Department of Veterans Affairs and the U.S. Department of Defense and which has become a particular focus with the return of military personnel who have lost limbs in Iraq or Afghanistan (Perlin, 2006; see also Chapter 10).

NIDRR funds a number of Rehabilitation Engineering Research Centers that conduct research and development related to specific populations,

---

[18]For drugs, Congress has defined a rare disease or condition to mean one that either affects less than 200,000 people in the United States or affects more people but for which there is "no reasonable expectation that the cost of developing and making available in the United States a drug for such disease or condition will be recovered from sales in the United States" (PL 97-414, Section 526 [360bb](a)(1)). For medical devices that require FDA approval, Congress created special exemptions from certain regulations for humanitarian use devices, which are "intended to benefit patients in the treatment or diagnosis of a disease or condition that affects or is manifested in fewer than 4,000 individuals in the United States per year" (21 CFR 814.3(n)). For a description of these provisions, see the report of FDA (2006.) These provisions affect very few devices.

technologies, or strategic issues (Box 7-2).[19] The centers may work on accessible mainstream technologies (e.g., household products and computers) as well as assistive technologies. Some centers focus on conditions (e.g., spinal cord injuries), some focus on technologies (e.g., wheelchairs), and some focus on environments (e.g., workplaces). Intensive consideration of assistive technologies in different environments may bring new and useful perspectives on environmental barriers to work and social life and on engineering strategies for removing or mitigating these barriers.

Total funding for the centers program was relatively steady at about $11 million in the late 1990s, but in FY 2000, the funding increased to more than $15 million and increased again in FY 2001 to more than $20 million as additional centers were funded (Arthur Sherwood, Science and Technology Advisor, NIDRR, personal communication, November 16, 2006). It has declined slightly since then. The funding for each center is modest, however, averaging less than $1 million per center per year.

Government support for research is not restricted to government and academic researchers. The U.S. Congress has specified that a portion of certain government agency budgets for assistive technology, science, or engineering research be allocated to support technological innovation in the small business community and to encourage commercial applications of technologies developed through government-supported research (SBA, 2001).

Involvement of Consumers at the Research and Development Stage

Although discussions of research and development focus on the roles of public- and private-sector organizations and funding, the development of a successful product—one that works and that is commercially feasible—often depends on consumer involvement, for example, through focus groups and evaluation of prototypes (see, e.g., Lane [1998] and Scherer [2005]). The 1997 IOM report *Enabling America* called for consumers with potentially disabling conditions to be involved in research and technology development and dissemination.

For certain products, the ability of companies to assess market demand and profit potential may be restricted by the limited market data on people with disabilities, including their numbers, their perceived needs and preferences for assistive and accessible products or services, and other characteristics. A recent national task force report recommended—and this committee endorses—government support for surveys and market research to help reduce the knowledge gap (NTFTD, 2004).

In some cases, companies could also benefit from information on the

---

[19]The Rehabilitation Act of 1973, which established NIDRR, provided for agency support for these centers, and the program began with five centers.

BOX 7-2
Focus of NIDRR-Supported Rehabilitation
Engineering Research Centers

Condition, impairment, or group characteristic
  Spinal cord injuries
  Low vision, blindness, and multisensory loss
  Children with orthopedic disabilities
  Technology access for land mine survivors
  Technology for successful aging

Technology
  Accessible medical instrumentation
  Wheeled mobility
  Prosthetics and orthotics
  Communication enhancement
  Telecommunications access
  Wireless technologies
  Universal interface and information technology access
  Universal design and the built environment
  Telerehabilitation
  Robotics and telemanipulation (machines that assist with recovery from
    stroke)
  Recreational technologies and exercise physiology

Other
  Workplace accommodations
  Accessible public transportation
  Wheelchair transportation safety
  Technology transfer

SOURCE: NARIC (2006b).

---

broader market, for example, how people without mobility or sensory limitations view various accessibility features for mainstream products. Even with a rapidly growing older population, companies may be concerned that people may avoid products that suggest disability, and firms may be unaware of universal design principles that include the attractiveness of a product to a broad range of users (Vanderheiden and Tobias, 2000).

A rather different way of involving consumers has to do with the development of technical standards that are appropriate for different populations. As noted in Chapter 6, the U.S. Department of Veterans Affairs—citing the average age of its population—has developed standards for its facilities that differ somewhat from the standards developed by the Access Board. Many of the data on human performance standards and guidelines were derived from studies that relied heavily on young male participants

(Gardner-Bonneau, 2007). If the average user of, for example, home medi-cal equipment is an older woman with mobility or sensory limitations, or both, then the development of equipment using standards derived from data based on a population that is quite different is not appropriate. Data on older populations and children are available but are not necessarily widely known. Designers and standard setters are, however, beginning to take note, as evidenced by the publication by the Access Board of ADA building accessibility guidelines relevant for children (Access Board, 1998; see also ISO [2001], Fisk et al. [2004], and Kroemer [2006]). (The U.S. Department of Justice has not yet adopted these guidelines as standards.)

Challenge of Technology Transfer and Commercial Application

A good product idea, design, or prototype is of little value to consum-ers if it does not lead to commercial production and distribution. Even when the federal government supports research and development in the area of assistive and accessible products, this support may not extend far enough into the next stage, that is, technology transfer for the purposes of commercial application (Wessner, 2006). One definition of technology transfer is the "process of converting scientific findings from [government or academic] research laboratories into useful products by the commercial sector" (NLM, 2006, unpaged). One of the recommendations (Recommen-dation 8.1) in the 1997 IOM report *Enabling America* implicitly defined technology transfer more broadly to include what this report characterizes as steps to increase consumer and professional awareness of the available technologies.

The gap between long-term, government-supported basic research and short-term product development by industry has been characterized as the "valley of death" (see, e.g., Fong [2001]). For example, in 1998, a congres-sional committee used that term to label a "widening gap between federally funded basic research and industry-funded applied research and devel-opment" (U.S. House of Representatives, Committee on Science, 1998, unpaged).

The U.S. Congress and federal agencies have taken some steps to pro-mote and monitor technology transfer from government research agencies to the private sector through research and development partnerships; the implementation of patenting, information disclosure, and licensing proce-dures; the provision of technical assistance; standards development; and other means (see, e.g., U.S. Department of Commerce [2006]). Unfortu-nately, the effectiveness of these steps in the area of assistive technology has been limited by the industry and market characteristics described above (Bauer, 2003). To encourage technology transfer, each of the previously mentioned Rehabilitation Engineering Research Centers is expected to produce some transfer of technology to the private sector. NIDRR has also funded a center (at the State University of New York at Buffalo) specifically to promote transfer for assistive technologies.

Even with government support for product development and applied research, product developers, governmental agencies, and advocates may have to invest considerable effort to identify and attract a private company that is prepared to manufacture and market a product. In the U.S. Department of Commerce survey cited earlier, almost two-thirds of the companies surveyed indicated that they were "passive in their pursuit of new ideas—or not interested at all" (Baker et al., 2003, unpaged). More positively, almost 60 percent said that they would be interested in working with government research and development agencies, although their lack of knowledge of these agencies and their procedures may impede collaboration.

Awareness, Adoption, and Maintenance of Available Technologies

Consumer Awareness

When suitable assistive or accessible products are commercially available, other barriers may still stand in the way of their effective use. At the most basic level, people with disabilities (and their family members) may not be aware of the availability of useful products. In addition, particularly in the case of older people who have gradually developed functional limitations, people may not recognize that they could benefit from assistance (Gitlin, 1995; NTFTD, 2004; Carlson et al., 2005). Also, people who acquire disabilities later in life and who have trouble accepting their situation may see some assistive technologies as stigmatizing, which points to an advantage of accessible mainstream products (NTFTD, 2004). As Caust and Davis (2006, unpaged) have observed, "[p]eople want to believe they are competent and capable and they are happy to ignore the safety risks associated with not using assistive technology, for the sake of appearing competent."

The University of Michigan survey of people with disabilities discussed earlier in this chapter reported that roughly half of the respondents reported that they had received little or no information about assistive technologies. This finding suggests that the needs for information about assistive technologies are going unmet. Among the respondents who did obtain information, about half mentioned health care professionals (e.g., occupational or physical therapists) as the source (Ehrlich et al., 2003). (Many of the technologies reported by respondents, e.g., wheelchairs and hearing aids, require a medical prescription or guidance.) About 15 percent mentioned family and friends as sources of information, and 13 percent mentioned vocational rehabilitation counselors.

At the time of the survey in 2001, less than 10 percent of the respondents mentioned the Internet as a source of information. With the explosion of Internet resources and increased computer use by older individuals and their family networks, the Internet would likely be cited more frequently today. Internet searches may lead people to resources such as ABLEDATA, Technology for Long-Term Care (www.techforltc.org, which was originally funded by the U.S. Department of Health and Human Services), and other information resources developed by governmental agencies, nonprofit organizations, and manufacturers.

Although NIDRR, which administers the Assistive Technology Act of 1998, supports activities to help increase consumer awareness of useful technologies, the agency's website is (in the committee's view) not easy to use as a resource to find information about assistive or accessible technologies. Government and support group websites are especially important resources for developing consumer awareness because company advertising and other promotional activities may be very limited for small markets.[20]

More can be done to ensure that people with disabilities and their families become aware of and educated about the range of technologies that are available to them to meet many of their specific needs. A national task force recently proposed a broad-ranging public awareness campaign "to communicate the existence and benefits of [assistive and accessible technologies], provide mechanisms for consumers to find accessibility features in [other] products, and showcase best practices" in universal design (NTFTD, 2004, p. 43). The committee offers a similar recommendation below.

In addition, further investigation of the extent and quality of Internet and other information resources (including support group and industry websites) would be helpful in developing strategies to improve the availability, reliability, and usefulness of the information available online. To the extent that the Internet is the focus of public education and information programs, it is important that policy makers and advocates be alert to gaps in Internet access and use among low-income and other consumers and that they investigate additional strategies that can be used to reach these groups.

---

[20]The direct-to-consumer television advertisements for scooters and power wheelchairs (which prominently mention Medicare coverage) are the exception rather than the rule, but they also contribute to government concerns about fraudulent and abusive marketing. These concerns have provoked various government efforts to curtail abuse; these efforts, in turn, have been criticized by consumer and suppliers as draconian (see, e.g., Jalonick [2006] and RESNA [2006]; see also Chapter 9).

Guidance for Health Professionals

The move from awareness to the acquisition and application of a technology may be as simple as going to a store, buying a new household gadget, and using it, possibly without the need for even simple instructions (e.g., as with an accessibly designed utensil that replaces a similar but less user-friendly device). In the case of advanced prosthetic devices and other technologies, the process may be complex, involving the expertise and guidance of highly trained medical and other specialists in the selection and individual fitting of equipment, the training of the consumer in its safe and effective use and ongoing maintenance, and periodic reevaluation of equipment performance and use.

Physicians who specialize in care for people with particular disabilities may be aware of products that require medical assessment and prescription, but they may not always be well informed about household and other products that could benefit their patients. For both simpler and more complex technologies, physicians and other health care professionals should be alert to their patients' ability to benefit from assistive technologies and be prepared to provide guidance and information or to refer them as appropriate to other information sources.

However, even with products requiring medical assessment and prescription, the rapid changes in some kinds of technologies and the introduction or disappearance of products or product models from the market may make it difficult for physicians to track and evaluate specific products. Thus, for example, instead of recommending a particular device, a clinician may determine that a consumer has impaired manual dexterity; evaluate what product features may be relevant, given the individual's fine motor skills; identify the need for products with features such as large control buttons; and then focus on products with the relevant features. For products that do not require a medical prescription, such as household products, the consumer or a family member may then take the lead in searching for products with the appropriate features.

For some types of assistive technologies, personnel who are trained and knowledgeable about product options and selection may be in short supply, as may be the physical locations where products can be viewed and tried. For example, the Rehabilitation Engineering and Assistive Technology Society of North America (RESNA) has stated that there are not enough occupational and physical therapists certified as assistive technology practitioners or certified suppliers with the expertise needed to serve people who need powered mobility devices (RESNA, 2005). Likewise the American Foundation for the Blind has stated that a "critical shortage of professionals who are qualified to provide specialized computer skills training to blind and visually impaired people significantly affects their viability in today's job market" (AFB, 2001, unpaged). In yet another arena, the National Council on Disability has observed that it means little to recommend that the role of assistive technologies be considered more fully in the development of individual education plans (under the Individuals with Disabilities Education Act) if no member of the team developing such plans "is familiar with the range of [technologies] available to address desired goals (NCD, 2000b, unpaged).

Some consumers find information through state programs that have been funded under the Assistive Technology Act to aid consumers in learning about and acquiring technologies. For example, in a report on state activities funded under the Assistive Technology Act, RESNA (2003) found that the 34 states that provided data reported that they supported or operated 109 assistive technology demonstration centers. States also reported providing information to consumers through the Internet, e-mail, regular telephone and text telephone, and regular mail.

Financial Access

Particularly for the more expensive assistive technologies, a lack of financial resources can be a significant barrier to the acquisition of an effective, recommended technology. According to the University of Michigan survey of people with disabilities, the percentage of respondents for whom assistive technologies were paid for through public or private insurance (38 percent) was about equal to those for whom their equipment was paid for personally or through family members (37 percent) (Carlson and Ehrlich, 2005). Six percent received their equipment at no cost to themselves. People with low incomes were far more likely than people with higher incomes to report unmet needs for technology.

About 23 percent of the survey respondents sought help from an agency in selecting or purchasing equipment, and about 19 percent reported receiving help from an agency (Carlson and Ehrlich, 2005). Most people believed that they did not need agency help, but some said that they did not know an agency to contact. This again suggests the need for a more intensive public awareness effort.

As discussed further in Chapter 9, Medicare and private insurance coverage of assistive technologies is limited and often complex. Medicaid programs, for those who qualify, tend to cover a wider range of assistive technologies. This coverage is sometimes provided under waiver programs that do not extend to all parts of a state or to all categories of Medicaid recipients. The rules are often complex for consumers, family members, and even professionals.

One option for improving access to assistive technologies is through innovative practices in leasing or rental arrangements. One example is a leasing arrangement developed by the Center for Assistive Technology at the University of Pittsburgh Medical Center (UPMC) in conjunction with the UPMC Health Plan, a manufacturer of costly power wheelchairs, and a local network of suppliers (Schmeler et al., 2003). The program is specifically designed to make the equipment quickly available to people with rapidly advancing health conditions (e.g., amyotrophic lateral sclerosis) whose use of the equipment may be limited to a period of months. Rather than the Health Plan purchasing a $25,000 power wheelchair for a consumer, the chair can be leased on a monthly basis for a reasonable fee. The fee includes the provision of all maintenance and upgrades as the person's condition changes. Once that person no longer uses the equipment, it is recycled and re-leased. With the program, people with these conditions have access to equipment much sooner and the health plan claims significant cost savings. The suppliers and the manufacturer do not consider the program to have interfered with their profit objectives because the equipment can be leased repeatedly over several years.

A particularly weak point in the chain of effective technology use is coverage for maintaining, repairing, and replacing an assistive technology when necessary. Some users may have the knowledge and physical abilities to repair simple products, but expert assistance will often be required, especially for complex and expensive equipment. In addition, when an effective product is prescribed and is then used and wears out, people often find that their insurance does not provide for replacement or does not provide for replacement frequently enough. Chapter 9 recommends revisions in health plan policies to increase access to assistive technologies and support their maintenance, replacement, and repair.

Although the committee did not locate specific documentation, committee members working in rehabilitation reported decreasing numbers of assistive technology clinics and programs within hospitals and reductions in the scope of programs related to reduced rates of reimbursement and other onerous provider payment policies. (See footnote 2 in Chapter 9 on the controversy about restrictions on reimbursements to inpatient rehabilitation facilities.) An analysis of the complex issues of payment for rehabilitation services was beyond the committee's resources. Still, without mechanisms in place to fit equipment and adapt or train individuals in its proper use, even a potentially very effective assistive technology can fail.

Through the Consumer's Eyes

One challenge for health care professionals, family members, and others who may be involved in discussions of assistive technologies is to consider outcomes "through the consumer's eyes" (see, e.g., Taugher [2004] and Lilja et al. [2003]). Each of these parties may have priorities different from those of the individual considering or using an assistive technology (Scherer, 2005).[21]

For example, from a user's perspective, a seemingly inferior device may be more practical to use and maintain, may be less obtrusive in social situations, or may otherwise be more acceptable, and thus more effective than a more sophisticated device. Seigle cites the case of a man who had lost both arms in an accident.

> *Robotic arms were created and fitted to the man, but because they were heavy and uncomfortable they stayed on the floor of his closet. When the man asked what he most wanted to do on his own, he answered that he just wanted to be able to go out to a restaurant and drink a beverage without someone having to hold the cup. . . . In this case, the best assistive technology solution was a long straw.*

Seigle (2001, unpaged)

In reality, although this anecdote highlights the mismatch between a technology and the user, a better solution for this individual would be prostheses that were lighter, more comfortable, and more functional. As described earlier, prostheses are the focus of considerable advanced research that has been given added impetus because of the wars in Iraq and Afghanistan, although cost will limit access to the more advanced devices for many individuals with limited or no insurance.

Research and experience suggest that consumer involvement in the selection process (rather than an essentially one-sided prescription by a health care professional) helps avoid later rejection or abandonment of the technology (see, e.g., Phillips and Zhao [1993], Gitlin [1995], and Riemer-Reiss and Wacker [2000]). Abandonment or nonuse of a technology, particularly an expensive one, is a costly and wasteful outcome that contributes to policy maker and insurer concerns about the provision of coverage for assistive technologies and to the adoption of restrictive coverage policies and practices. The committee found no evidence, however, that the rate of abandonment of assistive technologies is higher or even equal to the rate at which people fail to complete or maintain complex medication regimens.

RECOMMENDATIONS

Creating more accessible environments—whether through the provision of better assistive technologies and improved mainstream products or the removal of barriers in buildings and public spaces—is an important avenue

---

[21]Committee members reported hearing the label "inflictor" applied to professionals who prescribe or select assistive technologies without involving the consumer and considering that person's views about what will work in his or her own life.

to independence and community participation for people with disabilities. This chapter has identified needs in two broad areas: the development of new or improved technologies and the better use of existing technologies. The discussion below sets forth three recommendations related to these needs. Chapters 6 and 9 identify additional steps related to regulatory and financing policies.

Innovation and Technology Transfer

New and more effective assistive technologies are possible. For products with large markets, a good business case for investment in research, development, and production can often be made, although it may still be useful for consumers, policy makers, and others to become more articulate and persuasive in encouraging investment. Unfortunately, many types of assistive technology do not fit this model, and normal market processes fall short in meeting urgent consumer needs.

Tackling this shortfall is, however, complex. Although government efforts to promote assistive technology development and commercial applications do appear to have had positive results, the committee concluded that a more detailed exploration of obstacles, possible incentives, and even mandates would be useful. This exploration could build on the analyses cited in this chapter and other related work. It should involve a broad range of participants and should use subgroups as appropriate to investigate issues related to particular barriers, incentives, or product categories and to identify priorities for new public investments in the development and evaluation of assistive and accessible technologies. As recommended in Chapter 9, it is also important to undertake research to support coverage decisions for assistive technologies based on evidence of effectiveness.

> **Recommendation 7.1:** Federal agencies that support research on assistive technologies should collaborate on a program of research to improve strategies to identify, develop, and bring to market new or better assistive technologies for people with disabilities. Such research should involve consumers, manufacturers, medical and technical experts, and other relevant agencies and stakeholders.

As noted in this chapter, some helpful steps have been taken to increase government support for technology development and transfer. Funding for the Rehabilitation Engineering Research Centers program, for instance, almost doubled between FY 1999 and FY 2001 but has recently dropped back slightly. Additional research by NIDRR, units of the National Institutes of Health, the National Science Foundation, and other relevant agencies is needed to identify both new technologies and strategies for getting effective products to consumers.

Research into better methods to develop and bring to market effective new technologies needs to extend beyond "high-tech" technologies. Strategies to promote research and commercial development to improve relatively "low-tech" but common equipment, such as walkers, are also important.

Another topic for research is the role of legislation, including existing policies such as the ADA and Section 508 of the Rehabilitation Act, in providing incentives to industry by enlarging the market for accessible technologies. One study that examined patent applications in an attempt to assess the impact of the ADA on assistive technology development found that although references to civil rights laws were not typical in patent records, applications mentioning the ADA increased after passage of the act (Berven and Blanck, 1999). That study, which examined patent applications from 1976 through 1997, found a substantial increase in the numbers of patents related to various kinds of impairments over the entire period but did not note a particular spike after the passage of the ADA.

Accessible Mainstream Technologies

As described earlier in this chapter, public policies have sought to make some mainstream products more accessible, particularly telecommunications and other electronic and information technologies. Some of these policies apply only to government purchases. The ADA focused on reducing certain kinds of environmental barriers and setting standards for the accessibility of buildings, transportation systems, and other public spaces. Although that law and accompanying regulations covered some products that are often installed in buildings (e.g., ATMs), many other mainstream products that are not covered by the ADA or other policies also present substantial barriers to people with disabilities. With an aging population, inaccessible mainstream products will present increasing burdens and costs to individuals with disabilities in the form of reduced independence and reduced participation in the community. This, in turn, will create costs for family members and other caregivers and for society in general. As with the policies discussed in other chapters, further actions to remove barriers and expand access to helpful technologies will have to be assessed in relation to other pressing demands on public and private resources.

Recommendation 7.2: To extend the benefits of accessibility provided by existing federal statutes and regulations, the U.S. Congress should direct the Architectural and Transportation Barriers Compliance Board (the Access Board) to collaborate with relevant public and private groups to develop a plan for establishing accessibility standards for

important mainstream and general use products and technologies. The plan should

- propose criteria and processes for designating high-priority product areas for standard setting;
- identify existing public or private standards or guidelines that might be useful in setting standards; and
- include medical equipment as an initial priority area.

This recommendation proposes a priority-setting process to extend the accessibility policies of the federal government to new product areas. Such a process would take industry concerns as well as consumer and health professional concerns into account and would also consider technical issues in setting standards for different kinds of products. Taking into account the issues discussed in Chapter 6, the committee identified medical equipment as a priority area. It also identified home products and product packaging as particularly important for helping people maintain the most basic levels of independence in activities of daily living. Among the criteria that might be considered in a priority-setting process are the numbers of people likely to be affected by a product and related standards, the potential for standards to improve product accessibility, and the potential for standards to have unwanted effects, such as sharply increasing costs and discouraging innovation.

Increasing Public and Professional Awareness

Discussions of assistive technology generally focus on the development of new and better assistive and accessible technologies and on better insurance coverage. An equal need (also acknowledged in the 1991 IOM report on disabilities) exists to make sure that people with disabilities and those close to them are aware of existing products or product categories, especially products that may not be mentioned or prescribed by health care professionals. Increasing consumer and professional knowledge about assistive technologies should increase the use of the products, which should, in turn, make the market for such products more attractive to private companies, promote greater product diversification, reduce the costs of some products, and generally increase product availability.

The committee believes that a substantial national program to increase the awareness, availability, and acceptability of assistive technologies and accessible mainstream technologies is timely, given the demographic changes in the United States noted earlier in this report. The objectives would be to assist the people with disabilities, family members and friends, and health professionals in learning about (1) the existence and range of potentially beneficial mainstream and assistive technologies and (2) the ways in which consumers and professionals can obtain additional, up-to-date information about available technologies and products. A campaign can build on the information provision efforts already undertaken by NIDRR and other federal agencies and upon the particular expertise of the Centers for Disease Control and Prevention in developing and managing public and professional awareness programs. In addition, state public health programs are natural partners in developing and implementing an awareness campaign. The campaign can also build on ideas suggested by the National Task Force on Technology and Disability in its draft report (NTFTD, 2004).

> **Recommendation 7.3: The Centers for Disease Control and Prevention, working with the National Institute on Disability and Rehabilitation Research, should launch a major public health campaign to increase public and health care professional awareness and acceptance of assistive technologies and accessible mainstream technologies that can benefit people with different kinds of disabilities.**

Increasing Public Awareness

The consumer component of a public awareness campaign would target not only the lack of knowledge about available technologies but would also help people assess whether they have developed functional deficits for which helpful products exist. The campaign would include guidance for people on

- recognizing their potential needs for assistive technology;
- finding useful information about available technologies and their pluses and minuses;
  - identifying and evaluating specific products;
  - locating sources of financial assistance; and
  - working with health care professionals, suppliers, manufacturers, and others to obtain, maintain, adjust, repair, or replace equipment.

In some cases, people are aware of products but consider them unattractive or stigmatizing, which can be a major barrier to their use. A large-scale, long-term, repetitive public media campaign to increase the acceptance of assistive technologies can highlight what products are available to "make life easier" and convey that it is normal to use smart technologies. Promotions might show celebrities using technologies and natural-looking aids. Another strategy might be to persuade the producers of popular television programs to show the unobtrusive, routine use of assistive technologies. The idea is to help people feel more comfortable using technologies that may allow them to live independently longer or to stay with their families longer by reducing the amount of informal caregiving needed. If a public awareness campaign identifies unattractive product design as a problem, then that knowledge can also guide contacts with manufacturers and designers about how to modify the products to reduce this barrier to the use of helpful technologies.

Increasing Professional Awareness

In contrast to medications, getting assistive technologies to those who could benefit from them requires more than a physician's prescription. The process also involves the broader spectrum of rehabilitation professionals, such as physical and occupational therapists. Current data suggest that the primary source of information regarding assistive technologies is physicians and other medical personnel (Carlson and Ehrlich, 2005). It also suggests that many people are also unaware of their options.

Nonetheless, in the committee's experience, the lack of awareness by health care professionals (especially those who are not rehabilitation specialists) of the range of assistive technologies and their potential uses is a significant barrier to the wider and more effective use of these technologies. Remedying this lack of awareness will involve efforts on several fronts, including the undergraduate, graduate, and continuing education of health professionals. The committee recognizes that space is at a premium in heavily loaded and tightly structured professional training curricula. Strategies need to be identified to provide quick, interesting, and effective means of injecting information about helpful technologies and methods of assessing consumer needs into education programs.

Health care professionals themselves generally do not need to be experts in the technologies; rather, they need to know, in general, what exists that might help their patients or clients and what basic features of a technology are important for a given patient (e.g., features for people who lack fine motor skills). With this basic knowledge, physicians and other health care professionals may continue their education about particular technologies on their own, designate staff to become resources, or encourage their patients or clients to investigate technologies that do not require a physician prescription or particular professional assistance.

In sum, increasing consumer and professional awareness of useful assistive and accessible technologies should have a positive effect on the use of these technologies and, in turn, on people's functioning and independence. As noted throughout this chapter, the acquisition of useful technologies may be limited by a lack of insurance coverage or other financial access, particularly for people with modest or low incomes. The next two chapters discuss selected issues related to the financing of health care services for people with disabilities.

8

Access to Health Insurance and the Role of Risk-Adjusted Payments to Health Plans

I have to go down my list of medications and choose which pills I can take and which ones I can't. . . . Some months, I have a little extra money and I can take it, and other months I can't. . . . I've just been picking and choosing. . . . I haven't done myself any favors by doing that, but you have to do what you've got to do.

Maggie (woman with multiple sclerosis waiting for Medicare coverage)
Quoted by Williams et al. (2004)

Maggie had to make decisions about which medications to take and which to forego, which is a dangerous dilemma. In her case, these hard choices are necessary because she has just started receiving Social Security Disability Insurance (SSDI) benefits but will not become eligible for Medicare for 2 more years. In the interim, she has no health insurance. For others, the complexities of the Medicare prescription drug program or the state-federal Medicaid program can lead to interruptions in access to services or medications as program rules change or individual circumstances fluctuate. Yet others lose coverage when they lose their job or their employer stops offering health insurance. Although people with disabilities are somewhat more likely than other people to have insurance (especially public insurance), the consequences of a lack of insurance can be more severe for them because they often have more needs for health care (DeJong and Sutton, 1998).

In 1991, the Institute of Medicine (IOM) report *Disability in America* observed that "a system that provided accessible, affordable, quality health care for all would have enormous beneficial effect on the prevention of dis-

222

ability. Yet economic and political hurdles to that end are formidable, and a near-term solution is not in sight" (p. 281). Those observations about the obstacles to the creation of such a health system are as true today as they were 15 years ago. Recent renewed attention to the problem of uninsurance at the national level and the movement by some states toward universal coverage are encouraging (see, e.g., NCSL [2007]). Still, the barriers to affordable coverage for all Americans remain daunting. Moreover, as many have argued, even with better access to insurance, the American health care delivery and financing system was not and is not well designed to meet the needs of people with serious long-term health conditions or disabilities (see, e.g., Anderson and Knickman [2001], IOM [2001a,b], Wagner et al. [2001], DeJong et al. [2002], Vladeck [2002]. Eichner and Blumenthal [2003], Etheredge and Moore [2003], NCD [2005], Teitelbaum et al. [2005], Iezzoni and O'Day [2006], and Palsbo and Kailes [2006]). As the baby boom generation enters old age, these flaws in the design of the American health care delivery and financing system are likely to become even more troublesome—at the same time that general anxieties about the affordability and sustainability of the current acute and long-term care services grow.

A comprehensive discussion of the deficiencies of the current system of health insurance and directions for reform is beyond the scope of this report, but this chapter and the next chapter highlight certain shortfalls that seriously affect people with disabilities. Chapter 4 discussed the improvements in the organization and coordination of services that could be made for young people with disabilities as they move from pediatric to adult care. Most of those improvements involve changes that would be applicable to care for people of any age.

The charge to the IOM included two issues related to the financing of health care for people with disabilities. The first issue, which is discussed in this chapter, involves methods for adjusting Medicare, Medicaid, or employer payments to health maintenance organizations (HMOs) and other health plans to account fairly for the potentially high health care costs of health plan members with disabilities. The second issue, health insurance coverage of assistive technologies, is discussed in the next chapter, which also examines the coverage of personal assistance services. In addition, the next chapter reviews the fiscal context of decisions about expanding coverage, the constraints that rising costs place on policies to expand access to needed services, and the confusion surrounding complex federal and state changes in Medicaid.

This chapter begins by reviewing data on health insurance coverage by age and disability status. It notes some areas of concern, including the waiting period before SSDI-based Medicare coverage begins and the instability in children's enrollment in public insurance programs. The subsequent sections summarize the characteristics and complexities of health insurance markets as a source of coverage for people with disabilities and the threats to future coverage posed by competitive market dynamics, including the avoidance by health plans of people at risk for higher-than-average health care costs. The chapter discusses strategies to respond to the latter dynamic by risk adjusting payments to health plans. Appendix C includes a more detailed examination of risk adjustment methods. The chapter concludes with recommendations.

HEALTH INSURANCE COVERAGE FOR
PEOPLE WITH DISABILITIES

Today, as in 1991, when IOM published the report *Disability in America*, people with disabilities are somewhat more likely than people without disabilities to be insured. This is primarily because they are more likely to qualify for public health insurance, although insurance coverage status varies considerably among people with disabilities by age and type of disability. The major sources of health insurance for people with disabilities continue to be Medicare, Medicaid, and private employer-sponsored health plans. For many veterans with disabilities, especially those that are combat related, the Veterans Health Administration is an additional source of coverage.[1]

Nevertheless, as described below, depending on their age and type of disability, between 5 and 14 percent of people with disabilities who are under age 65 lack insurance. Lack of coverage creates a variety of problems for this population. For example, a survey reported by Hanson and colleagues (2003) found that people with disabilities who lacked insurance were more likely than their peers with insurance to have no regular physician, to have trouble finding physicians who understood their disabilities, and to have postponed or to have gone without care. Data on children with special health care needs likewise show higher rates of unmet needs among those without health insurance (see, e.g., Dusing et al. [2004] and Mayer et al. [2004]). Although it did not identify the health insurance status of the respondents, a 2004 Harris Poll found that 24 percent of respondents with severe disabilities, 11 percent of those with moderate or slight disabilities, and 7 percent of those reporting no disability reported going without needed health care (Harris Interactive, Inc., 2004a; see also Harris Interactive [2004b]). Beyond financial issues, these findings of unmet need

---

[1]Data indicate that in 1999 about half of veterans had Medicare coverage (most because they were over age 64 but others because of serious disability) (Hynes, 2002). A recent analysis of data on veterans who had received care for stroke found that 30 percent used services only through the Veterans Health Administration (Jia et al., 2006).

may also reflect barriers to access in health care facilities, transportation, and other aspects of the environment.

As discussed in the next chapter, even for people with insurance, the policies of Medicare, Medicaid, and private health plans often restrict access to assistive products and services that are particularly important to people with mobility, self-care, and certain other types of limitations. Moreover, individuals with disabilities are more likely than others to have low incomes that make deductibles, copayments, and coinsurance a burden, which may deter them from seeking these products and services.

Health Insurance for Older Adults with Disabilities

Approximately 36 million people age 65 or over are covered by the federal Medicare program without regard to their disability status or income (CMS, 2006a).[2] About 9 in 10 Medicare beneficiaries have some additional public or private coverage that pays for certain costs or services that Medicare does not cover (e.g., the deductible for inpatient care, which is $992 per episode of illness for 2007) (Super, 2002; CMS, 2006j). This additional coverage (with the exception of traditional Medicaid) generally does not fill the gaps in coverage of long-term institutional or personal care services.[3] The new Medicare drug program partly fills one major gap: the lack of coverage for drugs.

In 2003, more than 60 percent of older Medicare beneficiaries had either individually purchased "Medigap" policies or employer-sponsored supplemental insurance (or both) to help pay for the deductibles and other expenses not paid for by Medicare (CMS, 2005a). This figure was down from the more than 70 percent of beneficiaries who had such coverage in 1994 (CMS, 1994). Employer sponsorship of retiree health benefits has dropped in recent years (particularly for new retirees), and the costs to retirees with employer-sponsored coverage have increased (Fronstin, 2005; Kaiser Commission and Health Research and Educational Trust, 2005). As is the case for Medicare itself, neither employer-sponsored nor individu-

---

[2]Medicare eligibility depends on eligibility for Social Security, which is based on required payroll tax contributions to that system. National survey data show that nearly all (99 percent) of those over age 65 have health insurance. Other data suggest that perhaps 5 to 20 percent of older residents in some states may lack Medicare, although in New York City at least, the majority of those not covered by Medicare have private insurance or Medicaid coverage (Gray et al., 2006). Many, but not all, of those without Medicare coverage are immigrants.

[3]For the purposes of this report, long-term care refers to supportive health, personal care, and related services that are provided over an extended period to people who are limited in their ability to care for themselves as a result of a chronic condition. Care may be provided in institutions or in the community. Regular use of primary and specialist physician services or periodic short-term hospitalizations as a result of a chronic condition that does not limit self-care is usually not characterized as long-term care.

ally purchased supplemental insurance is particularly tailored to meet the needs of individuals with disabilities; coverage of long-term care services is minimal or absent (see the summary of Medigap plan options in CMS [2006b]).[4]

With some exceptions, federal and state rules generally allow insurers offering Medigap policies to charge higher premiums or restrict sales to people with health problems or disabilities. To simplify comparisons and to reduce marketing abuses and other problems, federal rules establish 12 different, standardized benefit options for these policies (CMS, 2006b).

In addition to employer-sponsored or individually purchased supplemental options, Medicare beneficiaries may also enroll in private Medicare Advantage (formerly Medicare+Choice) health plans. Although these plans vary, they generally offer extra benefits similar to those available in some or all Medicare supplemental policies. In 2005, approximately 5.5 million beneficiaries opted for these plans, which typically limit the choice of providers and are concentrated in urban areas (Gold, 2006). As discussed later in this chapter and in Appendix C, Medicare Advantage and other, similar health plans typically receive capitated payments (i.e., a per person payment for a defined time period) rather than per service payments.

Finally, more than 4.7 million low-income beneficiaries age 65 and over, including many with serious disabilities, have additional coverage through the federal-state Medicaid program (CMS, 2005a). More than 80 percent of these dually eligible beneficiaries receive assistance with Medicare Part B premiums and cost sharing; the rest receive either assistance with premiums only or assistance with both premiums and cost sharing (Peters, 2005; Kaiser Commission, 2006b). More than two-thirds of Medicaid spending for dually eligible beneficiaries goes for long-term care, including home care (Kaiser Commission, 2005).

In sum, nearly all adults age 65 and over have health coverage through Medicare, and most also have some form of supplemental private or public coverage. Those with very low incomes often have additional Medicaid coverage. The main concern for this group is the scope of coverage, for example, coverage of assistive technologies and personal care services, as discussed in Chapter 9.

---

[4]The market for private long-term care insurance is growing but is still small and not relevant for people with existing disabilities. As of 2002, an estimated 9 million long-term care insurance policies had been sold since 1987, and an estimated 70 percent of these policies were still in force (AHIP, 2004). Industry statistics do not report the number of policies held by people age 65 and over.

Health Insurance for Younger Adults with Disabilities

Health insurance coverage is more varied and uncertain for younger adults with disabilities than for older, Medicare-eligible adults. A recent analysis of data collected from 1997 to 2002 by Olin and Dougherty (2006) reported that people ages 18 to 64 who have functional or mobility limitations are more likely to have public insurance than people without such limitations and are slightly less likely to be uninsured altogether (Table 8-1). Nonetheless, more than 8 percent of people ages 18 to 64 who had difficulties with activities of daily living (ADLs) had neither public nor private insurance.

TABLE 8-1 Insurance Status of Adults Ages 18 to 64 with Physical, ADL or IADL Limitations, Civilian, Noninstitutional Population, Pooled Data for 1997 to 2002

Characteristic	Total	Ages 18–49	Ages 50–64
Population (in 1,000s) 18 to 64[a]	170,805	128,906	41,899
Limitation and insurance status			
Number (in 1,000s) with no limitation	156,380	121,286	35,095
Percent private insurance	79.0	77.3	84.8
Percent public insurance	5.7	6.0	4.5
Percent no insurance	15.3	16.7	10.7
Number (in 1,000s) with physical limitation	11,060	5,730	5,330
Percent private insurance	53.2	52.7	53.8
Percent public insurance	33.0	31.9	34.2
Percent no insurance	13.8	15.5	12.0
Number (in 1,000s) with IADLs	1,885	1,093	792
Percent private insurance	31.3	32.4	29.9
Percent public insurance	59.5	57.5	62.3
Percent no insurance	9.1	—	—
Number (in 1,000s) with any ADLs	1,480	798	682
Percent private insurance	32.9	33.3	32.6
Percent public insurance	58.8	60.3	57.1
Percent no insurance	8.3	—	—

NOTE: Any ADL = having activity of daily living limitations, regardless of other limitations; IADL = having instrumental activity of daily living (IADL) limitations but no ADLs; physical limitation = having no limitations in ADLs or IADLs, mobility limitations only; no limitation = having no activity or mobility limitations. Percentages may not add to 100 because of rounding. Dashes indicate less than 100 sample cases.

[a]The numbers of individuals for whom data on limitations were missing were not included in the population count.

SOURCE: Olin and Dougherty (2006). Data from Medical Expenditure Panel Survey, 1997 to 2002.

Using different classifications of impairments and data from a single year (2001), Iezzoni and O'Day (2006) reported higher levels of uninsurance for people with certain self-reported vision, hearing, and mobility impairments than for people with no impairment. For example, 21 percent of those with major vision loss lacked insurance. Iezzoni and O'Day also found that approximately 20 percent of people under age 65 with a major impairment had Medicaid coverage only, almost 11 percent had Medicare only, and about 6 percent were dually eligible for Medicaid and Medicare coverage. Other data show that in 2003 about 37 percent of all dually eligible individuals were under age 65 (CMS, 2005a, Section 8).

The analysis cited in Table 8-1 did not differentiate between employer-sponsored private insurance and individually purchased insurance. Companies that sell health insurance to individuals generally restrict the ability of people with serious chronic health conditions or disabilities to purchase coverage.[5] In the Medical Expenditure Panel Survey for 2004, only 13 individuals of the 7,000 adults under age 65 with a disability (broadly defined) in the 30,000-person sample reported having nongroup insurance (Jeffrey Rhoades, survey statistician, Agency for Healthcare Research and Quality, personal communication, August 30, 2006). (Given a policy that requires a minimum sample size of 100 for estimation purposes, the survey analysts did not generate a population estimate for this group.) Based on the same source, an estimated 3.9 percent of younger adults without disabilities have this kind of insurance.

As the severity of limitations increases, so does the percentage of expenses paid by Medicaid and Medicare (Table 8-2). For people ages 18 to 44 with disabilities, Medicaid is substantially more important as a source of payment than it is for people ages 45 to 64. Overall, about 8 million people between the ages of 18 and 64 who have disabilities are covered by Medicaid. They account for about 16 percent of total Medicaid program enrollment and about 43 percent of total expenditures (Kaiser Commission, 2005).

Employment-Based Insurance

For people with disabilities who are employed (and, often, for their family members), employer-based health insurance is an important resource that provides access to coverage that is often not available or not affordable in the market for individually purchased insurance. Individuals with

---

[5]Various federal and state policies, which are too complex for a brief summary, impose some limitations on private insurance practices related to the issuance, renewal, and pricing of insurance as they affect people with health conditions (see, e.g., Williams and Fuchs [2004] and Buchmueller and Liu [2005]).

TABLE 8-2 Sources of Payment by Age Group and Disability Status for Adults Ages 18 to 64 with Functional Limitations, U.S. Civilian, Noninstitutionalized Population, 1997 to 2002

Age (Years) and Limitation	Percent Distribution of Total Expenses by Source of Payment				
	Self	Medicare	Medicaid	Private	Other
Total[a]	23.5	4.8	10.1	52.0	9.6
All 18-49-year-olds	23.2	3.5	11.8	52.0	9.5
No limits	25.5	0.8	7.1	58.3	8.4
Physical limits	18.4	11.1	21.4	37.3	11.9
IADL only	14.8	10.2	31.2	25.5	18.4
Any ADL	9.2	15.7	39.0	23.2	12.9
All 50-64-year-olds	24.0	6.7	7.7	52.0	9.6
No limits	27.3	2.0	3.0	59.8	7.9
Physical limits	20.6	10.5	13.4	44.7	10.8
IADL only	19.4	16.4	19.1	33.9	11.2
Any ADL	13.5	22.4	16.9	30.2	17.0

NOTE: Any ADL = having activity of daily living limitations, regardless of other limitations; IADL only = having only instrumental activity of daily living limitations; physical limitation having no ADL or IADL limitations, i.e., mobility limitations only; no limitation having no activity or mobility limitations. Other category includes data for those with veterans' health benefits. Percentages may not add up to 100 because of rounding.

[a]Only individuals who had a medical event were included in the total. Data for individuals who had eyeglass expenditures were not included in this table.

SOURCE: Olin and Dougherty (2006). Data from Medical Expenditure Panel Survey, 1997 to 2002.

employer-provided health insurance who become disabled (or whose family member becomes disabled) generally do not face a higher premium or the loss of coverage, as long as they remain in the employer group. The loss of employment can result in the loss of affordable insurance for the worker and his or her family members, although people who stop working as a result of a disability may be able to pay for continued employer coverage for up to 18 months. (This continuation coverage is available—without employer subsidy of the premium—under provisions of the Consolidated Omnibus Budget Reconciliation Act of 1985. This coverage is often referred to as "COBRA coverage" for its legislation acronym.[6])

---

[6]If an individual without a disability qualifies for COBRA coverage as a result of job loss or reduction in hours and then becomes disabled under Social Security Administration criteria within the first 60 days of coverage, he or she can qualify for an additional 11 months of coverage (U.S. Department of Labor, 2007). This could bring that person nearly through the 29-month waiting period between becoming qualified for SSDI benefits and being eligible for Medicare.

Although employment-based health insurance has many advantages, especially in the present U.S. political culture, linking health insurance to employment can expose people with disabilities to an additional risk of discrimination. Notwithstanding antidiscrimination policies, employers, especially small employers, may be reluctant to hire people with disabilities or chronic health problems for fear of subsequent increases in health insurance premiums for their employees, although the policies of some states limit the size of yearly rate increases (see discussion below). Even large companies that self-fund most of their health plans' costs (and pay only for insurance administration and perhaps reinsurance against very costly claims) may be reluctant to hire individuals whom they believe would further increase their costs. Data suggest that the highest-cost 10 percent of adults with employment-based coverage accounted for 60 percent of the health care costs for that group (Merlis, 2005). In addition, workers who have family members with serious chronic conditions or disabilities may fear discrimination.

Employees with disabilities have some legal protections against certain kinds of discrimination, although discrimination can be hard to prove. Title I of the Americans with Disabilities Act (ADA) restricts an employer from discriminating in the "terms and conditions of employment," for example, refusing to hire people with disabilities or excluding them from health insurance plans. The boundaries of the ADA provisions are not clear, and differential coverage of health conditions is allowed under some circumstances (Mathis, 2004). For example, an employer's health insurance plan can generally exclude coverage for certain kinds of services (e.g., home health care), as long as the limitations apply to all plan members. In addition, as noted elsewhere in this report and in Appendix D, the U.S. Supreme Court has narrowly interpreted the ADA definition of disability so that fewer people are protected than lawmakers had anticipated when they passed the legislation. The ADA does not apply to discrimination against workers on the basis of the disability status of family members (Sara Rosenbaum, Hirsh Professor and Chair, Department of Health Policy, George Washington University, personal communication, December 18, 2006).

Title V of the ADA contains explicit limitations on the application of the law to health insurers. Six years after passage of the ADA, however, the Health Insurance Portability and Accountability Act (PL 104-191) added some restrictions on insurer group health plans. Unlike insurers selling coverage directly to individuals, these group plans cannot charge individuals higher premiums on the basis of their health status or history and generally cannot limit coverage of preexisting conditions for more than 12 months and (U.S. Department of Labor, 2004a). (A preexisting condition is a condition for which medical advice or medical care was provided or recommended during the 6 months before an individual's enrollment in a covered health plan.) In addition, the law includes "guaranteed issue" provisions that prohibit insurers from refusing to renew policies for small employer groups (those with 2 to 50 employees) and from refusing to offer coverage to these groups—if the employers are willing and able to pay the premium. Under federal law, insurers can, however, charge one employer more than another on the basis of the claims experience or health status of its employees (Merlis, 2005). Other laws (e.g., the Mental Health Parity Act of 1996) also limit certain kinds of discrimination in health insurance.

Insurance regulation has traditionally been the province of the states, and many states preceded the federal government in adopting policies similar to those cited above. Most states have also adopted other policies aimed at making health insurance more available, affordable, and stable for small employers and their employees, although assessments of their success vary (see, e.g., NAHU [2005], Chollet [2006], and Kofman and Pollitz [2006]).[7] For example, many states have policies that restrict the extent to which insurers can take employee characteristics (e.g., age and health status) into account in setting rates for small groups. Some states also regulate insurer marketing practices, for example, forbidding insurers from marketing only to low-risk groups.

Medicare and Medicaid

Although Medicare is generally thought of as a program for older individuals, Medicare covered some 6,700,000 people under age 65 in 2005 (CMS, 2006f). These younger adults, who became eligible for Medicare after they qualified for SSDI benefits, account for about 15 percent of all Medicare beneficiaries. An analysis of 1995 data reported that 37 percent of younger beneficiaries had mental retardation, severe mental illness, or dementia (Foote and Hogan, 2001). In 2003, about 5 percent of younger Medicare beneficiaries, mostly individuals with the diagnoses just mentioned, lived in institutions (CMS, 2005a). As noted earlier, Medicare coverage of long-term institutional care is very limited.

With few exceptions, adults under age 65 who qualify for SSDI benefits must wait 24 months after they start receiving benefits before they can enroll in Medicare.[8] (The exceptions allow benefits to start earlier for qualifying individuals who have been diagnosed with amyotrophic lateral

---

[7]The federal Employee Retirement Income Security Act restricts state regulation of large employers who use insurers to administer their insurance benefits but who self-insure the cost.

[8]In 1971, when the House Committee on Ways and Means recommended the extension of Medicare to working-age adults with disabilities, it explained that the waiting period served several purposes, including to "help keep the costs within reasonable bounds, avoid overlapping private health insurance protection, particularly where a disabled worker may continue his membership in a group insurance plan for a period of time following the onset of his disability and minimize certain administrative problems that might otherwise arise. . . . Moreover,

sclerosis or end-stage renal disease or individuals who have had a kidney transplant [Whittaker, 2005].) The waiting period for Medicare coverage is a serious hardship for many individuals, most of whom qualify for disability insurance in the first place because they have a serious medical condition that precludes working and is expected to end in death or to last at least 1 year.[9] One study estimated that approximately 400,000 of the 1.26 million individuals in the Medicare waiting period in 2002 lacked any form of health insurance (Dale and Verdier, 2003).[10] Others are covered by a family member's health plan or veterans health benefits, and some are able to pay for the continuation of employer-based coverage for up to 18 months under COBRA provisions.

Roughly 40 percent of those who qualify for SSDI also qualify for Supplemental Security Income (SSI) and are enrolled in Medicaid (Whittaker, 2005). SSI provides cash benefits for low-income individuals with disabilities. In most states, people who qualify for SSI are automatically qualified for Medicaid in the month that they apply for SSI (and sometimes retroactively), although some states require a separate Medicaid application (Lopez-Soto and Sheldon, 2005). The U.S. Congress has also provided that some former SSI recipients remain eligible for Medicaid under certain conditions.

Not surprisingly, interviews suggest that many SSDI beneficiaries who lack insurance during the Medicare waiting period forego necessary medical services, medications, and rehabilitation care (Williams et al., 2004). The final section of this chapter returns to the problems created by the SSDI waiting period and includes a recommendation for phasing it out.

Health Insurance for Children

As a group, children with disabilities are more likely than other children to be insured and are somewhat more likely than other children to have public insurance. In theory, children covered by Medicaid have more extensive coverage than adults through the Early Periodic Screening, Detection, and Treatment (EPSDT) program (see Chapters 4 and 9). Also, federal

---

this approach provides assurance that the protection will be available to those whose disabilities have proven to be severe and long lasting" (U.S. House of Representatives, Committee on Ways and Means, 1971, p. 67, as cited in Whittaker [2005]).

[9]Most recipients of SSDI benefits qualify on the basis of their own work experience, but some qualify as surviving disabled spouses or children of workers. In addition, adult children who become disabled before age 22 can obtain Social Security disability benefits if a parent who is retired, disabled, or deceased has paid qualifying amounts into the system (SSA, 2007b).

[10]Another study reported that during the waiting period, 12 percent of beneficiaries died but 2 percent recovered and left SSDI (Riley, 2004).

TABLE 8-3 Insurance Coverage for Children With and Without Special Health Care Needs (SHCN), by Type of Coverage, 2000

Insurance	All Children[a]	Children with SHCN	Children without SHCN
Any private	69.4	69.4	69.9
Public only	21.8	25.9	20.9
Uninsured	8.7	4.7	9.3

[a]Includes unknown special health care need status, which is not shown. In 2000, an estimated 3 percent of children had unknown special health care needs.

SOURCE: Chevarley (2006). Data from Household Component of the Medical Expenditure Panel Survey, 2000.

policies require school districts to pay for certain services and assistive technologies for children who need special education and related services.

An analysis of Medical Expenditure Panel Survey data for the year 2000 reported insurance data for children with and without special health care needs (Chevarley, 2006).[11] Reflecting their higher rate of Medicaid coverage, approximately 5 percent of children with special health care needs and 9 percent of children without special health care needs were uninsured at some time in the preceding year (Table 8-3). Almost 70 percent of children in both groups were, however, covered by private insurance. Data from the 2004 National Health Interview Survey show that 7.5 percent of children with activity limitations and 9.5 percent of children without such limitations were not insured (H. Stephen Kaye, Research Director, Institute for Health and Aging, University of California, San Francisco, personal communication, December 14, 2006). This survey showed lower levels of private health insurance for children with activity limitations (52 percent) than for children without such limitations (63 percent). For children overall (not only those with disabilities or special health care needs), data from the Current Population Survey show that in 2005 about 65 percent of children had private health insurance (92 percent of it employer based), 30 percent had public coverage, and 11 percent had no insurance (DeNavas-Walt et al., 2006). Other data indicate that in 2003 25 percent of children who were uninsured for all or part of a year and 12 percent of children who had insurance during the entire year received no care during the year (RWJF, 2006).

---

[11]About 16 percent of children are characterized as having special health care needs. As explained in Chapter 4, the Maternal and Child Health Bureau of the U.S. Department of Health and Human Services defines children with special health care needs as "those who have or are at increased risk for a chronic physical, developmental, behavioral, or emotional condition and who also require health and related services of a type or amount beyond that required by children generally" (McPherson et al., 1998, p. 137).

Analyses of data from the National Health Interview Survey show that the percentage of all children who lacked coverage for at least part of the past year dropped by almost one-third between 1997 and 2005 (Cohen and Martinez, 2006). This drop coincides with the introduction in 1997 of the State Child Health Insurance Program (SCHIP) (Hudson, 2005; RWJF, 2006). As discussed in Chapter 4, SCHIP is a source of public coverage for children under age 18 in low-income families with incomes that exceed the limits that qualify them for coverage through Medicaid. Although children who are covered by SCHIP have lower rates of disability than children enrolled in Medicaid, SCHIP still covers many children with special health care needs (Szilagyi et al., 2003). SCHIP benefits do *not* include the Medicaid EPSDT and long-term care benefits described in Chapter 9.

In 2003, children accounted for almost half of Medicaid enrollment and about 19 percent of program spending (Kaiser Commission, 2005). Children with disabilities accounted for about 75 percent of Medicaid spending for that population (Long and Coughlin, 2004–2005).

One problem for children and families is the instability of Medicaid, SCHIP, and other public insurance coverage. Children are frequently disenrolled and then reenrolled in one program option or another as a result of burdensome program requirements (e.g., requirements for periodic reenrollment or for the payment of premiums for some programs) or changes in family income or other family or child characteristics that determine whether a child is eligible for Medicaid, other public coverage, or no coverage (Dick et al., 2002; Summer and Mann, 2006). For example, studies of SCHIP indicate that requirements for frequent recertification and reenrollment contribute to high rates of disenrollment and that 25 percent of disenrolled children are reenrolled within 2 months (Dick et al., 2002). (During the period of disenrollment in SCHIP, some children will have become eligible for Medicaid and some will become covered by a parent's private health insurance, but specific information is lacking.)

These enrollment discontinuities affect children's access to timely and appropriate health care services, create difficulties for health care professionals and providers, and waste administrative resources. For example, children who are not continuously covered are more likely to delay care, have unfilled prescriptions, and go without needed services (Aiken et al., 2004; Olson et al., 2005). The loss of coverage, even if it is temporary, will disrupt the ongoing monitoring and assistance that children with certain conditions, for example, diabetes, require and that are provided in organized chronic care or disease management programs. Cumbersome administrative requirements also contribute to the fact that some 60 percent of children who remain uninsured are eligible for these programs but are not enrolled (Dorn and Kenney, 2006).

As discussed in Chapter 4, a prospective concern for poor children with disabilities who have qualified for Medicaid by virtue of qualifying for SSI is the requirement that at age 18 they undergo a new assessment to determine whether they meet the adult criteria for continued eligibility. Research suggests that young people who continue to receive SSI benefits after they reach age 18 are in poorer health and are less likely to be working than those who no longer receive benefits (Loprest and Wittenburg, 2005).

HEALTH INSURANCE MARKETS AND THEIR LIMITS FOR PEOPLE WITH DISABILITIES

Health insurance protects individuals and families from high health care costs. It has also become a positive means to encourage the timely use of beneficial health care services, in particular, relatively low-cost preventive services. The discussion below touches on only a few of the issues that are relevant to health insurance for people with disabilities. The focus is on certain aspects of health insurance markets that create difficulties for this population.

Standard Models of Insurance

Standard economic models of private health insurance build on the expectation that insurance is valuable to individuals because it mitigates the financial risk associated with medical care costs resulting from unpredictable illnesses or injuries (Phelps, 2003). The purchase of health insurance may also be viewed as an income transfer mechanism, whereby insurers transfer income from large numbers of mostly healthy purchasers of insurance to the small proportion of insured people who are ill and using medical care (see, e.g., Nyman [2005]).

The *insurable event* is a central concept in standard insurance models (see, e.g., Faulkner [1940], MacIntyre [1962], Donabedian [1976], and IOM [1993]). Conventionally, an insurable event is (1) individually unpredictable and unwanted, (2) relatively uncommon and costly, (3) precisely definable and measurable, (4) predictable for large groups, and (5) unlikely to occur to a large portion of the insured population simultaneously.

Violations of Standard Insurance Models in Health Care

Health insurance violates several of the just cited core principles of standard insurance models.[12] For example, unlike the events insured against by homeowners or automobile owners, health plans today frequently cover

---

[12]For a more comprehensive view of situations when insurance theory and actual realities diverge, see the work of Cutler and Zeckhauser (2004).

care for events that are clearly anticipated and even planned, such as pregnancy, childbirth, and vaccinations. Such practices can be explained, in part, by the view of public and private decision makers that insurance coverage is a reasonable vehicle to encourage the timely use of services that promote individual and public health.

Of greater relevance for this report is that insurance for much of the care used or needed by Americans who have serious chronic health conditions or disabilities does not fit the standard insurance model well. Certainly, some individuals with disabilities—for example, healthy young adults who have low vision or hearing—are not predictably high users of health care services. Nonetheless, for many people with disabilities or serious chronic illness, their future use of services is often fairly predictable. Individuals with progressive mobility impairments may, for instance, know or expect that they will soon need a wheelchair or some other assistive device. Similarly, people with certain disabling heart conditions know that they need ongoing drug therapy. As shown in Table 8-4, per person spending is substantially higher for people with serious disabilities than for others.

If people with chronic health conditions or disabilities are able to work—and particularly if they can work for a large employer—they can generally obtain private health insurance. If they must purchase private health insurance on an individual basis, they may find that no insurer will cover them or will do so only by charging them a premium that they cannot afford. The private market thus fails them. (As reported earlier, only 13 of the working-age adults with disabilities surveyed in the Medical Expenditure Panel Survey reported having nongroup health insurance.) Also, because health insurance is sold on a year-to-year basis, people with individually purchased insurance may find that they cannot renew the policy at an affordable price if they develop a serious chronic condition or disability during the course of a year.[13]

---

[13]As an alternative, some economists have proposed a kind of long-term health care insurance that people would buy when they are healthy and retain, possibly for decades, at premiums that would not change if an individual developed a chronic health condition or disability (see, e.g., Patel and Pauly [2002]). The approach is similar to that for long-term care insurance but would also apply to the kinds of acute and preventive care now covered under annual insurance policies. One concern under this model is that if an individual could not pay the premium at some point, then all the past payments would go for naught and the subsequent purchase of new coverage would be more costly than the old coverage. If that individual had developed health problems in the time since the original insurance purchase, he or she might not find an insurer willing to sell the individual coverage once he or she sought it anew. Also, at the time that people seek initial coverage, many who do not have chronic health conditions or disabilities can be identified through health questionnaires and screenings as being at moderate to high risk for these conditions, and thus not attractive prospects for this kind of insurance. No insurance company is marketing this kind of health insurance, which would (other things being equal) require a higher premium for the guarantee of renewability (Glied, 2005).

TABLE 8-4 Average Annual Expenditures for Health Care by Disability Status and Age Group for Working-Age Adults with Functional Limitations, Civilian Noninstitutional Population, Pooled Data, 1997 to 2002

Age (Years) and Limitation	Population Ages 18 to 64 (in 1,000s)	Total Expense ($, in millions)	Per Person with a Medical Event	
			Median Annual Expense ($)	Mean Annual Expense ($)
Total*a*	139,683	463,721	1,146	3,320
All 18-49 year-olds	102,059	268,196	883	2,628
No limits	94,909	204,343	816	2,153
Physical limits	5,329	37,963	3,115	7,124
IADL only	1,041	12,535	4,779	12,036
Any ADL	780	13,355	6,407	17,121
All 50-64 year-olds	37,623	195,525	2,198	5,197
No limits	31,037	118,518	1,834	3,819
Physical limits	5,148	50,083	5,293	9,729
IADL only	763	11,182	7,489	14,659
Any ADL	675	15,742	12,248	23,292

NOTE: Any ADL = having activity of daily living limitations, regardless of other limitations; IADL only = having only instrumental activity of daily living limitations; physical limitation = having no ADL or IADL limitations, i.e., mobility limitations only; no limitation = having no activity or mobility limitations.

*a*Only individuals who had a medical event (e.g., a hospitalization) were included in the total. Data for individuals who had eyeglass expenditures were not included in this table.

SOURCE: Olin and Dougherty (2006). Data from Medical Expenditure Panel Survey, 1997 to 2002.

Market Failure and Publicly Financed Health Insurance for Certain Groups

About 15 percent of the U.S. population lacks health insurance, and proposals to make insurance coverage universal through public programs or public subsidies have repeatedly failed. (One exception, which has yet to be fully implemented and proved, is the recent approval in Massachusetts of a plan to create ways for nearly all residents to obtain health insurance [Haislmaier and Owcharenko, 2006].) This response reflects the country's preference for private markets and its century-long reluctance to adopt—and pay taxes to finance—the kinds of universal or nearly universal publicly sponsored or supported health insurance programs that were adopted decades ago by virtually all economically developed countries.[14]

---

[14]This brief discussion draws from a large literature on the history of private and public health insurance—and uninsurance—in the United States (see, e.g., Somers and Somers [1961], Marmor [1973], Starr [1982], IOM [1993, 2004d], Berkowitz [2005–2006], Davis and Collins [2005–2006], and Moore and Smith [2005–2006]).

Nonetheless, despite the rapid growth of private, primarily employer-based health insurance during the 1940s and 1950s,[15] it was clear by 1960 that the private insurance market was limited in its ability to reach low-income groups and populations at high risk of incurring significant medical expenses. For example, in 1960, less than half of people age 65 or over had some form of private insurance. Those who did not have private insurance remained uninsured either because they could not afford it or because they were not considered insurable (Davis and Collins, 2005–2006).

With the passage of Medicare in 1965, policy makers opted for a public rather than a private insurance model for older people, who were covered without regard to income or health status. In 1972, the U.S. Congress extended Medicare to include a smaller group of younger Americans who had disabilities that severely limited their ability to work. As noted above, Medicare focuses on acute medical care and was not intended to finance the long-term institutional or personal care services needed by many beneficiaries with disabilities. Nonetheless, the program covers more non-acute care than is covered by private health insurance plans. From the outset, Medicare covered limited stays in skilled nursing homes and home health care visits after hospital stays (GAO, 1997). The rationale was that the provision of coverage for these services would be less costly than the provision of payment for inpatient services for beneficiaries recuperating after hospitalization (Kane et al., 1998). In 1980, the U.S. Congress eliminated the link to acute hospitalizations, but limits on the amounts of services remain (PL 96-499).

In creating Medicaid, the U.S. Congress established a different kind of program in which eligibility is, for the most part, limited to certain categories of poor or low-income individuals as well as those who have impoverished themselves in paying for long-term care (Moore and Smith, 2005–2006). Recognizing that poor people generally could not afford or budget for even relatively small expenses and that chronic illness and long-term care could threaten both poor and moderate-income people with destitution, policy makers included a wider range of services (e.g., medications, preventive services, eyeglasses, and long-term nursing home care) in Medicaid than in Medicare. Most beneficiaries do not pay premiums or copayments, although recent changes in federal law permit states to require such payments for an increasing number of Medicaid beneficiaries (see Chapter 9).

---

[15]During World War II, when wage and price controls were in effect, the U.S. Congress allowed employers to deduct payments for employee health insurance and certain other nonwage compensation. This helped spur the development of a strong basis for the group purchase of health insurance. The presence of large group purchasers that exist for purposes other than facilitating access to health insurance reduces the prospect that insurance will disproportionately be purchased by people at a high risk of needing health care.

Competition and Consumer Choice

In the past three decades, policy makers have strongly promoted competition and consumer choice among health plans, particularly within Medicare and Medicaid. Although consumers can benefit from having choices among qualified health care providers and health plans that compete on the basis of price and quality, this exercise of choice can, over time, seriously diminish the degree to which the burden of health care costs are shared between people who need few services and people with chronic health conditions who routinely need more services. Problems arise because people with chronic health conditions or disabilities are likely to want health plans with more extensive benefits (e.g., more choice of specialists, greater access to academic health centers, better drug or mental health care coverage, and lower deductibles and cost sharing) than people without disabilities (see, e.g., Kronick et al. [1996] and Batavia and DeJong [2001]).

Other things being equal, plans that offer benefits that disproportionately attract people with many health care needs will become disproportionately expensive. That is, they will require higher premiums than their benefit structure would imply if they had an "average" group of enrollees. Such premiums will, in turn, make these plans increasingly unattractive to healthier individuals so that their pool of enrollees becomes even more skewed and their premiums become even higher in relation to the actual benefits. The next section discusses this dynamic, its implications for health insurance markets, and methods for risk adjustment of payments to health plans to compensate them fairly for their enrollee population.

DISABILITY AND RISK ADJUSTMENT OF PAYMENTS TO HEALTH PLANS

The market dynamic just described is called "risk segmentation" or "risk selection."[16] The growth of employment-based health insurance and public insurance was a response to the insurance industry's understandable efforts to limit their exposure to this dynamic in the market for individual health insurance. Risk segmentation in health insurance markets undermines the sharing of financial risk among people with different levels of health care needs. Unless it is controlled or offset in some fashion, health

---

[16]The terms "risk selection" and "risk segmentation" are often used interchangeably. As used here, *risk selection* refers to the process by which people at higher risk of health care expenditures enroll in health plans different from those that people with lower risk enroll (IOM, 1993). *Risk segmentation* refers to the consequence of risk selection: health plans that differ systematically in the financial risk presented by their pools of enrollees. Risk segmentation may also be used to describe a health plan strategy or behavior aimed at selecting people who are good risks and avoiding people who are bad risks.

plans that attract disproportionate numbers of people with extensive health care needs (i.e., experience unfavorable selection) will become financially unsustainable. If these plans disappear but a subset of surviving plans then becomes particularly attractive to high-risk individuals, these plans, too, will become vulnerable. If the process successively drives all health plans to restrict coverage or charge exorbitant premiums to high-risk individuals (or go out of business), then only health plans with minimal benefits will survive, except perhaps for well-to-do or low-risk individuals. Given the subsidies and rules established by Medicare and Medicaid, program beneficiaries with disabilities are not at the same disadvantage as individuals trying to buy individual health insurance, but, as described below, they—and the system overall—can still encounter problems with competitive health plans.

The problem with the risk selection dynamic is not that some health plans do not survive. It is that the dynamic promotes a socially unproductive and inequitable competition for low-risk individuals rather than the efficient management of health care services that meet people's needs (GAO, 1991; Hall, 1992; Light, 1992; IOM, 1993; Kronick et al., 1996; Blumenthal et al., 2005). It particularly disadvantages people with serious chronic health conditions or disabilities. Policies and practices to control risk selection and minimize its harmful consequences are important to protect these groups.

The risk selection dynamic can be difficult to control. Governments, employers, and health plans themselves have devised a variety of strategies to try to manage risk selection or protect health plans or beneficiaries from significant negative risk selection. Strategies to protect health plans have ranged from the outrageous (e.g., Medicaid health plans that required in-person enrollment, which is more difficult for many people with disabilities) to the merely discouraging (e.g., excluding academic medical centers from provider panels) (see, e.g., Luft and Miller [1988] and Mehrotra et al. [2006b]). They also include a number of generally, if not universally, accepted practices, including employer or government limits on the number and types of plans that are offered and restrictions on the ways in which health plan features can differ. For example, as noted earlier, the Centers for Medicare and Medicaid Services (CMS) limits Medigap policies to 12 (formerly 10) standardized options (CMS, 2006b).

In the face of abuses, governments have also forbidden some discriminatory marketing, enrollment, and other practices. Other strategies used to manage risk (including risks from unexpected catastrophic care as well as from unfavorable risk selection) include stop-loss insurance or reinsurance (which protects health plans against extraordinary health care costs for one or several enrollees), risk corridors (which limit how much a plan can gain or lose), and risk pools (which provide for sharing of the financial risk across health plans) (see, e.g., Ladenheim et al. [2002], Palsbo and Post [2003], and Caterall et al. [2006]). In addition, the required collection and dissemination of risk- or case mix-adjusted information on the quality of services and outcomes for health plan members helps inform the decisions made by both health plan members and health plan sponsors. These and other administrative policies—which are important for health insurance programs that offer multiple health plans—attempt to focus plan competition on price and quality rather than risk selection. Each of these strategies has some value, but they do not substitute for a robust risk adjusted payment method that limits the pursuit and consequences of risk selection.

Risk adjustment methods seek to set payments to health plans on the basis of the health status or the health risk of plan enrollees so that plans are not penalized for disproportionately enrolling people with greater health care needs and thus are not encouraged to discriminate against this population. Appendix C provides a detailed discussion of these methods, the criteria used to evaluate them, and assessments of how well the existing methods meet these criteria. These methods have additional actual or potential uses in adjusting payments to health care providers, setting premiums for small employers in insurance purchasing pools, and improving the fairness of comparisons of provider costs and quality (see, e.g., Iezzoni [2003] and Martin et al. [2004]).

Interest in Risk Adjustment Methods

The federal government provided considerable impetus for the development and refinement of risk adjustment methods after it began to promote managed care and health plan competition within the Medicare program in the 1970s. Although some initially doubted the warnings of actuaries and others that these health plans could draw healthier beneficiaries away from the traditional Medicare program and lead to excess payments to health plans, most studies have reported favorable selection in the health plans (see, e.g., Luft [1987], Newhouse et al. [1989], Morgan et al. [1997], Iezzoni et al. [1998], Greenwald et al. [2000], and Zaslavsky and Buntin [2002]). That is, managed care plans were attracting individuals in better health with expected costs lower than provided for by Medicare's existing method of paying the plans, which relied primarily on demographic factors to adjust for risk. (Table 8-5 later in this chapter presents data comparing the original method to the current payment adjustment method.)

These results encouraged the federal government to support research to develop and test risk adjustment methods. In practice, however, state Medicaid programs initially led in adopting health-based risk adjustment methods (Martin et al., 2004). Not all states have adopted these methods, and many still contract with private health plans on bases that create incentives for health plans to avoid high-risk beneficiaries and also jeopardize plans that do not (Blumenthal et al., 2005). Palsbo and Post reported in 2003 that only 12 Medicaid programs were using advanced risk adjustment methods.

Private employers that offer multiple health plans to their employees also create the conditions for biased risk selection. Employees with chronic conditions may be disadvantaged by risk selection if the employer plans with more generous benefits are more costly, not just because they have more extensive benefits, but also because they have members with more chronic health problems. Also, if the process of risk selection contributes to the "natural" destruction of health plan options with more generous coverage, some employers may see the process as a means of reducing their costs that does not require an explicit decision to reduce benefits. A recent study found that the use of risk adjustment methods in the private sector is "uncommon and scattered" and that the methods used are sometimes proprietary and have not been subjected to the same kind of open validation process as methodologies used or considered by Medicare (Blumenthal et al., 2005; see also Keenan et al. [2001]).

Interest in risk adjustment methods that specifically consider disability is growing, not only because policy makers continue to be concerned about apparent overpayments to health plans by the current methods, but also because policy makers have been promoting Medicare special needs plans, which focus specifically on people with disabilities. The U.S. Congress has identified individuals with special needs as people who live in institutional settings, people who are dually eligible for Medicare and Medicaid, or people who have severe or disabling chronic conditions (Section 231 of the Medicare Modernization Act of 2003). Any health plan interested in serving these individuals—whether they are served under Medicare or state Medicaid rules, or both—would be particularly concerned about the accuracy of the government's risk adjustment method, including its accuracy for the entire group and particular subgroups within the population of those with special needs. Data show that health care expenditures are skewed even within groups of people with serious chronic health problems, although to a lesser degree than they are for the population overall (see, e.g., CBO [2005c]).

As of 2006, CMS had 226 special needs plans for people dually eligible for Medicare and Medicaid, 37 plans for institutionalized beneficiaries, and 13 plans for other beneficiaries with a specific severe or disabling chronic condition (Verdier and Au, 2006). Most of these plans have contracted with Medicare only, although approximately 40 also had contracts with state Medicaid programs (Verdier, 2006). The committee notes that the success of these plans and their pluses and minuses for people with disabilities will be affected by many factors, in addition to the adequacy of the risk-adjusted payment. These factors include Medicare and Medicaid administrative procedures, the complexities of integrating Medicare and Medicaid benefits, geographic differences in capitation rates, relationships with long-term care providers, and performance assessment methods and timetables (Verdier and Au, 2006). Many of the original special needs plans were sponsored by organizations that specialized in serving this group, but commercial HMOs have now set up many such plans.

Although it is important for all health plans, the addition of data and methods to assess the quality of care and outcomes is particularly important for special needs populations. For fairness, these methods—like those for plan payment—need to adjust for the risk presented by a health plan's membership (Iezzoni, 2003).

Desirable Characteristics of a Risk Adjustment Method

As Knutson writes in Appendix C, a perfect risk adjustment method would yield a health plan payment that "exactly fits the actual cost along the entire cost distribution for the population" with no systematic bias, only random sampling error (p. C-12). Under such conditions, more efficient plans should be able to serve their enrolled population at a cost below the cost projected by the risk adjustment model. Health plans would therefore not fear enrolling people with chronic conditions but might actually seek them both because they would bring in more income per enrollee and because they would offer more potential for profit through the efficient and economical management of services (especially if individuals were enrolling from fee-for-service Medicare).

Despite substantial improvements in methodology, this perfect risk adjuster does not exist. Each method in use or proposed has pluses and minuses related to accuracy and fairness, complexity, credibility to clinicians, cost of data collection, and susceptibility to manipulation or gaming by health plans. Box 8-1 lists several criteria for evaluating risk adjustment methods. It does not include political acceptability, but this is also an issue. Health plans that benefit from the current approach to risk adjustment tend not to support methods that would significantly reduce that benefit or require major changes in their operations.

In evaluations of various early risk adjustment methods, some analyses have considered risk selection and risk adjustment issues specific to people with disabilities (see, e.g., Lichtenstein and Thomas [1987], Tanenbaum and Hurley [1995], and Kronick and Drefus [1997]). Responding to the lack of disability-based adjustments, Kronick and colleagues (1996) developed the Disability Payment System and then the Chronic Illness and Disability Payment System (Kronick et al., 2000), which were created initially for Medicaid managed care programs serving people with disabilities and

---

BOX 8-1
Criteria for Assessing Risk Adjustment Methods

Predictive power: ability to accurately explain the variation in the expenses of a given population

Underlying logic: link to daily clinical practice and whether it is clinically meaningful to providers

Incentives: the behavior encouraged among providers and health plans in the short and long term

Resistance to "gaming": the degree to which providers and plans cannot manipulate the tool to their benefit, including an ability to verify and/or audit the results

Data availability: accessibility of the data upon which the tool is based, including the completeness, quality, and timeliness of the data

Transparency: ability of stakeholders to understand the basis and operation of the tool

Simplicity: how easy it is to implement and use

Reliability: how stable the risk scores are over time and with data from different health plans

Cost: monetary and non-monetary expense of the tool and of acquiring data.

SOURCE: Martin et al. (2004).

---

which were subsequently adapted to incorporate diagnoses (e.g., pregnancy) that are important to the general Medicaid population. The Chronic Illness and Disability Payment System method appears to be the most widely used method among the states that use risk adjustment (AHRQ, 2002; Martin et al., 2004). (Like the method recently adopted by Medicare, this method relies on diagnosis codes rather than measures of impairment or activity limitations as such.)

Evolution of Risk Adjustment Methods

Medicare's early efforts to adjust health plan payments to reflect the financial risk presented by their enrollees were rudimentary. The initial method computed an average adjusted per capita cost (AAPCC) that relied primarily on easily available demographic data: age, sex, institutional status, and, for noninstitutionalized individuals, their welfare status (plus county of residence). For policy reasons (e.g., to avoid disincentives for health plans to manage or control health care use), Medicare did not want to factor in the past use of health services, a primary variable that private health insurers use to establish "experience-rated" premiums for employer-based health plans. As noted above, a variety of early analyses showed that the use of demographic adjusters was not sufficient to compensate for risk selection. It resulted in overpayments to health plans with favorable selection (disproportionate enrollments of healthier individuals) and underpayments to plans with unfavorable selection.

The payment implications of the failure of risk adjustment methods to consider health risk are illustrated by an analysis by Manton and Stallard (1992). They used disability data from the National Long-Term Care Survey to compare the Medicare risk adjustment method then in place with an alternative that included data on limitations in ADLs. The researchers reported that when a Medicare HMO enrolled only "nondisabled (noninstitutional)" beneficiaries, its expected profit would be $300 per person per year, whereas the enrollment of "the noninstitutional disabled" would lead to a loss of $1,957 per person per year.

Acknowledging the inadequacies in the AAPCC, the U.S. Congress included in the Balanced Budget Act of 1997 provisions that directed the Health Care Financing Administration (which is now CMS) to take beneficiary health status into account in setting payments to managed care plans (Martin et al., 2004; Pope et al., 2004). In 2000, as a first step, CMS adopted the Principal Inpatient Diagnosis-Diagnostic Cost Group model. Then, in 2004, it switched to a 4-year phased-in implementation of the CMS Hierarchical Conditions Categories model (CMS-HCC). As described by its developers (Pope et al., 2004, pp. 122–123), the original classification system

> first classifies each of over 15,000 ICD-9-CM [*International Classification of Diseases*, 9th edition, Clinical Modification] codes into 804 diagnostic groups, or DxGroups. Each ICD-9-CM code maps to exactly one Dx-Group, which represents a well-specified medical condition, such as Dx-Group 28.01 Acute Liver Disease. DxGroups are further aggregated into 189 Condition Categories, or CCs. CCs describe a broader set of similar diseases, generally organized into body systems, somewhat like ICD-9-CM major diagnostic categories. Although they are not as homogeneous as DxGroups, CCs are both clinically- and cost-similar. An example is CC 28 Acute Liver Failure/Disease that includes DxGroups 28.01 and 28.02 Viral Hepatitis, Acute or Unspecified, with Hepatic Coma. Hierarchies are imposed among related CCs, so that a person is only coded for the most severe manifestation among related diseases. . . . Although HCCs reflect hierarchies among related disease categories, for unrelated diseases, HCCs accumulate. For example, a male with heart disease, stroke, and cancer has (at least) three separate HCCs coded, and his predicted cost will reflect increments for all three problems.

In response to concerns from health plans, the model modified for use by CMS cut the number of condition categories to 70, among other adjustments. Although the model improved the cost predictions for all beneficiaries by about 25 percent, it still underpredicted the costs for high-cost beneficiaries in the range of 12 to 15 percent. In addition to diagnostic information, the model also incorporates information about a beneficiary's age, sex, Medicaid status, and basis of qualifying for Medicare, specifically, qualifying on the basis of disability rather than age.

During the development of the current methodology, the analysts considered but rejected the inclusion of data on the rates of use of home health care services and durable medical equipment (Pope et al., 2000, 2004). These data, which take into account services disproportionately used by people with disabilities, improved the accuracy of the model but raised concerns about data reliability, possible manipulation by providers, and the administrative costs of collecting and auditing the data. The model does, however, take into account whether a beneficiary originally qualified for Medicare by virtue of disability (under SSDI).

As discussed in Appendix C, the addition of information about an individual's functional status adds modestly to the predictive power of methods that use diagnostic categories, primarily for individuals age 55 or over living in the community. One practical problem with using functional status information is that it is not routinely available for Medicare beneficiaries, for example, in claims data (Walsh et al., 2003; Kautter and Pope, 2004). Functional status information for the frailty adjuster discussed below must be collected through surveys of health plan participants.

The new health-based risk adjustment methods are a significant improvement over the original AAPCC, but they still allow overpayment for healthy individuals and underpayment for people with chronic health conditions or disabilities. For example, Hwang and colleagues compared demographic adjustment with four different diagnosis-based adjustment methods using data for children with chronic health conditions enrolled in Maryland's Medicaid program (Hwang et al., 2001). Although the researchers found that all four measures resulted in substantial improvement in accuracy over the demographic adjustment, they also found that all diagnosis-based methods had projected underpayments when the proportion of total health plan enrollment of children with chronic conditions reached 80 percent. The errors ranged from 5 to 10 percent. Kuhlthau and colleagues (2005) found similar results in an analysis of Medicaid data for three states and concluded that no method worked equally well in all situations.

Similarly, a recent analysis by the Medicare Payment Advisory Commission (MedPAC, 2005a) described the new risk adjustment methodology as a substantial improvement over demographic adjustments. Nonetheless, it also found that the method overpredicts payments for beneficiaries in better health and underpredicts the costliness of care for those in poorer health, as indicated by selected diagnoses or use of inpatient care or costliness in a previous year. Table 8-5 shows examples of how much Medicare overpaid or underpaid providers for different categories of beneficiaries. (For example, the new system overpaid by about 34 percent for the least costly 20 percent of beneficiaries and underpaid by about 17 percent for the most costly 20 percent.) As is typical of most analyses, the analysis did not consider predictions for beneficiaries by level of functional limitation or other indicator of disability.

For certain community-based demonstration programs serving Medicare beneficiaries with significant functional impairments, CMS has included—in addition to the basic risk adjustment used for all plans (see below)—a "frailty adjuster" (measured at the organizational level). It is intended to adjust for costs that the basic method does not consider. As implied by the label, the target population for method is the frail older person with "age-related physiologic vulnerability" (Kautter and Pope, 2004). The adjuster for a health plan starts with information about a person's difficulty

TABLE 8-5 Prediction of Medicare Beneficiary Costliness by Risk Adjustment Method

| Beneficiary Group | Predictive Ratios from Two Risk Adjusters | |
	CMS-HCCs	Age and Sex Only
Quintile of costliness in 2001		
Lowest	1.34	2.53
Second	1.30	1.96
Third	1.19	1.47
Fourth	0.98	0.96
Highest	0.83	0.44
Number of impatient stays in 2001		
Zero	1.07	1.38
One	0.96	0.65
Two	0.92	0.49
Three or more	0.80	0.29
Conditions diagnosed in 2001		
Alcohol or drug dependence	0.99	0.39
Congestive heart failure	0.90	0.50
Chronic obstructive pulmonary disease	0.93	0.67
Cerebral hemorrhage	1.09	0.65
Hip fracture	1.08	0.80

NOTE: Predictive ratio for a group = the group's mean costliness predicted by a risk adjuster divided by the mean of the group's actual costliness. If a risk adjuster predicts a group's costliness perfectly, predicted costliness equals actual costliness and the predictive ratio equals 1.0.
SOURCE: MedPAC (2005a).

with the performance of ADLs collected from a sample survey of the beneficiaries in each health plan residing in the community. CMS is considering whether to apply this additional adjustment to all health plans, whether or not they specialize in care for frail populations (Verdier, 2006). One concern is whether the frailty adjuster designed for a frail elderly population is appropriate for other populations. For example, some research suggests cost-relevant (and thus payment-relevant) differences in frailty and disability (see, e.g., Fried et al. [2004] and Bringewatt [2006]).

The issue of fair payment for health plan enrollees with disabilities remains a concern, despite analyses showing that, overall, Medicare is now paying Medicare Advantage plans considerably more per beneficiary than it would pay under fee for service (Biles et al., 2006; MedPAC, 2006). For example, one analysis estimated that Medicare's additional payments to these plans averaged 12.4 percent more than the costs for beneficiaries in the traditional program, for a total of $5.2 billion in extra costs overall—or $922 in extra costs per health plan enrollee (Biles et al., 2006). The higher payments are not unintentional. The Congress sharply increased payments to plans after previous payment changes (which are no longer in place) had led some plans to leave Medicare.

Even if Medicare is paying health plans generously overall, the additional payments to health plans do not correct the inaccuracies in risk adjustment methods, and thus they leave in place incentives to avoid high-risk individuals. Plans still profit more from enrolling healthier beneficiaries. Moreover, even if the new payment method reduces the disadvantage to plans that disproportionately enroll people with disabilities, those plans may still do poorly if they must compete against plans that seek or attract the people who are the best risks. In general, it is easier to profit from attracting low-risk individuals than from efficiently managing the care of those with chronic illnesses, and many health plans are responsible to shareholders for their financial performance. Thus, in addition to methods of adjusting health plan payments, it would be desirable to have risk-adjusted measures of the quality of care provided by health plans.

RECOMMENDATIONS

Improving Risk Adjustment Methods

The committee recognizes the long history of work by CMS to develop methods for paying health plans that do not encourage plans to favor healthier Medicare beneficiaries over beneficiaries who have more serious health conditions. The analyses cited above indicate that recent changes in Medicare's payment methods have significantly improved on previous demographic-based methods and have reduced the degree of underpayment for beneficiaries with costly health conditions. Nonetheless, it appears that the current method still substantially overpays for the least costly beneficiaries and modestly underpays for the most costly. To the extent that the medical home and chronic care models discussed in Chapter 4 work most easily in organized systems of care and under capitated payment arrangements that allow flexibility in the use of clinical and other resources, inadequate risk adjustment methods are a particular threat to the potential of these plans to improve health care for people with disabilities.

Although policy makers should be commended for their support of improved risk adjustment methods, they should not assume that improvements in risk adjustment methods are sufficient to the task of fairly paying health plans that serve people with disabilities and protecting the options of people with disabilities. As recommended below, they should continue to support research and data collection efforts to evaluate current and alternative methods and strategies to improve their accuracy and practicality. Evaluations of the effects of alternative payment methods (e.g., use of the frailty adjuster for different populations) and health plan designs (e.g., special needs plans of different kinds) on the quality of care for beneficiaries with disabilities are also important.

Because state Medicaid programs are also primary promoters of enrollment of Medicaid beneficiaries (including people with disabilities) in private health plans and because many states appear not to be using contemporary risk adjustment techniques, it would be prudent for CMS to commission an evaluation of the potential consequences of different state approaches to health plan payment, including the potential effects on both health plans and beneficiaries with disabilities and the rationale for the U.S. Congress to require the use of health-based risk adjustment.

> **Recommendation 8.1: The U.S. Congress should support continued research and data collection efforts to**
>
> • **evaluate and improve the accuracy and fairness of methods of risk adjusting payments to health plans serving Medicare and Medicaid beneficiaries;**
>
> • **assess how these methods affect the quality of health care for people with disabilities, including those enrolled in special needs plans; and**
>
> • **evaluate differences in the risk adjustment methods that state Medicaid programs use to pay health plans that enroll people with disabilities.**

Risk adjustment does not stand by itself as a means of limiting the negative consequences of risk selection in a competitive market. For example, policy makers also need to consider limiting the diversity of choices offered to consumers to make comparisons of health plans easier and to restrict health plan tactics to attract low-cost enrollees and discourage high-cost enrollees through benefit features. (As noted earlier, Congress has acted to standardize the options available in the Medigap policies.) Likewise, to supplement comparisons of plan price and features, consumers and policy makers need comparative information on the quality of plan processes and outcomes.

Although the committee did not examine the use of risk adjustment methods for other purposes, such as assessing and comparing the quality of care offered by health plans or health care providers, the continued refinement of methods for health plan payment purposes will likely be useful for these purposes. In addition, risk-adjusted information on the characteristics of those disenrolling from different plans is another element of a comprehensive approach to limiting and monitoring the negative consequences of risk selection.

The possible utility of including additional clinical information in risk adjustment tools is yet another issue for further evaluation. Inclusion of such information will likely require better health information systems. As noted in Chapter 4, the use of electronic medical records to support the coordination and evaluation of chronic care is still disappointingly limited.

One further issue that the committee did not examine in depth but that requires careful attention is whether Medicare and Medicaid should consider explicitly promoting and supporting health plans that truly specialize in the care of people with disabilities and that are, in a sense, "health plans of excellence" for this population. Several possible strategies or tools to implement such an option exist, including devising special payment arrangements, quality management mechanisms, administrative rules, and qualifying requirements. Risk adjustment methods might serve various purposes for payment, quality, and performance management in this environment. In any case, evaluation of special needs plans and changes in policies related to such plans is important to gauge their effects on people with disabilities.

Other Issues in Medicare and Medicaid

Although this committee supports the extension of health insurance to all people with serious chronic health conditions or disabilities, recommendations for achieving this goal are beyond its charge. The committee commends the principles for extending coverage that were set forth by a recent IOM committee that examined uninsurance in America (see Box 9-5 in Chapter 9). Lack of insurance is a particularly serious problem for people with disabilities.

On the basis of the review of coverage earlier in this chapter, the committee proposes more limited, albeit expensive, policy changes related to the SSDI-Medicare waiting period, incentives for work, and interruptions in SCHIP coverage. Chapter 9 includes additional recommendations related to coverage for assistive technologies and personal care services. It also suggests the value of formally monitoring changes in the Medicaid program that may negatively affect beneficiaries with disabilities.

Recommendation 8.2: To improve access to health insurance for people with disabling or potentially disabling health conditions, the U.S. Congress should
  • adopt a phased-in or selective elimination of the 24-month waiting period for Medicare eligibility for people who have newly qualified for Social Security Disability Insurance;
  • encourage continued testing of methods to reduce disincentives in public insurance programs for people with disabilities to return to work; and
  • direct states to limit recertification and reenrollment for the State Children's Health Insurance Program to no more than once a year for children with disabilities.

Members of the U.S. Congress have introduced various proposals to reduce or eliminate the 24-month waiting period for all or some SSDI beneficiaries (e.g., terminally ill individuals or those with conditions that could prove fatal without treatment) (see, e.g., Whittaker [2005]). Most recently, in 2001, Congress authorized an exception for people with amyotrophic lateral sclerosis (PL 106-554).

The primary current obstacle to the complete removal of the 24-month waiting period between the start of SSDI benefits and Medicare eligibility is cost. Dale and Verdier (2003) estimated that elimination of the waiting period at the start of 2002 would have cost Medicare $8.7 billion that year (for those qualifying on the basis of their own work records, in 2000 dollars). Some offsetting federal (and state) savings would accrue in the Medicaid program, but the estimated $2.5 billion in federal Medicaid savings would not offset the additional federal costs (the net cost to Medicare would thus have been $6.2 billion).

Short of eliminating the waiting period, the Social Security Administration is conducting demonstration projects that would allow the agency, under certain circumstances, to provide medical benefits to people in the waiting period and, in some situations, to provide benefits to SSDI applicants (SSA, 2006d). For example, the Accelerated Benefits Demonstration project will provide immediate health benefits to new SSDI beneficiaries who have medical conditions that are expected to improve or that might improve if they obtain appropriate medical care. The project will also include employment supports. A primary objective of the demonstration is to help individuals improve their health and functioning enough that they might "improve their self-sufficiency through employment" (SSA, 2006d). The agency is considering another demonstration project that would provide interim medical benefits to certain applicants for SSDI who have no insurance, whose health would likely improve with treatment, and for whom additional medical information would assist the disability adjudication process.

The committee strongly encourages the agency to pursue these demonstration projects and other strategies that would help reduce the features of the program that discourage work and thereby undermine the goals of independence and community participation that are the hallmarks of modern disability policies. Nonetheless, these approaches will affect only a subset of individuals, a subset that is likely to have the best chance of recovery, and will exclude the most vulnerable. In the absence of a complete phase out of the waiting period, the Congress could consider the expanded use of exceptions or other strategies that would target particularly vulnerable groups.

The Congress has created some options for states to provide Medicaid coverage for certain low-income people with disabilities who have qualified for SSDI or SSI but who can work (Lopez-Soto and Sheldon, 2002; Teitelbaum et al., 2005). For example, among other provisions, the Ticket to Work and Work Incentives Improvement Act of 1999 enhances earlier legislation that allows states to continue Medicaid benefits for individuals with disabilities who enter or reenter the workforce and who meet certain income and asset criteria. Eligible individuals may, however, have to pay premiums ("buy in") or cover other costs (e.g., make copayments for services). The legislation also extends to 8.5 years the period of premium-free Medicare Part A coverage for people receiving SSDI who return to work. As useful as these federal and state programs may be for some people, they lack the reach of federal and state policies that have extended insurance coverage for children. It is important that policy makers continue to develop and evaluate policies that remove or reduce economic and other barriers to work for people with disabilities, including barriers related to eligibility requirements for public insurance.

Notwithstanding the successful expansion of health insurance for children through the SCHIP program, interruptions in coverage are a problem in this program. As discussed earlier in this chapter, studies have identified administrative practices that increase such interruptions, in particular, requirements for active recertification and reenrollment every 6 months. Requiring recertification no more often than every 12 months would reduce administrative barriers to continuing enrollment in SCHIP of children with disabilities or special health care needs.

As noted above, Chapter 9 includes recommendations related to Medicare and Medicaid coverage for assistive technologies and personal care services. In addition, it cites examples of troubling and complicated actions taken by state Medicaid programs that may seriously affect people with disabilities, even when protections for this group supposedly exist.

9

Coverage of Assistive Technologies and Personal Assistive Services

After retiring a few years ago, Mr. B led a vigorous independent life until he experienced a major stroke. Paralyzed on his right side, he now needs a wheelchair to move around his house, where he has lived alone since his wife died. The contractor who processes Medicare claims for this kind of medical equipment approved a manual wheelchair, but with his paralyzed right arm, Mr. B cannot self-propel it. He has asked for approval for a power wheelchair, but the contractor—citing Medicare rules—insists on additional documentation that the more expensive equipment is required. All this is time-consuming, complex, and frustrating, even though Mr. B's rehabilitation team is helping. In the meantime, Mr. B is having difficulty getting around at home, and he and his daughter are worrying about what he will do if his request is not approved.

This story—recounted by an airline employee to a committee member who uses a scooter—illustrates the hurdles that individuals often face in trying to obtain coverage from a public or a private health plan for wheelchairs and other mobility assistive devices. Persistence in appealing denials and assistance from professionals in navigating complex policies and procedures are often necessary when someone wishes to have coverage for particular assistive devices and services approved—and even then, success is not assured.

This chapter focuses on the second issue in health care financing included in the committee's charge: health insurance coverage of assistive technologies. Because personal assistance services sometimes serve similar purposes for people with disabilities, this chapter also examines coverage of these services. The discussion begins with a brief, general overview of the types of coverage policies and limitations that may affect access to services important to people with disabilities. The subsequent two sections describe insurance coverage of assistive technologies and services. A short section on access to services or equipment through programs not based on insurance follows. The chapter then considers the challenges of expanding coverage in an environment of high and increasing health care costs. The final section presents recommendations.

Overall, the committee found that many of the health plan coverage policies identified in the 1991 Institute of Medicine (IOM) report *Disability in America* continue to be targets of criticism more than 15 years later. The concept and interpretation of medical necessity remain controversial, as do statutory and regulatory limits on coverage for assistive technologies and personal care services. In many areas, health care financing policies have not evolved to support the independence and community participation of people with disabilities. One major exception is the expanded use by states of waivers of certain Medicaid regulations to cover a wider range of "home- and community-based" services as alternatives to institutional care. For the most part, as also described in Chapters 4, 6, and 8, this nation's system of health care financing and delivery is not well designed to meet the needs of people with chronic health conditions or disabilities.

The question of whether a technology or service is covered by a health plan arises only for people who are insured. As described in the preceding chapter, although Medicare covers virtually all older adults, almost 14 percent of younger adults with a physical limitation and 8 percent of those with a limitation in activities of daily living (ADLs) are uninsured, as are almost 5 percent of children with special health care needs. For people who are uninsured or whose health plans do not pay for assistive technologies or personal assistance services, the options include going without; paying for the item personally (often called "out-of-pocket payment" or "self-payment"); or securing assistance from vocational rehabilitation, assistive technology, or other special public or private programs, some of which are described below.

Neither this chapter nor the previous one offers a comprehensive examination of health care financing issues relevant to people with disabilities, a task that would demand a report in itself. For example, this chapter does not examine coverage of occupational and physical therapy, including the concerns that have been raised that Medicare payment caps on these services could harm patients with mobility and other impairments.[1] It

---

[1]Responding to rising costs and evidence of improper billing, the Balanced Budget Act of 1997 provided for two dollar-amount caps per beneficiary for outpatient therapy services that were not provided in a hospital outpatient setting: one cap for occupational therapy and another cap for physical therapy services and speech language pathology services combined (GAO, 2005). Although the Centers for Medicare and Medicaid Services is supposed to develop an outpatient therapy payment system that recognizes patient needs and justifies individual waivers of the caps, the agency has, according to the Government Accountability Office (GAO, 2005), lacked the data necessary to do so. The U.S. Congress has provided temporary moratoria on the caps for most of the period since they were implemented in 1999. The Deficit Reduction Act of 2005 (which was enacted in February 2006) provided that exceptions to the

also does not consider controversies over payment rules for specialized inpatient rehabilitation facilities that critics argue will deny many people with disabilities the appropriate intensity of care because the rules rely on an outdated or questionable set of diagnoses to define the patient mix that facilities must have to qualify for payment (see, e.g., Hackbarth [2003] and Thomas [2005]).[2] The committee recognizes that inadequate provider payments levels and methods can affect the availability and quality of services and health care. Along with inadequate professional education, they can contribute to the problems that people with disabilities often report in finding health care professionals who understand their medical condition and its nonmedical dimensions, who appreciate their need for routine health promotion and primary care services, and who have accessible facilities and equipment.

The committee also recognizes that rising health care costs, particularly costs for Medicare and Medicaid, make some of the changes proposed in this chapter difficult. Decisions to pay for such changes by reducing spending elsewhere or by increasing taxes will present policy makers with hard choices—particularly in the context of pressure to control overall spending growth in federal health care programs. Successful steps to make health care services more efficient and to control fraudulent and abusive practices by providers and suppliers will help reduce spending but, in the committee's view, are unlikely to suffice.

TYPES OF LIMITATIONS ON COVERAGE

For an insured individual, coverage of any service or product depends on the answers to several questions. First, is the product or service explic-

---

cap could be granted for medically necessary services under certain circumstances for calendar year 2006 (CMS, 2006i; Vettleson, 2006). For example, certain conditions or diagnoses, such as hip replacement or aphasia, qualify for an automatic exception to the therapy caps when they are supported by a documented need for services exceeding the cap. The act provided for a manual exception process for beneficiaries who have conditions or diagnoses that are not covered by the automatic exception and who also have a documented need for services exceeding the cap amount.

[2] Medicare rules require that 75 percent of the admissions of inpatient rehabilitation facilities be concentrated in 1 of 10 diagnoses (the "75 percent rule"). Full implementation of the rules has been delayed, but the rules are set to go into effect fully in 2007. Providers have argued that the 10 diagnoses (which were defined in 1983 as a way of excluding these facilities from application of the rules of the hospital prospective payment system) are no longer sufficient to describe the core patient population needing their services. Advocates for people with disabilities have argued that the rule will force many people into settings where they receive less intensive health care, such as nursing homes (Thomas, 2005). In 2003, the Medicare Payment Advisory Commission (Hackbarth, 2003) reported that more than 85 percent of facilities were estimated to be out of compliance with the requirement.

itly covered (or excluded), or if it is not, is it covered (or excluded) under a broad category of services or products? Second, what general additional criteria or conditions apply to coverage? Third, does a given individual's specific situation meet the requirements for coverage? The answers to these questions are not always easy for a patient, family member, or health care provider to determine. The answers may vary depending on the source of insurance and the specific type of assistive service or technology.

Medical Necessity and Coverage

By statute, Medicare is prohibited (unless it is explicitly authorized) from paying for services and items that are not "reasonable and necessary for the diagnosis or treatment of illness or injury or to improve the functioning of a malformed body member" (42 CFR 1395y(a)(1)(A)). The U.S. Congress has made certain statutory exceptions to the diagnosis and treatment restrictions, for example, by authorizing coverage of selected preventive services such as screening mammography. Otherwise, this "medical necessity" provision provides the basis both for decisions about coverage of whole categories of technologies or services (e.g., personal care services) and for decisions about coverage in individual cases. For example, a service or product may be covered for one individual and denied for another because the service or item was judged to be not reasonable and necessary given the latter individual's diagnosis and condition (e.g., a power wheelchair for someone who can operate a manual wheelchair). (See also the discussion in Appendix D.)

Medical necessity criteria have proved particularly troublesome for people with disabilities seeking coverage of assistive technologies and personal care services. They may be invoked to deny payment for nonmedical services, such as assistance with bathing, or products, such as bathroom grab bars, that help people manage daily life or protect their health (e.g., by avoiding falls). Because the rules and procedures are complex, otherwise approvable claims may also be denied because beneficiaries or their providers did not correctly document the case for coverage or because the organizations administering claims for services applied policies inconsistently or incorrectly. Denials of claims for certain assistive technologies and services based on the failure to meet medical necessity criteria are disheartening and confusing and reduce people's ability to function at home and in the community (Iezzoni and O'Day, 2006).

Federal law does not define medical necessity for the Medicaid program, and state definitions vary and may be broader than the Medicare definition (Rosenbaum et al., 2002; Perkins et al., 2004).[3] Connecticut's language is particularly broad, covering health care that is provided "to correct or diminish the adverse effects of a medical condition or mental illness; to assist an individual in attaining or maintaining an optimal level of health; [or] to diagnose a condition or prevent a medical condition from occurring" (Connecticut Department of Social Services, 2003, p. 2). A number of states refer to services for conditions that may cause or worsen a disability or that may prevent deterioration of a health condition (Rosenbaum et al., 2005).

Definitions of medically necessary care also vary for private health plans. Many use definitions and interpretations similar to those governing Medicare.

Medicare administrators have devoted considerable effort to developing guidance for providers and consumers about when a service will or will not be covered (CMS, 2006e). The decision memo on assistive mobility technologies discussed later in this chapter is in an example. Nonetheless, the great range of individual care needs and circumstances makes it difficult to eliminate subjective decision making and variability.

Other Coverage Limitations

Even if a service or a product is not excluded for lack of medical necessity, various provisions of public or private health plans may limit access. Examples include

- restrictions that apply temporarily or indefinitely to someone with a preexisting condition (but the federal rules described in Chapter 8 limit the length of such restrictions in group insurance policies);
- limits on the number of services (e.g., 20 home visits) that will be reimbursed;
- caps on total reimbursement (e.g., $1,000 for home medical equipment);
- restrictions on who can provide a service (e.g., excluding coverage for personal care provided by a family member); and
- widespread requirements that individuals pay part of the cost of a service or product.

---

[3]One exception to the discretion of states to define medical necessity is the legislation that created the Early Periodic Screening, Diagnostic, and Treatment benefit for children. It specifies that children are entitled to "necessary . . . diagnostic services, treatment and other measures . . . to correct or ameliorate defects and physical and mental illnesses and conditions discovered by the screening services" (Section 1905(r)(5) of the Social Security Act, cited by Peters [2006]).

Most such restrictions are intended to control programs costs. The intent may be to discourage spending on services of minimal benefit or to limit fraudulent or abusive practices by health care providers and vendors.[4] Some coverage restrictions have quality-of-care objectives. For example, coverage of complex, high-risk procedures may be limited to specifically approved facilities (e.g., a Medicare-approved center for heart or lung transplantation). Likewise, as described in Chapter 7, coverage and marketing of complex medical equipment may require U.S. Food and Drug Administration approval on the basis of evidence of safety and perhaps effectiveness. The rejection of a service or product for coverage on the basis of evidence of harm or ineffectiveness also serves quality-of-care objectives.[5] Yet another example of a coverage-related policy that serves quality objectives is the recently issued quality standards for suppliers of durable medical equipment, prosthetics, orthotics, and medical supplies (CMS, 2006c).

COVERAGE OF ASSISTIVE TECHNOLOGIES

Chapter 7 defined assistive technologies, consistent with the Assistive Technology Act of 1998, as any item, piece of equipment, or product system, whether it is acquired commercially, modified, or customized, that is used to increase, maintain, or improve the functional capabilities of individuals with disabilities. It also noted that the broad legislative language intentionally permitted programs created by the legislation to cover general use products if, for a given individual, such a product worked as well as or better than for a specially designed product. That breadth does not extend to federal or private health insurance plans.

As described by Iezzoni and O'Day (2006), assistive technology "re-

---

[4]A recent Government Accountability Office report cited an estimate by the Centers for Medicare and Medicaid services that Medicare made about $700 million in improper payments for durable medical equipment, prostheses, orthotics, and supplies between April 1, 2005, and March 31, 2006 (GAO, 2007). The report defined improper payments as resulting from clerical errors, the misinterpretation of program rules, fraud ("an intentional act or representation to deceive with knowledge that the action or representation could result in gain"), and abuse (which "typically involves actions that are inconsistent with acceptable business and medical practices and result in unnecessary cost") (p. 1).

[5]Consistent with the Medicare statute, those administering Medicare and other health insurance programs have increasingly sought evidence of effectiveness before covering new procedures (e.g., lung volume reduction surgery) or products (e.g., implantable automatic defibrillators) (Strongin, 2001; IOM, 2000a; CMS, 2005c, 2006e). Only limited evidence supporting the effectiveness of existing covered services may be available, but a lack of evidence is typically a more prominent issue for new technologies. In some cases, coverage may be restricted to those participating in a clinical trial that is intended to provide evidence that Medicare can use to make a coverage decision. Coverage approval criteria for Medicare do not include evidence of cost-effectiveness, although the implementation of such a criterion has been proposed (CMS/HCFA, 2000; Garber, 2004; Neumann et al., 2005).

sides at that fractious border between covered and uncovered benefits" (p. 150). Wolff and colleagues (2005) observed that, although most health plans cover some assistive technology, "its predominant use in daily functioning rather than for therapeutic purposes has contributed to ambiguity in health insurance coverage. Coverage policies are typically stringent, and coverage disputes in this area are among the most common and problematic" (Wolff et al., 2005, p. 1140).

A 2001 University of Michigan survey of people with disabilities found that approximately 40 percent of people who obtained assistive technologies paid for them out of pocket (Carlson and Berland, 2002).[6] Private health insurance and Medicare were the primary third-party sources of payment, and each was mentioned as a source of payment by between 15 and 20 percent of respondents. Free provision, Medicaid, and the U.S. Department of Veterans Affairs were each mentioned as a source of payment by between 5 and 10 percent of respondents. As reported in Chapter 7, about 40 percent of respondents reported that the use of assistive technologies had reduced their need for help from another person. Nevertheless, the users of assistive technologies cite a lack of funding and a lack of information about appropriate technologies as barriers to access (NCD, 2000b).

Freiman and colleagues (2006) recently reviewed public funding for an array of assistive technologies. Table 9-1 summarizes their conclusions about the extent of public insurance coverage of several kinds of technologies. It shows a very mixed pattern of coverage with the U.S. Department of Veterans Affairs most consistently offering coverage (see also PAI [2002]).

Medicare

Medicare covers certain medically necessary assistive technologies under its statutory benefits for durable medical equipment, prosthetic devices, and orthotic devices (42 U.S.C. 1395(k), (m), and (x)). It specifically excludes coverage of certain assistive items, notably, hearing aids and eyeglasses (except that one pair of glasses is covered following cataract surgery) (42 U.S.C. 1395y). The statutory definition of durable medical equipment includes some items, such as oxygen tents, that are not usually considered assistive technologies.

The federal officials and private contractors who administer Medi-

---

[6]The Medical Expenditure Panel Survey, which is used for many purposes, divides spending on assistive technologies in ways that make it difficult to determine the source of payment in any comprehensive way (Freiman et al., 2006). For example, Medicaid spending through home- and community-based service waivers (including payments for assistive technologies) is categorized under "other personal health care," and other spending may be included in either the durable medical equipment category or the other medical equipment category, both of which include items other than assistive technologies.

TABLE 9-1 Summary of Public Health Plan Coverage of Assistive Technology

Assistive Technology Category	Coverage Provided by:			
	Medicare[a]	Medicaid State Plans[a,b]	Medicaid Waivers[b]	VA
Personal ATs for ADLs	Some	Yes	Some	Yes
Personal mobility ATs	Yes	Yes	Some	Yes
Orthotics and prostheses	Yes	Yes	Some	Yes
Hearing, vision, and speech ATs and augmentative communication	Little	Some	Some	Yes
Cognitive ATs	No	No	Some	No
Transportation ATs	No	No	No	Yes
Home modifications	No	No	Some	Yes

NOTE: Medicaid state plans = benefits included in a state's approved plan, including optional benefits that states choose to provide, must be provided statewide and cannot be capped; a provision of the Deficit Reduction Act of 2005, adopted since the data for this table were collected, makes exceptions for certain home-and community-based services that previously required waivers. Medicaid waivers = benefits approved as part of an approved waiver may be capped, targeted to specific groups (e.g., individuals with brain injuries), and limited to certain geographic areas of a state; some = although some items are covered, a significant portion of the assistive technologies in this category are not covered; ADL = Activities of daily living; AT = assistive technology; VA = U.S. Department of Veterans Affairs.

[a]Coverage needs to meet medical necessity criteria.

[b]Due to state-by-state coverage variations, the information in this column roughly represents the modal coverage by the states.

SOURCE: Freiman et al. (2006 [used with permission]).

care have developed interpretations of statutes and regulations to guide decisions about coverage in individual cases. Examples of assistive items excluded under such guidance as *not* meeting the criteria for coverage are bath seats, grab bars, humidifiers, home elevators, and wheelchair ramps (*Medicare Carriers Manual*, Section 2100.1). They are considered convenience items, not medical items, even though some of this equipment may help prevent falls and otherwise protect an individual's health.

One critical statutory requirement is that durable medical equipment must involve use in the home. Based on the statute, regulations define durable medical equipment as "equipment furnished by a supplier or a home health agency that: (1) can withstand repeated use; (2) is primarily and customarily used to serve a medical purpose; (3) generally is not useful to an individual in the absence of an illness or injury; and (4) *is appropriate for use in the home*" (42 CFR 414.202) (emphasis added).[7] As discussed below,

---

[7]In 2001, approximately 6.5 percent of Medicare beneficiaries living in the community used the durable medical equipment benefit to obtain a mobility-related assistive device: 2.6 percent

the home use provision has been restrictively interpreted to limit coverage of mobility assistive equipment that helps beneficiaries get around outside the home. Coverage may require a prescription, and repairs to equipment are usually covered only if the equipment is rented (DATI, 2005).

A recent example of administrative guidance on coverage determinations involved a 2005 decision memorandum that was intended to clarify the interpretation of the statute and regulations related to mobility assistive devices, including manual and power wheelchairs (CMS, 2005b). It replaced a more restrictive proposal that had been prompted by concerns about rapidly increasing spending for power wheelchairs and specific instances of fraud and abuse (see, e.g., GAO [2004]).[8] Although the memorandum liberalized the policy in some respects, it left critical restrictions in place, as described below. The document, which was developed with the involvement of other governmental agencies and outside experts, cited evidence identified through a literature review that the equipment was reasonable and necessary for beneficiaries with mobility limitations. The memorandum stressed that determinations of coverage should include assessment of "the technology that most appropriately addresses the beneficiary's needs as determined by the coverage criteria" (CMS, 2005b, p. 9). Clearly, such an assessment involves subjective judgments that can lead to variations in individual coverage decisions.

Unfortunately, based on the statutory reference to durable medical equipment used in the home, the memorandum focused on individual needs related to ADLs, which are primarily performed in the home, rather than instrumental activities of daily living, which include some activities (e.g., shopping and traveling) that occur outside the home. Thus a power wheelchair would be covered for an individual who needs the device both for personal care activities in the home and for travel outside the home but not for an individual who requires the device only outside the home. A person might also be denied coverage if the device could not actually be used in the home because of the home's small size or floor plan. Furthermore, on the basis of a particularly restrictive interpretation of the home use criterion, coverage may be limited to a type of wheelchair or other equipment that will not allow people to travel easily or safely outside the home. Thus the statutory and regulatory criteria for coverage of assistive technologies are quite different from those for coverage of surgical and medical interventions. For example, hip replacement surgery would not be challenged

---

for a manual wheelchair, 2.4 percent for a walker, 1.0 percent for a cane, and 0.5 percent for a power wheelchair (Wolff et al., 2005). Beneficiaries obtaining wheelchairs were younger and had more limitations in ADLs than beneficiaries obtaining canes or walkers but were less likely to have been hospitalized.

[8]The new policy replaced the past policy that limited coverage to individuals who were "bed or chair confined."

for individuals simply because pain limited their activities outside but not inside their home.[9] (The necessity of surgery might still be challenged for other reasons.)

The "use-in-the-home" language of the statute has become a central issue in efforts to revise Medicare policies on durable medical equipment. Critics of current interpretations argued that the language was intended to distinguish between equipment suitable for home use and equipment that required an institutional setting. As one advocacy group has argued: "[t]he intent of the 'in the patient's home' clause was not to make elderly and disabled persons prisoners in their own homes" (UCP, 2006, unpaged).

Clearly, the "use-in-the-home" restriction, especially as it is now interpreted, is inconsistent with the values of independence and community participation that have become widely recognized elsewhere in federal health and social policies since Medicare was enacted. Nonetheless, efforts to change the statute have, to date, not succeeded. Also, although the Centers for Medicare and Medicaid Services (CMS) was to consider the appropriateness of the "in-home" criterion as part of President George W. Bush's New Freedom Initiative and in light of efforts to promote work and community living, CMS action seems to be limited to congressionally directed demonstration projects (DHHS, 2002).[10]

The evidence base for many assistive technologies and services important to people with disabilities is limited, which points to the need for more research in this area (Clancy and Andresen, 2002). In a paper that outlines the many financial obstacles to accessible assistive technologies, the American Academy of Physical Medicine and Rehabilitation observed that "to be fair, Medicare is often asked to approve coverage and reimbursement of assistive technology with little clinical data [or] outcomes studies" (AAPM&R/FPM&R, 2003, p. 5). As noted above, CMS judged that the evidence base supported the coverage of much mobility assistive equipment for people with limitations in ADLs.

Criticism is often directed at government officials and Medicare contractors for their restrictive coverage decisions, but certain coverage restrictions appear to be so firmly based in the Medicare statute that statutory change is needed to permit easier access to assistive technologies that support independence and productivity. The home use criterion for durable medical equipment is one example, at least as it relates to durable medical

---

[9]Also, as pointed out by the American Academy of Physical Medicine and Rehabilitation (AAPM&R/FPM&R, 2003), the home use criterion is not found in the statutory discussion of prosthetics.

[10]CMS was also to consider allowing trial rental periods for expensive equipment that is usually purchased and allowing equipment to be furnished to people in skilled nursing facilities for up to 1 month prior to discharge to provide time for equipment adjustments, training, and practice in using the equipment (DHHS, 2002).

equipment that cannot actually be used inside the home but that can help people get around in the community. The statutory language related to medically necessary care is another example. Given the statute, more expansive administrative interpretations can only go so far.

Medicaid Coverage

Medicare is a national program, despite some variability in interpretation of Medicare coverage policies or guidelines by the private contractors who administer the program.[11] Medicaid, in contrast, operates under federal standards that give states considerable authority to determine whether individuals should have access to assistive technologies. Under federal law, home health services are a required element of state Medicaid programs, and certain medical equipment and supplies are a required part of home health care coverage (42 CFR 440.70). Even when a Medicaid program covers assistive technologies, it may still impose various restrictions, such as caps on the amount that will be paid for equipment.

Some items, such as hearing aids and prosthetic devices, are optional for most adults but are required for children under the Medicaid's Early Periodic Screening, Detection, and Treatment (EPSDT) benefit. (The State Children's Health Insurance Program [SCHIP] option, which covers many children with special health care needs, does not include EPSDT benefits as such.) As summarized in Box 9-1, the EPSDT benefit covers an extensive array of services for children, including health care that "must be made available for treatment or other measures to correct or ameliorate defects and physical and mental illnesses or conditions discovered by the screening services" (CMS, 2005e, unpaged; see also the discussion of EPSDT in Chapters 4 and 8). Many of these services are particularly relevant for children with disabilities (see, e.g., Smith et al. [2000]). As described later in this chapter, the passage of the Deficit Reduction Act of 2005 has raised some concerns about children's continued access to EPSDT services.

As discussed further in the section on personal assistance services, the U.S. Congress has authorized waivers of certain Medicaid requirements in a variety of situations. Nearly all states have received waivers for home- and community-based service programs that are intended to facilitate care in the community for people who would otherwise be at high risk of needing institutional care. Most waiver programs for adults age 65 and over include some coverage of home modifications (e.g., installation of grab bars and widening of doors to accommodate wheelchairs) and some products (e.g.,

---

[11]Medicare policies do, however, differ in a number of respects for beneficiaries enrolled in the traditional fee-for-service program and those enrolled in Medicare-approved private health plans, in that the latter may choose to cover some services not usually covered.

BOX 9-1
Medicaid's Early Periodic Screening,
Detection, and Treatment Benefits
(as required under Section 1905(r) of the Social Security Act)

Screening Services (all of the following):
- Comprehensive health and developmental history (physical and mental health);
- Comprehensive unclothed physical exam;
- Appropriate immunizations;
- Laboratory tests;
- Lead toxicity screening;
- Health education (for parents and children);
- Vision services (including diagnosis and treatment for defects in vision, including eyeglasses);
- Dental services (including relief of pain and infections, restoration of teeth and maintenance of dental health);
- Hearing services (include diagnosis and treatment for defects in hearing, including hearing aids); and
- Other necessary health care to correct or ameliorate defects, and physical and mental illnesses and conditions discovered by the screening services.

Diagnosis
When a screening examination indicates the need for further evaluation of an individual's health, provide diagnostic services. The referral should be made without delay and follow-up to make sure that the recipient receives a complete diagnostic evaluation. If the recipient is receiving care from a continuing care provider, diagnosis may be part of the screening and examination process. States should develop quality assurance procedures to assure comprehensive care for the individual.

Treatment
Health care must be made available for treatment or other measures to correct or ameliorate defects and physical and mental illnesses or conditions discovered by the screening services.

Any additional diagnostic and treatment services determined to be medically necessary must also be provided to a child diagnosed with an elevated blood lead level.

SOURCE: CMS (2005e).

---

personal emergency response systems) that are excluded under conventional Medicaid coverage guidelines (Freiman et al., 2006).

Although most discussions of assistive technologies focus on people living in the community, these technologies may also benefit people living in residential care facilities, including nursing homes. Examples range from wheelchairs and hearing aids to products that assist with cognition and "wander management" systems for people with dementia. A recent report identified several barriers to the use of such technologies in institutions, including a perceived lack of financial resources (Freedman et al., 2005a). It noted that Medicaid and Medicare do not specifically reimburse organizations for the devices that they supply to the residents of nursing homes, although the programs do pay for covered devices that individuals obtain directly from equipment vendors.

Private Health Insurance

The committee found little specific information on private health plan coverage of different kinds of assistive technologies.[12] In general, people covered by private health plans will often encounter problems with coverage restrictions and medical necessity determinations similar to those that that Medicare beneficiaries face (Iezzoni, 2003; Iezzoni and O'Day, 2006).

A few states have mandates that require private insurance plans to cover certain assistive technologies, primarily hearing aids and prostheses, subject to various restrictions. For example, seven states (Connecticut, Kentucky, Louisiana, Maryland, Minnesota, Missouri, and Oklahoma) require coverage of hearing aids for children and one (Rhode Island) requires coverage for children and adults (ASHA, 2007). The reach of these mandates is, however, limited by federal law that exempts self-insured employer health plans from such mandates and from many other state regulations (Mendelsohn, 2006).

In addition to outright exclusions, private health plans often place fairly low limits (e.g., $1,500) on the maximum amount that they will pay for assistive equipment during a year. They may also limit how often they will pay for an item (e.g., once every 5 years) (Iezzoni, 2003).

COVERAGE OF PERSONAL ASSISTANCE SERVICES

Even with advances in the value, availability, and use of assistive technologies that can reduce the need for some kinds of caregiving, human caregiving remains a crucial resource that allows many people, particularly those with serious disabilities, to live independently and to participate in

---

[12]A survey by McManus (2001) of 98 private health plans (half health maintenance organizations and half preferred provider organizations) of coverage of hearing services for children found that only 11 percent explicitly covered hearing aids (and most had cost caps or other limits) and more than 80 percent specifically excluded them. Two plans covered assistive communication devices under a state-mandated benefit for early intervention services, but most other plans included no specific information about coverage.

community life. In a 2004 Harris poll, of the respondents who reported the need for personal assistance, 77 percent reported that they relied on family or friends and 29 percent reported that they relied on paid assistance (Harris Interactive, 2004b). In 2005, about 7 percent of all kinds of paid home care (including skilled care) was paid for out of pocket and another 7 percent was covered by private insurance; Medicare paid for about 27 percent, and Medicaid paid for 55 percent (Komisar and Thompson, 2007).

LeBlanc and colleagues have observed that "personal care is a complex construct, known by a variety of names, overlapping with existing service systems, blurring the lines between skilled and unskilled, and between formal and informal home care . . . [and] . . . evolving in different ways across the States, many of which continually make changes in their programs" (LeBlanc et al., 2001 p. 2). The term "personal assistance" seems to be preferred by consumer groups, but Medicare and Medicaid policies generally refer to personal care services or personal care attendants. As used here, personal assistance services or personal care services support individuals who are limited in their ability to perform basic daily activities such as bathing, eating, and dressing. Such services may also include assistance with shopping, light housekeeping, meal preparation, bill paying, and other activities.

Medicare and Private Insurance

Medicare does not cover personal assistance or personal care services as such. Nonmedical personal care services may, however, be provided by home health aides in the course of providing covered home health services (Box 9-2). Such care can be provided *only* if beneficiaries are also receiving skilled services, which, in turn, are available only if beneficiaries are determined to be homebound. Medicare rules define homebound to mean that a beneficiary has "a normal inability to leave home," such that trips outside the home require "a considerable and taxing effort by the individual" (such as relying on personal assistance or assistive technology) and are "infrequent or of relatively short duration" (see 42 U.S.C. 1395n(a)(2)(F)). Legislation passed in 2000 provided that absences for health care treatment (including services at day care centers) will not disqualify a beneficiary from being considered homebound under Medicare, Medicaid, and SCHIP.[13]

During the early 1990s, the use of the Medicare home health benefit increased significantly, particularly the use of home health aide services. In

---

[13]In 2002, CMS issued guidance that provided additional examples of acceptable trips outside the home and emphasized that the person's situation should be considered "over a period of time rather than for short periods within the home health stay" (*Medicare Home Health Agency Manual*, §§204.1-204.2) (CMS, 2002).

BOX 9-2
Medicare Coverage of Personal Care
Services as a Home Health Service

• Home health services are covered under Medicare Parts A and B.

• To qualify for home health care, a person must need skilled care, be home-bound, and have a plan of care ordered by a physician.

• Home health services include intermittent or part-time skilled nursing care, physical therapy, speech therapy, occupational therapy, medical social services, and home health aide services.

• Home health aide services, which may include personal care services such as help with eating and dressing, are limited to beneficiaries who are also getting skilled nursing or therapy services.

• Medicare is conducting three two-year demonstration projects to assess the provision and costs of services to people with certain chronic conditions who would not qualify as homebound.

SOURCES: CMS (2004a,c) and GAO (2000).

---

the words of the Medicare Payment Assessment Commission, the benefit "increasingly began to resemble long-term care" rather than care covered under other Medicare benefits for post-acute care (MedPAC, 2004, p. 142).[14] Reflecting concern about the sharply increased expenditures and allegations of fraud and abuse by home health care providers, the U.S. Congress changed provider payment methods and eligibility criteria. Spending dropped substantially after the implementation of these changes. The Medicare home health benefit now involves "less of the maintenance of chronically ill or disabled people over time" at a low intensity of care (MedPAC, 2004, pp. 145–146).

Private coverage of personal care services is also limited. Some (but not all) private Medicare supplemental insurance policies will pay for a limited number of "at-home recovery" visits to help beneficiaries with ADLs after an illness, injury, or surgery (CMS, 2006b).

The committee found no systematic information on employer-sponsored or private health insurance coverage of personal assistance services. Private long-term care insurance may cover personal care services, but, again, the

---

[14]In contrast to the limits on the number of days of care in skilled nursing facilities that Medicare covers, the Medicare statute sets no numerical limit on the number of home health visits.

committee found no systematic information on the extent of such coverage. Again, much personal care is provided by family members on an unpaid basis or is paid for out of pocket by individuals or family members.

Medicaid

Home health care is a required benefit under Medicaid (Box 9-3), but personal care services for adults are an optional benefit that many states offer.[15] As of 2004, 26 states and the District of Columbia covered personal care services as an optional benefit under their Medicaid state plans (Summer and Ihara, 2005). Any optional benefit included in a state plan must be available statewide to "categorically needy" beneficiaries.[16] States may also cover personal care services under special waiver arrangements that encourage home- and community-based services as an alternative to institutional care. Use of such waivers has expanded substantially since publication of the 1991 IOM report, in part as a result of the U.S. Supreme Court's 1999 decision in *Olmstead v. L.C.* That decision held that states may have to provide community-based services for people with disabilities rather than care in less integrated institutional settings (see Appendix D). For children, personal care services are covered under the EPSDT benefit (Smith et al., 2000). In 1988, the U.S. Congress required that Medicaid pay for covered services provided to eligible children in public schools (Herz, 2006).[17] The variety of ways that states can cover personal assistance services and the frequency of state coverage changes make it difficult to summarize state policies on these services.

A 2004 survey of the states that offer personal care services as an optional Medicaid benefit found that 4 of 24 responding states limited coverage to the home (Summer and Ihara, 2005). Policies in other states varied, with some states covering services in day care settings, relatives' homes, and workplaces. All states offering the benefit included assistance with dressing,

---

[15]Personal care services are defined in the *State Medicaid Manual* (LeBlanc et al., 2001).

[16]Under the statute, state programs must cover "categorically needy" groups, which include people who met requirements for the Aid to Families with Dependent Children program as of 1996, children under age 6 whose family income is at or below 133 percent of the federal poverty level and children ages 7 to 18 in families with incomes at or below the poverty level, Supplemental Security Income recipients in most states, the recipients of adoption or foster care assistance under Title IV of the Social Security Act, and certain low-income Medicare beneficiaries. States have the option of providing Medicaid coverage for an extensive list of other groups, including certain working-age individuals with disabilities (CMS, undated).

[17]This provision has generated considerable controversy, some of which is related to conflicting regulations from the U.S. Department of Education and the Centers for Medicare and Medicaid Services on whether Medicaid is the payer of first or last resort. In fiscal year 2005, Medicaid paid about $2.1 billion for school-based services and another $0.8 billion for school administrative expenses (Herz, 2006).

**BOX 9-3
Personal Assistance Services and
Medicaid Home Health Benefits**

- Federal policy requires that state Medicaid plans include home health services for eligible people age 21 and over who qualify for nursing home care.

- The Medicaid statute, unlike the Medicare statute, does not explicitly define home health services as services provided in a place of residence.

- Required home health services include skilled nursing care, home health aide services, medical supplies, and medical equipment.

- Optional home health services include occupational therapy, physical therapy, audiology services, and speech pathology services.

- Personal care services are also optional but are not categorized as home health services. Personal care is considered a required benefit for children under the provisions of EPSDT. Personal care services may be provided as part of Home- and Community-Based Service waivers.

SOURCES: CMS (2005d) and Smith et al. (2000).

---

bathing, laundry, and toileting. Most states covered assistance with eating, meal preparation, grooming, mobility, shopping, and housekeeping. Fifteen of the responding states limited the number of hours of covered services.

In addition, seventeen of the states had some provision for a consumer to direct the services that he or she receives, for example, by preparing service plans or supervising workers (Summer and Ihara, 2005). Three states provided consumers with an individual budget for services and allowed them to purchase services within that budget. Most states (21) had training programs for personal care workers, and a majority (16) reported shortages of such workers. Three-quarters of states allowed payments for services provided by family members (conditioned on the receipt of training). The estimated cost per beneficiary ranged from less than $1,500 in two states to more than $10,000 in eight states.

When states cover personal assistance services under a Medicaid waiver, they may depart from certain Medicaid rules that apply to required or optional benefits, for example, rules that require coverage for categorically needy individuals in the entire state and all categorically needy beneficiaries. The Home- and Community-Based Service (HCBS) waiver program, which was authorized in 1981 under Section 1915c of the Social Security Act, encourages states to cover alternatives to institutional long-term care for beneficiaries who meet the admission criteria for such care (or who would do so in the absence of home- and community-based services). The alternative services are supposed to be cost neutral, which is defined to mean that the average cost per participant is not to exceed the average cost of nursing home care for a person with similar needs. According to CMS, 48 states and the District of Columbia have at least one HCBS waiver, and an additional state has a similar program operating under another waiver authority (CMS, 2007). Many states have several waivers, and the total number of programs exceeds 285. In 1998–1999, 45 states included some coverage of personal care services under at least one HCBS waiver program (Le Blanc et al., 2001). Waiver-based programs may also cover other nonmedical services, for example, home modifications and respite care.

Waiver-based programs can set caps on spending and on the number of people to be served (slots). In 2002, slightly more than 400,000 slots were available across all states, but this amount is less than the number of people wishing to participate (Reester et al., 2004). Of 171 programs, 69 programs had waiting lists totaling more than 155,000 people. The waiting times for people with traumatic brain injuries and children with special needs averaged over 20 months.

Collectively, HCBS waivers accounted for 30 percent of Medicaid long-term care spending in 2001 (up from 15 percent in 1992) and 66 percent of spending on community-based services (up from 37 percent in 1992) (Reester et al., 2004). Much of the growth in the HCBS waiver program is due to the extension of home- and community-based services to people with mental retardation or developmental disabilities, who accounted for 38 percent of the program participants and almost 75 percent of the spending in 2001 (compared with approximately two-thirds of spending in 1991) (Litvak and Kennedy, 1991; Reester et al., 2004). As noted above, the U.S. Supreme Court's decision in *Olmstead v. L.C.* has helped spur this growth, although the growth began before that 1999 decision was handed down. People with other disabilities and beneficiaries age 65 and over together accounted for 54 percent of participants and 21 percent of HCBS waiver program spending.

In addition to the programs described above, the Tax Equity and Financial Responsibility Act of 1982 gave states the option of providing community-based services to children with physical or mental disabilities if the children would be eligible for Medicaid institutional services but could be cared for at home at a cost that does not exceed the estimated cost of institutional care (Bazelon Center for Mental Health Law, 2002). A child who qualifies receives a Medicaid card and is eligible for regular Medicaid child services. States cannot set caps on the number of children who can be served under the waiver or limit coverage to children with certain diagnoses or children in certain geographic areas. In 2002, 20 states had programs under this option (often called the Katie Beckett option after the child whose situation prompted the provision) (Peters, 2005). Ten states did not include children with diagnoses of mental disabilities, despite federal requirements prohibiting such limitations (Peters, 2005). (Some children may also be eligible for direct services under the Maternal and Child Health Bureau's Title V state grants program [Markus et al., 2004].)

A recent review of evaluations of the benefits and costs of home- and community-based services reported that the programs tended to increase both costs and benefits (Grabowski, 2006). (The statutes creating the programs emphasize cost neutrality, hence the emphasis on costs as well as benefits in the evaluations.) Benefits included increased social activity and interaction, greater caregiver and recipient satisfaction, and reduced levels of unmet needs. The costs increased because the savings achieved from the substitution of less expensive services for some nursing home residents (or potential nursing home residents) were offset by the increased spending for people who likely would not have received nursing home care in the absence of the program. The review noted that achieving program savings has become harder as noninstitutional care has become more common, thereby shrinking the pool of people for whom institutional care costs can be reduced. On the basis of recent evaluations, the review concluded that, overall, the evidence about program cost-effectiveness was relatively weak (because of the use of research designs that did not adequately control for nonrandom selection into intervention and comparison groups) and accumulating slowly. The author of the review argued against cutbacks in home- and community-based services, given the strong consumer and public preference for noninstitutional care, but he also proposed the use of research strategies that would better identify efficient program and policy strategies.

An evaluation of North Carolina's waiver program attempted to control for selection effects (e.g., the choice of participants on the basis of their expected costs) through the use of a complex statistical analysis (Van Houtven and Domino, 2005). The analysts concluded that the program decreased nursing home and hospital costs (which are not always considered in cost neutrality assessments) for participants compared with those for nonparticipants. It had no effect on total costs, once differences in health status were taken into account.

Despite some concerns about the quality of care and program oversight,[18] the U.S. Congress included provisions to expand coverage for certain Medicaid home- and community-based services in the Deficit Reduc-

---

[18]Given the rapid growth of the HCBS waiver programs, it is perhaps not surprising that a 2003 government report identified quality-of-care problems, including a failure to provide needed services and inadequate case management (GAO, 2003b; see also GAO [2002]). The report also criticized the oversight provided by CMS.

tion Act of 2005. The law now permits states to provide all services allowed under the HCBS waiver program without getting a formal waiver when the services are for people age 65 and over or for people with disabilities who have incomes up to 150 percent of the poverty level (Crowley, 2006). Beneficiaries do not have to meet the criteria for institutional care. The services do not have to be provided statewide, and enrollment can be capped.

In addition, the act allows states to undertake "cash and counseling" programs without obtaining a waiver (Crowley, 2006). The details may vary among the programs in different states, but these programs usually give a consumer (or a representative) a cash allowance or budget based on a needs assessment. They allow the consumer to direct his or her own personal care and certain other services. The programs also provide consumer counseling and other assistance (e.g., provision of an independent service that actually manages the payments to workers and monitors use). Researchers have evaluated the first three states to implement cash and counseling demonstration projects (before the waiver was implemented).[19] One evaluation reported "unambiguous evidence that Cash and Counseling improved the amount and quality of paid personal assistance from the perspective of consumers, with no discernible adverse effects on safety or health" (Carlson et al., 2005). A companion evaluation reported that the costs per beneficiary were 15 to 20 percent higher than the costs for each individual in the control group, in part because individuals in the intervention groups were more likely to receive services for which they were eligible (Dale and Brown, 2005). In two of three states, the costs for the intervention group were not significantly different from those projected if the individuals had received the agency services authorized in their baseline care plan.

Although the Deficit Reduction Act included features that may benefit people with disabilities, it also included several provisions that may shift costs to Medicaid beneficiaries, potentially limiting their access to needed services (Kaiser Commission, 2006a). Almost all of the expected savings (deficit reductions) in the legislation would come from cuts in benefits or from higher beneficiary costs in the form of premiums and copayments. Before passage of the law, states could not require premium payments for most Medicaid beneficiaries nor impose more than nominal copayments.

---

[19]These demonstrations were conducted under the Medicaid research and demonstration waiver program, which is authorized under Section 1115 of the Social Security Act (Kaiser Commission, 2001). The cash and counseling demonstration projects and evaluations were jointly sponsored by the Office of the Assistant Secretary for Planning and Evaluation, U.S. Department of Health and Human Services and the private Robert Wood Johnson Foundation (RWJF, 2004). People were randomly assigned to receive a cash allowance for personal care services or to have services provided and reimbursed by an agency.

Up to 9 million beneficiaries (half of them children) now could face such new costs. Although beneficiaries with disabilities and those who are dually eligible for Medicare and Medicaid are exempt, the legislation also allows states to offer alternatives to the traditional Medicaid coverage that may have less extensive rehabilitation benefits. Concerns about this legislation are discussed further below.

ACCESS TO ASSISTIVE TECHNOLOGIES AND SERVICES THROUGH NONINSURANCE PROGRAMS

To various degrees, depending on an individual's age, place of residence, type of disability, and other characteristics, people who need assistive technologies or services may find noninsurance programs helpful. Some of these programs are privately sponsored. Others are funded by federal or state governments.

For children, the Individuals with Disabilities Education Act (IDEA), as amended, includes important provisions related to assistive technology (Hager and Smith, 2003). In essence, IDEA requires that if states and school districts accept federal education funds, they must make available to children with disabilities a free, appropriate public education, including special education and related services that allow a child to benefit from such education (see Chapter 4). Each child is to have an individual education program or plan that identifies the services that need to be provided without charge, as determined on a case-by-case basis. Covered devices (e.g., specially adapted laptop computers) may sometimes be used at home as well as at school if that is educationally necessary. The school district often retains ownership of assistive devices that have not been personally prescribed, which means that a young person may lose access to the technology once he or she graduates from high school. The "related services" provision of IDEA also extends to personal care services. In 2004, more than 6.8 million children ages 3 to 21 received services under IDEA (U.S. Department of Education, 2005).

The federal Assistive Technology Act does not directly fund the provision of equipment but, rather, supports technology development, training for rehabilitation engineers and technicians, technical assistance and advocacy, and research on needs for assistive technology. In addition, it requires states that receive grants under the act (as all states do) support awareness programs, provide outreach, provide loans, and engage in certain other activities to promote assistive technologies.

Other programs, including Vocational Rehabilitation programs, may also provide access to assistive technologies, as summarized in Table 9-2. These programs generally do not have assistive technology as their primary focus (Freiman et al., 2006). In addition to the programs listed, state work-

TABLE 9-2 Summary of Financial Assistance for Assistive Technology in Selected Federal Programs

Category of Assistive Technology[a]	Older Americans Act	Selected Housing Programs	Supplemental Security Income IRWE and PASS[b]	Vocational Rehabilitation
Personal ATs for activities of daily living	No		Yes	Yes
Personal mobility ATs	No		Yes	Yes
Orthotics and prostheses	No		Yes	Yes
Hearing, vision, and speech ATs; and augmentative communication	No		Yes	Yes
Cognitive ATs	No		Yes	Yes
Transportation ATs	No		Yes	Yes
Home modifications	Yes	Yes	Yes	Yes

[a]AT = assistive technology.

[b]IRWE = Impaired Related Work Expenses program; PASS = Plan for Achieving Self-Support (if the equipment may enable the person to work). These provisions, in effect, subsidize assistive technologies for some individuals who have qualified for Social Security Income.

SOURCE: Freiman et al. (2006 [used with permission]).

ers' compensation programs require coverage of some assistive technologies, although the details vary (Allen, 1998).

The committee did not locate a similar overview of programs that support financial access to personal assistance services. It did identify a number of federal and state programs that include some direct or indirect support for such services, usually as part of a broader program of home- and community-based services. Box 9-4 lists some examples. In addition, the National Institute on Disability and Rehabilitation Research has funded a number of relevant research and data collection programs, including the Center for Personal Assistance Services at the University of California at San Francisco (UCSF, undated).

In addition, nearly all states have programs that use "state-only" funds (i.e., funds not used to obtain federal matching funds) to support home- and community-based services that supplement and fill gaps in Medicaid services (Kitchener et al., 2006). Most programs are relatively small but provide more flexibility than has been allowed under Medicaid rules and waivers.

A patchwork of charitable, advocacy, and other private organizations (many of which receive support from the federal government or state governments) also help people obtain assistive technologies and, less often, personal care services. Some, such as most Centers for Independent Living,

---

BOX 9-4
Examples of Federal Programs (Other Than
Medicare and Medicaid) That Provide Some
Support for Personal Assistance Services

• The Aid and Attendance program and the Homebound program of the U.S. Department of Veterans Affairs allow veterans to receive a cash benefit to pay for personal care and other assistive services, including housekeeping and shopping (Rosenkranz, 2005). For a single veteran, the maximum yearly payment for the aid and attendance benefit in 2006 was approximately $18,200 (VA, 2006c).

• As one of five primary goals, the Social Services Block Grant program (Title XX of the Social Security Act) funds services to prevent inappropriate institutionalization by supporting community- or home-based care (total spending on the program was limited to $1.7 billion in 2003) (U.S. House of Representatives, Committee on Ways and Means, 2003).

• Title III of the Older American's Act funds assistance to people age 60 or over whose incomes exceed the income limits that allow them to qualify for Medicaid. Federal spending on personal care services under this legislation is quite small: $13 million in 2002, plus $33 million for chores and homemaker services and $193,000 for home delivery of meals (Kassner, 2004).

• CMS provides infrastructure grants to states to help establish personal care programs and train workers (CMS, 2005g).

• The Office of Civil Rights in the U.S. Department of Health and Human Services has investigated and intervened in cases involving complaints about a lack of access to community-based services that would prevent or allow an individual to transfer from institutional care to home. Some cases were resolved when states agreed to cover personal care services (DHHS, 2006a).

• In 2001, as part of the New Freedom Initiative, Executive Order 13217 (Community-Based Alternatives for Individuals with Disabilities) directed six federal agencies to evaluate their policies and programs to determine how they might better support states in implementing the *Olmstead v. L.C.* decision. One area to be evaluated was personal assistance and direct care services (DHHS, 2001).

---

encompass a range of conditions. Others focus on particular chronic conditions or disabilities, such as spinal cord injuries, multiple sclerosis, and cerebral palsy. One example is The Wheelchair Recycler, whose founder received Christopher Reeve's first wheelchair from the Christopher Reeve Foundation and recycled the parts to at least three different people whose chairs needed replacement parts and repairs (New Mobility Magazine, 2006).

RISING COSTS AND THE CHALLENGE OF EXPANDING COVERAGE OF ASSISTIVE SERVICES AND TECHNOLOGIES

As discussed in Chapter 8, the future will bring increasing stresses on this country's system of financing health care services for individuals with and without disabilities. The specter of rising costs is a major constraint on proposals to expand coverage of assistive services and technologies and, indeed, poses the threat of cutbacks in public and private health care programs that may particularly affect people with disabilities.

For all the difficulties and problems that have thus far confronted this country's system of financing health care services, including services for individuals with disabilities, the situation will surely become more challenging in the future. Although some challenges stem from those with philosophical opposition to government- or employer-based health insurance programs, the most widely understood threat relates to health care costs that continue to rise at rates higher than general inflation. Other problems stem from the link between employment and health insurance and from competitive market dynamics that discourage insurers from offering coverage to people with higher-than-average health care costs.

Rising Costs

For decades, health care costs per capita have grown faster than the gross domestic product (GDP), and these costs have thus consumed an ever larger share of GDP—with an increase from 7.2 percent of GDP in 1979 to 16 percent in 2004 (Smith et al., 2006). By 2015 the share of the GDP accounted for by health care spending is projected to reach 20 percent (Borger et al., 2006). In addition, Medicare and Medicaid account for an increasing share of federal spending, and this shift will accelerate as the baby boom generation becomes eligible for Medicare (CBO, 2005a). Policy makers will eventually have to confront growing deficits that are, among other consequences, projected to exhaust the Medicare Part A Trust Fund by 2018 (CMS, 2006a).

Among the states, Medicaid is consuming an increasing share of state budgets, 22 percent in fiscal year 2004, which is an amount that slightly exceeds state spending for elementary and secondary education (NASBO, 2006). Most of the projected growth in Medicaid expenditures is linked to spending for older people and people with disabilities (Ku, 2003).

Health care expenditures will continue to rise for several reasons. As described in Chapter 1, the aging of the population will lead to a substantial increase in the number of people who are in the age group that is at the highest risk of disability. Even if rates of disability continue to decline modestly in the future (and this is hardly assured, as discussed in Chapter

3), total spending for Medicare beneficiaries is likely to continue to increase (Chernew et al, 2005b; see also Cutler and Meara [1999] and CMS [2006g]). The pace of expensive innovation in medical care is more likely to continue or increase than abate. Although the aging of the population, price inflation, and other factors contribute to increased health care expenditures, advances in medicine are generally viewed as the strongest force behind the growth in health care spending—one that has proved difficult to constrain in the long term through cost control strategies (see, e.g., Newhouse [1992], Cutler [1995], Chernew et al. [2004], and Bodenheimer [2005]).

Responses to Rising Costs and Implications for People with Disabilities

Since the enactment of Medicare, rising costs have limited policy makers' willingness to expand Medicare coverage to new groups (e.g., those ages 55 to 64) or a broader range of services (e.g., personal assistance services). The recent extension of Medicare coverage to include prescription drugs is one of the few expansions since the program's start. (Other expansions include benefits for hospice care and benefits for specified preventive services, such as certain kinds of cancer screening.)

Currently, actions or proposals to increase or establish cost sharing for Medicaid beneficiaries are generating controversy, as are a range of other cutbacks in Medicaid programs that may have a disproportionate impact on people with disabilities. Given the number of states, the number of options, the complexity of the policies and proposals (at both the federal and the state levels), and the early stage of implementation, it is very difficult to gauge or even catalog what is happening across the states. One suggestion at the end of this chapter is for more systematic tracking of changes in federal and state Medicaid policies and programs that may affect adults and children with disabilities.

Examples of a few worrisome developments in the Medicaid program include provisions in the Deficit Reduction Act of 2005 that removed the general prohibition against the imposition of premiums and cost sharing on Medicaid beneficiaries (Kaiser Commission, 2006a). For families with incomes over 150 percent of the federal poverty level, the total can reach 5 percent of the family's income in a month or a fiscal quarter. (For a family of four, the poverty level in 2006 was $20,000 [DHHS, 2006b].) Although children (under age 18) who are in mandatory Medicaid categories are exempt, adult beneficiaries with disabilities may be affected.

The Deficit Reduction Act also allows the mandatory or voluntary enrollment of beneficiaries in "benchmark" health plans that are not required to offer the benefits traditionally required for Medicaid beneficiaries. In violation of statutory requirements, it appears that some states have been enrolling beneficiaries who are exempt from mandatory Medicaid enrollment in benchmark plans without offering them a choice or a clear explanation of the differences between the regular Medicaid benefits and those offered by the benchmark plan (Solomon, 2006). A benchmark plan can be "modeled on (or equivalent to) benefit options offered to state and federal employees or the benefits provided by the state's largest HMO [health maintenance organization]" or simply be approved as "appropriate" by the secretary of the U.S. Department of Health and Human Services (Solomon, 2006, p. 2). The state employee plan could, in principle, be a bare bones option created by the state to provide a minimal benefit benchmark plan for Medicaid beneficiaries (Mann and Guyer, 2005). Given that a significant proportion of Medicaid beneficiaries with disabilities may not be in the categories theoretically exempt from enrollment in benchmark plans (Rosenbaum, 2006) and given concerns about the adequacy of enforcement of protections by CMS, beneficiaries with disabilities may be more vulnerable to benefit reductions than an initial review of the legislation would suggest.

Another worrisome action is the implementation by the state of Tennessee of a new, highly restrictive definition of medical necessity that appears to allow managed care plans great leeway in disapproving services on the basis of their costs (see, e.g., Mann [2005] and Cha [2006]). To cite one more example, CMS has approved a West Virginia plan that could reduce or eliminate Medicaid benefits for beneficiaries who fail to keep medical appointments, do not follow treatment regimens, and otherwise fail to take "personal responsibility" for their health (Bishop and Brodkey, 2006; Eckholm, 2006). How transportation difficulties, mental health problems, disagreements between the patient and the physician, and other common complications will be considered is not clear. It also not clear how the program might affect beneficiaries with disabilities, including those who are supposed to be exempt from the requirements.

Beyond these public-sector responses, health care cost inflation has also contributed to a decline in the percentage of employers offering health insurance, although employer decisions are also sensitive to the health of the overall U.S. or state economy, labor markets, and other conditions (Kaiser Commission and Health Research and Educational Trust, 2005). The decline has been most significant for smaller employers, which, in any case, have been less likely to offer health insurance than large companies (Gencarelli, 2005; Kaiser Commission and Health Research and Educational Trust, 2005). (In 2005, 98 percent of firms with 200 or more workers offered employee health insurance, whereas 59 percent of smaller firms did so.) A recent analysis suggested that "more than half of the decline in [health insurance] coverage rates experienced over the 1990s is attributable to the increase in [private] health insurance premiums" (Chernew et al., 2005a, p. 1021). As discussed above, employees with chronic health conditions or disabilities who must seek individually purchased insurance are very likely to find that coverage is either unaffordable or unavailable.

As health insurance coverage costs have grown, employers have also shifted more of the costs to employees.[20] Between 2001 and 2005, average premium payments by employees increased from $30 to $51 per month for individual coverage and from $149 to $226 per month for family coverage (Kaiser Commission and Health Research and Educational Trust, 2005). For most health plan options, average annual deductibles more than doubled during this 5-year period, reaching average levels of nearly $325 for preferred provider plans and more than $600 for conventional health plans. The percentage of employers who offered what are termed high-deductible health plans (a deductible of $1,000 or more for an individual plan) grew from 5 percent in 2003 to 20 percent in 2005 The average deductible in these plans was $1,870 for single coverage and nearly $3,700 for family coverage.

High-deductible plans—or even an end to employer-based health insurance—have been promoted by some as a way of increasing personal responsibility for one's health and health care use. For people with moderate to significant health care needs and low or modest incomes, the burden of increased cost sharing can be substantial. For example, one analysis estimated that with a $500 deductible, almost one-quarter of hospitalized patients would have out-of-pocket costs that exceeded 10 percent of their income; a $2,500 deductible would lead to that result for approximately two-thirds of patients (Trude, 2003, as analyzed by Davis [2004]).

Beyond simply transferring some costs from the insurer to the insured, increased cost sharing is expected to reduce the amount of health care that people use. Unfortunately, research suggests that cost sharing decreases the use of beneficial as well as nonbeneficial or unnecessary services (see, e.g., Newhouse [1993] and Tamblyn et al. [2001]). For people with chronic conditions who need medications, physician management, and other services, cost sharing may reduce patient adherence to medication regimens and compromise other management of these conditions (see, e.g., Dor and Encinosa [2004] and Federman et al. [2001]). Such a reduction in adherence could lead to worse outcomes for individuals with disabilities and could increase the incidence or severity of disabilities in individuals with chronic diseases.

Various strategies have been proposed and, to a limited degree, implemented or tested as alternatives to strategies that simply increase the financial burdens on people with serious chronic conditions or disabilities.

---

[20]Blumenthal (2006, p. 196) has observed that "the ultimate form of cost shifting to employees is to drop health insurance altogether." As described above, the percentage of employers (especially small employers) offering health insurance coverage has dropped in recent years.

The promotion of Medicare, Medicaid, and private managed care plans, particularly in the 1980s and 1990s, is an example. These plans often have broader coverage (e.g., including prescription drugs) than other health plans but usually place restrictions on the patient's choice of health care provider. Analysts and advocates have expressed concerns that health plans restrict access to services important to people with disabilities to control costs and discourage enrollment by higher-risk individuals (see, e.g., DeJong and Sutton [1998] and Beatty et al. [2005]). Some cite a backlash against managed care controls on access to providers and services as one reason for the renewed interest in cost sharing as a cost containment strategy (see, e.g., Robinson [2002]).

More recently, the use of disease management programs have been promoted as a way to improve outcomes and reduce costs for people with specific chronic health conditions that collectively account for a significant share of health care costs.[21] The programs, which are quite variable, typically emphasize education and other means to increase patient adherence to diet, medication, exercise, or other regimens supported by clinical evidence. To date, evidence of the effectiveness of such disease management programs in improving outcomes or reducing costs is limited and uneven, and observers have expressed concern that the emphasis on limiting costs may undercut the programs' potential to improve health outcomes (Short et al., 2003; Brown and Chen, 2004; CBO, 2004; Gold et al., 2005). The federal government has a number of disease management demonstration projects under way, and these may provide findings to help guide the design of successful programs (CMS, 2005f).[22] Even if the adoption of such programs improves health status and reduces the progression of a chronic condition to a disability, the effects on health status and costs are not likely to offset the demographic trends cited elsewhere in this report.

Another proposed approach, under the rubric of "value-based insurance design," has sought to relate the level of patient cost sharing to the

---

[21]"Disease management is a system of coordinated health care interventions and communications for populations with conditions in which patient self-care efforts are significant. Disease management supports the physician or practitioner/patient relationship and plan of care, emphasizes prevention of exacerbations and complications utilizing evidence-based practice guidelines and patient empowerment strategies, and evaluates clinical, humanistic, and economic outcomes on an going basis with the goal of improving overall health" (CBO, 2004, p. 19).

[22]Depending on their structure and incentives, disease management programs may be an example of a so-called pay-for-performance program. This label covers a number of initiatives that provide financial incentives for health care providers to meet patient outcome, efficiency, or other goals (e.g., adoption of electronic patient information systems) (see, e.g., CMS [2005f], MedPAC [2005b], and Rosenthal [2005]). Notwithstanding the considerable enthusiasm for pay-for-performance programs, evidence about their effects on people with disabilities or potentially disabling conditions is still accumulating.

benefit of a drug or other service for a particular category of patients (see, e.g., Fendrick and Chernew [2006]). For example, the cost sharing required for a particular service would be lower for people with conditions for which research on the condition has documented that the service provides value but would be higher for other people with other conditions. The goal would be to constrain the inappropriate use of services by some people and increase the appropriate of services by others. Discussions of this strategy have focused on people with chronic conditions, but the approach could be extended to people with high-cost disabilities.

Rising costs for health care clearly do not preclude expansions in covered services or in covered populations, especially in good economic times. A case in point is SCHIP, as is the extension of Medicare coverage to prescription drug benefits noted earlier in this chapter. Notwithstanding these policy changes, rising health care costs will make it increasingly difficult to expand access to coverage for the services needed by individuals with disabilities and may in fact threaten the existing coverage provided through SCHIP and other programs (see, e.g., Broaddus and Park [2007] and Kenney and Yee [2007]).

As health care costs continue to increase and the population grows older, the United States will face several important and difficult trade-offs. First, decisions about the share of societal resources that should be allocated to publicly funded health insurance programs such as Medicare and Medicaid are critical and are intimately related to overall tax and fiscal policies. In addition to the direct taxes that help support Medicare and Medicaid, tax subsidies for private health insurance and health care in general must be considered as part of the total resource allocation picture for governments. Although an increasing share of the country's resources has been going to health care, this cannot continue without limit.

Second, within the health care sector, decisions will have to be made about how to allocate resources among alternative uses or needs. The offsetting of increases in spending for one group (e.g., children) with decreases in spending for other groups (e.g., working-age adults) is hardly new, but the future is likely to bring more difficult trade-offs, often in the face of limited evidence about the potential consequences. Generational stresses are likely to become even more apparent. A recent assessment of the value of the increased medical spending in the United States between 1960 and 2000 concluded that "the money spent has provided good value" but noted that the cost per additional year of life achieved has increased sharply for older age groups compared with that for newborns and children (Cutler et al., 2006, p. 926).

Third, in the private sector, continued or accelerated cost escalation could see an unraveling of employer-sponsored private health insurance. As noted in Chapter 8, fewer employers are offering health insurance benefits, and the percentage of working-age people without health insurance has been increasing.

This is the environment in which people with disabilities and their advocates seek to protect and expand access to important services simultaneously, particularly within Medicare and Medicaid. Certainly, disagreements exist about the role of governments in spreading the cost burdens of chronic illness and disability, but the major constraint on the expansion—and, indeed, the maintenance—of covered services for people with disabilities is anxiety about costs. This anxiety—combined with disappointment at the checkered history of various cost-containment strategies—stands as a barrier to expansive policy changes for public and private insurance programs.

Assessing Expansions of Coverage in the Context of Rising Costs

Policy makers, advocates for people with disabilities, economists, health care services researchers, and others explicitly or implicitly apply various criteria in proposing what services and products should be covered by Medicare, Medicaid, or other private health care plans. A thorough discussion of principles for assessing (and, more controversially, ranking or setting priorities for) coverage of health care and related services is beyond the scope of this report (see, e.g., Patrick and Erickson [1993] and IOM [2000a]). Box 9-5 lists several commonly cited criteria for evaluating or determining coverage of specific services or products.

The list of coverage criteria does not include political acceptability. As a practical matter, however, public officials are sensitive to voter and interest group views. Government officials have proposed making cost-effectiveness a consideration in Medicare decision making but have, so far, put the proposal aside after negative public reaction. Acceptability is, to various degrees, an issue for employers who see health insurance as a recruitment and employee relations asset (as well as a cost).

Turning the criteria listed above into a workable decision-making process about coverage is not easy. Particularly for a well-accepted service for which coverage has not traditionally been questioned, a lack of positive evidence of effectiveness is generally not regarded as a barrier to coverage. Indeed, for such services, policy makers may be unresponsive or may even reject evidence of harm or ineffectiveness in response to objections from consumers or providers.

In any case, many widely used and accepted services have not been assessed in any rigorous way or have not been assessed for all the conditions and patient populations for which they are used. Testing existing as well as new technologies and services would require extremely large increments in research budgets, assuming that valid, feasible, and ethical evaluations could be constructed for all such services.

BOX 9-5
Criteria Used to Determine Coverage of
Specific Services or Products

- Evidence of effectiveness in improving health and well-being.

- Evidence of cost-effectiveness (generally or practically interpreted to mean that the cost associated with an additional year of life or some other desired outcome measure is judged to be reasonable in light of the cost-effectiveness of other well-accepted services).

- Evidence of cost savings (meaning that the costs of coverage are offset by reduced costs to the payer or society).

- Sensitivity to patient preferences, including quality-of-life preferences (although services shown to be harmful or of marginal benefit might be excluded or otherwise limited).

- Social equity, including protection of vulnerable and disadvantaged populations.

- Contribution to public health (e.g., for services that might otherwise be seen as not appropriate for insurance because they are predictable, low in cost, and recommended for provision to large segments of the population).

Finally, although the committee did not examine the principles that should be used to determine the expansion of health insurance coverage more generally, it notes that another recent IOM report set forth such principles (IOM, 2004d). Box 9-6 lists the principles. These principles address a number of concerns identified in this and the preceding chapter—for example, discontinuous coverage and affordability—that are particularly serious for people with serious chronic health conditions or disabilities. The committee recognizes that these principles represent aspirations that may be difficult to fulfill, given the cost pressures discussed above and competing political interests and priorities.

RECOMMENDATIONS

The 1991 IOM report on disability singled out limited coverage of assistive technologies and personal care services as major shortcomings in the ability of the American health care financing system to meet the needs of people with disabilities. It particularly cited Medicare's "outmoded" concepts of medical necessity as it applied to these services (IOM, 1991, p. 257). Consistent with the 1991 report's focus on the primary prevention of disability, its recommendations about health care financing focused on

---

BOX 9-6
Key Principles to Guide the Extension
of Health Insurance Coverage

1. Health care coverage should be universal.

2. Health care coverage should be continuous.

3. Health care coverage should be affordable to individuals and families.

4. The health insurance strategy should be affordable and sustainable for society.

5. Health insurance should enhance health and well-being by promoting access to high-quality care that is effective, efficient, safe, timely, patient centered, and equitable.

SOURCE: IOM (2004d).

---

expanded services for mothers and children and on the development of new models of health promotion appropriate for people with disabilities.

For the most part, the problems identified in 1991 continue. Interpretations of medical necessity still do not recognize the special health care needs of many people with disabilities. Likewise, the statutory requirements that durable medical equipment be suitable for "use in the home" and its narrow interpretation by CMS are inconsistent with the emphasis on independence and community integration exemplified in the Americans with Disabilities Act and other policies.

At the same time, as described in this chapter and Chapter 8, recent years have brought some progress in expanding health insurance coverage of assistive services and technologies. For example, the expansion of Medicaid home- and community-based services has increased resources for services that support independence and participation and that help people avoid institutional care. SCHIP, a federal-state program, has increased the number of children with public insurance coverage. The committee commends state and federal policy makers and those who have worked to achieve the goals of these policy changes.

Many of the restrictions on assistive services and technologies appear to stem in part from concerns about instances of fraud by health care providers and vendors and, to a lesser extent, the abandonment of equipment by consumers. Concerns about fraud in certain areas are legitimate, as are the positive objectives of providing care that is cost-effective and no more costly than necessary. Excessive attention to program integrity can, however, lead to barriers to beneficial services and to avoidable suffering, loss of independence, and restricted lives. Efforts to link expanded access to net cost savings (as in some Medicaid waiver programs) have been difficult to construct in ways that actually produce such savings. The broad challenge is to find better ways to remove harsh restrictions on assistive services and technologies without offering the proverbial "blank check."

Although this country's current health care financing system is not one that policy makers would likely design if they were starting anew, the system as it currently exists is a political and practical reality. Many people with disabilities and their advocates may seek broad reform or radical change (e.g., universal health coverage, the elimination of the employment-insurance link, and the federalization of Medicaid), but they also advocate for more modest or incremental changes, for example, steps to improve access to assistive services and technologies through health insurance and other programs and evaluations to assess the cost-effectiveness of different ways of improving access and outcomes. The innovative wheelchair leasing arrangement described in Chapter 7 is an example of the kinds of innovative approaches that need more systematic attention and evaluation.

The committee encourages the U.S. Congress to take a new look at how the statutory provisions on medically necessary care and their interpretation might be updated in light of scientific and technological advances and new understandings of health and disability. It also encourages continuing research to support clinical practice and coverage decisions based on evidence of effectiveness. At the same time that outmoded restrictions are discarded, continued efforts to prevent and detect fraudulent wasteful practices by providers and vendors remain important, but such efforts must be made with care to avoid actions that limit access. This committee's recommendations are directed primarily at the Medicare and Medicaid programs, but the committee encourages private health plans to make similar adjustments in their policies relating to durable medical equipment.

Recommendation 9.1: The U.S. Congress and the U.S. Department of Health and Human Services should begin a process of revising Medicare and Medicaid laws and regulations and other relevant policies to make needed assistive services and technologies more available to people with disabilities and to put more emphasis on beneficiaries' functional capacities, quality of life, and ability to participate in work, school, and other areas of community life. Priorities include

- eliminating or modifying Medicare's "in-home-use" requirement for durable medical equipment and revising coverage criteria to consider the contribution of equipment to an individual's independence and participation in community life;
- evaluating new approaches for supplying assistive technologies

(such as time-limited rentals and recycling of used equipment) and providing timely and appropriate equipment repairs; and

• continuing research to assess and improve the appropriateness, quality, and cost-effectiveness of the assistive services and technologies provided to people with disabilities.

In addition to concerns about Medicare, the committee was concerned about the flood of changes in state Medicaid programs noted earlier in this chapter. Tracking Medicaid policies and practices is difficult, especially given the complexity of the changes directed or permitted under the Balanced Budget Act of 2003 and the Deficit Reduction Act of 2005. Analyzing the potential effects of these and other changes on people with disabilities (including changes that come with intended safeguards for this population) adds further complexity. Nonetheless, systematic tracking and analysis are important, given the particular vulnerability of Medicaid beneficiaries with disabilities—both children and adults—to reductions in coverage and increases in beneficiary (or parent) responsibilities for understanding and following complex rules.

Much research on strategies to balance access, quality, and costs has focused on care for people with high-cost chronic illnesses. These strategies include the disease management and value-based insurance strategies described earlier in this chapter and the chronic care programs discussed in Chapter 4. This research and these programs could be refined to consider more explicitly and fully the relevance and consequences of such strategies for people with various degrees of physical, mental, and cognitive impairment. The special needs plans described in Chapter 8 constitute one narrowly targeted approach, but less restrictive approaches also need to be evaluated.

This chapter and preceding chapters have suggested a number of specific topics for research. The next chapter considers more generally the organization and financing of disability and rehabilitation research. It reiterates the messages of the 1991 IOM report on disability that research in this area is underfunded and inadequately coordinated.

10

Organization and Support
of Disability Research

Previous chapters have discussed the scope and magnitude of the issues related to disability that are facing U.S. society. These issues present broad and costly challenges, but delays in tackling them will only exacerbate the challenges and increase the costs of action in the future. Although many steps suggested earlier can be taken on the basis of current knowledge or the analysis of existing data, further research on disability can help refine policies and practices and assess their relative costs and benefits. Research is also needed to generate new and more effective policies and practices based on a better understanding of the nature of disability; the factors that contribute to its creation or reversal over time; and the clinical, environmental, and other actions and interventions that can prevent or mitigate impairments, activity limitations, and participation restrictions.

Consistent with the charge to the Institute of Medicine (IOM), preceding chapters have proposed directions for research and conceptual clarification in several specific areas. Reflecting the complex, dynamic, and diverse nature of disability, the proposed research involves a wide range of clinical, health services, engineering, epidemiological, behavioral, and environmental questions. In this chapter, the first section reviews the federal government's major disability research programs and describes some developments related to these programs in the decade since publication of the IOM report *Enabling America* (IOM, 1997). The second section discusses a number of current and future challenges of organizing and conducting disability research. The last two sections present recommendations and concluding comments.

Unfortunately, although the committee's review suggests that progress has been made since publication of the 1997 report, many of the same problems of limited visibility and poor coordination continue to characterize the organization and funding of federal disability research. The enterprise is still substantially underfunded, given the individual and population impact of disability in America, which will grow as the population of those most at risk of disability increases substantially in the next 30 years.

For purposes of this discussion, disability-related research is construed quite broadly to encompass research with the ultimate goals of restoring functioning, maintaining health and preventing secondary conditions, and understanding the factors that contribute to impairments, activity limitations, and participation restrictions.[1] This research takes many forms, including classical clinical trials, observational and epidemiological studies, engineering research, health services research, survey research on many topics, other kinds of social science and behavioral studies, the development of measures and research tools, and research training and other capacity-building activities. Investment in each of these areas is important to guide clinicians, public agencies, private organizations, families, and individuals with disabilities in making and implementing choices that promote independence, productivity, and community participation.

---

[1] The 1997 IOM report focused more specifically on rehabilitation research. It defined *rehabilitation science* as "the study of *movement among states* [that is, pathology, impairment, functional limitation, and disability] in the enabling-disabling process" (emphasis added) (IOM, 1997, p. 25). Such research involves "fundamental, basic, and applied aspects of the health sciences, social sciences, and engineering as they relate to (1) the restoration of functional capacity in a person and (2) the interaction of that person with the surrounding environment" (p. 25). The report defined *rehabilitation engineering research* as involving "devices or technologies applicable to one of the rehabilitation states" (p. 249). *Disability research*, as it is used in the 1997 IOM report, focused on the interaction between individual characteristics and environmental factors that influence whether a potentially disabling condition or impairment actually limits an individual's participation in society. Consistent with the discussion in Chapter 2, this report uses "disability research" as an umbrella term for research related to impairment, activity limitations, and participation restrictions. It includes but is not limited to rehabilitation and rehabilitation engineering research.

FEDERAL DISABILITY RESEARCH PROGRAMS

Developing a comprehensive and detailed picture of the changes in federally supported disability research that have occurred in the past decade is not an easy task. No agency within the federal government maintains a government-wide database on federally supported or federally conducted disability research (i.e., research that has been completed, that is in progress, or that is planned) or its funding. The committee could not identify any government-wide definition or categorization of the domain of disability research and could not always get information about the definitions of disability research that specific federal agencies use. The issue of defining and categorizing disability research is considered in the Recommendations section of this chapter.

One consequence of the broad scope and dispersed conduct of federal research and the lack of a database on federal research activities is that the committee often found it difficult to determine whether projects that might help answer some of the questions that it identified in other chapters of this report were under way. For example, research on sensory-related assistive technologies or environmental factors might be funded by units within the U.S. Department of Health and Human Services (DHHS), the National Science Foundation (NSF), the U.S. Department of Education, the U.S. Department of Transportation, the U.S. Department of Veterans Affairs (VA), or the U.S. Department of Defense—and by other agencies as well.

Box 10-1 lists the three major federal agencies that have disability research as their primary missions: the National Institute on Disability and Rehabilitation Research (NIDRR), the National Center for Medical and Rehabilitation Research (NCMRR), and Department of Veterans Affairs Rehabilitation Research and Development Service (VA RR&D). It also lists several other agencies with broader research missions that include disability research. In the latter category are several units of the National Institutes of Health (NIH), in addition to NCMRR, that fund primarily biological and clinical research related to a wide range of health conditions that contribute to disability.

Overall, since the publication of the 1997 IOM report, the basic organization of federal disability and rehabilitation research appears to have remained largely the same. Funding levels for research have increased modestly in some agencies but are still inadequate to the need. Little has changed with respect to two of the 1997 report's major critiques: the limited visibility that disability research programs have within their respective parent agencies in the federal government and the lack of coordination to set and assess the implementation of broad priorities for the productive use of limited research resources. The Recommendations section of this chapter returns to these concerns.

BOX 10-1
Federal Sponsors of Disability Research

Major Disability-Focused Sponsors of Research

- National Institute on Disability and Rehabilitation Research, U.S. Department of Education
- National Center for Medical and Rehabilitation Research, National Institute of Child Health and Human Development, U.S. Department of Health and Human Services
- Rehabilitation Research and Development Service, U.S. Department of Veterans Affairs

Selected Other Sponsors of Disability Research

- National Science Foundation
- Centers for Disease Control and Prevention, U.S. Department of Health and Human Services
- Other institutes and centers of the National Institutes of Health: National Institute on Aging; National Institute of Neurological Disorders and Stroke; National Heart, Lung, and Blood Institute; National Institute of Arthritis and Musculoskeletal and Skin Disease; National Institute of Mental Health; National Institute of Deafness and Other Communication Disorders; National Eye Institute; and Physical Disabilities Branch
- Other components of the U.S. Department of Health and Human Services: Agency for Health Care Research and Quality; Maternal and Child Health Bureau; Substance Abuse and Mental Health Administration; and Office of Disability, Aging, and Long-Term Care Policy
- Other components of the U.S. Department of Education: Rehabilitation Services Administration and Office of Special Education Programs
- U.S. Census Bureau, U.S. Department of Commerce
- Office of Research, Evaluation, and Statistics, Social Security Administration
- Office of Disability Employment Policy, U.S. Department of Labor
- Office of Policy Development and Research, U.S. Department of Housing and Urban Development
- Federal Transit Administration and Research and Innovative Technology Administration, U.S. Department of Transportation
- Army Medical Research and Materiel Command, U.S. Department of Defense
- Architectural and Transportation Barriers Compliance Board (the Access Board)

Figure 10-1 shows the funding trends for the three largest disability-focused research units in the federal government. The increase in funding during the late 1990s and early 2000s is encouraging, but the more recent leveling off of funding (except for a recent upturn for NCMRR) means that past gains will soon be dissipated by inflation.

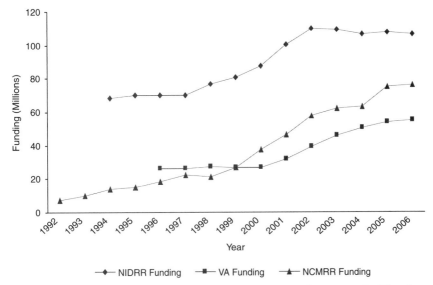

FIGURE 10-1 Funding trends for NIDRR, NCMRR, and VA RR&D. The data are in real, not constant, dollars. The data for NCMRR do not include costs for grant administration and review, which are borne by its parent agency, the National Institute of Child Health and Human Development, or by the NIH Center for Scientific Review (Michael Weinrich, Director, NCMRR, personal communication, September 8, 2006). The data for VA RR&D are for direct costs only. About 20 percent of NIDRR's budget is spent on knowledge translation and dissemination, capacity building, interagency activities, grant review, and other nonresearch purposes (Arthur Sherwood, Science and Technology Advisor, NIDRR, personal communication, September 5, 2006). The data for VA do not include rehabilitation research conducted elsewhere in the department.

SOURCES: for NCMRR through 2005, NCMRR, 2006; for NCMRR in 2006, Michael Weinrich, Director, NCMRR, personal communication, December 15, 2006; for NIDRR, Robert Jaeger, Executive Secretary, Interagency Committee on Disability Research, personal communication, February 27, 2006 (and confirmed by other NIDRR staff); for VA RR&D, Patricia Dorn, Deputy Directory, VA Rehabilitation Research and Development Service, personal communication, December 21, 2006.

Status of Federal Disability Research Efforts

National Institute on Disability and Rehabilitation Research

NIDRR stands out among federal research agencies for its focus on research that addresses the activity and participation dimensions of disability and health. As directed by the U.S. Congress, NIDRR administers

research and related activities "to maximize the inclusion and social integration, employment, and independent living of individuals of all ages
with disabilities," with an emphasis on people with serious disabilities
(NIDRR, 2006, p. 8168).[2] The latest 5-year plan for fiscal years 2005 to
2009 (NIDRR, 2006) lists the emphases or major domains of the agency's
research program as

- employment,
- participation and community living,
- health and function,
- technology for access and function, and
- disability demographics.

To build research capacity and innovation, NIDRR supports investigator-initiated projects, fellowships, rehabilitation research training, and
small business projects. Beyond supporting research, the Congress also
directed NIDRR to disseminate the knowledge generated by the research
and provide practical information to professionals, consumers, and others;
to promote technology transfer; and to increase opportunities for researchers with disabilities.[3]

After a period of budget stagnation in the mid-1990s, the agency saw
moderate funding increases between 1998 and 2002, followed by slight
reductions in funding in more recent years (Figure 10-1). This recent trend
is particularly troubling because NIDRR is the primary base of federal
support for research related to activity and participation. Again, taking
inflation into account, even stable funding means an effective decrease in
resources.

For the years from 1997 to 2004, approximately 80 percent of NIDRR
funding supported research and research capacity building. Of this amount,
approximately 92 percent was allocated for research, exclusive of training support (NIDRR, 2005). Approximately 19 percent supported model
systems of care that are, to various degrees, involved in treatment-related
research. More than 60 percent of the research spending was allocated to
centers through the request for applications (RFA) mechanism. One char-

---

[2]In 1978, the U.S. Congress amended the Rehabilitation Act of 1973 to create the National
Institute of Handicapped Research (which is now NIDRR). Two years later the agency moved
from what is now the U.S. Department of Health and Human Services to the newly created
U.S. Department of Education as part of the Office of Special Education and Rehabilitative
Services. The director of NIDRR chairs the Interagency Committee on Disability Research,
which is discussed later in this chapter.
[3]Outside the research arena, the agency funds several technical assistance centers and projects designed to help organizations understand and meet their obligations under the Americans
with Disabilities Act.

acteristic of the RFA strategy is that it helps develop over time knowledge in defined areas that reflect agency rather than investigator priorities.[4]

In 2006, NIDRR funded 27 Rehabilitation Research and Training Centers and 21 Rehabilitation Engineering Research Centers (Arthur Sherwood, Science and Technology Advisor, NIDRR, personal communication, March 19, 2007; see also NARIC [2006b,c]). (A few additional centers were operating on no-cost extensions of earlier awards.) These centers undertake projects in areas identified by the agency, such as community living, employment outcomes, universal design, disability statistics, personal assistance services, children's mental health, rural communities, accessible medical instrumentation, cognitive technologies, wheeled mobility, and workplace accommodations. Some centers focus on specific health conditions, for example, multiple sclerosis and substance abuse. In addition to the centers, NIDRR supports 14 model programs for spinal cord injuries, 16 model programs for traumatic brain injuries, and 4 model programs for burns.

NIDRR engages in a small amount of collaborative research with other federal agencies. It has worked with the U.S. Department of Labor on employment research and has collaborated on various studies with the Agency for Healthcare Research and Quality, the Centers for Disease Control and Prevention, NIH, the Substance Abuse and Mental Health Services Administration, and other components of DHHS. The amount of research funded through interagency agreements that transfer resources to or from NIDRR in support of these projects was approximately $3.8 million in fiscal year (FY) 2005 (Arthur Sherwood, Science and Technology Advisor, NIDRR, personal communication, September 5, 2006).

After acknowledging NIDRR's unique focus on the interaction of the person and the environment as a strength of the agency, the 1997 IOM report on disability cited criticisms from past agency directors and staff and from the General Accounting Office (GAO; now the Government Accountability Office) related to agency operations. These criticisms focused

---

[4]In general, funds targeted by a funding agency for a particular research purpose (i.e., issued through an RFA) tend to encourage capacity building and to focus attention on a particular area of investigation. Funds awarded through investigator-initiated mechanisms tend to reward the science that is the most well developed and methodologically sound, irrespective of the topic. This is particularly true within the NIH system, which has a peer-review system that is largely independent from priority setting and thus is not strongly influenced by those strategic decisions. NIDRR is primarily oriented toward earmarked funding, while NCMRR and other NIH agencies emphasize investigator-initiated funding. Both emphases present risks. Targeted funding may focus on topics that are important but not "ripe" for exploration, given limitations related to the number of experienced investigators, the state of supporting theory, and the availability of suitable research tools. Investigator-initiated funding may focus on topics for which the methods are well developed but may overlook areas in major need of new investment.

on poorly developed peer-review processes, insufficient personnel, and lack of authority. (Criticisms related to the coordinating role of Interagency Committee on Disability Research [ICDR], which NIDRR staffs, are discussed below.)

The GAO report (1989) attributed many of the agency's problems to the policies and infrastructure of the parent department, the U.S. Department of Education. The IOM report stated that the U.S. Department of Education neglected NIDRR. With respect to review procedures specifically, the report noted criticisms that the review panels were too small, reviewed field initiated research only once a year, occasionally did not get grant applications in advance of meetings, and generally lacked the continuity of standing review panels or study sections.

The 1997 IOM report recommended that NIDRR be moved from the U.S. Department of Education to DHHS to serve as the foundation for the creation of a new agency, the Agency on Disability and Rehabilitation Research. It argued that the research activity would have a more nurturing environment at DHHS and that the move would make disability and rehabilitation research more visible and would also allow the better coordination of research activities. The recommendations section of this chapter revisits the proposal to relocate NIDRR.

Since publication of the 1997 report, NIDRR and the U.S. Department of Education have taken important steps to improve the agency's peer-review processes, and additional planned changes are described in the agency's current long-range plan (NIDRR, 2006a). NIDRR has created standing review panels for field-initiated proposals and the Small Business Innovation Research Program (SBIR) but not for the centers grants. Given the pattern of 5-year funding for centers-based grants and the large numbers of applicants for those grants, standing panels for that program may not be feasible because it would be difficult to predict which members of a standing committee would be from institutions that would not be applying for grants.

As part of its long-range plan, the agency "envisions a standardized peer review process across NIDRR's research portfolio, with standing panels servicing many program funding mechanisms" (NIDRR, 2006a, p. 8178). The stated objective is to create a more consistent, higher-quality process that will, in turn, encourage the submission of stronger proposals with respect both to their substance and to their methodological rigor. In addition, the agency is implementing a fixed schedule for grant competitions that is intended to make it easier to recruit, train, use, and maintain review panel members. One stated objective of the panels continues to be the involvement of people with disabilities on the panels.

The committee believes that some additional measures could further strengthen the review process and help with capacity development. These would include explicit consideration of the past performance of those submitting proposals in the evaluation criteria for new applications; the creation of a mechanism to allow revision and resubmission for investigator-initiated proposals; the assignment of proposal scores based on the quality of the entire proposal, similar to the approaches taken by NIH and NSF; limiting reviews by the lay consumer members of review panels to the non-technical aspects of proposals; and providing more educational feedback on the reviews, especially for young or first-time investigators. The committee understands the funding constraints and legislatively specified funding directives that influence NIDRR's priorities, but it nonetheless believes that a larger field-initiated research program with possibly two review cycles per year might help develop new and younger researchers and open up new areas of research.

National Center for Medical Rehabilitation Research

In 1990, the same year that it passed the Americans with Disabilities Act, the U.S. Congress created NCMRR as a unit within the National Institute of Child Health and Human Development (NICHD) at NIH. The legislation that created NCMRR also created an Advisory Council and a Medical Rehabilitation Coordinating Committee, which includes representatives from 12 other units within NIH. Although the U.S. Congress has established freestanding NIH centers, the legislative creation of a center within an NIH institute was unusual (Verville and DeLisa, 2003).

NCMRR describes its mission as supporting the "development of scientific knowledge needed to enhance the health, productivity, independence, and quality of life of persons with disabilities" through research focused on the "functioning of people with disabilities in daily life" (NCMRR, 2006, p. 2). Early in its existence, NCMRR established seven priority areas for research or the support of research (NIH, 1993). These areas, which still apply, are

- improving functional mobility;
- promoting behavioral adaptation to functional losses;
- assessing the efficacy and outcomes of medical rehabilitation therapies and practices;
- developing improved assistive technology;
- understanding whole-body-system responses to physical impairments and functional changes;
- developing more precise methods of measuring impairments, disabilities, and societal and functional limitations; and
- training research scientists in the field of rehabilitation.

NCMRR administers programs in five areas: traumatic brain injury and stroke rehabilitation, biological science and career development, behavioral sciences and rehabilitation engineering technologies, spinal cord and musculoskeletal disorders and assistive devices, and pediatric critical care and rehabilitation.[5] After comments about the important but seemingly peripheral relationship of the pediatric critical care research to the center's research portfolio (NCMRR, 2002), the center pointed to the need for collaboration between pediatric critical care and pediatric rehabilitation because many critical care patients are children with disabilities.[6]

Recently, NCMRR defined the areas in which it saw the greatest opportunities for research in the next 5 years, given a more constrained future funding environment (NCMRR, 2006). For investigator-initiated research, the emphases are (1) translation research (from the laboratory bench to the community), (2) basic research to advance rehabilitation, (3) plasticity and adaptation of tissue in response to activities and the environment, and (4) the reintegration of people with disabilities into the community. It also defined what it described as cross-cutting objectives: developing mechanisms to support new investigators, enhancing consumer input and outreach, and extending the interdisciplinary model from basic research through applied research and community studies.

NCMRR has funded specific programs intended to develop technical expertise and infrastructure for rehabilitation research. Among other things, these programs are intended to attract basic scientists into the rehabilitation arena and promote greater communication between basic scientists and those studying applied rehabilitation topics. It will be important to gauge the impact of efforts such as these on the progress of rehabilitation research development.

Because NCMRR is not an independent center and does not have its own appropriation separate from NICHD, the amount of funding that is devoted to rehabilitation research primarily depends on how rehabilitation research proposals are scored in relation to proposals on other topics of interest to NICHD (e.g., prematurity and reproductive health). As shown

---

[5]In addition, within NIH, NICHD joined with the NIH Clinical Center in 2001 to create the Physical Disabilities Branch, which includes the goal of reducing the costs of health care as well as improving the lives of people with disabilities (Physical Disabilities Branch, undated). The unit, which is located within the Rehabilitation Medicine Department of the Clinical Center, describes the focus of its research as increasing the capacity of individuals with disabilities to perform activities of daily living. It assists other NIH units with research that involves Clinical Center patients, for example, by administering measures of functional outcomes.

[6]As implied by its label, the pediatric critical care and rehabilitation research supported by NCMRR includes some research (e.g., research on cerebral edema in pediatric diabetic ketoacidosis and research to develop a new type of pediatric heart valve) that does not fit the definition of disability-related research offered earlier in this chapter because the focus is acute care.

earlier in Figure 10-1, funding for NCMRR was very limited during its first few years of existence, amounting to less than $15 million in FY 1995. From FY 1999 through FY 2003, when the U.S. Congress doubled the budget of NIH overall, NCMRR funding more than doubled—from $26.8 million in FY 1999 to $62.5 million in FY 2003 (NCMRR, 2006). NCMRR saw a subsequent increase in funding to $75.4 million in FY 2005, but for FY 2006 the figure was almost the same, at $76.1 million. The funding trajectory for NCMRR before 2003 was encouraging, but the shift to essentially flat or slightly decreasing spending for NIH will mean a loss of the momentum achieved in earlier years.[7] To put NCMRR's program in context, the total FY 2005 NIH budget for research and development was almost $28 billion (AAAS, 2006c).

For FY 2004, about 65 percent of NCMRR's total research and training budget was allocated to investigator-initiated research of various kinds (NCMRR, 2006). The remainder was devoted to training, career development, methods development, and other capacity-building activities. Among the priority areas for research, the largest shares of funding for the period from FY 2001 to FY 2005 went to assessing the efficacy and outcomes of rehabilitation therapies (22 percent) and developing improved assistive devices (17 percent). Thirty-five percent of the NCMRR research funding involved mobility limitations, 18 percent involved cognitive limitations, 18 percent involved bowel and bladder conditions, and 11 percent supported participation research or health services research.

The priorities and portfolios of NCMRR and NIDRR overlap in several areas. For example, both have made significant investments in medical rehabilitation research on spinal cord injuries and traumatic brain injuries, with minimal attempts to coordinate their activities, as described below.

The 1997 IOM report on disability observed that NCMRR's medical orientation—a function of its organizational home in NIH—is perceived to be a strength by some but is perceived to be a potential weakness by those who contend that the medical theory of disability "frequently loses sight of the person" (IOM, 1997, p. 254). The report concluded that NCMRR—like NIDRR—suffered from its parent agency's (in this case, NIH) inattention to disability research. One consequence of its organizational location within an institute of NIH is a limited ability to plan and set spending priorities strategically. For example, research proposals with the highest scores within

---

[7]According to an analysis of the final 2006 budget by the American Association for the Advancement of Science, NIH overall has "a declining budget for the first time since 1970 [and] [a]fter adjusting for inflation, FY 2006 is the first time in 24 years that the NIH R&D [research and development] portfolio falls behind inflation in the economy as a whole, after just barely staying ahead of inflation in 2004 and just matching it in 2005. . . . The 2006 budget cut is steep enough to bring NIH R&D below the 2003 funding level in real terms, erasing the increases of the last two years" (AAAS, 2006b, unpaged; see also AAAS [2006a]).

the various divisions of NICHD must be funded (within the available resources), even if they do not support NCMRR's stated priorities. The report noted that the Medical Rehabilitation Coordinating Committee had "no effective mechanisms for tracking [rehabilitation-related research across NIH] or raising priorities within other Institutes, . . . [which results in] a discordant effort in which even the definitions of rehabilitation research vary among the Institutes" (IOM, 1997, p. 251). To provide NCMRR with more visibility and control over its planning and strategic priority setting, the 1997 IOM report proposed that NCMRR be elevated to the status of a freestanding center or institute within NIH. This recommendation is revisited later in this chapter.

The 1997 IOM report on disability viewed the rigor of the NIH peer-review process and the scientific standards for the conduct of research as strengths of NCMRR. It noted, however, that rehabilitation research lacked a dedicated application review study section. One benefit of making NCMRR a freestanding NIH institute was that it "could then form one or more special emphasis review committees managed by the Division of Research Grants" (IOM, 1997, p. 291). Such a group would review training grants, applications in response to RFAs, and certain other projects tightly linked to the agency's missions.

The NCMRR review process has, however, changed since publication of the 1997 IOM report. All applications for training awards, major center grants, small grants (R03 grants), and awards for which applications have been requested are now reviewed by a peer review group constituted by NICHD (Michael Weinrich, Director, NCMRR, personal communication, November 9, 2006).[8] Unsolicited applications for research project grants (R01 grants) go to the Center for Scientific Review (CSR).[9] CSR manages the peer-review groups or study sections that evaluate the majority of NIH research grant applications. One question of concern to those involved in disability and rehabilitation research is whether CSR study sections tend to equate scientific rigor with a range of research designs that are more easily applied to medical and impairment interventions or studies than to psychosocial and participation research. A related and more general issue is whether the expertise represented in the study sections truly provides informed peer review of disability-related research proposals, especially those that focus more on psychosocial questions. In 2003, CSR created the

---

[8]R03 grants support small research projects that investigators can complete with limited resources in a short period of time (NIH, 2006b).

[9]Research project (R01) grants support specific studies to be performed by a named investigator(s) involving a topic related to the investigator's specific interest and competencies and NIH priorities (NIH, 2006b). They can be initiated by investigators or submitted in response to a program announcement or RFAs.

Musculoskeletal Rehabilitation Sciences study section, in which a majority of the members are rehabilitation and disability researchers.

VA Rehabilitation Research and Development Service

In 1948, the U.S. Congress authorized the Veterans Administration (now the U.S. Department of Veterans Affairs) to undertake rehabilitation research and engineering projects with an initial emphasis on prosthetics (Reswick, 2002). Today, the mission of the VA RR&D is to support research relevant to veterans with chronic impairments that may lead to disability. Demands on the VA rehabilitation research program have recently increased as a result of the war in Iraq,[10] and the system as a whole is facing significant financial challenges (see, e.g., Edsall [2005]).

Although veterans do not represent the full spectrum of people with disabilities or potentially disabling conditions (notably, children), nonveterans may also benefit from the knowledge generated by VA research. The areas of focus of the VA RR&D program include vocational, cognitive, visual, motor, sensory, amputation, cardiopulmonary, and general medical rehabilitation (VA, 2006b).

The VA RR&D program is one of four units in the Medical and Prosthetic Research program. The other units are the Clinical Science Research and Development Service, the Health Services Research and Development Service, and the Biomedical Laboratory Research and Development Service. (The funding for the Biomedical Laboratory Research program is larger than that for the first three programs combined [AAAS, 2006c].) Some disability-related research is undertaken in the Health Services Research and Development Service program.

VA RR&D is an intramural program, which means that it funds only the research conducted by VA employees (many of whom have joint appointments with academic institutions). VA scientists can, however, compete for research funding from NIH and other public and private sources. The program publishes the *Journal of Rehabilitation Research and Development*. The program supports 13 research centers of excellence. Some

---

[10]Because of faster and better medical treatment and other developments, the proportions of casualties accounted for by injuries rather than deaths has shifted significantly from the Vietnam War (73 percent injured and 27 percent killed) to the Iraq War (88 percent injured and 12 percent killed) (CNN, 2006; LSU, 2006). The absolute numbers of affected military personnel are far smaller in the Iraq War than the numbers affected in the Vietnam War; but the severe injuries that they have experienced, especially severe brain injuries and amputations, still constitute a stimulus for advances in rehabilitation research. The initial responsibility for acute care and post-acute care for wounded military personnel lies with the U.S. Department of Defense. Aspects of this care, particularly outpatient rehabilitation, have recently been the focus of intense scrutiny (see, e.g., Priest and Hull [2007a, b]).

are identified with health conditions (e.g., spinal cord injuries and brain injuries), whereas others are linked to assistive and other technologies (e.g., wheelchairs and functional electrical stimulation) (VA, 2006b). One center, which is sponsored jointly with the VA Health Services Research and Development Service program, focuses broadly on rehabilitation outcomes research for veterans with central nervous system damage.

One particular asset of the VA rehabilitation research program continues to be its association with a nationwide integrated health care system with strong patient and financial information systems (Perlin et al., 2004). The VA system can support large clinical trials involving multiple centers or sites across the country. The 1997 IOM report noted that "no other health care system, public or private, has a similar unified research program with the breadth and depth" of the VA program (p. 263). Because the VA combines a broad service mission and a research mission in a single agency and research is conducted by VA staff, the VA rehabilitation research program has a strong relationship with the population that it is intended to serve.

As Figure 10-1 shows, the budget for the VA rehabilitation research program was flat during the 1990s but increased from FY 2001 to FY 2005 as part of a general increase in agency spending on research and development. Investigator-initiated research projects account for about 54 percent of the total spending, and research centers account for about 27 percent (Ruff, 2006).

The 1997 IOM report noted no specific weakness in the VA rehabilitation research program and made no explicit recommendations for changes in the program. A 2004 Office of Management and Budget (OMB) review of the VA research and development overall described the research proposal review process as rigorous and managed "to assure scientific quality and fiscal soundness" (OMB, 2004, p. 38; see similar conclusions made by OMB [2005]). OMB (2004) also observed that the programs of research duplicated the activities of other public and private programs, but overall, it gave the VA research program good marks for research management and quality and compared it favorably with other similar programs. The committee is aware of criticisms of the research environment at VA, including excessive bureaucratic requirements, disincentives for outside researchers to collaborate with VA researchers, and workload concerns; but it was unable to investigate these issues.

Other Sponsors of Disability Research

As indicated above in Box 10-1, many federal agencies that do not have a specific mission to support disability do fund some disability research activities. The rest of this section briefly discusses a few of the more significant supporters of disability research among agencies that are not primarily focused on such research. Other chapters have cited the research and data collection efforts supported by the U.S. Census Bureau, the U.S. Department of Transportation, the Social Security Administration, the U.S. Department of Housing and Urban Development, and the U.S. Department of Labor.

Centers for Disease Control and Prevention

CDC is the federal government's lead public health agency. In 1988, the U.S. Congress created the Disability and Health Program within the CDC's National Center for Environmental Health and provided it with an appropriation of $3.8 million for activities related specifically to "the prevention of disabilities." Today, the unit primarily responsible for broad disability issues, the Disability and Health Team, is lodged within the CDC's National Center on Birth Defects and Developmental Disabilities (NCBDDD), which, in turn, is part of Coordinating Center for Health Promotion.[11]

This placement represents a major organizational change since publication of the 1997 IOM report on disability. The change was required under the Children's Health Act of 2000, which created NCBDDD and directed that it include, among other programs, the programs related to disability prevention that were formerly within the National Center for Environmental Health (42 U.S.C. 247b-4; CDC, 2001). Many of the staff and other resources were transferred from the Disabilities Prevention Program in the latter center. Because the Disability and Health Team is located within the CDC's NCBDDD, no major CDC center or office currently focuses on disability across the life span as a primary topic.

Notwithstanding its location, the Disability and Health Team is concerned with the health of people with disabilities throughout the life span and gives its attention to health promotion, the prevention of secondary conditions, and access to preventive health care, as well as supports for family caregivers. It works with state health departments, universities, and national health and consumer organizations to develop and implement programs in these areas. For many years, it has particularly encouraged research and other attention to the understanding and prevention of secondary conditions as a source of increased disability and a target of rehabilitation interventions. The unit's research also emphasizes health disparities among people with and without disabilities. It has funded re-

---

[11]CDC has four coordinating centers (each of which coordinates subsidiary centers or offices) and two coordinating offices, as well as the National Institute for Occupational Health and Safety. Research is dispersed throughout these centers and offices. Although CDC funds some investigator-initiated research, funding tends to "track categorical program dollars" rather than be driven by a separate assessment of population needs (Green, 2003, p. 5).

search to develop measures of environmental factors affecting people with disabilities, work that is consistent with efforts recommended in Chapters 2 and 5 of this report. CDC and NIDRR jointly support monitoring of the objectives in *Healthy People 2010* related to disability and secondary conditions (DHHS, 2000a).

Core funding for the Disability and Health Team in FY 2006 totaled just under $10.6 million, down from $12.6 million in 1996 (John Crews, Lead Scientist, Disability & Health Program Team, personal communication, November 8, 2006).[12] About $3 million was allocated for research specifically. Overall, the funds support program and scientific staff, 16 state programs, the American Association for Disability and Health, 11 research projects, and one information center. In addition to core funding, the unit is responsible for nearly $18 million to support several congressionally mandated programs, including the Amputee Coalition of America, the Special Olympics, and the Christopher and Dana Reeve Paralysis Resource Center.

For CDC as a whole, it is difficult to characterize research spending trends accurately or even to identify the total spending on disability research across all parts of the agency. Certainly, other parts of the agency support disability research. In any case, the level of funding for the research that is the focus of the Disability and Health Team has been and remains quite small.

Some other areas of CDC support research related to disability, most of which is focused on primary prevention. Within NCBDDD, the developmental disabilities program supports several centers of excellence for autism and developmental disabilities research. The Center for Injury Prevention and Control is funding a study of chronic pain prevention following spinal cord injury or limb loss (CDC, undated). Overall, CDC devotes about 8 percent of its funding to research of all kinds, about two-thirds of which supports extramural research (Spengler, 2005). (CDC's total appropriation for FY 2006 was $6.2 billion, and funding from all sources was $8.5 billion, including funding from the U.S. Department of Defense for activities required to prepare for a possible influenza pandemic [CDC, 2006b].)

In report language for the 2005 appropriations bill for the U.S. Department of Health and Human Services and other agencies, the Senate Appropriations Committee urged "the CDC to significantly expand and strengthen its investment in the public health research, surveillance activities, and dissemination of scientific and programmatic health promotion and

---

[12]The 1997 IOM report stated that CDC disability prevention program spending on rehabilitation-related research (not including primary prevention research) amounted to $9 million in 1995. A review of the associated discussion in the report suggests, however, that much of this funding actually supported public education or other nonresearch activities.

wellness information for children and adults with disabilities" (U.S. Senate, Committee on Appropriations, 2004, p. 81). Unfortunately, the Congress did not allocate any funds specifically to support such an expansion.

As in 1997, the strengths of the Disability and Health Team remain its population-based approach to disability research and its persistence in directing attention to understanding and preventing secondary conditions. CDC overall continues to be a major actor in disability surveillance through the National Center for Health Statistics. Chapter 2 includes recommendations for improvements in this area.

The 1997 IOM report on disability noted that the Disability and Health Team's lack of visibility within its parent organization was a weakness shared with other agencies. If anything, the organizational changes since 1997 appear to have further diminished the visibility of disability research within CDC or have at least obscured the unit's concern with adult as well as childhood disability. The broader reorganization within CDC (e.g., the creation of four coordinating centers), whatever its merits, has in some respects further submerged chronic conditions and disabilities as areas of concern. The 1997 IOM report pointed to the need for more involvement in disability research by other parts of CDC, a view that this committee also supports.

National Science Foundation

NSF supports disability research in a number of areas, including assistive technologies, medical rehabilitation, prosthetic devices, universal access and universal design, sensory impairment, and mobility impairments (Devey, 2002; NSF, 2005). Within the Chemical, Bioengineering, Environmental, and Transport Systems Division, the Research to Aid Persons with Disabilities program specifically supports research and development that will lead to improved devices or software for people with physical or mental disabilities. It also funds projects that enlist students in the design of technologies to aid people with disabilities. The Research in Disabilities Education program, which is part of NSF's Division of Human Resource Development, makes resources available to increase the levels of participation and achievement of people with disabilities in science, technology, engineering, and mathematics education and careers. The program funds a broad range of projects to make education in these areas accessible and increase the quantity and quality of students with disabilities completing associate, baccalaureate, and graduate degrees in these fields.

Much of the research supported by NSF involves the development, evaluation, and refinement of both basic and sophisticated basic technologies. Examples of the latter include noise reduction techniques that may improve hearing aids, retinal prostheses for those with complete vision loss, and "aware home" technologies that use sensors and sensor systems to support people with disabilities with independent living and the avoidance of institutionalization (Sanders, 2000; Devey, 2002, NSF, 2005).[13]

NSF did not supply yearly or trend data for disability research funding. A draft analysis prepared in 2002 by the NSF liaison to ICDR estimated that from FY 1998 to FY 2002, NSF supported 148 disability-related projects with funding of almost $73 million—an average of not quite $15 million per year (Devey, 2002). The Research in Disabilities Education program budget averaged $5 million per year from FY 2002 to FY 2006. For comparison purposes, the total NSF budget for FY 2002 was almost $4.8 billion (NSF, 2001).

The 1997 IOM report on disability noted a lack of coordination of NSF programs with other federal programs, "thus limiting the potential synergy among the projects being supported by other agencies" (p. 269). In the committee's judgment, despite some improvement, this continues to be the case. The former executive secretary of ICDR recently moved to NSF, which could improve coordination.

Units of NIH Other than NCMRR

Beyond NCMRR, other institutes and centers of NIH support a range of disability research, although such research is not their primary focus. It is, however, difficult to identify the full array of disability and rehabilitation research funded throughout all the units of NIH. This may become easier in the future. The NIH Reform Act, which the U.S. Congress passed late in 2006, requires the NIH director to report to the Congress every 2 years on the state of biomedical and behavioral research. Among other information, the report is to include a catalog of research activities as well as a summary of research in several key areas, one of which is life stages, human development, and rehabilitation. In addition, the legislation provides for the creation of a research project data system that uniformly codes research grants and activities at NIH and that is searchable by public health area of interest.

NIH is also funding the development of the Patient-Reported Outcomes Measurement Information System (generally referred to as PROMIS) to

---

[13]NSF sponsors several Engineering Research Centers (ERCs) to promote interdisciplinary research and collaboration with industry (ERCA, 2006). The ERC for Biomimetic MicroElectronic Systems conducts research with the ultimate goal of developing implantable or portable microelectronic devices to treat blindness, paralysis, and memory loss. The mission of the ERC for Quality of Life Technology is improve quality of life by creating "a scientific and engineering knowledge base" for developing "human-centered intelligent systems that co-exist and co-work with people, particularly people with impairments" (Quality of Life Technology Center, 2006; see http://www.qolt.org/).

improve measures of patient-reported symptoms and other health outcomes and make them more easily and widely used in clinical research and practice. For example, one goal is "to build an electronic Web-based resource for administering computerized adaptive tests, collecting self-report data, and reporting instant health assessments" (NIH, undated, unpaged; see also Fries et al. [2005]). The first areas identified for measurement development include pain, fatigue, emotional distress, physical functioning, and social role participation. (The initiative relied on the World Health Organization's domains of physical, mental, and social health as its organizing framework.)

Several examples of important rehabilitation research at NIH outside NCMRR can be cited. Through its intramural Laboratory of Epidemiology, Demography and Biometry, the National Institute on Aging (NIA) has long supported research on the consequences of diseases on functioning and independence and the risk factors for disability, especially mobility disability (NIA, 2004; Guralnik, 2006). NIA's extramural Behavioral and Social Science Research Program supports research and the collection of data on the individual and social dimensions of aging. It may be a model for supporting research within NIH that is not narrowly limited to a medical model of disability. The program funds research on the implications of population aging for health, retirement, disability, and families through its Centers on the Demography of Aging. It supports translational research on the health and well-being of older people and their families through its Roybal Centers. NIA has also funded national panel surveys related to disability, such as the National Long Term Care Survey and the Health and Retirement Study (see Chapter 2).

A number of other institutes also fund some disability research. A few additional examples include the following:

- The National Institute of Nursing Research has funded research on formal and informal caregiving for people with chronic health conditions, and it sponsored a state-of-the-science meeting on informal caregiving in 2001 (NINR, 2001).
- The National Institute on Deafness and Other Communication Disorders supports work to develop assistive devices for people with impaired sensory and communications functions and to characterize and develop treatments for aphasia.
- The National Institute of Biomedical Imaging and Bioengineering includes biomechanics and rehabilitation research among its extramural research program areas.
- The National Institute of Neurological Disorders and Stroke funds research on rehabilitation as well as research on the prevention and treatment of stroke, brain injuries, and various neuromuscular conditions.

• The National Heart, Lung, and Blood Institute has supported a number of clinical trials to test exercise training for cardiac rehabilitation.

Some NIH research, especially in the area of assistive technologies, is funded through the SBIR program, a competitive research award program that was created by the U.S. Congress in 1982 to stimulate technological innovation in the small business community (SBA, 2001). DHHS is 1 of 11 agencies that are required to have this kind of small business research support program. The U.S. Department of Education and NSF also participate. Another program, the Small Business Technology Transfer Program, emphasizes the successful movement of innovations from the research setting to the marketplace.

For the NIH overall, the NIH website reports that FY 2005 spending on rehabilitation research was $305 million of the total NIH budget for research and development of almost $28 billion (NIH, 2006a). (The NIH budget office did not respond to questions from the committee about how it developed these figures.) By way of additional context, NIH lists FY 2005 spending on aging at $2,415 million, spending on attention deficit disorder at $105 million, spending on multiple sclerosis at $110 million, and spending on obesity at $519 million NCMRR accounted for about a quarter of the 2005 NIH rehabilitation research spending.

In 1995, NIH identified that it spent $158 million on rehabilitation research. Given the amount of $305 million spent on rehabilitation research in FY 2005, the data suggest that, overall, rehabilitation research has not fully participated in the more than doubling of research funding that NIH has experienced since 1999.

The 1997 IOM report on disability developed an independent estimate of overall NIH funding of rehabilitation research.[14] That estimate of $206 million for individual project funding was $46 million higher than the $158 million that NIH identified.[15] This discrepancy likely reflects both the breadth and volume of NIH-sponsored research and the lack of a well-accepted and understood conceptualization of disability and rehabilita-

---

[14]The committee for the 1997 IOM report reviewed and categorized approximately 2,000 research abstracts collected either from individual agencies directly or through a computerized database on extramural and intramural research funded by the U.S. Public Health Service.

[15]In some cases the 1997 IOM estimates of funding for specific institutes were considerably higher than the NIH figures; for example, IOM calculated funding of $36 million for NHLBI but NIH reported funding of $17.8 million. In a few cases, however, the figure calculated by IOM was lower. For example, IOM calculated funding of $20 million for NCI but NIH reported funding of $23.5 million. The 1997 IOM report also identified almost $126 million in funding for "rehabilitation-related activities" in "broader-based center grants and community clinical oncology programs" (IOM, 1997, p. 251). The abstract identification and evaluation process used for the 1997 IOM report unavoidably had a subjective dimension, and others might have come to somewhat different judgments.

tion research within NIH. Some units of NIH may not have viewed their research projects as rehabilitation related. An appendix to the 1997 IOM report observed that "agencies seemed unsure of their own rehabilitation efforts, much less those of other agencies" (IOM, 1997, p. 326). Altogether, it is not possible to obtain a coherent picture of NIH disability research activities or trends, given the information currently available either from NIH itself or through ICDR (as discussed further below). This gap is addressed by the recommendations presented at the end of this chapter.

Other Units of the U.S. Department of Health and Human Services

A number of other units within DHHS undertake or support some disability research, although the committee found no systematic accounting of such work and was not able to assess the changes that have taken place since 1997. Examples of other units within DHHS that undertake or support disability research follow:

• Agency for Healthcare Quality and Research (AHRQ). AHRQ funds health services and policy research, technology assessments, data collection, and other work in a variety of areas. When the agency was reauthorized in 1999, the U.S. Congress included, as a priority area for attention, individuals with special health care needs, including individuals with disabilities and individuals who need chronic care or end-of-life health care (Clancy and Andresen, 2002). Projects have included studies of the effects of managed care on children with chronic conditions, determinants of disability in people with chronic renal failure, and the levels of satisfaction with health care quality and access among people with disabilities. Several years of flat funding for this agency have limited its work in this and other priority areas.

• Maternal and Child Health Bureau. This unit within the Health Resources and Services Administration funds data collection, research, and demonstration activities related, in particular, to children with special health care needs (see Chapter 4).

• Centers for Medicare and Medicaid Services. Chapters 8 and 9 described a number of this agency's disability-related research projects.

• Office of Disability, Aging, and Long-Term Care Policy in the Office of the Assistant Secretary for Planning and Evaluation. This office is responsible for a program of health services research and policy analysis to support the development and evolution of policies and programs that promote "the independence, productivity, health, and long-term care needs of children, working-age adults, and older persons with disabilities" (ASPE, 2005). The office supported the cash and counseling demonstration projects discussed in Chapter 9. It recently funded an assessment of access to assistive technologies in long-term care facilities.

U.S. Department of Defense

The U.S. Department of Defense sponsors some research focused on the short- and long-term rehabilitation needs of military personnel, particularly those who have experienced spinal cord injuries, amputations, and traumatic brain injuries. For example, under the label "revolutionizing prosthetics," the Defense Advanced Research Projects Agency has initiated a project to "provide fully integrated limb replacements that enable victims of upper body limb loss to perform arm and hand tasks with [the] strength and dexterity of the natural limb," based on advances in neural control, sensing, and other mechanisms that engage or mimic natural biological processes (Ling, 2005).

To cite another example, as part of a much broader portfolio of research, the Telemedicine and Advanced Technology Research Center (TATRC), a unit of the United States Army Research and Materiel Command, manages several projects related to advanced prosthetics, orthotics, and rehabilitation through partnerships with federal agencies, academic institutions, and commercial firms (Kenneth Curley, Chief Scientist, TATRC, personal communication, November 8, 2006; see also http://www.tatrc.org). Projects range from a study of sports and quality of life for veterans with disabilities to an evaluation of amputee rehabilitation at the Walter Reed Army Medical Center to a more typical project on powered foot and ankle prostheses to improve maneuverability and reduce the effort required to operate the prostheses. The program recently assumed responsibilities for technology transfer to move program knowledge into the private sector.

CHALLENGES OF ORGANIZING AND COORDINATING DISABILITY RESEARCH

As illustrated throughout this report, disability is a broad domain ranging from physiological processes to social participation and government policies. Research on this domain cannot, therefore, realistically be within the purview of a single research funding agency. With so many agencies sponsoring some disability research, however, the lack of coordination in establishing and implementing priorities for the use of federal research resources is a continuing concern. The 1997 IOM report on disability argued that perhaps the single greatest consequence of disjointed federal research efforts was "the lack of an appropriate emphasis on disability research per se, that is, [research focused on] the interaction of the person and the physical and social environment" (p. 278).

Efforts to develop and coordinate a coherent program of disability research across federal agencies encounter a number of barriers. First, differences in agency missions and organizational cultures (e.g., the professional training and experience of staff and grantees) can make communication, cooperation, and priority setting difficult. The classic example of a culture gulf is between agencies informed by a medical model of disability and agencies informed by a social or environmentally determined model of disability.

Second, in advocating for research funding, sponsoring agencies typically "claim" the accomplishments of their particular research programs and projects. The competitive budget process thus provides incentives to maintain both the program applications and the funding within agency boundaries. In contrast, the incentives for productive coordination and collaboration are weak to nonexistent.

Third, the development and implementation of long-range strategic plans are, for the most part, conducted separately across agencies. In addition, research funding mechanisms, application deadlines, peer-review processes, and progress reporting and performance evaluation procedures differ across agencies. All of these differences make it complicated and frustrating to even attempt collaborative priority setting and to achieve adequate and timely funding of collaborative research initiatives.

In addition to coordination among research agencies that fund disability and rehabilitation research, coordination between agencies that fund disability and rehabilitation research and those that fund treatment and support services for individuals with disabilities is important if research that informs health care policy is to be planned and conducted efficiently. Although Medicare has adopted policies that allow it to pay for the routine clinical care provided during certain clinical trials,[16] federal research agencies may still find it difficult to secure program payment for such care. For example, it may be difficult to coordinate coverage of routine care costs for a study that compares the care provided in a covered inpatient setting

---

[16]In 2000, in response to an executive memorandum that directed Medicare to pay for routine patient costs in certain clinical trials, the Health Care Financing Administration (now the Centers for Medicare and Medicaid Services [CMS]) issued a policy on such payments (CMS/HCFA, 2000). CMS is now considering a policy on the provision of payment for routine services in studies other than clinical trials and for services for which the evidence of effectiveness is promising but not yet sufficient to justify national approval for Medicare payment (CMS, 2006h). According to Tunis (2005), CMS applies a relatively broad interpretation of "routine costs," paying for all clinical costs for these patients unless a service would clearly have been provided only to patients participating in the clinical trial. In some cases, CMS has covered the experimental intervention itself. An example is the National Emphysema Treatment Trial (1996 to 2003), which evaluated lung volume reduction surgery (National Emphysema Treatment Trial Research Group, 2003). (The study was funded by NIH and AHRQ, except that Medicare paid the clinical costs.)

with the care provided in an outpatient setting where the services would not normally be covered. Waivers have, however, been authorized for a number of demonstration projects testing payment mechanisms, coordinated care arrangements, and other purposes.[17]

Weak Coordinating Mechanisms

When the U.S. Congress created NIDRR, it also created ICDR, which had as its mission promoting the "coordination and cooperation among Federal departments and agencies conducting rehabilitation research programs" (ICDR, 2005). ICDR is housed within the U.S. Department of Education and is chaired by the director of NIDRR. It has 12 statutory members, including its chair, and representatives of 18 other agencies also attend meetings (ICDR, 2006).[18] ICDR also has five subcommittees: Disability Statistics (1982), Technology (1996), Medical Rehabilitation (1997), Employment (2005), and New Freedom Initiative (2002). One goal of the medical rehabilitation subcommittee is to survey all federal medical rehabilitation projects, which would potentially help identify gaps in rehabilitation research and unproductive duplication.

The 1997 IOM report on disability noted "the ineffectiveness of ICDR as a federal coordinating body" (p. 259) and observed that it "has no staff, budget, or real control, and thus does not have the ability to carry out its stated mission" of coordinating federal disability research (p. 261). The Rehabilitation Act did not give ICDR the tools or the financial resources that it needs to compel or entice cooperation.

ICDR's situation appears to have improved only modestly in recent years. Beginning in 2002, ICDR received funding for specific work to establish priorities for assistive and universally designed technologies and to promote collaborative public-private projects in these areas (ICDR, 2005). One product is the assistive technology report discussed in Chapter 7. In responses to questions from the committee, the director of NIDRR stated

---

[17]For example, in the Medicare Modernization Act of 2003 (Section 702), the Congress authorized the waiver of Medicare rules for a project to study the benefits and cost of allowing Medicare beneficiaries with severe, chronic conditions to be "deemed homebound for the purposes of remaining eligible for Medicare home health services even though they leave home more than would be allowed under the usual Medicare rules" (CMS, 2004a).

[18]The 12 statutory members are the director of NIDRR (chair), the commissioner of the Rehabilitation Services Administration, the assistant secretary for the Office of Special Education and Rehabilitative Services, the secretary of the U.S. Department of Education, the secretary of the U.S. Department of Veterans Affairs, the director of NIH, the director of the National Institute of Mental Health, the administrator of the National Aeronautics and Space Administration, the secretary of the U.S. Department of Transportation, the assistant secretary of the U.S. Department of the Interior for Indian Affairs, the director of the Indian Health Service, and the director of NSF.

that ICDR had produced more than 70 internal reports and literature reviews to assist its members in planning and coordinating priorities for their future research (Steven James Tingus, Chair, ICDR, and Director, NIDRR, personal communication, July 19, 2006.). In addition, ICDR is now meeting quarterly, and the level of attendance by member agencies has increased from an average of 13 per meeting from 1998 to 2003 to 17 per meeting from 2004 to 2006. The unit's annual reports for the years 2004 and 2005 are, however, overdue, although the committee understands that the delay reflects, in part, clearance delays within the U.S. Department of Education.

In 2003, ICDR revised its administrative structure and resources (ICDR, 2005). For example, it created an internal website (an intranet) to support communications among committee and subcommittee members. It is also attempting to design an Internet-based system to simplify the collection of information from different federal agencies about their research portfolios that would help to identify research gaps and duplication and to coordinate research in different areas. This work is ongoing but has not reached the point of allowing ICDR to generate an accurate and comprehensive federal government-wide compilation of disability research and research funding. Nonetheless, although the work is only a small part of the larger problem of inadequate information and coordination, the movement is in the right direction.

Within NIH, the role of the NCMRR Medical Rehabilitation Coordinating Committee likewise does not match its title. A 1993 research plan for NCMRR said that the coordinating committee "will work to develop a method of reporting, coordinating and developing medical rehabilitation research initiatives at the NIH" (NICHD, 1993). That early objective has not been met. The 1997 IOM report stated that "meaningful coordination seems to be lacking" at NIH, resulting in "a discordant effort in which even the definitions of rehabilitation-related research vary among the institutes" (p. 251).

A few single or multiagency coordinating committees are concerned with particular health conditions, for example, autism and muscular dystrophy. The narrower focus of such groups might plausibly make their coordinating task somewhat easier, but this is speculative.

In the face of the barriers described above, ICDR fails as an instrument for coordinating disability research across federal agencies. As described above, it lacks the authority or incentives to command or entice attention and cooperation from powerful agencies such as NIH and VA. It serves largely as a communication conduit for agencies to learn more about each other's research activities and areas of mutual interest or complementary expertise. This is a worthy function but a weak coordination tool. Within

NIH, the Medical Rehabilitation Coordinating Committee appears to be even less significant as a means of coordinating disability research.

ICDR's recent acquisition of resources to undertake some data collection and analytical work is helpful. It is, however, likely to be useful mainly as an educational tool—absent any incentives for agencies to cooperate if problems of duplication or insufficient attention to research areas are identified. In this context of interdepartmental relationships, information does not equal power. One bright spot elsewhere is the recent legislative mandate described above for NIH to create an improved research database.

In discussing the advantages of the recommended move of NIDRR to DHHS, the 1997 IOM report noted that this step would move the program closer to NIH and CDC. The report also recommended the creation within the relocated agency of a "coordination and linkage division" that would assume the responsibilities of ICDR and that would also be funded and authorized to support collaborative research.

As discussed further below, the current committee recommends reinforcing ICDR's responsibilities for collecting and analyzing information on the federal government-wide disability research portfolio. Additional information does nothing directly about the structural barriers to coordination, but it provides a basis for a more informed discussion about the appropriate distribution of the research effort.

A recent example may illustrate a lost opportunity for interagency collaboration and may suggest a strategy that could be used to enhance such collaboration in the future. For many years, NIDRR has funded the Traumatic Brain Injury Model System program, in which a set of centers collects longitudinal data on individuals with moderate and severe brain injuries. This program has gathered a cadre of investigators interested in the condition, has established a research and data collection infrastructure, and has developed a registry of affected individuals for whom a set of standardized severity information is available. Funding for these grants is, however, insufficient to support ambitious clinical trials. In 2001, NCMRR announced a competition for the Traumatic Brain Injury Clinical Trials Network (NCMRR, 2001). That program sought to establish a set of centers that could enroll individuals with moderate and severe brain injuries in clinical trials of acute care and rehabilitation. Its development and implementation included no systematic collaboration with NIDRR, even though five of the eight funded centers were also NIDRR-funded model systems. The NCMRR system developed a separate data collection infrastructure. The lack of collaboration meant that some institutions competed for patients for separately funded protocols and also had to support some redundancy in administrative infrastructure. Strategic collaboration and coordination could have yielded at least two more-efficient or productive alternative arrangements. For example, the two agencies could have agreed that NIDRR would continue to fund the research infrastructure and that NCMRR funds would be used to support costly clinical trials conducted within the model system structure. Alternatively, the agencies could have agreed that the field needed a larger set of clinical trial sites with a different research focus, leading to specific efforts to fund appropriate sites that were not already model systems.

Continued Need for Capacity Building

As it is understood broadly, *research capacity* consists of several inter-related elements. They are (1) researchers in sufficient numbers and with appropriate experience and skills to conduct socially valued and ethically sound research, (2) educational programs that produce these researchers, (3) research and analytical methods and ethical standards suitable for the problems to be investigated, (4) institutional settings with the necessary administrative and physical resources to manage research and with the necessary leadership to stimulate good science and attract and retain good investigators, (5) mechanisms of accountability for research conduct, and (6) public and private funding and policies to support the enterprise. Given the importance of interdisciplinary collaboration in disability research, mechanisms of support for such collaborative research can be viewed as another element of research capacity. The support for translational research mentioned at the end of this section is an example.

Although this committee did not have the resources required to update the work of the 1997 IOM committee on research capacity, a recent rehabilitation research summit identified a number of problems that echo many of those identified in the 1997 report and that are likewise consistent with this committee's experience (Frontera et al., 2006). Summit participants, who included rehabilitation researchers, research funders, professional organizations, consumer representatives, and others, cited the following problems:

- Insufficient numbers of adequately prepared rehabilitation researchers
- Minimal recognition of the value of scientific research by relevant professional and clinical organizations and academic rehabilitation institutions
- Inadequate funding to support superior rehabilitation research education programs and training opportunities
- Limited models of interdisciplinary collaboration, which is important, given the diversity of people, interventions, and environments that are the subject of rehabilitation (disability) research
- Weak partnerships with different professional and academic groups and consumer groups

• A lack of an effective strategy of advocacy to build support for rehabilitation research from government agencies and academic institutions

Although the emphasis of the summit meeting was on rehabilitation research, many of the issues—including the continuing difficulties in defining disability and its dimensions—extend to other areas of disability research.

Implicit in much of the summit's discussion of shortfalls was a concern that research on disability—especially research focused on social integration and participation—is not valued within the larger research and academic communities and is valued more in word than in deed by policy makers and the public. The latter gap shows itself in the public funding of disability research, which is dwarfed by the funding for basic and clinical research on medical conditions.

Although infrequently recognized as such, rehabilitation science is a fertile domain for translational research. The breadth of the domain, as described earlier, requires collaborative "team science" across the domains of disability. Advances in basic fields such as neuroscience and tissue engineering provide new tools, but the notion of "translation" needs to be broadened beyond molecular medicine to include the translation of basic research on learning processes, behavioral adaptation, and a variety of other domains into day-to-day clinical decision making and practice and into relevant public and private programs. Chapter 7 described the limitations of current translation research efforts related to assistive and accessible technologies.

RECOMMENDATIONS

Directions for Research

This chapter has focused on the organization and funding of disability research. Earlier chapters discussed research on topics covered in the committee's charge.

The 1991 IOM report on disability presented a research agenda that emphasized the primary prevention of developmental, injury-related, and aging-related chronic conditions that contribute to disability. It also discussed research on the tertiary prevention of secondary health conditions related to chronic health conditions. Since publication of the 1991 report, research has advanced in these and other areas, including the understanding of risk factors related to the onset of disability at birth and throughout the life span.

For example, investigators have identified environmental risk factors—such as living in socioeconomically disadvantaged families and in households with exposures to environmental toxins—for childhood disability (see, e.g., Hogan et al. [2000]). In late life, researchers have identified potentially modifiable risk factors for functional decline, including a low frequency of social contacts, a low level of physical activity, smoking, and vision impairment (see, e.g., Stuck et al. [1999]). Researchers have also identified some promising interventions to limit disability in late life, including chronic disease self-management programs, physical activity programs, and multifactor fall prevention interventions (Center for the Advancement of Health, 2000a,b).

Still, earlier chapters of this report make it clear that many gaps remain in the knowledge base for practices and programs that reduce environmental barriers that restrict the independence, productivity, and participation in community life of people with disabilities. In addition, translating the findings of social and behavioral research into practice remains a formidable challenge in this and other areas (IOM, 2000b). Determining how best to promote activity and participation for people of all ages and abilities will require resources to develop, test, and disseminate promising interventions, practices, and programs. Given the disincentives to private investment described in Chapter 7, the federal government has a central role to play in developing and implementing an intervention research agenda focused on activity limitations, participation restrictions, and quality of life for people with disabilities. It will be important for the process to involve people with disabilities as well as private companies and foundations.

> Recommendation 10.1: Federal agencies should invest in a coordinated program to develop, test, and disseminate promising interventions, practices, and programs to minimize activity limitations and participations restrictions and improve the quality of life of people with disabilities.

Increasing the Funding and Visibility of Federal Disability Research

The 1997 IOM report on disability bluntly stated that the combined federal research effort was not adequate to address the needs of people with disabilities and that more funding would be required to expand research to meet these needs. Despite modest increases in funding during the late 1990s, the situation remains essentially the same 10 years later.

Disability research is a miniscule item in the federal government's research budget; and the federal government's funding for disability research is not in line with the current and, particularly, the future projected impact of disability on individuals, families, and American society. This committee reiterates the call in the 1997 IOM report for increased funding for disability research, which is becoming increasingly urgent in light of the approaching large increase in the numbers of people at highest risk of disability, as described in Chapter 1.

An overarching recommendation—and appeal—in the 1997 IOM report was that "rehabilitation science and engineering should be more widely recognized and accepted as an academic and scientific field of study" (p. 297). The research funding provided by the federal government is a powerful indicator of a field's recognition and acceptance. Since 1997, the field of rehabilitation research—and, more broadly, the field of disability research—has made a few gains in research funding at the federal level, but the overall federal funding picture remains as muddled and murky as it was in 1997.

Likewise, disability research still lacks adequate visibility and recognition within the federal bureaucracy. In fact, for most federal agencies, the committee discovered that it was extremely challenging to even identify the level and extent of disability research being supported by each agency. Therefore, this committee reiterates the call made in the 1997 IOM report for actions to be taken to increase the visibility of federal rehabilitation and disability research within federal research agencies. It again proposes that the U.S. Congress consider elevating NCMRR to the level of an independent center or freestanding institute within NIH. Doing so will create a much more visible entity within NIH that has disability and rehabilitation research as its primary mission and that appropriately occupies an organizational level that is comparable to that of the other institutes.

The committee is aware that the National Institutes of Health Reform Act of 2006, passed in December 2006 (3 months after the committee's last meeting), capped the number of freestanding NIH institutes and centers at 27 (the existing number). Although the new legislation is understandable in the larger context of research policy, it places a powerful and discouraging constraint on efforts to give disability and rehabilitation research a greater presence and independence in NIH and in the larger research community as well.

The committee also reiterates the suggestion in the 1997 IOM report for the creation of an Office of Disability and Health (similar to the Office of Minority Health and the Office of Women's Health) in the Director's Office at CDC to promote integration of disability issues into all CDC programs. Disability is an issue that crosses all age, gender, racial, and geographic groups and all dimensions of public health, a reality that is confused by the current location of the Disability and Health Team within a center focused on birth defects and developmental disabilities. Creating a presence within the Director's Office should help direct attention to disability issues across CDC and thereby support the Disability and Health Team.

As in 1997, the weak position of NIDRR in the U.S. Department of Education continues to be a source of concern. The committee considered reiterating the recommendation made in the 1997 report that NIDRR be moved out of the U.S. Department of Education into DHHS (as the Agency on Disability and Rehabilitation Research). Still, the committee recognizes the improvements undertaken and planned in the NIDRR review process and encourages continued efforts to build on these improvements and address continuing shortcomings in the process. Given the constructive steps at NIDRR in its current location and given the agency's unique focus on research that addresses the interaction of the person and the environment as strengths of the agency, the committee does not repeat the 1997 recommendation to move NIDRR out of the U.S. Department of Education. Rather, it calls for the department to support the agency's efforts to strengthen the quality and scope of its research portfolio.

As in 1997, the committee does not recommend the creation of a new umbrella agency that consolidates all rehabilitation research. Such a step would now, as then, require "uprooting and displacing many meritorious programs" and would reduce the variety of perspectives and approaches to disability issues found in existing agencies (IOM, 1997, p. 280).

Recommendation 10.2: To support a program of disability research that is commensurate with the need for better knowledge about all aspects of disability at the individual and societal level, Congress should increase total public funding for disability research. To strengthen the management and raise the profile of this research, Congress should also consider

• elevating the National Center for Medical Rehabilitation Research to the status of a full institute or free standing center within the National Institutes of Health with its own budget;

• creating an Office of Disability and Health in the Directors Office at the Centers for Disease Control and Prevention to promote integration of disability issues into all CDC programs; and

• directing the Department of Education to support the National Institute on Disability and Rehabilitation Research in continuing to upgrade its research review process and grants program administration.

Improving Disability Research Coordination and Collaboration

The inadequate coordination of disability research was highlighted in the 1997 IOM report on disability, and it remains a persistent problem today. With tightening federal budgets, the advantages of coordination—to avoid neglect or an insufficient emphasis on important issues, wasteful duplication, and the inefficient use of resources—are even more important today than they were in 1997. More than 30 years after amendments to the Rehabilitation Act of 1973 promoted the coordination of federal disability research, it is lamentable that it remains difficult to determine even the amount and the type of disability research being conducted by programs scattered across multiple federal departments.

It is also dismaying that the ICDR, which has the congressionally established responsibility of coordinating disability research, remains a weak instrument for this purpose. The U.S. Congress and the U.S. Department of Education have made some extra resources available to ICDR in recent years, and the unit is taking steps to identify and describe federal disability research activities in selected areas. Nonetheless, further action is needed to improve coordination.

The committee recognizes the challenges of coordination, especially coordination involving multiple federal departments and independent agencies with diverse missions. Indeed, coordination is difficult even within single agencies, especially those in large and complex organizations like NIH that have components with substantial independence. Like reorganization, coordination is not cost free. It is often (sometimes correctly) perceived as a largely symbolic or wishful exercise that absorbs time and energy with minimal benefit. The committee also acknowledges the lack of response to the 1997 IOM report's recommendation to relocate NIDRR and strengthen the resources for coordination available to the relocated agency. Nonetheless, an adequately funded mechanism to undertake certain basic coordination tasks is important for the reasons outlined earlier in this chapter.

> **Recommendation 10.3: To facilitate cross agency strategic planning and priority setting around disability research and to expand efforts to reduce duplication across agencies engaged in disability research, Congress should authorize and fund the Interagency Committee on Disability Research to**
>
> • **undertake a government-wide inventory of disability research activities using the International Classification of Functioning, Disability and Health;**
>
> • **identify underemphasized or duplicative areas of research;**
>
> • **develop priorities for research that would benefit from multi-agency collaboration;**
>
> • **collaborate with individual agencies to review, fund, and administer this research portfolio; and**
>
> • **appoint a public-private advisory committee that actively involves people with disability and other relevant stakeholders to advise on the above activities.**

As recommended above, one mundane but important task of a better-resourced ICDR would be to inventory and categorize government research activities and funding. One activity of the public-private advisory group convened by ICDR could be to advise agencies on the development of definitions and metrics that agencies could use to identify disability and rehabilitation research and then categorize this research by purpose, population, outcomes measures, research strategy, focus on disability or function states (*International Classification of Functioning, Disability and Health* components), and other useful characteristics. (This process would need to take into account the creation of the NIH research database mentioned earlier.) The recommendation calls for the Congress to provide the authority and resources for ICDR to administer a portfolio of such high-priority, multiagency collaborative research. The 1997 IOM report suggested that if $100 million in additional funding were available, $25 million should be devoted to coordination and linkage activities, including multiagency projects. The committee recognizes the constrained fiscal environment in which decisions about research funding are being made and understands that the decisions to increase funding in one area may imply reduced funding in another area or increased taxes or increased deficits. Although it would like to see substantially increased *total* funding for disability research, including additional collaborative research, the committee believes that encouraging collaborative research is sufficiently important to warrant the use of other alternatives if new funds are not appropriated. For example, drawing on the successes of other efforts to fund collaborative research, such as the NIH Roadmap Initiative, the Congress might consider a mechanism for earmarking contributions (e.g., a percentage of each agency's budget) from research agencies to develop and support multiagency collaborations in high-priority areas of disability research.

The committee recognizes that, although NCMRR has a key role in disability research within NIH, much additional, important disability-related research is undertaken or supported elsewhere in that organization. The whole NIH research portfolio in this area could benefit from greater coordination, including coordination in the planning of new initiatives. One strategy would be for the director of NIH to establish disability and rehabilitation as a cross-cutting priority within NIH to be promoted through interagency mechanisms such as the NIH Roadmap Initiative. The director could also develop a more significant role for the Medical Rehabilitation Coordinating Committee, for example, in promoting research on the environmental and personal factors that contribute to activity limitations and participation restrictions, as well as research on interventions that may alter these factors or their effects.

FINAL THOUGHTS

Research clearly has a critical role to play in developing and evaluating a national strategy to prevent the primary and secondary health conditions that contribute to disability and to improve the overall health, well-being, independence, and productivity of people with existing disabilities. Previous chapters of this report have detailed projections of a significant increase in the number of people at the highest risk of disability and have discussed the scope and magnitude of issues related to disability that are facing this country. These issues present broad and costly challenges to Americans, but a delay in tackling these issues will only exacerbate the problems and increase the costs of future actions.

Evidence continues to grow that disability is not an unavoidable consequence of injury and chronic disease but results, in part, from actions that society takes—both in the public arena and in commerce and other private domains. This report argues that American society should take explicit responsibility for defining the future of disability in this country. How it does so will reflect the country's deepest values. The record of the past 17 years offers reasons for serious concern, especially given the cost projections for public programs that are critical to people with disabilities and their families.

Although they are not comprehensive, this report presents a varied set of recommendations for improving the future health and well-being of people with disabilities and for preventing many of the health and environmental conditions that contribute to disability. Some recommendations are new, whereas others recall recommendations in earlier reports that remain compelling. Taken together, they challenge Americans to commit to fully integrating people with disabilities into community life and to making the investments that will generate the knowledge, policies, technologies, and public understanding needed to support that goal.

References

AAAS (American Association for the Advancement of Science). 2006a. *AAAS R&D Funding Update January 4, 2006, FY 2006 Final Appropriations (Part 2 of 2)—Tables.* [Online]. Available: http://www.aaas.org/spp/rd/upd1205tb.htm [accessed April 27, 2007].

AAAS. 2006b. Part 2: agency R&D budgets. In: *Congressional Action on Research and Development in the FY 2006 Budget.* [Online]. Available: http://www.aaas.org/spp/rd/ca06ag.htm#nih [accessed April 27, 2007].

AAAS. 2006c. *VA R&D Remains Flat in 2007 Budget.* [Online]. Available: http://www.aaas.org/spp/rd/va07p.pdf [accessed April 27, 2007].

AAMC (Association of American Medical Colleges). 2006. *New AAMC Grants Will Redesign Chronic Care Education.* [Online]. Available: http://www.aamc.org/newsroom/pressrel/2006/061002.htm [accessed April 27, 2007].

AAP (American Academy of Pediatrics). 1995. Informed consent, parental permission, and assent in pediatric practice. *Pediatrics* 95(2):314–317. [Online]. Available: http://aappolicy.aappublications.org/cgi/reprint/pediatrics;95/2/314.pdf [accessed April 27, 2007].

AAP. 1997. *State Children's Health Insurance Program (SCHIP) Medicaid Provisions of the Balanced Budget Act of 1997 (PL 105-33).* [Online]. Available: http://www.aap.org/advocacy/schippro.htm#reim [accessed April 27, 2007].

AAP. 1999a. Care coordination: integrating health and related systems of care for children with special health care needs. *Pediatrics* 104(4):978–981. [Online]. Available: http://aappolicy.aappublications.org/cgi/reprint/pediatrics;104/4/978.pdf [accessed April 27, 2007].

AAP. 1999b. The pediatrician's role in development and implementation of an Individual Education Plan (IEP) and/or an Individual Family Service Plan (IFSP). *Pediatrics* 104(1):124–127. [Online]. Available: http://aappolicy.aappublications.org/cgi/reprint/pediatrics;104/1/124.pdf [accessed April 27, 2007].

AAP. 2000. The role of the pediatrician in transitioning children and adolescents with developmental disabilities and chronic illnesses from school to work or college. *Pediatrics* 106(4):854–856. [Online]. Available: http://aappolicy.aappublications.org/cgi/reprint/pediatrics;106/4/854.pdf [accessed April 27, 2007].

AAP. 2001. Health supervision for children with Down syndrome. *Pediatrics* 107(2):442–449. [Online]. Available: http://pediatrics.aappublications.org/cgi/reprint/107/2/442 [accessed March 27, 2007].

AAP. 2002. Policy statement: the medical home. *Pediatrics* 110(1):184–186. [Online]. Available: http://aappolicy.aappublications.org/cgi/reprint/pediatrics;110/1/184.pdf [accessed April 27, 2007].

AAP. 2004. Policy statement: application of the resource-based relative value scale system to pediatrics. *Pediatrics* 113(5):1437–1440. [Online]. Available: http://aappolicy.aappublications.org/cgi/reprint/pediatrics;113/5/1437.pdf [accessed April 27, 2007].

AAP. 2005a. Care coordination in the medical home: integrating health and related systems of care for children with special health care needs. *Pediatrics* 116(5):1238–1244. [Online]. Available: http://aappolicy.aappublications.org/cgi/reprint/pediatrics;116/5/1238.pdf [accessed April 27, 2007].

AAP. 2005b. *The National Center of Medical Home Initiatives for Children with Special Needs: About Us.* [Online]. Available: http://www.medicalhomeinfo.org/about/index. html [accessed April 27, 2007].

AAP. 2006. *Coding and Reimbursement for CSHCN: Key to Solving Reimbursement Problems.* [Online]. Available: http://www.medicalhomeinfo.org/tools/coding.html [accessed April 27, 2007].

AAP, American Academy of Family Physicians, and American College of Physicians–American Society of Internal Medicine. 2002. A consensus statement on health care transitions for young adults with special health care needs. *Pediatrics* 110(6):1304–1306. [Online]. Available: http://aappolicy.aappublications.org/cgi/content/full/pediatrics;110/6/S1/1304 [accessed March 22, 2007].

AAPM&R/The Foundation for PM&R (American Academy of Physical Medicine and Rehabilitation/The Foundation for Physical Medicine and Rehabilitation). 2003. *Access to Assistive Technologies: Improving Health and Well-Being for People with Disabilities.* [Online]. Available: http://www.aapmr.org/zdocs/hpl/atoutcomes0503.pdf [accessed April 27, 2007].

AARP. 2006. *Home Design.* [Online]. Available: http://www.aarp.org/families/home_design/ [accessed April 27, 2007].

ABLEDATA. 2006. *Welcome to ABLEDATA.* [Online]. Available: http://www.abledata.com/ [accessed April 27, 2007].

Access Board (Architectural and Transportation Barriers Compliance Board). 1998. Americans with Disabilities Act (ADA) accessibility guidelines for buildings and facilities: building elements designed for children's use; final rule. *Federal Register* 63(8):2060–2091. [Online]. Available: http://www.access-board.gov/Adaag/kids/final.pdf [accessed April 27, 2007].

Access Board. 2004. *ADA and ABA Accessibility Guidelines for Buildings and Facilities.* [Online]. Available: http://www.access-board.gov/ada-aba/final.htm [accessed April 27, 2007].

Access Board. 2005. *ADA and ABA Accessibility Guidelines for Buildings and Facilities.* [Online]. Available: http://www.access-board.gov/ada-aba/final.htm#pgfId-1010761 [accessed April 27, 2007].

Access Board. Undated. *Uniform Federal Accessibility Standards (UFAS)*. [Online]. Available: http://www.access-board.gov/ufas/ufas-html/ufas.htm#intro [accessed April 27, 2007].

Acemoglu D, Angrist JD. 2001. Consequences of employment protection? The case of the Americans with Disabilities Act. *Journal of Political Economy* 109(5):915–957.

ACF/DHHS (Administration for Children and Families, U.S. Department of Health and Human Services). 2006. *The AFCARS Report*. [Online]. Available: http://www.acf.hhs.gov/programs/cb/stats_research/afcars/tar/report11.htm [accessed April 27, 2007].

ACGME (Accreditation Council for Graduate Medical Education). 2006a. *Introduction to Competency-Based Education*. [Online]. Available: http://www.acgme.org/outcome/e-learn/21M1_FacManual.pdf [accessed April 27, 2007].

ACGME. 2006b. *Program Requirements for Residency Education in Pediatrics*. [Online]. Available: http://www.acgme.org/acWebsite/resident_survey/res_index.asp [accessed April 27, 2007].

ACP (American College of Physicians). 2004. *Patient-Centered, Physician-Guided Care for the Chronically Ill: The American College of Physicians Prescription for Change*. ACP 2004 Public Policy Paper. Philadelphia, PA: ACP. [Online]. Available: http://www.acponline.org/hpp/patcen_chronill.pdf [accessed April 27, 2007].

ACP. 2006. *The Advanced Medical Home: A Patient-Centered, Physician-Guided Model of Health Care*. ACP 2006 Policy Monograph. Philadelphia, PA: ACP. [Online]. Available: http://www.acponline.org/hpp/adv_med.pdf [accessed April 27, 2007].

Adams PF, Barnes PM. 2006. Summary health statistics for the U.S. population: National Health Interview Survey, 2004. National Center for Health Statistics. *Vital and Health Statistics* 10(229). [Online]. Available: http://www.cdc.gov/nchs/data/series/sr_10/sr10_229.pdf [accessed April 27, 2007].

Adaptive Environments. 1995. *The Americans with Disabilities Act: Checklist for Readily Achievable Barrier Removal*. [Online]. Available: http://www.usdoj.gov/crt/ada/racheck.pdf [accessed April 27, 2007].

Adolescent Transition Project. Undated. *Health Care Skills Checklist*. University of Washington Computing and Communications. [Online]. Available: http://depts.washington.edu/healthtr/Checklists/health_care.htm [accessed April 27, 2007].

AFB (American Foundation for the Blind). 2001. *Wired to Work: An Analysis of the Reported Crisis in Access Technology Training for People with Visual Impairments*. [Online]. Available: http://www.afb.org/Section.asp?Documentid=1508#intro [accessed April 27, 2007].

Agree EM. 1999. The influence of personal care and assistive devices on the measurement of disability. *Social Science & Medicine* 48(4):427–443.

Agree EM, Freedman VA. 2000. Incorporating assistive devices into community-based long-term care: an analysis of the potential for substitution and supplementation. *Journal of Aging and Health* 12(3):426–450.

Agree EM, Freedman VA. 2003. A comparison of assistive technology and personal care in alleviating disability and unmet need. *Gerontologist* 43(3):335–344.

Agree EM, Freedman VA, Cornman JC, Wolf DA, Marcotte JE. 2005. Reconsidering substitution in long-term care: when does assistive technology take the place of personal care? *The Journals of Gerontology, Series B: Psychological Sciences and Social Sciences* 60(5): S272–S280.

AHIP (America's Health Insurance Plans). 2004. *Research Findings: Long-Term Care Insurance in 2002*. [Online]. Available: http://www.ahipresearch.org/pdfs/18_LTC2002.pdf [accessed April 27, 2007].

AHRQ (Agency for Healthcare Research and Quality, U.S. Department of Health and Human Services). 2002. *Designing Systems of Care That Work for Children with Special Health Care Needs: A Workshop Brief for State and Local Policymakers*. [Online]. Available: http://www.ahrq.gov/news/ulp/childneeds/ulpneeds.htm [accessed April 27, 2007].

AHRQ. 2005. *HCUP Fact Book No. 6: Hospitalization in the United States, 2002.* [Online]. Available: http://www.ahrq.gov/data/hcup/factbk6/factbk6b.htm#common [accessed April 27, 2007].

AIA (The American Institute of Architects). 2006. *Guidelines for Design and Construction of Health Care Facilities.* [Online]. Available: http://www.aia.org/aah_gd_hospcons [accessed April 27, 2007].

Aiken KD, Freed GL, Davis MM. 2004. When insurance status is not static: insurance transitions of low-income children and implications for health and health care. *Ambulatory Pediatrics* 4(3):237–243.

ALA (American Lung Association). 2002. *Trends in Chronic Bronchitis and Emphysema: Morbidity and Mortality.* [Online]. (The link is no longer available. For the most recent data, go to http://www.lungusa.org/site/pp.asp?c=dvLUK9O0E&b=33347 [accessed April 27, 2007]).

Alecxih L. 2006. *Nursing Home Use by "Oldest Old" Sharply Declines.* Presentation by the Lewin Group, November 21. [Online]. Available: http://www.lewin.com/NR/rdonlyres/9A0A92A2-4D76-4397-A0A2-04EB20700795/0/NursingHomeUseTrendsPaper.pdf [accessed April 27, 2007].

Allen J. 1998. *Workers' Compensation: An Old Model Revisited.* Arlington, VA: National Assistive Technology Technical Assistance Partnership (NATTAP). [Online]. Available: http://www.resna.org/taproject/goals/other/healthcare/comp.html [accessed April 27, 2007].

Allen SM. 2001. Canes, crutches and home care services: the interplay of human and technological assistance. *Policy Brief (Center for Home Care Policy and Research)* Fall;(4):1–6.

Allison DB, Gomez JE, Heshka S, Babbitt RL, Geliebter A, Kreibich K, Heymsfield SB. 1995. Decreased resting metabolic rate among persons with Down syndrome. *International Journal of Obesity and Related Metabolic Disorders* 19(12):858–861.

Altman BM, Barnartt SN, Hendershot GE, Larson SA, eds. 2003. *Research on Social Science and Disability,* Vol. 3. *Using Survey Data to Study Disability: Results from the National Health Interview Survey on Disability.* Amsterdam, The Netherlands: Elsevier Science Ltd.

Altman BM, Brown S, Hendershot G, Larson S, Weathers B, Chevarley F. 2006a. *From Theories to Questions: Considerations of Disability Definition and Survey Purpose in Survey Implementation.* Presented at the ISDS State of the Art Conference: Developing Improved Disability Data, July 12–13.

Altman BM, Rasch E, Madans J. 2006b. Disability Measurement Matrix: a tool for the coordination of measurement purpose and instrument development. *Research in Social Science and Disability* 4:263–284.

Anderson DH. 1938. Cystic fibrosis of the pancreas and its relation to celiac disease: a clinical and pathological study. *American Journal of Diseases of Children* 56:344–399.

Anderson DL, Flume PA, Hardy KK, Gray S. 2002. Transition programs in cystic fibrosis centers: perceptions of patients. *Pediatric Pulmonology* 33(5):327–331.

Anderson G, Knickman JR. 2001. Changing the chronic care system to meet people's needs. *Health Affairs (Millwood)* 20(6):146–160.

Andersson C and Mattsson E. 2001. Adults with Cerebral Palsy: A Survey Describing Problems, Needs, and Resources, with Special Emphasis on Locomotion. *Developmental Medicine and Child Neurology* 43(2):76–82.

Ando N, Ueda S. 2000. Functional deterioration in adults with cerebral palsy. *Clinical Rehabilitation* 14(3):300–306.

Andresen EM, Fitch CA, McLendon PM, Meyers AR. 2000. Reliability and validity of disability questions for U.S. Census 2000. *American Journal of Public Health* 90(8):1297–1299.

Andresen EM, Vahle VJ, Lollar D. 2001. Proxy reliability: health-related quality of life measures for people with disability. *Quality of Life Research* 10:609–619.

Andresen EM, Tang J, Barney KF. 2006. The importance of scholarly work in occupational therapy health services research. *Occupational Therapy Journal of Research* 26: 108–116.

Anie KA, Telfair J. 2005. Multi-site study of transition in adolescents with sickle cell disease in the United Kingdom and the United States. *International Journal of Adolescent Medicine & Health* 17(2):169–178.

Antonelli RC, Antonelli DM. 2004. Providing a medical home: the cost of care coordination services in a community-based, general pediatric practice. *Pediatrics* 113(5):1522–1528.

APA (American Psychiatric Association). 2000. *Diagnostic and Statistical Manual of Mental Disorders*, 4th ed., text revision (DSM-IV-TR). Arlington, VA: American Psychiatric Association.

Apling RN, Jones NL. 2005. *Individuals with Disabilities Education Act (IDEA): Analysis of Changes Made by P.L. 108-446*. CRS Report for Congress. [Online]. Available: http://www.cec.sped.org/Content/NavigationMenu/PolicyAdvocacy/IDEAResources/CRS AnalysisofNewIDEAPL108-446.pdf [accessed April 27, 2007].

Ardoin SP, Schanberg LE. 2005. The management of pediatric systemic lupus erythematosus. *Nature Clinical Practice Rheumatology* 1(2):82–92.

ASHA (American Speech-Language-Hearing Association). 2007. *State Insurance Mandates for Hearing Aids*. [Online]. Available: http://www.asha.org/about/legislation-advocacy/state/ issues/ha_reimbursement.htm [accessed April 27, 2007].

ASPE (Office of the Assistant Secretary for Planning and Evaluation, Department of Health and Human Services). 2005. *Office of Disability, Aging, and Long-Term Care Policy*. [Online]. Available: http://aspe.hhs.gov/_/office_specific/daltcp.cfm [accessed May 30, 2007].

Aston JW. 1992. Post-polio syndrome. An emerging threat to polio survivors. *Postgraduate Medicine* 92(1):249–256.

ATAP (Assistive Technology Act Programs). 2006. *Association of Assistive Technology Act Programs & 2007 Appropriations for the Assistive Technology Act of 1998, as Amended*. [Online]. Available: http://www.ataporg.org/ATAPFY07AppropriationsFinal.doc [accessed April 27, 2007].

Autor D, Dugan M. 2003. The rise in disability recipiency and the decline in unemployment. *Quarterly Journal of Economics* 118(1):157–205.

Baker S, Cahill M, Teeple-Low S. 2003. *Technology Assessment of the U.S. Assistive Technology Industry*. [Online]. Available: http://bxa.doc.gov/DefenseIndustrialBasePrograms/ OSIES/DefMarketResearchRpts/assisttechrept/index.htm [accessed April 27, 2007].

Banks J, Kapteyn A, Smith J, Van Soest A. In press. Work Disability is a Pain in the *****, especially in England, The Netherlands, and the United States. In: Cutler DM, Wise DA, eds. *Health in Older Ages: The Causes and Consequences of Declining Disability Among the Elderly*. Chicago, IL: The University of Chicago Press. [Online]. Available: http://www.nber.org/books/disability/index.html [accessed April 27, 2007].

Barbaresi WJ, Katusic SK, Colligan RC, Weaver AL, Jacobsen SJ. 2005. The incidence of autism in Olmsted County, Minnesota, 1976–1997: results from a population-based study. *Archives of Pediatrics & Adolescent Medicine* 159(1): 37–44.

Barbero G. 1982. Leaving the pediatrician for the internist. *Annals of Internal Medicine* 96(1):673–674.

Barker DJ. 1997. Fetal nutrition and cardiovascular disease in later life. *British Medical Journal* 53(1):96–108.

Barral C. 2004. ICF: Internal and external obstacles to implementation. Presentation at the 10th Annual NACC Conference on ICF: Halifax, Nova Scotia, Canada, June 1–4. [Online]. Available: http://www.cihi.ca/cihiweb/en/downloads/Catherine_Barral.pdf [accessed April 27, 2007].

Batavia AI, DeJong G. 2001. Disability, chronic illness, and risk selection. *Archives of Physical Medicine & Rehabilitation* 82(4):546–552.

Batavia AI, Hammer GS. 1990. Toward the development of consumer-based criteria for the evaluation of assistive devices. *Journal of Rehabilitation Research and Development* 27(4):425–436.

Bauer SM. 2003. Demand pull technology transfer applied to the field of assistive technology. *Journal of Technology Transfer* 28(3–4):285–303.

Bauman W. 2006. Secondary conditions with spinal cord injury. In: Field MJ, Jette AM, Martin L, eds. *Workshop on Disability in America: A New Look.* Washington, DC: The National Academies Press. Pp. 222–233.

Bayley JC, Cochran TP, Sledge CB. 1987. The weight bearing shoulder. The impingement syndrome in paraplegics. *Journal of Bone and Joint Surgery* 69(5):676–678.

Bazelon Center for Mental Health Law. 2002. *Fact Sheet: States Using the TEFRA Option for Children with Serious Mental Disorders.* [Online]. Available: http://www.bazelon. org/issues/children/publications/TEFRA/fact2.htm [accessed April 27, 2007].

Beatty P, DeJong G, Dhont K. 2005. *To Your Health! An Overview of Health and Managed Care Issues.* Houston, TX: Independent Living Research Utilization. [Online]. Available: http://www.ilru.org/html/training/webcasts/handouts/2002/07-31-PB/article2.html [accessed April 27, 2007].

Beneficial Designs, Inc. 1999. Disability rights legislation and accessibility guidelines and standards in the United States. In: *Designing Sidewalks and Trails for Access, Part I. Review of Existing Guidelines and Practices.* Federal Highway Administration, U.S. Department of Transportation. [Online]. Available: http://www.fhwa.dot.gov/environment/sidewalks/ chap1.htm [accessed April 27, 2007].

Bennett DL, Towns SJ, Steinbeck KS. 2005. Smoothing the transition to adult care. The most important need is for a change of attitude and approach. *The Medical Journal of Australia* 182(18):373–374.

Berenson RA. 2006. *Challenging the Status Quo in Chronic Care: Seven Case Studies.* The Urban Institute. [Online]. Available: http://www.chcf.org/documents/chronicdisease/ ChallengingStatusQuoCaseStudies.pdf [accessed April 27, 2007].

Berkowitz E. 2000. *Disability Policy and History.* Statement before the Subcommittee on Social Security of the Committee on Ways and Means, U.S. House of Representatives, July 13. [Online]. Available: http://www.socialsecurity.gov/history/edberkdib.html [accessed April 27, 2007].

Berkowitz E. 2005–2006. Medicare and Medicaid: the past as prologue. *Health Care Financing Review* 27(2):11–23.

Berven HM, Blanck PD. 1999. Assistive technology patenting trends and the Americans with Disabilities Act. *Behavioral Sciences & the Law* 17(1):47–71.

Bhattacharya J, Cutler D, Goldman DP, Hurd MD, Joyce GF, Lakdawalla DN, Panis CW, Shang B. 2004. Disability forecasts and future Medicare costs. In: Cutler DM, Garber AM, eds. *NBER Frontiers in Health Policy Research.* Cambridge, MA: The MIT Press. Pp. 75–94.

Bhattacharya J, Choudhry K, Lakdawalla D. 2006. Chronic disease and trends in severe disability in working-age populations. In: Field MJ, Jette AM, Martin L, eds. *Workshop on Disability in America: A New Look.* Washington, DC: The National Academies Press. Pp. 113–142.

Biles B, Nicholas LH, Cooper BS, Adrion E, Guterman S. 2006. *The Cost of Privatization: Extra Payments to Medicare Advantage Plans—Updated and Revised*. The Commonwealth Fund Publication No. 970. [Online]. Available: http://www.cmwf.org/usr_doc/Biles_costprivatizationextrapayMAplans_970_ib.pdf [accessed April 27, 2007].

Bingham SC, Beatty PW. 2003. Rates of access to assistive equipment and medical rehabilitation services among people with disabilities. *Disability and Rehabilitation* 25(9):487–490.

Birk T. 1993. Poliomyelitis and the post-polio syndrome: exercise capacities and adaptation—current research, future directions, and widespread applicability. *Medicine and Science in Sports and Exercise* 25(4):466–472.

Bishop G, Brodkey AC. 2006. Personal responsibility and physician responsibility—West Virginia's Medicaid plan. *New England Journal of Medicine* 355(8):756–758.

Blanck P, Song C. 2003. 1109 "Never forget what they did here": Civil War pensions for Gettysburg Union Army veterans and disability in the nineteenth-century America. *William and Mary Law Review*. [Online]. Available: http://www.cpe.uchicago.edu/publication/lib/Blanck_Song_WillMary.doc [accessed April 27, 2007].

Blessing C. 2003. *Integrating Essential Elements of Person-Centered Transition Planning Practices Into the Development of the Individualized Education Program with All Students with Disabilities*. Ithaca, NY: Cornell University, School of Industrial and Labor Relations. [Online]. Available: http://digitalcommons.ilr.cornell.edu/cgi/viewcontent.cgi?article=1105&context=edicollect [accessed April 27, 2007].

Bloom B, Dey AN. 2006. Summary health statistics for U.S. children: National Health Interview Survey, 2004. National Center for Health Statistics. *Vital and Health Statistics* 10(227). [Online]. Available: http://www.cdc.gov/nchs/data/series/sr_10/sr10_227.pdf [accessed April 27, 2007].

BLS (Bureau of Labor Statistics). 2005. The NLSY97—Chapter 2 (National Longitudinal Survey of Youth 1997). In: *NLS Handbook 2005*. Washington, DC: U.S. Department of Labor. [Online]. Available: http://www.bls.gov/nls/handbook/2005/nlshc2.pdf [accessed April 27, 2007].

Blum RW, Resnick MD, Nelson R, St Germaine A. 1991. Family and peer issues among adolescents with spina bifida and cerebral palsy. *Pediatrics* 88(2):280–285.

Blumenthal D. 2006. Employer-sponsored insurance—riding the health care tiger. Health policy report. *New England Journal of Medicine* 355(2):195–202.

Blumenthal D, Weissman JS, Wachterman M, Weil E, Stafford RS, Perrin JM, Ferris TG, Kuhlthau K, Kaushal R, Iezzoni LI. 2005. The who, what, and why of risk adjustment: a technology on the cusp of adoption. *Journal of Health Politics, Policy, and Law* 30(3):453–473.

Bodenheimer T. 2005. High and rising health care costs. Part 2. Technologic innovation. *Annals of Internal Medicine* 142(11):932–937.

Bonomi AF, Patrick DL, Bushnell PM, Martin M. 2000. Validation of the United States version of the World Health Organization Quality of Life (WHOQOL) instrument. *Journal of Clinical Epidemiology* 53(1):1–12.

Borger C, Smith S, Truffer C, Keehan S, Sisko A, Poisal J, Clemens M. 2006. Health spending projections through 2015: changes on the horizon. *Health Affairs, Web Exclusive* (February 22):61–73. [Online]. Available: http://content.healthaffairs.org/cgi/reprint/hlthaff.25.w61v1.pdf [accessed April 27, 2007].

Bosma GP, van Buchem MA, Voormolen JH, van Biezen FC, Brouwer OF. 1999. Cervical spondylarthrotic myelopathy with early onset in Down's syndrome: five cases and a review of the literature. *Journal of Intellectual Disability Research* 43(4):283–288.

Bottos M, Feliciangeli A, Sciuto L, Gericke C, Vianello A. 2001. Functional status in adults with cerebral palsy and its implications for treatment of children. *Developmental Medicine and Child Neurology* 43:516–528.

Bound J, Burkhauser RV. 1999. Economic analysis of transfer programs targeted on people with disabilities. In: Ashenfelter O, Card D, eds. *Handbook of Labor Economics*, Vol. 3. New York: Elsevier Science. Pp. 3417–3528.

Bound J, Waidmann T. 2002. Accounting for recent declines in employment rates among the working-aged disabled. *Journal of Human Resources* 37(2):231–250.

Brandt I, Sticker EJ, Lentze MJ. 2003. Catch-up growth of head circumference of very low birth weight, small for gestational age preterm infants and mental development to adulthood. *Pediatrics* 142(5):463–468.

Branum AM, Collman GW, Correa A, Keim SA, Kimmel CA, Klebanoff MA, Longnecker MP, Rigas M, et al. 2003. The National Children's Study of environmental effects on child health and development. *Environmental Health Perspectives* 111(4):642–646. [Online]. Available: http://www.pubmedcentral.nih.gov/picrender.fcgi?artid=1241458&blobtype= pdf [accessed April 27, 2007].

Breslow L. 2006. On "public health aspects of weight control." *International Journal of Epidemiology* 35:12–14.

BRFSS (Behavioral Risk Factor Surveillance System, Centers for Disease Control and Prevention). 2006. *Questionnaires—English Versions.* [Online]. Available: http://www.cdc.gov/brfss/questionnaires/english.htm [accessed April 27, 2007].

Bringewatt R. 2006. *Special Needs Plans: Building a Successful Care System for High-Risk Beneficiaries.* Washington, DC: National Health Policy Group. [Online]. Available: http://www.nhpg.org/content/Files/Building%20Successful%20Care%20System.pdf [accessed April 27, 2007].

Broaddus M, Park E. 2007. *Freezing SCHIP Funding in Coming Years Would Reverse Recent Gains in Children's Health Coverage.* Washington, DC: Center on Budget and Policy Priorities. [Online]. Available: http://www.cbpp.org/6-5-06health.htm [accessed April 27, 2007].

Bronner E. 2004. A quote from Marla Salmon from "The Teaching Nursing Home Program." In: Isaacs S, Knickman J. *To Improve Health and Health Care*, Vol. VII. San Francisco, CA: Jossey-Bass. [Online]. Available: http://www.rwjf.org/files/publications/books/2004/ index.html [accessed April 27, 2007].

Brown R, Chen A. 2004. *Disease Management Options: Issues for State Medicaid Programs to Consider.* Issue Brief No. 3. Mathematica Policy Research, Inc. [Online]. Available: http://www.mathematica-mpr.com/publications/PDFs/diseaseman.pdf [accessed April 27, 2007].

Broyles RS, Tyson JE, Heyne ET, Heyne RJ, Hickman JF, Swint M, Adams SS, West LA, Pomeroy N, Hicks PJ, et al. 2000. Comprehensive follow-up care and life-threatening illnesses among high-risk infants: a randomized controlled trial. *The Journal of the American Medical Association* 284(16):2070–2076.

Buchmueller TC, Liu S. 2005. *Health Insurance Reform and HMO Penetration in the Small Group Market.* NBER Working Paper 11446. Cambridge, MA: National Bureau of Economic Research. [Online]. Available: http://papers.nber.org/papers/w11446.pdf [accessed April 27, 2007].

Burkhauser RV, Houtenville AJ. 2004. Did the employment of those with disabilities fall in the 1990s and was the ADA responsible? A replication and robustness check of Acemoglu and Angrist (2001). Unpublished manuscript. Ithaca, NY Cornell University.

Burkhauser RV, Daly MC, Houtenville AJ, Nargis N. 2002. Self-reported work-limitation data: what they can and cannot tell us. *Demography* 39(3):541–555.

Byrd RS. 2002. *The Epidemiology of Autism in California: A Comprehensive Pilot Study.* M.I.N.D. Institute of the University of California, Davis. [Online]. Available: http://www.dds.ca.gov/autism/pdf/study_final.pdf [accessed April 27, 2007].

Cabana MD, Rand CS, Powe NR, Wu AW, Wilson MH, Abboud PC, Rubin HR. 1999. Why don't physicians follow clinical practice guidelines? *The Journal of the American Medical Association* 282(15):1458–1465.

Callahan ST, Cooper WO. 2006. Access to health care for young adults with disabling chronic conditions. *Archives of Pediatrics & Adolescent Medicine* 160:178–182.

Campbell AT. 2004. State regulation of medical research with children and adolescents: an overview and analysis. In: Field MJ, Behrman RE, eds. *Ethical Conduct of Clinical Research Involving Children.* Washington, DC: The National Academies Press. Pp. 320–375.

Campbell CC, Koris MJ. 1996. Etiologies of shoulder pain in cervical spinal cord injury. *Clinical Orthopaedics and Related Research* (322):140–145.

Campbell ML. 1993. *Aging with a Disability: A Life Course Perspective.* School of Public Health and Health Professions, University of Buffalo. [Online]. Available: http://codi.buffalo.edu/graph_based/.aging/.conf/.life.htm [accessed April 27, 2007].

Carandang R, Seshadri S, Beiser A, Kelly-Hayes M, Kase CS, Kannel WB, Wolf PA. 2006. Trends in incidence, lifetime risk, severity, and 30-day mortality of stroke over the past 50 years. *The Journal of the American Medical Association* 296(24):2939–2946.

CARF (Commission on Accreditation of Rehabilitation Facilities). 2004. *CARF Guide to Accessibility.* Tucson, AZ: CARF.

Carlson B, Dale S, Foster L, Brown R, Phillips B, Schore J. 2005. *Effect of Consumer Direction on Adults' Personal Care and Well-Being in Arkansas, New Jersey, and Florida.* Princeton, NJ: Mathematica Policy Research, Inc. [Online]. Available: http://www.mathematica-mpr.com/publications/pdfs/consumerdirection3states.pdf [accessed April 27, 2007].

Carlson D, Berland B. 2002. *Highlights from the NIDRR/RESNA/University of Michigan Survey of Assistive Technology and Information Technology Use and Need by Persons with Disabilities in the United States.* [Online]. Available: http://www.resna.org/taproject/library/bibl/highlights.html [accessed April 27, 2007].

Carlson D, Ehrlich N. 2005. *Assistive Technology and Information Technology Use and Need by Persons with Disabilities in the United States, 2001.* Washington, DC: National Institute on Disability and Rehabilitation Research, U.S. Department of Education. [Online]. Available: http://www.ed.gov/rschstat/research/pubs/at-use/at-use-2001.pdf [accessed April 27, 2007].

Carmeli E, Kessel S, Bar-Chad S, Merrick J. 2004. A comparison between older persons with Down syndrome and a control group: clinical characteristics, functional status and sensorimotor function. *Down's Syndrome, Research and Practice* 9(1):17–24.

Castro L, Yolton K, Haberman B, Roberto N, Hansen NI, Ambalavanan N, Vohr BR, Donovan EF. 2004. Bias in reported neurodevelopmental outcomes among extremely low birth weight survivors. *Pediatrics* 114(2):404–410.

Catterall G, Chimento L, Sethi R, Maughan B. 2006. *Rate Setting and Actuarial Soundness in Medicaid Managed Care.* Association for Community Affiliated Plans & Medicaid Health Plans of America. [Online]. Available: http://mhpa.org/pdf/misc/ACAP_MHPOAreport.pdf [accessed April 27, 2007].

CBO (Congressional Budget Office). 1999. *Projections of Expenditures for Long-Term Care Services for the Elderly.* [Online]. Available: http://www.cbo.gov/showdoc.cfm?index=1123&sequence=0 [accessed April 27, 2007].

CBO. 2004. *An Analysis of the Literature on Disease Management Programs.* [Online]. Available: http://www.cbo.gov/showdoc.cfm?index=5909&sequence=0 [accessed April 27, 2007].

CBO. 2005a. Summary. In: *The Budget and Economic Outlook: Fiscal Years 2006 to 2015.* Pp. xiii–xviii. [Online]. Available: http://www.cbo.gov/showdoc.cfm?index=6060&sequence=1[accessed April 27, 2007].

CBO. 2005b. *CBO March 2005 Baseline: Old Age and Survivors Insurance.* [Online]. Available: http://www.cbo.gov/ftpdocs/63xx/doc6323/03-OASDI.pdf [accessed April 27, 2007].

CBO. 2005c. *High-Cost Medicare Beneficiaries.* [Online]. Available: http://www.cbo.gov/ftpdocs/63xx/doc6332/05-03-MediSpending.pdf [accessed April 27, 2007].

CDC (Centers for Disease Control and Prevention). 1997. Trends in the prevalence and incidence of self-reported diabetes mellitus—United States, 1980–1994. *Morbidity and Mortality Weekly Report* 46(43):1014–1018.

CDC. 2000a. Measuring childhood asthma prevalence before and after the 1997 redesign of the National Health Interview Survey—United States. *Morbidity and Mortality Weekly Report* 49(40):908–911. [Online]. Available: http://www.cdc.gov/mmwr/preview/mmwrhtml/mm4940a2.htm [accessed April 27, 2007].

CDC. 2000b. State-specific prevalence of disability among adults—11 states and the District of Columbia. *Morbidity and Mortality Weekly Report* 49(31):711–714. [Online]. Available: http://www.cdc.gov/MMWR/preview/mmwrhtml/mm4931a2.htm [accessed April 27, 2007].

CDC. 2001. *New Center on Birth Defects and Disabilities Launches Today at CDC: Interim Director and Senior Management Official Named.* Press release. [Online]. Available: http://www.cdc.gov/ncbddd/press/center.htm [accessed April 27, 2007].

CDC. 2004. *Preventing Lead Exposure in Young Children: A Housing-Based Approach to Primary Prevention of Lead Poisoning.* Atlanta, GA: CDC. [Online]. Available: http://www.cdc.gov/nceh/lead/publications/Primary%20Prevention%20Document.pdf [accessed April 27, 2007].

CDC. 2005a. *Centers for Disease Control and Prevention Health-Related Quality-of-Life 14-Item Measure.* National Center for Chronic Disease Prevention and Health Promotion. [Online]. Available: http://www.cdc.gov/hrqol/hrqol14_measure.htm [accessed April 27, 2007].

CDC. 2005b. *Prevalence of Overweight Among Children and Adolescents: United States, 1999–2002.* [Online]. Available: http://www.cdc.gov/nchs/products/pubs/pubd/hestats/overwght99.htm [accessed April 27, 2007].

CDC. 2006a. *The Disability and Health State Chartbook—2006 Profiles of Health for Adults with Disabilities.* Atlanta, GA: CDC.

CDC. 2006b. *FY 2006 CDC/ATSDR Appropriation Fact Sheet.* [Online]. Available: http://www.cdc.gov/fmo/PDFs/FY06AppropFactsheet.pdf [accessed April 27, 2007].

CDC. 2007. Surveillance summaries—prevalence of autism spectrum disorders. *Morbidity and Mortality Weekly Report* 56(SS-1). [Online]. Available: http://www.cdc.gov/mmwr/pdf/ss/ss5601.pdf [accessed April 27, 2007].

CDC. Undated. *Acute Health Care, Rehabilitation and Disability Prevention Research: Grantee Abstracts-Project Title: Chronic Pain Prevention after Spinal Cord Injury (SCI) and Limb Loss.* National Center for Injury Prevention and Control. [Online]. Available: http://www.cdc.gov/ncipc/profiles/acutecare/default.htm [accessed April 27, 2007].

Center for the Advancement of Health. 2000a. *Selected Evidence for Behavioral Approaches to Chronic Disease Management in Clinical Settings: Cardiovascular Disease.* Washington, DC: Center for the Advancement of Health. [Online]. Available: http://www.cfah.org/pdfs/health_topic_cardio.pdf [accessed April 27, 2007].

Center for the Advancement of Health. 2000b. *Selected Evidence for Behavioral Approaches to Chronic Disease Management in Clinical Settings: Physical Activity.* Washington, DC: Center for the Advancement of Health. http://www.cfah.org/pdfs/health_topic_physical.pdf [accessed April 27, 2007].

Center for Universal Design. 1997. *Universal Design Principles.* Compiled by Connell B, Jones M, Mace R, Mueller J, Mullick A, Ostroff E, Sanford J, Steinfeld E, Story M, Vanderheiden G. [Online]. Available: http://www.design.ncsu.edu/cud/about_ud/udprinciples.htm [accessed April 27, 2007].

Center for Universal Design and North Carolina Office on Disability and Health. Undated. *Removing Barriers to Health Care: A Guide for Health Professionals.* [Online]. Available: http://www.fpg.unc.edu/~NCODH/RBar/ [accessed April 27, 2007].

CESSI (Cherry Engineering Support Services, Inc.). 2003. *Federal Statutory Definitions of Disability.* [Online]. Available: http://www.icdr.us/documents/definitions.htm#table1 [accessed April 27, 2007].

Cha SS. 2006. *Defining "medical necessity" in TennCare.* Electronic letter in response to an article by James C. Robinson, "The best of times and the worst of times: a conversation with Vicky Gregg," *Health Affairs* Web Exclusive, November 29, 2005. [Online]. Available: http://content.healthaffairs.org/cgi/eletters/hlthaff.w5.558v1 [accessed April 27, 2007].

Champagne FA, Meaney MJ. 2006. Stress during gestation alters postpartum maternal care and the development of the offspring in a rodent model. *Biological Psychiatry* 59(12): 1227–1235.

Chan F, Wang M, Thomas KR, Chan CCH, Wong DW, Lee G, Liu K. 2002. Conjoint analysis in rehabilitation counseling research. *Rehabilitation Education* 16(2):179–195.

Chan L, Doctor JN, MacLehose RF, Lawson H, Rosenblatt BA. 1999. Do Medicare patients with disabilities receive services? *Archives of Physical Medicine & Rehabilitation* 80(6):642–646.

Chan L, Shumway-Cook A, Yorkston KM, Ciol MA, Dudgeon BJ, Hoffman JM. 2005. Design and validation of a methodology using the International Classification of Diseases, 9th revision, to identify secondary conditions in people with disabilities. *Archives of Physical Medicine & Rehabilitation* 86(5):1065–1069.

CHDD (Center on Human Development and Disability). Undated. *Adolescent Autonomy Checklists: Introduction and Contents.* University of Washington. [Online]. Available: http://depts.washington.edu/healthtr/Checklists/intro.htm [accessed April 27, 2007].

Chernew M, Jacobson PD, Hofer TP, Aaronson KD, Fendrick AM. 2004. Barriers to constraining health care cost growth. *Health Affairs (Millwood)* 23(6):122–128.

Chernew M, Cutler D, Kennan PS. 2005a. Increasing health insurance costs and the decline in insurance coverage. *Health Services Research* 40(4):1021–1039.

Chernew M, Goldman D, Pan F, Shang B. 2005b. Disability and health care spending among Medicare beneficiaries. *Health Affairs (Millwood)* 24(Suppl 2, W5):R42–R52.

Chevarley FM. 2006. *Utilization and Expenditures for Children with Special Health Care Needs.* Research Findings No. 24. Agency for Healthcare Research and Quality. [Online]. Available: http://www.meps.ahcpr.gov/mepsweb/data_files/publications/rf24/rf24.pdf [accessed April 27, 2007].

Children's Hospital Boston. Undated. *Transitions: Managing My Own Health Care.* Checklist developed as part of the Massachusetts Initiative for Youth with Disabilities. [Online]. Available: http://www.bostonleah.org/PDF/transitions_questions.pdf [accessed April 27, 2007].

Chollet D. 2006. *State Regulation and Initiatives to Expand Small Group Coverage.* Mathematica Policy Research, Inc. [Online]. Available: http://www.allhealth.org/BriefingMaterials/CholletTestimony-120.pdf [accessed April 27, 2007].

Clancy C, Andresen E. 2002. Commentary: meeting the health care needs of people with disabilities. *Milbank Quarterly* 80(2):381–391.

Clark DO. 1997. US trends in disability and institutionalization among older blacks and whites. *American Journal of Public Health* 87(3):438–440.

CMS (Centers for Medicare & Medicaid Services). 1994. *The Health and Health Care of the Medicare Population*. Data from the 1994 Medicare Current Beneficiary Survey. [Online]. Available: http://198.232.249.10/mcbs/PubHHC94.asp [accessed April 27, 2007].

CMS. 2002. *Medicare Acts to Protect Coverage for Homebound Beneficiaries*. [Online]. Available: http://www.hhs.gov/news/press/2002pres/20020726d.html [accessed April 27, 2007].

CMS. 2004a. *Letter to Home Healthcare Providers from Stuart Gutterman, Director, CMS Office of Research, Development and Information*. October 8. [Online]. Available: http://www.cms.hhs.gov/DemoProjectsEvalRpts/downloads/MMA702_Home_Health_Provider_Letter_p.pdf [accessed April 27, 2007].

CMS. 2004b. *Medicare and Home Health Care*. [Online]. Available: http://www.medicare.gov/Publications/Pubs/pdf/10969.pdf [accessed April 27, 2007].

CMS. 2004c. *Revision of CR 3269 for the Demonstration Project to Clarify the Definition of Homebound (Homebound Demonstration)*. [Online]. Available: http://www.cms.hhs.gov/transmittals/downloads/R6DEMO.pdf [accessed April 27, 2007].

CMS. 2005a. *The Characteristics and Perceptions of the Medicare Population Series: Data from the 2003 Medicare Current Beneficiary Survey*. [Online]. Available: http://198.232.249.10/mcbs/PubCNP03.asp.

CMS. 2005b. *Decision Memo for Mobility Assistive Equipment (CAG-00274N)*. [Online]. Available: http://www.cms.hhs.gov/mcd/viewdecisionmemo.asp?id=143 [accessed April 27, 2007].

CMS. 2005c. *Draft Guidance for the Public, Industry, and CMS Staff: Factors CMS Considers in Making a Determination of Coverage with Evidence Development*. [Online]. Available: http://www.cms.hhs.gov/coverage/download/guidanceced.pdf [accessed April 27, 2007].

CMS. 2005d. *Medicaid At-a-Glance: A Medicaid Information Source*. [Online]. Available: http://www.cms.hhs.gov/MedicaidGenInfo/Downloads/MedicaidAtAGlance2005.pdf [accessed April 27, 2007].

CMS. 2005e. *Medicaid Early & Periodic Screening & Diagnostic Treatment Benefit: EPSDT Benefits*. [Online]. Available: http://www.cms.hhs.gov/MedicaidEarlyPeriodicScrn/02_Benefits.asp#TopOfPage [accessed April 27, 2007].

CMS. 2005f. *Medicare "Pay for Performance (P4P)" Initiatives*. [Online]. Available: http://www.cms.hhs.gov/apps/media/press/release.asp?Counter=1343 [accessed April 27, 2007].

CMS. 2006a. *The 2006 Annual Report of the Boards of Trustees of the Federal Hospital Insurance and Federal Supplementary Medical Insurance Trust Funds*. [Online]. Available: http://www.cms.hhs.gov/ReportsTrustFunds/downloads/tr2006.pdf [accessed April 27, 2007].

CMS. 2006b. *Choosing a Medigap Policy: A Guide to Health Insurance for People with Medicare*. [Online]. Available: http://www.medicare.gov/Publications/Pubs/pdf/02110.pdf [accessed April 27, 2007].

CMS. 2006c. *Competitive Acquisition for DMEPOS: New Quality Standards*. [Online]. Available: http://www.cms.hhs.gov/CompetitiveAcqforDMEPOS/04_new_quality_standards.asp [accessed April 27, 2007].

CMS. 2006d. *Decision Memorandum for the INDEPENDENCE 4000 iBOT Mobility System—Scope of Benefits §1862(a)(1)(A)*. [Online]. Available: http://www.cms.hhs.gov/mcd/ncpc_view_document.asp?id=5#dm [accessed April 27, 2007].

CMS. 2006e. *Guidance for the Public, Industry, and CMS Staff: Factors CMS Considers in Opening a National Coverage Determination*. [Online]. Available: http://www.cms.hhs.gov/mcd/ncpc_view_document.asp?id=6 [accessed April 27, 2007].

CMS. 2006f. *Medicare Enrollment: National Trends 1966–2005.* [Online]. Available: http://www.cms.hhs.gov/MedicareEnRpts/Downloads/HISMI05.pdf [accessed April 27, 2007].

CMS. 2006g. *National Health Expenditure Projections 2006–2016.* [Online]. Available: http://www.cms.hhs.gov/NationalHealthExpendData/downloads/proj2006.pdf [accessed April 27, 2007].

CMS. 2006h. *NCA Tracking Sheet for Clinical Trial Policy* (CAG-00071R). [Online]. Available: http://www.cms.hhs.gov/mcd/viewtrackingsheet.asp?id=186 [accessed April 27, 2007]

CMS. 2006i. *Outpatient Therapy Caps: Exceptions Process Required by the DRA.* Press release, February 15, CMS Office of Public Affairs. [Online]. Available: http://www.cms.hhs.gov/apps/media/press/release.asp?Counter=1782 [accessed April 27, 2007].

CMS. 2006j. *Update to Medicare Deductible, Coinsurance, and Premium Rates for 2006.* [Online]. Available: http://www.cms.hhs.gov/MLNMattersArticles/downloads/MM4132.pdf [accessed April 27, 2007].

CMS. 2007. *HCBS Waivers—Section 1915.* [Online]. Available: http://www.cms.hhs.gov/MedicaidStWaivProgDemoPGI/05_HCBSWaivers-Section1915(c).asp [accessed April 27, 2007].

CMS. Undated. *Technical Summary. Medicaid Program—General Information.* [Online]. Available: http://www.cms.hhs.gov/MedicaidGenInfo/03_TechnicalSummary.asp#TopOfPage [accessed April 27, 2007].

CMS/HCFA (Health Care Financing Administration). 2000. Medicare Program; Criteria for Making Coverage Decisions, Notice of Intent to develop a proposed rule. *Federal Register* 65(95):31124–31125.

CNN. 2006. *Forces: U.S. & Coalition/Casualties.* CNN.com war in Iraq main page. [Online]. Available: http://www.cnn.com/SPECIALS/2003/iraq/forces/casualties/ [accessed April 27, 2007].

Coble-Temple A. 2002. CDIP update: understanding the differences between worksite personal assistance services (PAS) and personal PAS on the job: why this is important to rehabilitation? In: *Rehabilitation Psychology News*, 29(4), Newsletter for Division 22 of the APA. Summer Convention. [Online]. Available: http://www.apa.org/divisions/div22/Summer-Conv2002news.html [accessed April 27, 2007].

Cohen R, Martinez M. 2006. *Health Insurance Coverage: Estimates from the National Health Interview Survey, 2005.* [Online]. Available: http://www.cdc.gov/nchs/data/nhis/early release/insur200606.pdf [accessed April 27, 2007].

Cohen SM, Labadie RF, Dietrich MS, Haynes DS. 2004. Quality of life in hearing-impaired adults: the role of cochlear implants and hearing aids. *Otolaryngology—Head and Neck Surgery* 131(4):413–422.

Cohen WI, Patterson B, eds. 1999. Health care guidelines for individuals with Down syndrome 1999 revision: Down syndrome preventive medical checklist. *Down Syndrome Quarterly* 4(3):1–15.

Cole J, Illis L, Sedgwick E. 1991. Intractable pain in spinal cord injury is not relieved by spinal cord stimulation. *Paraplegia* 29:167–172.

Colker R. 2000. ADA Title III: a fragile compromise. *Berkeley Journal of Employment and Law* 21:377–412.

Connecticut Department of Social Services. 2003. *The Definition of and the Determination of Medical Necessity for Durable Medical Equipment (DME).* [Online]. Available: http://www.ctmedicalprogram.com/bulletin/pb03_113.pdf [accessed April 27, 2007].

Connolly BH. 2006. Issues in aging in individuals with life long disabilities. *Revista Brasiliera de Fisioterapia, São Carlos* 10(3):249–262.

CSCM (Consortium for Spinal Cord Medicine). 1999. *Neurogenic Bowel: What You Should Know.* Washington, DC: Paralyzed Veterans of America. [Online]. Available: http://www.pva.org/site/DocServer/BWLC.pdf?docID=621 [accessed April 27, 2007].

CSCM. 2000. *Pressure Ulcer Prevention and Treatment Following Spinal Cord Injury: A Clinical Practice Guideline for Health-Care Professionals.* Washington, DC: Paralyzed Veterans of America. [Online]. Available: http://www.pva.org/site/DocServer/PU.pdf?docID=688 [accessed April 27, 2007].

CSCM. 2002. *Pressure Ulcers: What You Should Know.* Washington, DC: Paralyzed Veterans of America. [Online]. Available: http://www.pva.org/site/DocServer/PUC.pdf?docID=702 [accessed April 27, 2007].

CSCM. 2005a. *Preservation of Upper Limb Function Following Spinal Cord Injury: A Clinical Practice Guideline for Health-Care Professionals.* Washington, DC: Paralyzed Veterans of America. [Online]. Available: http://www.pva.org/site/DocServer/upperlimb.pdf?docID=705 [accessed April 27, 2007].

CSCM. 2005b. *Respiratory Management Following Spinal Cord Injury: A Clinical Practice Guideline for Health-Care Professionals.* Washington, DC: Paralyzed Veterans of America. [Online]. Available: http://www.pva.org/site/DocServer/resmgmt.pdf?docID=703 [accessed April 27, 2007].

CSCM. 2006. *Bladder Management for Adults with Spinal Cord Injury: A Clinical Practice Guideline for Health-Care Providers.* Washington, DC: Paralyzed Veterans of America. [Online]. Available: http://www.pva.org/site/DocServer/Bladder.WEB.pdf?docID=1101 [accessed April 27, 2007].

Cooley WC, Committee on Children with Disabilities. 2004. Providing a primary care medical home for children and youth with cerebral palsy. *Pediatrics* 114(4):1106–1113.

Cooper RA, Spaeth DM, Jones DK, Boninger ML, Fitzgerald SG, Guo S. 2002. Comparison of virtual and real electric powered wheelchair driving using a position sensing joystick and an isometric joystick. *Medical Engineering and Physics* 24(10): 703–708.

Cornman JC, Freedman VA, Agree EM. 2005. Measurement of assistive device use: implications for estimates of device use and disability in late life. *Gerontologist* 45(3):347–358.

Cortiella C. 2005. *IDEA 2004 Close Up: Transition Planning.* [Online]. Available: http://www.schwablearning.org/articles.asp?r=998 [accessed April 27, 2007].

Couriel J. 2003. Asthma in adolescence. *Pediatric Respiratory Reviews* 4(1):47–54.

Courthouse Access Advisory Committee (Architectural and Transportation Barriers Compliance Board). 2006. *Justice for All: Designing Accessible Courthouses: Recommendations from the Courthouse Access Advisory Committee.* [Online]. Available: http://www.access-board.gov/caac/report.htm [accessed April 27, 2007].

Covinsky KE, Palmer RM, Fortinsky RH, Counsell SR, Stewart Al, Kresevic D, Burant CJ, et al. 2003. Loss of independence in activities of daily living in older adults hospitalized with medical illness: increased vulnerability with age. *Journal of the American Geriatrics Society* 51(4):451–458.

Covinsky KE, Hilton J, Lindquist K, Dudley RA. 2006. Development and validation of an index to predict activity of daily living dependence in community-dwelling elders. *Medical Care* 44(2):149–157.

CPPP (Center for Public Policy Priorities). 2001. *All Grown Up, Nowhere to Go: Teens in Foster Care Transition.* CPPP, Texas Foster Care Transitions Project [Online]. Available: http://www.cppp.org/files/4/all%20grown%20up.pdf [accessed April 27, 2007].

Cremers MJ, Bol E, de Roos F, Van Gijn J. 1993a. Risk of sports activities in children with Down's syndrome and atlantoaxial instability. *Lancet* 342(8870):511–514.

Cremers MJ, Ramos L, Bol E, vanGijn J. 1993b. Radiological assessment of the atlantoaxial distance in Down's syndrome. *Archives of Disease in Childhood* 69(3):347–350.

Crimmins E. 2004. Trends in the health of the elderly. *Annual Review of Public Health* 25(1):79–99.

Crimmins E, Saito Y. 2000. Change in the prevalence of diseases among older Americans: 1984–1994. *Demographic Research* (Online Journal) 3(9). [Online]. Available: http:// www.demographic-research.org/Volumes/Vol3/9/3-9.pdf [accessed April 27, 2007].

Crowley J. 2006. *Medicaid Long-Term Services Reforms in the Deficit Reduction Act.* Kaiser Commission on Medicaid and the Uninsured. [Online]. Available: http://www.ihcs.msu. edu/ltc/Commission/DRA%20summary%205-16-05.pdf [accessed April 27, 2007].

Crowley J, Elias R. 2003. *Medicaid's Role for People with Disabilities.* The Kaiser Commission on Medicaid and the Uninsured. [Online]. Available: http://www.kff.org/medicaid/ upload/Medicaid-s-Role-for-People-with-Disabilities.pdf [accessed April 27, 2007].

Curtis KA, Roach KE, Applegate EB, Amar T, Benbow CS, Genecco TD, Gualano J. 1995. Reliability and validity of the Wheelchair User's Shoulder Pain Index (WUSPI). *Paraplegia* 33(10):595–601.

Curtis KA, Drysdale GA, Larnza RD, Kolber M, Vitolo RS, West MR. 1999a. Shoulder pain in wheelchair users with tetraplegia and paraplegia. *Archives of Physical Medicine & Rehabilitation* 80(4):453–457.

Curtis KA, Tyner TM, Zachary L, Lentell G, Brink D, Didyk T, Gean K, Hall J, Hooper M, Klos J, et al. 1999b. Effect of a standard exercise protocol on shoulder pain in long-term wheelchair users. *Spinal Cord* 37(6):421–429.

Cutler DM. 1995. Technology, health costs and the NIH. Paper prepared for the National Institutes of Health Economics Roundtable on Biomedical Research, Cambridge, MA, September.

Cutler DM. 2001. Declining disability among the elderly. *Health Affairs (Millwood)* 20(6): 11–27.

Cutler DM. 2003. Intensive medical technology and the reduction of disability. In: Wise D, ed. *Analyses in the Economics of Aging.* Chicago, IL: University of Chicago Press.

Cutler DM, Meara E. 1999. *The Concentration of Medical Spending: An Update.* NBER Working Paper 7279. Cambridge, MA: National Bureau of Economic Research. [Online]. Available: http://www.nber.org/papers/W7279 [accessed April 27, 2007].

Cutler DM, Wise DA, eds. In press. *Health in Older Ages: The Causes and Consequences of Declining Disability Among the Elderly.* Chicago, IL: The University of Chicago Press. [Online]. Available: http://www.nber.org/books/disability/index.html [accessed April 27, 2007].

Cutler DM, Zeckhauser R. 2004. *Extending the Theory to Meet the Practice of Insurance.* Harvard University Economics Department. [Online]. Available: http://post.economics. harvard.edu/faculty/dcutler/papers/cutler_zeckhauser_theory_and_practice_of_insurance. pdf [accessed April 27, 2007].

Cutler DM, Rosen AB, Vijan S. 2006. The value of medical spending in the United States, 1960–2000. *New England Journal of Medicine* 355(9):920–927. [Online]. Available: http://content.nejm.org/cgi/content/abstract/355/9/920 [accessed April 27, 2007].

Dale S, Brown R. 2005. *The Effect of Cash and Counseling on Medicaid and Medicare Costs: Findings for Adults in Three States.* Princeton, NJ: Mathematica Policy Research, Inc. [Online]. Available: http://www.mathematica-mpr.com/publications/pdfs/ cashandcounseling3states.pdf [accessed April 27, 2007].

Dale S, Verdier J. 2003. *Elimination of Medicare's Waiting Period for Seriously Disabled Adults: Impact on Coverage and Costs.* The Commonwealth Fund Publication No. 660. Mathematica Policy Research, Inc. [Online]. Available: http://www.cmwf.org/usr_ doc/660_Dale_elimination.pdf [accessed April 27, 2007].

Darer JD, Hwang W, Pham HH, Bass EB, Anderson G. 2004. More training needed in chronic care: a survey of US physicians. *Academic Medicine* 79(6):541–548.

DATI (Delaware Assistive Technology Initiative). 2005. *Guide to Funding Resources for Assistive Technology in Delaware*. [Online]. Available: http://www.dati.org/funding/Funding_Guide_PrintVersion.pdf [accessed April 27, 2007].

Davidoff A. 2004. Insurance for children with special health care needs: patterns of coverage and burden on families to provide adequate insurance. *Pediatrics* 114(2):394–403.

Davidoff A, Kennedy G. 2005. *Uninsured Americans with Chronic Health Conditions: Key Findings from the National Health Interview Survey*. Robert Wood Johnson Foundation. [Online]. Available: http://www.urban.org/UploadedPDF/411161_uninsured_americans.pdf [accessed April 27, 2007].

Davis K. 2004. *Will Consumer Directed Health Care Improve System Performance?* The Commonwealth Fund Publication No. 773. [Online]. Available: http://www.cmwf.org/usr_doc/davis_cdhc-hsr_ib_773.pdf [accessed April 27, 2007].

Davis K, Collins S. 2005–2006. Medicare at forty. *Health Care Financing Review* 27(2): 53–62.

Davis R, Lentini R. 1975. Transcutaneous nerve stimulation for treatment of pain in patients with spinal cord injury. *Surgical Neurology* 4(1):100–101.

Day JC. 1996. Projections of the number of households and families in the United States: 1995 to 2010, U.S. Census Bureau. *Current Population Reports*, P 25-1129. Washington, DC: U.S. Government Printing Office. [Online]. Available: http://www.census.gov/prod/1/pop/p25-1129.pdf [accessed April 27, 2007].

Dean E, Ross J. 1988. Modified aerobic walking program: effect on patients with postpolio syndrome symptoms. *Archives of Physical Medicine & Rehabilitation* 69(12):1033–1038.

Decker FH. 2005. *Nursing Homes, 1977–99: What Has Changed, What Has Not?* Hyattsville, MD: National Center for Health Statistics. [Online]. Available: http://www.cdc.gov/nchs/data/nnhsd/NursingHomes1977_99.pdf [accessed April, 27, 2007].

DeJong G, Sutton J. 1998. Managed care and catastrophic injury: the case of spinal cord injury. *Topics in Spinal Cord Injury Rehabilitation* 3(4):1–16.

DeJong G, Palsbo SE, Beatty PW, Jones GC, Kroll T, Neri MT. 2002. The organization and financing of health services for persons with disabilities. *Milbank Quarterly* 80(2): 261–301.

DeLeire T. 2000. The wage and employment effects of the Americans with Disabilities. *Journal of Human Resources* 35:693–715.

Dell S, To T. 2001. Breastfeeding and asthma in young children: findings from a population-based study. *Archives of Pediatrics & Adolescent Medicine* 155(11):1261–1265.

DeNavas-Walt C, Proctor B, Lee C. 2006. Income, poverty, and health insurance coverage in the United States: 2005. U.S. Census Bureau. In: *Current Population Reports*. [Online]. Available: http://www.census.gov/prod/2006pubs/p60-231.pdf [accessed April 27, 2007].

Desai M, Pratt LA, Lentzner H, Robinson KN. 2001. Trends in vision and hearing among older Americans. *Aging Trends* Mar(2):1–8. [Online]. Available: http://www.cdc.gov/nchs/data/achd/agingtrends/02vision.pdf [accessed April 27, 2007].

Devey G. 2002. National Science Foundation disability research. Working Draft. Unpublished staff paper. Arlington, VA: Biomedical Engineering Program, Research to Aid Persons with Disabilities Program, National Science Foundation.

DHHS (U.S. Department of Health and Human Services). 1990. *Healthy People 2000: National Health Promotion and Disease Prevention Objectives*. Washington, DC: U.S. Government Printing Office.

DHHS. 2000a. Disability and secondary conditions. In: *Healthy People 2010: Understanding and Improving Health*, 2nd ed. Washington, DC: U.S. Government Printing Office. [Online]. Available: http://www.healthypeople.gov/document/HTML/Volume1/06Disability.htm [accessed April 27, 2007].

DHHS. 2000b. *Healthy People 2010: Understanding and Improving Health*, 2nd ed. Washington, DC: U.S. Government Printing Office. [Online]. Available: http://www.healthypeople.gov/Document/tableofcontents.htm#volume1 [accessed April 27, 2007].

DHHS. 2001. *Delivering on the Promise: Preliminary Report: Federal Agency Actions to Eliminate Barriers and Promote Community Integration.* [Online]. Available: http://www.hhs.gov/newfreedom/prelim/assist.html [accessed April 27, 2007].

DHHS. 2002. *Delivering on the Promise: Self-Evaluation to Promote Community Living for People with Disabilities.* Report to the President on Executive Order 13217. [Online]. Available: http://www.hhs.gov/newfreedom/final/pdf/hhs.pdf [accessed April 27, 2007].

DHHS. 2004. *The National Survey of Children with Special Health Care Needs Chartbook 2001.* Rockville, MD: U.S. Department of Health and Human Services. [Online]. Available: http://mchb.hrsa.gov/chscn [accessed May 30, 2007].

DHHS. 2006a. *Delivering on the Promise: OCR's Compliance Activities Promote Community Integration.* [Online]. Available: http://www.hhs.gov/ocr/complianceactiv.html [accessed April 27, 2007].

DHHS. 2006b. Notice: annual update on the HHS poverty guidelines. *Federal Register* 71(15):3848–3849. [Online]. Available: http://aspe.hhs.gov/poverty/06fedreg.pdf [accessed April 27, 2007].

DHHS. 2006c. *Strategic Plan FY 2004–2009.* [Online]. Available: http://aspe.hhs.gov/hhsplan/2004/hhsplan2004.pdf [accessed April 27, 2007].

DHHS. Undated. *Healthy People 2010 Midcourse Review: Focus Area 6, Disability and Secondary Conditions.* [Online]. Available: http://www.healthypeople.gov/data/midcourse/comments/facontents.asp?id=6 [accessed April 27, 2007].

DHHS/U.S. Department of Labor. 2003. *The Future Supply of Long-Term Care Workers in Relation to the Aging Baby Boom Generation.* Report to Congress. [Online]. Available: http://aspe.hhs.gov/daltcp/reports/ltcwork.pdf [accessed April 27, 2007].

Diab ME, Johnston MV. 2004. Relationships between level of disability and receipt of preventive health services. *Archives of Physical Medicine & Rehabilitation* 85(5):749–757.

Dick AW, Allison RA, Haber SG, Brach C, Shenkman E. 2002. Consequences of states' policies for SCHIP disenrollment. *Health Care Financing Review* 23(3):65–88.

Dickens C, Creed F. 2001. The burden of depression in patients with rheumatoid arthritis. *Rheumatology (Oxford)* 40(12):1327–1330.

Dole, R. 1999. Forward. In: *Just as I Am: Americans with Disabilities.* Sherer C, Dossett E. 1999. Birmingham, AL: Crane Hill Publishers.

Donabedian A. 1976. *Benefits in Medical Care Programs.* Cambridge, MA: Harvard University Press.

Dor A, Encinosa W. 2004. *Does Cost Sharing Affect Compliance? The Case of Prescription Drugs.* NBER Working Paper 10738. Cambridge, MA: National Bureau of Economic Research. [Online]. Available: http://papers.nber.org/papers/w10738.pdf [accessed April 27, 2007].

Dorn S, Kenney G. 2006. *Automatically Enrolling Eligible Children and Families into Medicaid and SCHIP: Opportunities, Obstacles, and Options for Federal Policymakers.* Commonwealth Fund Publication No. 931. [Online]. Available: http://www.cmwf.org/usr_doc/Dorn_auto-enrollingchildren_931.pdf [accessed April 27, 2007].

DRA (Disability Rights Advocates). 2006. *The Briefcase. Disability Rights Advocates' Semi-Annual Newsletter: Sidewalk Accessibility.* [Online]. Available: http://www.dralegal.org/briefcase/ [accessed April 27, 2007].

Dusing SC, Skinner AC, Mayer ML. 2004. Unmet need for therapy services, assistive devices, and related services: data from the national survey of children with special health care needs. *Ambulatory Pediatrics* 4(5):448–454.

Eckel R. 2005. Obesity. *Circulation* 111:257–259. [Online]. Available: http://circ.ahajournals. org/cgi/reprint/111/15/e257 [accessed April 27, 2007].

Eckholm E. 2006. Medicaid plan prods patients toward health. *The New York Times*, December 1. [Online]. Available: http://www.nytimes.com/2006/12/01/us/01medicaid.html?_ r=1&oref=slogin [accessed April 27, 2007].

Edsall T. 2005. Funds for health care of veterans $1 billion short. *The Washington Post*, June 24, p. A29. [Online]. Available: http://www.washingtonpost.com/wp-dyn/content/ article/2005/06/23/AR2005062301888.html [accessed April 27, 2007].

EEOC (U.S. Equal Employment Opportunity Commission). 2002. *Federal Laws Prohibiting Job Discrimination Questions and Answers.* [Online]. Available: http://www.eeoc.gov/ facts/qanda.html [accessed April 27, 2007].

Ehrlich NJ, Carlson D, Bailey N. 2003. Sources of information about how to obtain assistive technology: findings from a national survey of persons with disabilities. *Assistive Technology* Summer; 15(1):28–38.

Eichner J, Blumenthal D, eds. 2003. *Medicare in the 21st Century: Building a Better Chronic Care System.* Washington, DC: National Academy of Social Insurance. [Online]. Available: http://www.nasi.org/usr_doc/Chronic_Care_Report.pdf [accessed April 27, 2007].

Einarsson G. 1991. Muscle conditioning in late poliomyelitis. *Archives of Physical Medicine & Rehabilitation* 72(1):11–14.

Elborn JS, Shale DJ, Britton JR. 1991. Cystic fibrosis: current survival and population estimate to the year 2000. *Thorax* 46:881–885.

Engel JM, Kartin D, Jensen MP. 2002. Pain treatment in persons with cerebral palsy: frequency and helpfulness. *American Journal of Physical Medicine & Rehabilitation* 81(4): 291–296.

Engel JM, Petrina TJ, Dudgeon BJ, McKearnan KA. 2005. Cerebral palsy and chronic pain: a descriptive study of children and adolescents. *Physical & Occupational Therapy in Pediatrics* 25(4):73–84.

English A, Moreale MC, Larsen J. 2003. Access to health care for youth leaving foster care: Medicaid and SCHIP. *Journal of Adolescent Health* 32S:53–69.

English A, Stinnett AJ, Dunn-Georgiou E. 2006. *Health Care for Adolescents and Young Adults Leaving Foster Care: Policy Options for Improving Access.* Center for Adolescent Health and the Law. [Online]. Available: http://www.cahl.org/PDFs/FCIssueBrief.pdf [accessed April 27, 2007].

ERCA (Engineering Research Centers Association). 2006. *About the ERC's.* [Online]. Available: http://www.erc-assoc.org [accessed April 27, 2007].

Erlandson RE, Enderle JD, Winters JM. 2007. Educating engineers in universal and accessible design. In: Winters JM, Story MF, eds. *Medical Instrumentation: Accessibility and Usability Considerations.* Boca Raton, FL: CRC Press. Pp. 101–118.

Ernstoff B, Wetterqvist H, Kvist H, Grimby G. 1996. Endurance training effect on individuals with postpoliomyelitis. *Archives of Physical Medicine & Rehabilitation* 77(9):843–848.

Escobedo EM, Hunter J, Hollister M, Patten RM, Goldstein B. 1997. MR imaging of rotator cuff tears in individuals with paraplegia. *American Journal of Roentgenology* 168(4):919–923.

Estes JP, Deyer CA, Hansen RA, Russell JC. 1991. Influence of occupational therapy curricula on students' attitudes toward persons with disabilities. *American Journal of Occupational Therapy* 45(2):156–159.

Etheredge L, Moore J. 2003. A new Medicaid program. *Health Affairs, Web Exclusive* (August 27):426–439. [Online]. Available: http://content.healthaffairs.org/cgi/content/abstract/ hlthaff.w3.426v1 [accessed March 27, 2007].

Ettinger WH, Fried LP, Harris T, Shemanski L, Schulz R, Robbins J. 1994. Self-reported causes of physical disability in older people: the Cardiovascular Health Study. *Journal of the American Geriatric Society* 42(10):1035–1044.

Ettner S, Kuhlthau K, McLaughlin TJ, Perrin J, Gortmaker S. 2000. Impact of expanding SSI on Medicaid expenditures of disabled children. *Health Care Financing Review*, Spring 2000. [Online]. Available: http://www.findarticles.com/p/articles/mi_m0795/is_3_21/ai_69434517 [accessed April 27, 2007].

Evans PM, Alberman E. 1991. Certified cause of death in children and young adults with cerebral palsy. *Archives of Disease in Childhood* 66(3):325–329.

Eyman RK, Grossman HJ, Chaney RH, Call TL. 1990. The life expectancy of profoundly handicapped people with mental retardation. *New England Journal of Medicine* 323(9): 584–589.

Farbu E, Gilhus N, Barnes M, Borg K, de Visser M, Driessen A, Howard R, Nollet, Opara J, Stalberg E. 2006. EFNS guideline on diagnosis and management of post-polio syndrome. Report of an EFNS task force. *European Journal of Neurology* 13(8):795–801.

Farkas M, Jette AM, Tennstedt S, Haley SM, Quinn V. 2003. Knowledge dissemination and utilization in gerontology: an organizing framework. *Gerontologist* 43(1):47–56.

Faulkner E. 1940. *Accident-and-Health Insurance.* New York: McGraw-Hill Book Company, Inc.

FDA (Food and Drug Administration). 1993. *FDA Plans to Strengthen Hearing Aids Rules.* [Online]. Available: http://www.fda.gov/bbs/topics/ANSWERS/ANS00507.html [accessed April 27, 2007].

FDA. 1999. *Regulation of Medical Devices: Background Information for International Officials.* [Online]. Available: http://www.fda.gov/cdrh/manual/ireas.pdf [accessed April 27, 2007].

FDA. 2003. *Summary of Safety and Effectiveness Data.* [Online]. Available: http://www.fda.gov/cdrh/pdf2/P020033b.pdf [accessed April 27, 2007].

FDA. 2006. *Humanitarian Device Exemption (HDE) Regulation: Questions and Answers.* [Online]. Available: http://www.fda.gov/cdrh/ode/guidance/1381.pdf [accessed April 27, 2007].

Federal Interagency Forum on Child and Family Statistics. 2005. *America's Children: Key National Indicators of Well-Being, 2005.* [Online]. Available: http://www.childstats.gov/amchildren05/index.asp [accessed April 27, 2007].

Federman AD, Adams AS, Ross-Degnan D, Soumerai SB, Ayanian JZ. 2001. Supplemental insurance and use of effective cardiovascular drugs among elderly Medicare beneficiaries with coronary heart disease. *The Journal of the American Medical Association* 286(14):1732–1739.

Fendrick AM, Chernew ME. 2006. Value-based insurance design: aligning incentives to bridge the divide between quality improvement and cost containment. *American Journal of Managed Care* 12(Special Issue):SP1–SP6.

Ferrucci L, Guralnik JM, Simonsick E, Salive ME, Corti C, Langlois J. 1996. Progressive versus catastrophic disability: a longitudinal view of the disablement process. *The Journals of Gerontology, Series A: Biological Sciences and Medical Sciences* 51(3):M123–M130.

Fishman E. 2001. Aging out of coverage: young adults with special health needs. *Health Affairs (Millwood)* 20(6):254–266.

Fisk AD, Rogers WA, Charness N, Czaja SJ, Sharit J. 2004. *Designing for Older Adults: Principles and Creative Human Factors Approaches.* Boca Raton, FL: CRC Press.

Fitzgerald SG, Arva J, Cooper RA, Dvorznak MJ, Spaeth DM, Boninger ML. 2003. A pilot study on community usage of a pushrim-activated, power-assisted wheelchair. *Assistive Technology* 15(2):113–119.

Flegal K, Carroll M, Ogden C, Johnson C. 2002. Prevalence and trends in obesity among U.S. adults, 1999-2000. *The Journal of the American Medical Association* 288(14): 1723-1727.

Flegal K, Graubard B, Williamson D, Gail M. 2005. Excess deaths associated with underweight, overweight, and obesity. *The Journal of the American Medical Association* 293:1861-1867.

Flume PA, Taylor LA, Anderson DL, Gray S, Turner D. 2004. Transition programs in cystic fibrosis centers: perceptions of team members. *Pediatric Pulmonology* 37(1):4–7.

Foltz A. 1982. *An Ounce of Prevention: Child Health Politics Under Medicaid.* Cambridge, MA: The MIT Press.

Fombonne E. 2002. Epidemiological trends in rates of autism. *Molecular Psychiatry* 7(Suppl 2):S4–S6.

Fong GR. 2001. Repositioning the advanced technology program. *Issues in Science and Technology* 18(1):65–70.

Foote SM, Hogan C. 2001. Disability profile and health care costs of Medicare beneficiaries under age sixty-five. *Health Affairs (Millwood)* 20(6):242–253.

Forrest CB, Riley AW. 2004. Childhood origins of adult health: a basis for life-course health policy. *Pediatrics* 23(5):155–164.

Fougeyrollas P. 1995. Documenting environmental factors for preventing the handicap creation process: Quebec contributions relating to ICIDH and social participation of people with functional differences. *Disability and Rehabilitation* 17(3–4):145–153.

Fougeyrollas P, Noreau I, St Michel G, Boschen K. 1997. Measure of the quality of the environment. *ICIDH and Environmental Factors International Network* 9(1):32–39.

Fougeyrollas P, Noreau L, Bergeron H, Cloutier R, Dion SA, St-Michel G. 1998. Social consequences of long term impairments and disabilities: conceptual approach and assessment of handicap. *International Journal of Rehabilitation Medicine* 21(2):127–141.

Fox HB, Newacheck PW. 1990. Private health insurance of chronically ill children. *Pediatrics* 85(1):50–57.

Fox HB, McManus MA, Reichman MB. 2002. *The Strengths and Weaknesses of Private Health Insurance Coverage for Children with Special Health Care Needs.* Washington, DC: MCH Policy Research Center. [Online]. Available: http://www.mchpolicy.org/publications/pdfs/phi.pdf [accessed April 27, 2007].

Freedman VA. 2006. Late-life disability trends: an overview of current evidence. In: Field MJ, Jette AM, Martin L, eds. *Workshop on Disability in America: A New Look.* Washington, DC: The National Academies Press. Pp. 101–112.

Freedman VA, Martin LG. 1998. Understanding trends in functional limitations among older Americans. *American Journal of Public Health* 88(10):1457–1462.

Freedman VA, Martin LG. 1999. The role of education in explaining and forecasting trends in functional limitations among older Americans. *Demography* 36(4):461–473.

Freedman VA, Martin LG. 2000. Contribution of chronic conditions to aggregate changes in old-age functioning. *American Journal of Public Health* 90(11):1755–1760.

Freedman VA, Martin LG, Schoeni R. 2002. Recent trends in disability and functioning among older adults in the United States: a systematic review. *The Journal of the American Medical Association* 288:3137–3146.

Freedman VA, Crimmins EM, Schoeni RF, Spillman BC, Aykan H, Kramarow E, Land K, Lubitz J, Manton KG, Martin LG. 2004a. Resolving inconsistencies in trends in old-age disability: report from a technical working group. *Demography* 41(3):417–441.

Freedman VA, Martin LG, Schoeni RF. 2004b. Disability in America. Population Reference Bureau. *Population Bulletin* 59(3):1–32. [Online]. Available: http://findarticles.com/p/articles/mi_qa3761/is_200409/ai_n9432640/pg_1 [accessed April 27, 2007].

Freedman VA, Calkins M, DeRosiers R, Van Haitsma K. 2005a. *Barriers to Implementing Technology in Residential Long-Term Care Settings.* Office of the Assistant Secretary for Planning and Evaluation, U.S. Department of Health and Human Services. [Online]. Available: http://aspe.hhs.gov/daltcp/reports/techbarr.pdf [accessed April 27, 2007].

Freedman VA, Waidmann T, Spillman B. 2005b. *Opportunities for Improving Survey Measures of Late-Life Disability. Part II. Workshop Summary.* Washington, DC: Office of the Assistant Secretary for Planning and Evaluation, U.S. Department of Health and Human Services. [Online]. Available: http://aspe.hhs.gov/daltcp/reports/2006/survmeasII. pdf [accessed April 27, 2007].

Freedman VA, Agree EM, Martin LG, Cornman JC. 2006. Trends in the use of assistive technology and personal care for late-life disability, 1992–2001. *Gerontologist* 46(1):124–127.

Freiman M, Mann W, Johnson J, Lin S, Locklear C. 2006. *Public Funding and Support of Assistive Technologies for Persons with Disabilities.* [Online]. Available: http://assets.aarp. org/rgcenter/il/2006_04_assist.pdf. [accessed April 27, 2007].

Fried LP, Young Y, Rubin G, Bandeen-Roche K, WHAS II Collaborative Research Group. 2001. Self-reported preclinical disability identifies older women with early declines in performance and early disease. *Journal of Clinical Epidemiology* 54(9):889–901.

Fried LP, Ferrucci L, Darer J, Williamson JD, Anderson G. 2004. Untangling the concepts of disability, frailty, and comorbidity; implications for improved targeting and care. *The Journals of Gerontology, Series A: Biological Sciences and Medical Sciences* 59(3): 255–263.

Friedland R. 2004. Caregivers and long-term care needs in the 21st century: will public policy meet the challenge? *Long-Term Care Financing Project, Georgetown University.* [Online]. Available: http://ltc.georgetown.edu/pdfs/caregiversfriedland.pdf [accessed April 27, 2007].

Friedman JM. 2001. Racial disparities in median age at death of persons with Down syndrome—United States, 1968–1997. *Morbidity and Mortality Weekly Report* 50(22):463–465.

Fries JF. 1980. Aging, natural death and the compression of morbidity. *New England Journal of Medicine* 303(3):130–135.

Fries JF, Bruce B, Cella D. 2005. The promise of PROMIS: using item response theory to improve assessment of patient-reported outcomes. *Clinical and Experimental Rheumatology* 23(5 Suppl 39):S53–S57.

Fronstin P. 2005. *The Impact of the Erosion of Retiree Health Benefits on Workers and Retirees.* EBRI Issue Brief No. 279. [Online]. Available: http://www.ebri.org/pdf/briefspdf/ 0305ib.pdf [accessed April 27, 2007].

Frontera WR, Fuhrer MJ, Jette AM, Chan L, Cooper RA, Duncan PW, Kemp JD, Ottenbacher KJ, Peckham PH, Roth EJ, et al. 2006. Rehabilitation Medicine Summit: building research capacity—executive summary. *Assistive Technology* 18(1):2–14.

FTA (Federal Transit Administration). 2005. *ADA Compliance Review Final Reports.* [Online]. Available: http://www.fta.dot.gov/civilrights/ada/civil_rights_3899.html [accessed April 27, 2007].

Fuhrer MJ, Jutai JW, Scherer MJ. 2003. A framework for the conceptual modelling of assistive technology device outcomes. *Disability and Rehabilitation* 18(25):1243–1251.

Fuji T, Yonenobu K, Fujiwara K, Yamashita K, Ebara S, Ono K, Okada K. 1987. Cervical radiculopathy or myelopathy secondary to athetoid cerebral palsy. *Journal of Bone and Joint Surgery* 69(6):815–821.

Fujiura GT. 2001. Emerging trends in disability. *Population Today* 29(August/September): unpaged. [Online]. Available: http://www.prb.org/pdf/PT_augsep01.pdf [accessed April 27, 2007].

GAO (General Accounting Office). 1989. *Department of Education: Management of the Office of Special Education and Rehabilitative Services*. Report to the Chairman, Subcommittee on Select Education, Committee on Education and Labor, U.S. House of Representatives. [Online]. Available: http://archive.gao.gov/d26t7/140122.pdf [accessed April 27, 2007].

GAO. 1991. *Private Health Insurance: Problems Caused by a Segmented Market*. Report GAO/HRD-91-114. Washington, DC: GAO.

GAO. 1993. *Americans with Disabilities Act: Initial Accessibility Good but Important Barriers Remain*. Report to the Chairman, Subcommittee on Select Education and Civil Rights, Committee on Education and Labor, U.S. House of Representatives. [Online]. Available: http://archive.gao.gov/t2pbat5/149390.pdf [accessed April 27, 2007].

GAO. 1994a. *Americans with Disabilities Act: The Effects of the Law on Access to Goods and Services*. Washington, DC: GAO. [Online]. Available: http://archive.gao.gov/t2pbat2/152169.pdf [accessed April 27, 2007].

GAO. 1994b. *Social Security: Rapid Rise in Children on SSI Disability Rolls Follows New Regulations*. Report GAO/HEHS-225. Washington, DC: GAO. [Online]. Available: http://archive.gao.gov/t2pbat2/152512.pdf [accessed April 27, 2007].

GAO. 1997. *Cost Growth and Proposals to Manage It Through Prospective Payment and Other Controls*. Statement of William J. Scanlon to the Committee on Finance, U.S. Senate. [Online]. Available: http://www.gao.gov/archive/1997/he97106t.pdf [accessed April 27, 2007].

GAO. 2000. *Medicare Home Health Care: Prospective Payment System Could Reverse Recent Declines in Spending*. Report to the Chairman, Subcommittee on Health, Committee on Ways and Means, U.S. House of Representatives. [Online]. Available: http://www.gao.gov/new.items/he00176.pdf [accessed April 27, 2007].

GAO. 2001a. *Medicaid: Stronger Efforts Needed to Ensure Children's Access to Health Screening Services*. Report to congressional requesters. [Online]. Available: http://www.gao.gov/new.items/d01749.pdf [accessed April 27, 2007].

GAO. 2001b. *SSA Disability: Other Programs May Provide Lessons for Improving Return-to-Work Efforts*. Report to congressional requesters. [Online]. Available: http://www.gao.gov/new.items/d01153.pdf [accessed April 27, 2007].

GAO. 2002. *Long Term Care: Availability of Medicaid Home and Community Services for Elderly Individuals Varies Considerably*. Report to the Chairman, Special Committee on Aging, U.S. Senate. [Online]. Available: http://www.gao.gov/new.items/d021121.pdf [accessed April 27, 2007].

GAO. 2003a. *Transportation-Disadvantaged Populations*. [Online]. Available: http://www.gao.gov/new.items/d03697.pdf [accessed April 27, 2007].

GAO. 2003b. *Federal Oversight of Growing Medicaid Home and Community-Based Waivers Should be Strengthened*. [Online]. Available: http://www.gao.gov/new.items/d03576.pdf [accessed April 27, 2007].

GAO (Government Accountability Office). 2004. *Medicare: CMS's Program Safeguards Did Not Deter Growth in Spending for Power Wheelchairs*. Report GAO-05-43. [Online]. Available: http://www.gao.gov/new.items/d0543.pdf [accessed April 27, 2007].

GAO. 2005. *Medicare: Little Progress Made in Targeting Outpatient Therapy Payments to Beneficiaries' Needs*. Report to congressional requesters. [Online]. Available: http://www.gao.gov/new.items/d0659.pdf [accessed April 27, 2007].

GAO. 2006. *Federal Information Collection: A Reexamination of the Portfolio of Major Federal Household Surveys Is Needed*. Report for congressional requesters. [Online]. Available: http://www.gao.gov/new.items/d0762.pdf [accessed April 27, 2007].

GAO. 2007. *Medicare Improvements Needed to Address Improper Payments for Medical Equipment and Supplies.* Report to the ranking minority member, Committee on Finance, U.S. Senate. [Online]. Available: http://www.gao.gov/new.items/d0759.pdf [accessed April 27, 2007].

Garber A. 2004. Cost-effectiveness and evidence evaluation as criteria for coverage policy. *Health Affairs, Web Exclusive* (May 19):284–296. [Online]. Available: http://content. healthaffairs.org/cgi/reprint/hlthaff.w4.284v1 [accessed April 27, 2007].

Gardner-Bonneau D. 2007. Accessibility standards and their application to medical device accessibility. In: Winters JM, Story MF, eds. *Medical Instrumentation: Accessibility and Usability Considerations.* Boca Raton, FL: CRC Press. Pp. 259–269.

Geenen SJ, Powers LE, Sells W. 2003. Understanding the role of health care providers during the transition of adolescents with disabilities and special health care needs. *Journal of Adolescent Health* 32(3):225–233.

Gelijns AC, Killelea B, Vitale M, Mankad V, Moskowitz A. 2005. Appendix C: The dynamics of pediatric device innovation: putting evidence in context. In: Field MJ, Tilson H, eds. *Safe Medical Devices for Children.* Washington, DC: The National Academies Press.

Gellman H, Sie I, Waters RL. 1988. Late complications of the weight-bearing upper extremity in the paraplegic patient. *Clinical Orthopaedics and Related Research* 223:132–135.

Gencarelli D. 2005. *Health Insurance Coverage for Small Employers.* National Health Policy Forum Background Paper. Washington, DC: The George Washington University. [Online]. Available: http://www.nhpf.org/pdfs_bp/BP_SmallBusiness_04-19-05.pdf [accessed April 27, 2007].

Gerber E, Kirchner C. 2003. Livable communities throughout the life course. *Disability Studies Quarterly* 23(2):41–57.

Gething L. 1992. Nurse practitioners' and students' attitudes towards people with disabilities. *The Australian Journal of Advanced Nursing* 9(3):25–30.

Gill CJ. 1993. When is a woman not a woman. *The Disability Rag & Resource.* May/June: 26–29.

Gill TM, Kurland B. 2003. The burden and patterns of disability in activities of daily living among community-living older persons. *The Journals of Gerontology, Series A: Biological Sciences and Medical Sciences* 58(1):70–75.

Gill TM, Robinson JT, Tinetti ME. 1997. Predictors of recovery in activities of daily living among disabled older persons living in the community. *Journal of General Internal Medicine* 12(12):757–762.

Gill TM, Allore HG, Hardy SE, Guo Z. 2006. The dynamic nature of mobility disability in older persons. *Journal of the American Geriatrics Society* 54(2):248–254.

Gillberg C, Wing L. 1999. Autism: not an extremely rare disorder. *Acta Psychiatrica Scandinavica* 99(6):399–406.

Gitler J. 1998. *Title V of the Social Security Act and State Programs for Children with Special Health Care Needs—Legislative History.* [Online]. Available: http://www2.sph.unc.edu/toolbox/tech_support/TitleV.pdf [accessed April 27, 2007].

Gitlin LN. 1995. Why older people accept or reject assistive technology. *Generations* 19: 41–47.

Gitlin LN, Winter L, Dennis MP, Corcoran M, Schinfeld S, Hauck WW. 2006. A randomized trial of a multicomponent home intervention to reduce functional difficulties in older adults. *Journal of the American Geriatrics Society* 54(5):809–816.

Glied S. 2005. The employer-based health insurance system. In: Mechanic D, Rogut L, Colby D, Knickman J, eds. *Policy Challenges in Modern Health Care.* New Brunswick, NJ: Rutgers University Press. Pp 37–52.

Gold M. 2006. *The Growth of Private Plans in Medicare, 2006.* Henry J. Kaiser Family Foundation. [Online]. Available: http://www.kff.org/medicare/upload/7473.pdf [accessed April 27, 2007].

Gold M, Lake T, Black W, Smith M. 2005. Challenges in improving care for high-risk seniors in Medicare. *Health Affairs, Web Exclusive* (April 26):199–211. [Online]. Available: http://content.healthaffairs.org/cgi/reprint/hlthaff.w5.199v1 [accessed March 16, 2007].

Gorman Health Group. 2006. *Special Needs Plans.* [Online]. Available: http://www.gormanhealthgroup.com/consult-spcl.needs.plans.asp [accessed April 27, 2007].

Gortmaker SL, Perrin JM, Weitzman M, Homer CJ, Sobol AM. 1993. An unexpected success story: transition to adulthood in youth with chronic physical health conditions. *Journal of Research on Adolescence* 3(3):317–336.

Grabois EW, Nosek MA, Rossi CD. 1999. Accessibility of primary care physicians' offices for people with disabilities: an analysis of compliance with the Americans with Disabilities Act. *Archives of Family Medicine* 8(1):44–51.

Grabowski D. 2006. The cost-effectiveness of noninstitutional long-term care services: review and synthesis of the most recent evidence. *Medical Care Research and Review* 63(1):3–28.

Gray BH, Scheinmann R, Rosenfeld P, Finkelstein R. 2006. Aging without Medicare? Evidence from New York City. *Inquiry* 43(3):211–221.

Green LW. 2003. *CDC's Initiatives in Public Health and Health Systems Research.* Academy Health 20th Annual Research Conference, June 27, Nashville, TN. [Online]. Available: http://www.academyhealth.org/2003/presentations/green.pdf [accessed April 27, 2007].

Greenwald LM, Levy JM, Ingber MJ. 2000. Favorable selection in the Medicare+Choice program: new evidence. *Health Care Financing Review* 21(3):127–134.

Grimby G, Einarsson G. 1991. Post-polio management. *CRC Critical Reviews in Physical Rehabilitation Medicine* 2:189–200.

Grosse SD, Waitzman NJ, Romano PS, Mulinare J. 2005. Re-evaluating the benefits of folic acid fortification in the United States: economic analysis, regulation, and public health. *American Journal of Public Health* 95(11):1917–1922.

Guralnik JM. 2006. Aspects of disability across the lifespan: risk factors for disability in late life. In: Field MJ, Jette AM, Martin L, eds. *Workshop on Disability in America: A New Look.* Washington, DC: The National Academies Press. Pp. 157–165.

Guralnik JM, Fried LP, Simonsick EM, Kasper JD, Lafferty ME eds. 1995. *The Women's Health and Aging Study: Health and Social Characteristics of Older Women with Disability.* NIH Publication No. 95-4009. Bethesda, MD: National Institute on Aging.

Guralnik JM, Ferrucci L, Balfour JL, Volpato S, Di Iorio A. 2001. Progressive versus catastrophic loss of the ability to walk: implications for the prevention of mobility loss. *Journal of the American Geriatrics Society* 49(11):1463–1470.

Gurney JG, Fritz MS, Ness KK, Sievers P, Newschaffer CJ, Shapiro EG. 2003. Analysis of prevalence trends of autism spectrum disorder in Minnesota. *Archives of Pediatrics & Adolescent Medicine* 157(7):619–621.

Hack M, Youngstrom E, Carter L, Schluchter M, Taylor HG, Flannery D, Klein N, Borawski E. 2004. Behavioral outcomes and evidence of psychopathology among very low birth weight infants at age 20 years. *Pediatrics* 11(4):932–940.

Hackbarth GM (Chair, Medicare Payment Advisory Committee). 2003. *Letter to Thomas Scully, Administrator Centers for Medicare & Medicaid Services.* July 7. [Online]. Available: http://www.medpac.gov/publications/other_reports/70703_rehab_SK_comment.pdf [accessed April 27, 2007].

Hager R, Smith D. 2003. *The Public School's Special Education System as an Assistive Technology Funding Source: The Cutting Age,* 2nd ed. Washington, DC: National Association of Protection & Advocacy Systems. [Online]. Available: http://www.nls.org/pdf/special-ed-booklet-03.pdf [accessed April 27, 2007].

Haislmaier EF, Owcharenko N. 2006. The Massachusetts approach: a new way to restructure state health insurance markets and public programs. *Health Affairs (Millwood)* 25(6):1580–1590.

Hall MA. 1992. Reforming the health insurance market for small businesses. *New England Journal of Medicine* 326(8):566–570.

Halstead LS, Rossi CD. 1985. New Problems in old polio patients: results of a survey of 539 polio survivors. *Orthopedics* 8(7):845–850.

Halstead LS, Rossi CD. 1987. Post-polio syndrome: clinical experience with 132 consecutive outpatients. *Birth Defects Original Article Series* 23(4):12–26.

Hammel J, Lai JS, Heller T. 2002. The impact of assistive technology and environmental interventions on function and living situation status with people who are ageing with developmental disabilities. *Disability and Rehabilitation* 24(1-3):93–105.

Hansen NS, Forchheimer M, Tate DG, Luera, G. 1998. Relationships among community reintegration, coping strategies, and life satisfaction in a sample of persons with spinal cord injury. *Top Spinal Cord Injury Rehabilitation* 4(1)56–72.

Hanson K, Neuman P, Dutwin D, Kasper J. 2003. Uncovering the health challenges facing people with disabilities: the role of health insurance. *Health Affairs, Web Exclusive* (November 19):552–565. [Online]. Available: http://content.healthaffairs.org/cgi/reprint/hlthaff.w3.552v1 [accessed April 27, 2007].

Hardy SE, Gill TM. 2004. Recovery from disability among community-dwelling older persons. *The Journal of the American Medical Association* 291(13):1596–1602.

Hardy SE, Gill TM. 2005. Factors associated with recovery of independence among newly disabled older persons. *Archives of Internal Medicine* 165(1):106–112.

Hardy SE, Dubin JA, Holford TR, Gill TM. 2005. Transitions between states of disability and independence among older persons. *American Journal of Epidemiology* 161(6): 575–584.

Harris F, Sprigle S. 2003. Cost analyses in assistive technology research. *Assistive Technology* 15(1):16–27.

Harris Interactive Inc. 2004a. *Key "Indicators" by Severity of Disability* (Exhibits 2, 3, and 4). [Online]. Available: http://www.nod.org/Resources/harris2004/harris2004_summ.doc [accessed April 27, 2007].

Harris Interactive Inc. 2004b. *2004 Gaps Survey.* [Online]. Available: http://www.nod.org/Resources/harris2004/harris2004_data.doc [accessed April 27, 2007].

Harrison T. 2002. Has the Americans with Disabilities Act made a difference? A policy analysis of quality of life in the post-Americans with Disabilities Act era. *Policy, Politics, & Nursing Practice* 3(4):333–347.

Harrison T, Stuifbergen. 2001. Barriers that further disablement: a study of survivors of polio. *Journal of Neuroscience Nursing* 33(3):160–166.

Hauser ES, Dorn L. 1999. Transitioning adolescents with sickle cell disease to adult-centered care. *Pediatric Nursing* 25(5):479–488.

Hauser RM. 2002. Investments in longitudinal surveys, databases, advanced statistical research, and computation technology. In: Perkman L, ed. *Through the Kaleidoscope: Viewing the Contributions of the Behavioral and Social Sciences to Health—The Barbara and Jerome Grossman Symposium.* Washington, DC: National Academy Press. Pp. 36–41.

Hemming K, Hutton JL, Colver A, Platt M. 2005. Regional variation in survival of people with cerebral palsy in the United Kingdom. *Pediatrics* 116(6):1383–1390.

Hemming K, Hutton JL, Pharoah PO. 2006. Long-term survival for a cohort of adults with cerebral palsy. *Developmental Medicine and Child Neurology* 48(2):90–95.

Hendershot G. 2005. *Statistical Analyses Based on the National Health Interview Survey on Disability: A Bibliography and Summary of Findings.* [Online]. Available: http://rtc.umn.edu/docs/NHIS-DBibliography.pdf [accessed April 27, 2007].

Herz E. 2006. *The Link Between Medicaid and the Individuals with Disabilities Education Act (IDEA): Recent History and Current Issues.* CRS Report for Congress. [Online]. Available: http://www.opencrs.com/rpts/RS22397_20060309.pdf [accessed April 27, 2007].

Herz E, Chawla A, Gavin N. 1998. Preventive services for children under Medicaid, 1989 and 1992. *Health Care Financing Review* 19(4):25–44.

Hintz SR, Kendrick DE, Vohr BR, Poole WK, Higgins RD. 2005. Changes in neurodevelopmental outcomes at 18 to 22 months' corrected age among infants of less than 25 weeks' gestational age born in 1993–1999. *Pediatrics* 115(6):1645–1651.

Hobbs N, Perrin JM, Ireys HT. 1985. *Chronically Ill Children and Their Families.* San Francisco, CA: Jossey-Bass.

Hoenig H, Taylor DH, Sloan FA. 2003. Does assistive technology substitute for personal assistance among the disabled elderly? *American Journal of Public Health* 93(2):330–337.

Hogan DP, Rogers ML, Msall ME. 2000. Functional limitations and key indicators of well-being in children with disability. *Archives of Pediatrics & Adolescent Medicine* 154(10): 1042–1048.

Holliday PJ, Mihailidis A, Rolfson R, Fernie G. 2005. Understanding and measuring powered wheelchair mobility and maneuverability. Part I. Reach in confined spaces. *Disability and Rehabilitation* 27(16):939–949.

Holman H. 2004. Chronic disease—the need for a new clinical education. *The Journal of the American Medical Association* 292(9):1057–1059.

Houlihan CM, O'Donnell M, Conaway M, Stevenson RD. 2004. Bodily pain and health-related quality of life in children with cerebral palsy. *Developmental Medicine and Child Neurology* 46(5):305–310.

Houtenville AJ. 2006. *2005 Disability Status Reports: United States.* Ithaca, NY: Rehabilitation Research and Training Center on Disability Demographics and Statistics, Cornell University. [Online]. Available: http://digitalcommons.ilr.cornell.edu/edicollect/1236 [accessed April 27, 2007].

Houtenville AJ, Burkhauser RV. 2004. *Did the Employment of People with Disabilities Decline in the 1990's, and was the ADA Responsible? A Replication and Robustness Check of Acemoglu and Angrist (2001).* Ithaca, NY: Employment and Disability Institute, Cornell University. [Online]. Available: http://digitalcommons.ilr.cornell.edu/cgi/viewcontent.cgi?article=1090&context=edicollect

Hoyert D, Anderson R. 2001. Age-adjusted death rates: trend data based on the year 2000 standard population. *National Vital Statistics Report* 49:1–8. [Online]. Available: http://www.cdc.gov/nchs/data/nvsr/nvsr49/nvsr49_09.pdf [accessed April 27, 2007].

Hoyert D, Kung H, Smith B. 2005. Deaths: preliminary data for 2003. *National Vital Statistics Report* 53:1–48. [Online]. Available: http://www.cdc.gov/nchs/data/nvsr/nvsr53/nvsr53_15.pdf [accessed April 27, 2007].

HRSA (Health Resources and Services Administration). 2004. *The National Survey of Children with Special Needs Chartbook 2001.* Rockville, MD: U.S. Department of Health and Human Services.

HRSDC (Human Resources and Social Development Canada). 2005. *Advancing the Inclusion of Persons with Disabilities 2005.* [Online]. Available: http://www.hrsdc.gc.ca/en/hip/odi/documents/advancingInclusion05/chap2.shtml [accessed April 27, 2007].

HRTWNC (Healthy and Ready to Work National Resource Center). Undated. *About HRSA/ MCHB and Title V CSHCN.* [Online]. Available: https://www.hrtw.org/systems/aboutprg.html [accessed April 27, 2007].

Hudson J. 2005. *Trends in Children's Health Insurance Coverage for Families with Children, 1996-2002 (First Half).* Statistical Brief No. 99, Medical Expenditure Panel Survey. Agency for Healthcare Research and Quality. [Online]. Available: http://www.meps.ahcpr.gov/papers/st99/stat99.pdf [accessed April 27, 2007].

Hungerford D, Cockin J. 1975. Fate of the retained lower limb joints in Second World War amputees. *Journal of Bone & Joint Surgery* 57(1):111.

Hwang W, Ireys HT, Anderson GF. 2001. Comparison of risk adjusters for Medicaid-enrolled children with and without chronic health conditions. *Ambulatory Pediatrics* 1(4):217–224.

Hynes DM. 2002. Veterans' use of Medicare and VA health care services by VISN. Paper presented at 2002 National VA HSR&D Service Meeting, Washington, DC, February.

ICDR (Interagency Committee on Disability Research). 2003. *Federal Statutory Definitions of Disability*. McLean, VA: CESSI. [Online]. Available: http://www.icdr.us/documents/definitions.htm#table1 [accessed April 27, 2007].

ICDR. 2005. *2003 Annual Report to the President and Congress*. [Online]. Available: http://www.icdr.us/pubs/ICDR03AnnRpt-Final.doc [accessed April 27, 2007].

ICDR. 2006. *About the ICDR: Members*. [Online]. Available: http://www.icdr.us/membership.html [accessed April 27, 2007].

ICDRI (The International Center for Disability Resources on the Internet). 2006. *Bank of America: 2006 Addendum to Settlement Agreement*. [Online]. Available: http://www.icdri.org/Assistive%20Technology/ATMs/bank_of_america_addendum_to_settlement.htm [accessed April 27, 2007].

IDEAdata. 2005. *Data Tables for OSEP [Office of Special Education Programs, U.S. Department of Education] State Reported Data*. [Online]. Available: https://www.ideadata.org/arc_toc6.asp#partbCC [accessed April 27, 2007].

Iezzoni LI. 2003. *When Walking Fails: Mobility Problems of Adults with Chronic Conditions*. Berkeley, CA: University of California Press.

Iezzoni LI, O'Day BR. 2006. *More Than Ramps: A Guide to Improving Health Care Quality and Access for People With Disabilities*. New York: Oxford University Press.

Iezzoni LI, Ayanian JZ, Bates DW, Burstin HR. 1998. Paying more fairly for Medicare capitated care. *New England Journal of Medicine* 339(26):1933–1938.

Iezzoni LI, McCarthy EP, Davis RB, Harris-David L, O'Day B. 2001. Use of screening and preventive services among women with disabilities. *American Journal of Medical Quality* 16(4):135–144.

IOM (Institute of Medicine). 1988. *The Future of Public Health*. Washington, DC: National Academy Press.

IOM. 1990a. *Clinical Practice Guidelines: Directions for a New Program*. Washington, DC: National Academy Press.

IOM. 1990b. *Healthy People 2000: Citizens Chart the Course*. Washington, DC: National Academy Press.

IOM. 1991. *Disability in America: Toward a National Agenda for Prevention*. Washington, DC: National Academy Press.

IOM. 1992. *Guidelines for Clinical Practice: From Development to Use*. Washington, DC: National Academy Press.

IOM. 1993. *Employment and Health Benefits: A Connection at Risk*. Washington, DC: National Academy Press.

IOM. 1995. *Setting Priorities for Clinical Practice Guidelines*. Washington, DC: National Academy Press.

IOM. 1997. *Enabling America: Assessing the Role of Rehabilitation Science and Engineering*. Washington, DC: National Academy Press.

IOM. 2000a. *Extending Medicare Coverage for Preventive and Other Services*. Washington, DC: National Academy Press.

IOM. 2000b. *Promoting Health: Intervention Strategies from Social and Behavioral Research*. Washington, DC: National Academy Press.

IOM. 2001a. *Coverage Matters: Insurance and Health Care*. Washington, DC: National Academy Press.

IOM. 2001b. *Crossing the Quality Chasm: A New Health System for the 21st Century.* Washington, DC: National Academy Press.

IOM. 2001c. *Improving the Quality of Long-Term Care.* Washington, DC: National Academy Press.

IOM. 2002. *The Dynamics of Disability: Measuring and Monitoring Disability for Social Security Programs.* Washington, DC: National Academy Press.

IOM. 2003a. *Childhood Cancer Survivorship: Improving Care and Quality of Life.* Washington, DC: The National Academies Press.

IOM. 2003b. *Priority Areas for National Action: Transforming Health Care Quality.* Washington, DC: The National Academies Press.

IOM. 2004a. *Children's Health, the Nation's Wealth: Assessing and Improving Child Health.* Washington, DC: The National Academies Press.

IOM. 2004b. *Ethical Conduct of Clinical Research Involving Children.* Washington, DC: The National Academies Press.

IOM. 2004c. *Immunization Safety Review: Vaccines and Autism.* Washington, DC: The National Academies Press.

IOM. 2004d. *Insuring America's Health: Principles and Recommendations.* Washington, DC: The National Academies Press.

IOM. 2005a. *Preventing Childhood Obesity: Health in the Balance.* Washington, DC: The National Academies Press.

IOM. 2005b. *Safe Medical Devices for Children.* Washington, DC: The National Academies Press.

IOM. 2006a. *Preterm Birth: Causes, Consequences, and Prevention.* Washington, DC: The National Academies Press.

IOM. 2006b. *Workshop on Disability in America: A New Look.* Washington, DC: The National Academies Press.

ISO (International Standards Organization). 2001. *ISO Guide 71: Guidelines for Standards Developers to Address the Need of Older Persons and Persons with Disabilities.* Geneva, Switzerland: ISO.

ITEM Coalition (Independence Through Enhancement of Medicare and Medicaid Coalition). 2006. ITEM Coalition Blasts Medicare's Coverage Decision for iBOT Mobility System. [Online]. Available: http://www.itemcoalition.org/press/pr/pr_07-31-06.htm [accessed April 27, 2007].

Jahnsen R, Villien L, Stanghelle JK, Holm I. 2003. Fatigue in adults with cerebral palsy in Norway compared with the general population. *Developmental Medicine and Child Neurology* 45(5):296–303.

Jahnsen R, Villien L, Aamodt G, Stanghelle JK, Holm I. 2004. Musculoskeletal pain in adults with cerebral palsy compared with the general population. *Journal of Rehabilitation and Medicine* 436(2):78–84.

Jalonick MC. 2006. *Medicare Cuts Hurt Wheelchair Suppliers.* October 18. [Online]. Available: http://www.washingtonpost.com/wp-dyn/content/article/2006/10/18/AR2006101801369.html [accessed April 27, 2007].

Jans L, Stoddard S. 1999. *Chartbook on Women and Disability in the United States.* An InfoUse Report. Washington, DC: National Institute on Disability and Rehabilitation Research. [Online]. Available: http://www.infouse.com/disabilitydata/womendisability/ [accessed April 27, 2007].

Jans L, Stoddard S, Graus L. 2004. *Chartbook on Mental Health and Disability in the United States.* An InfoUse Report. Washington, DC: National Institute on Disability and Rehabilitation Research. [Online]. Available: http://www.infouse.com/disabilitydata/mental-health/ [accessed April 27, 2007].

JCAHO (The Joint Commission on Accreditation of Healthcare Organizations). Undated. *Setting the Standard: The Joint Commission & Health Care Safety and Quality.* [Online]. Available: http://www.jointcommission.org/NR/rdonlyres/6C33FEDB-BB50-4CEE-950B-A6246DA4911E/0/setting_the_standard.pdf [accessed April 27, 2007].

Jeffrey AE, Newacheck PW. 2006. Role of insurance for children with special health care needs: a synthesis of the evidence. *Pediatrics* 118(4):e1027–e1038.

Jensen MP, Engel JM, Hoffman AJ, Schwartz L. 2004. Natural history of chronic pain and pain treatment in adults with cerebral palsy. *American Journal of Physical Medicine & Rehabilitation* 83(6):439–445.

Jette AM, Badley E. 2002. Conceptual issues in the measurement of work disability. In: Wunderlich G, Rice D, Amado N, eds. *The Dynamics of Disability.* Washington, DC: National Academy Press. Pp. 183–210.

Jette AM, Haley SM, Kooyoomjian JT. 2003. Are the ICF activity and participation dimensions distinct? *Journal of Rehabilitation Medicine* 35(3):145–149.

Jha AK, Ferris TG, Donelan K, DesRoches C, Shields A, Rosenbaum S, Blumenthal D. 2006. How common are electronic health records in the United States? A summary of the evidence. *Health Affairs, Web Exclusive* (October 11):496–W507. [Online]. Available: http://content.healthaffairs.org/cgi/reprint/25/6/w496 [accessed April 27, 2007].

Jia H, Zheng E, Cowper DC, Wu SS, Vogel WB, Duncan PW, Reker DM. 2006. How veterans use stroke services in the VA and beyond. *Federal Practitioner* 23(6):21–24.

Jolls C, Prescott J. 2004. *Disaggregating employment protection: the case of disability discrimination.* National Bureau of Economic Research Working Paper 10740. Cambridge, MA: National Bureau of Economic Research.

Jonasson G, Carlsen KH, Sodal A, Jonasson C, Mowinckel P. 1999. Patient compliance in a clinical trial with inhaled budesonide in children with mild asthma. *The European Respiratory Journal* 14(1):150–154.

Jones A. 2002. The National Nursing Home Survey: 1999 Summary. National Center for Health Statistics. *Vital and Health Statistics* 13(152). [Online]. Available: http://www.cdc.gov/nchs/data/series/sr_13/sr13_152.pdf [accessed April 27, 2007].

Jones DR, Speier J, Canine K, Owen R, Stull GA. 1989. Cardiorespiratory responses to aerobic training by patients with post-poliomyelitis sequelae. *The Journal of the American Medical Association* 261(22):3255–3258.

Jones NL. 2003. *The Americans with Disabilities Act (ADA): Statutory Language and Recent Issues.* Report to Congress from the Congressional Research Service. [Online]. Available: http://usinfo.state.gov/usa/infousa/society/rights/ada.pdf [accessed April 27, 2007].

Jubelt B, Cashman NR. 1987. Neurological manifestation of the post-polio syndrome. *Critical Reviews in Neurobiology* 3(3):199–220.

Jutai JW, Fuhrer MJ, Demers L, Scherer MJ, DeRuyter. 2005. Toward a taxonomy of assistive technology device outcomes. *American Journal of Physical Medicine & Rehabilitation* 84(4):294–302.

Kailes JI. 2006. A user's perspective on midlife (ages 18 to 65) aging with disability. In: Field MJ, Jette AM, Martin L, eds. *Workshop on Disability in America: A New Look.* Washington, DC: The National Academies Press. Pp. 194–204.

Kailes JI. 2007. The patient's perspective on access to medical equipment. In: Winters JM, Story MF, eds. *Medical Instrumentation: Accessibility and Usability Considerations.* Boca Raton, FL: CRC Press. Pp. 3–14.

Kailes JI, MacDonald. 2004. *Tax Incentives for Improving Accessibility.* [Online]. Available: http://www.cdihp.org/briefs/brief6-tax-incentives.html#sect3 [accessed April 27, 2007].

Kaiser Commission (Kaiser Commission on Medicaid and the Uninsured). 2001. *Section 1115 Waivers in Medicaid and the State Children's Health Insurance Program: An Overview.* Washington, DC: KFF Publications. [Online]. Available: http://www.kff.org/medicaid/upload/Section-1115-Wiavers-in-Medicaid-and-the-State-Children-s-Health-Insurance-Program-An-Overview.pdf [accessed April 27, 2007].

Kaiser Commission. 2002. Appendix 1: Medicaid legislative history, 1965–2000 In: Schneider A, Elias R, Garfield R, Rousseau D, Wachino V. *The Medicaid Resource Book.* Washington, DC: Kaiser Family Foundation. [Online]. Available: http://www.kff.org/medicaid/loader.cfm?url=/commonspot/security/getfile.cfm&PageID=14266 [accessed April 27, 2007].

Kaiser Commission. 2003. *Understanding the Health-Care Needs and Experiences of People with Disabilities: Findings from a 2003 Survey.* [Online]. Available: http://www.kff.org/medicare/upload/Understanding-the-Health-Care-Needs-and-Experiences-of-People-with-Disabilities-Findings-from-a-2003-Survey.pdf [accessed April 27, 2007].

Kaiser Commission. 2005. *The Medicaid Program at a Glance. Key Facts: Medicaid and the uninsured.* [Online]. Available: http://www.kff.org/medicaid/upload/The-Medicaid-Program-at-a-Glance-Fact-Sheet.pdf [accessed April 27, 2007].

Kaiser Commission. 2006a. *Deficit Reduction Act of 2005: Implications for Medicaid.* [Online]. Available: http://www.aucd.org/medicaid/docs/kaiser_medicaid_uninsured.pdf [accessed April 27, 2007].

Kaiser Commission. 2006b. *Dual Eligibles and Medicare Part D.* [Online]. Available: http://www.kff.org/medicaid/upload/7454.pdf [accessed April 27, 2007].

Kaiser Commission and Health Research and Educational Trust. 2005. *Employer Health Benefits—2005 Summary of Findings.* [Online]. Available: http://www.kff.org/insurance/7315/upload/7315.pdf [accessed April 27, 2007].

Kane RA, Kane RL, Ladd R. 1998. *The Heart of Long-Term Care.* New York: Oxford University Press.

Kapteyn A, Smith J, Soest A. 2004. *Self-reported work disability in the US and The Netherlands.* Working Paper No. WR-206.Labor and Population Division, Santa Monica, CA: RAND.

Kautter J, Pope GC. 2004. CMS frailty adjustment model. *Health Care Financing Review* 26(2):1-19.

Kaye HS. 2002. *Activity Limitation in the National Health Interview Survey: Effect of the 1997 Revision on Measuring Disability.* Institute for Health and Aging: University of California, San Francisco.

Kaye HS. 2003. *Improved Employment Opportunities for People with Disabilities.* Disability Statistics Center, University of California, San Francisco. [Online]. Available: http://dsc.ucsf.edu/pub_listing.php?pub_type=report.

Kaye HS. 2005. *Community-Level Influences on Disability Rates Among Working-Age Adults.* Working Paper No. 0501. Disability Statistics Center, University of California, San Francisco. [Online]. Available: http://www.dri.uiuc.edu/research/p04-06c/Kaye%20Revised%20Final%20Report%20in%20response%20to%20SSA%20comments.doc [accessed pril 27, 1007].

Kaye HS, Chapman S, Newcomer R, Harrington C. 2006. The personal assistance workforce: trends in supply and demand. *Health Affairs (Millwood)* 25(4):1113–1120.

Keenan PS, Buntin MJ, McGuire TG, Newhouse JP. 2001. The prevalence of formal risk adjustment in health plan purchasing. *Inquiry* 38(3):245–259.

Kelly AM, Kratz B, Bielski M, Rinehart PM. 2002. Implementing transitions for youth with complex chronic conditions using the medical home model. *Pediatrics* 110(6):1322–1327.

Kemp BJ. 2006. Depression as a secondary condition in people with disabilities. In: Field MJ, Jette AM, Martin L, eds. *Workshop on Disability in America: A New Look.* Washington, DC: The National Academies Press. Pp. 234–250.

Kemp BJ, Campbell M. 1993. *Health, Functioning and Psychosocial Aspects of Aging with Disability, Final Report.* Downey, CA: Rehabilitation Research and Training Center on Aging, Rancho Los Amigos Medical Center.

Kemp BJ, Mosqueda L, eds. 2004. *Aging with a Disability: What the Clinician Needs to Know.* Baltimore, MD: The Johns Hopkins University Press.

Kemp BJ, Adams B, Campbell M. 1997. Depression and life satisfaction in aging polio survivors versus age-match controls. *Archives of Physical Medicine & Rehabilitation* 78(2):187–192.

Kenney G, Yee J. 2007. SCHIP at a crossroads: experiences to date and challenges ahead. *Health Affairs (Millwood)* 26(2):356–369. [Online]. Available: http://content.healthaffairs.org/cgi/reprint/26/2/356.pdf [accessed April 27, 2007].

Keysor J. 2006. How does the environment influence disability? Examining the evidence. In: Field MJ, Jette AM, Martin L, eds. *Workshop on Disability in America: A New Look.* Washington, DC: The National Academies Press. Pp. 88–100.

Kidron D, Steiner I, Melamed E. 1987. Late-onset progressive ariculomyelopathy in patients with cervical athetoid-dystonic cerebral palsy. *European Neurology* 27(3):164–166.

Kinne S, Patrick DL, Doyle DL. 2004. Prevalence of secondary conditions among people with disabilities. *American Journal of Public Health* 94(3):443–445.

Kipps S, Bahu T, Ong K, Ackland FM, Brown RS, Fox CT, Griffin NK, Knight AH, Mann NP, Neil HAW, et al. 2002. Current methods to transfer of young people with Type 1 diabetes to adult services. *Diabetic Medicine* 19:649–654.

Kirkpatrick A, Rutter R, Heilmann C, Thatcher J, Waddell C. 2006. *Web Accessibility: Web Standards and Regulatory Compliance.* New York: Friends of ED.

Kitchener M, Willmott M, Harrington C. 2006. *Home and Community-Based Services: State-Only Funded Programs.* Center for Personal Assistance Services, University of California, San Francisco. [Online]. Available: http://www.pascenter.org/state_funded/ [accessed April 27, 2007].

Kivivuori SM, Rajantie J, Siimes MA. 1996. Peripheral blood cell counts in infants with Down's syndrome. *Clinical Genetics* 49(1):15–19.

Klein MG, Whyte J, Keenan MA, Esquenazi A, Polansky M. 2000. The relationship between lower extremity strength and shoulder overuse symptoms: a model based on polio survivors. *Archives of Physical Medicine & Rehabilitation* 81(6):789–795.

Kofman M, Pollitz K. 2006. *Health Insurance Regulation by States and the Federal Government: A Review of Current Approaches and Proposals for Change.* Georgetown University Health Policy Institute. [Online]. Available: http://www.pbs.org/now/politics/Healthinsurancereportfinalkofmanpollitz.pdf [accessed April 27, 2007].

Komisar HL, Thompson LS. 2007. *National Spending for Long-Term Care: Updated Fact Sheet.* Georgetown University Long-Term Care Financing Project. [Online]. Available: http://ltc.georgetown.edu/pdfs/natspendfeb07.pdf [accessed April 27, 2007].

Krahn Gl. 2003. Survey of physician wellness practices with persons with disabilities. In: *Changing Concepts of Health and Disability: State of Science Conference & Policy Forum 2003.* RRTC Health and Wellness Consortium. Portland, OR: Oregon Health and Sciences University. Pp. 47–51.

Krause JS, Adkins RH. 2004. Methodological issues. In: Kemp B, Mosqueda L, eds. *Aging with a Disability: What the Clinician Needs to Know.* Baltimore, MD: The Johns Hopkins University Press. Pp. 237–261.

Krause JS, Bell RB. 1999. Measuring quality of life and secondary conditions: experiences with spinal cord injury. In: Simeonsson R, McDevitt L, eds. *Issues in Disability and Health: The Role of Secondary Conditions and Quality of Life.* Chapel Hill: University of North Carolina Press.

Krause L, Stoddard S, Gilmartin. 1996. *Chartbook on Disability in the United States, 1996.* An InfoUse Report. Washington, DC: National Institute on Disability and Rehabilitation Research. [Online]. Available: http://www.infouse.com/disabilitydata/disability/ [accessed May 30, 2007].

Kreamer BR, McIntyre LL, Blacher J. 2003. Quality of life for young adults with mental retardation during transition. *Mental Retardation* 41(4):250–262.

Kroemer JH. 2006. *"Extra-ordinary" Ergonomics: How to Accommodate Small and Big Persons, the Disabled and Elderly, Expectant Mothers, and Children.* Boca Raton, FL: CRC Press.

Kronick R, Drefus T. 1997. *The Challenge of Risk Adjustment for People with Disabilities: Health-Based Payment for Medicaid Programs.* Center for Health Care Strategies, Inc. [Online]. Available: http://www.chcs.org/usr_doc/The_Challenge_of_Risk_Adjustment. pdf [accessed April 27, 2007].

Kronick R, Dreyfus T, Lee L, Zhou Z. 1996. Diagnostic risk adjustment for Medicaid: the Disability Payment System. *Health Care Financing Review* 17(3):7–33.

Kronick R, Gilmer T, Dreyfus T, Lee L. 2000. Improving health-based payment for Medicaid beneficiaries: CDPS. *Health Care Financing Review* 21(3):29–64. [Online]. Available: http://www.cms.hhs.gov/apps/review/00spring/00Springpg29.pdf [accessed April 27, 2007].

Kruse D, Schur L. 2003. Employment of people with disabilities following the ADA. *Industrial Relations* 42(1):31–64.

Ku L. 2003. *The Medicaid-Medicare Link: State Medicaid Programs Are Shouldering a Greater Share of the Costs of Care for Seniors and People with Disabilities.* Washington, DC: Center on Budget and Policy Priorities. [Online]. Available: http://www.cbpp.org/2-25-03health2.pdf [accessed April 27, 2007].

Kudrjavcev T, Schoenberg BS, Kurland LT, Groover RV. 1985. Cerebral palsy: survival rates, associated handicaps, and distribution by clinical subtype (Rochester, MN, 1950–1976). *Neurology* 35(6):900–903.

Kuh D, Ben-Shlomo Y, eds. 1997. *A Life Course Approach to Chronic Disease Epidemiology: Tracing the Origins of Ill-Health from Early to Adult Life.* Oxford, United Kingdom: Oxford University Press.

Kuhlthau K, Ferris TG, Davis RB, Perrin JM, Iezzoni LI. 2005. Pharmacy-and diagnosis-based risk adjustment for children with Medicaid. *Medical Care* 43(11):1155–1159.

Ladenheim K, Farmer C, Folkemer D, Fox-Grage W, Horahan K, Scanlon A, Straw T. 2002. *Medicaid Cost Containment: A Legislator's Tool Kit.* National Conference of State Legislatures. [Online]. Available: http://www.ncsl.org/programs/health/forum/cost/ containment.htm#ackbot [accessed April 27, 2007].

Lahiri K, Vaughn DR, Wixon B. 1995. Modeling SSA's sequential disability determination process using matched SIPP data. *Social Security Bulletin* 58(4):3–42.

Laine L, Bombardier C, Hawkey CJ, Davis B, Shapiro D, Brett C, Reicin A. 2002. Stratifying the risk of NSAID-related upper gastrointestinal clinical events: results of a double-blind outcomes study in patients with rheumatoid arthritis. *Gastroenterology* 123(4):1006–1012.

Lakdawalla D, Goldman D, Shang B. 2005. The health and cost consequences of obesity among the future elderly. *Health Affairs, Web Exclusive* W5:R30–R41. [Online]. Available: http://content.healthaffairs.org/cgi/reprint/hlthaff.w5.r30v1 [accessed April 27, 2007].

Lal S. 1998. Premature degenerative shoulder changes in spinal cord injury patients. *Spinal Cord* 36(3):186–189.

Lane JP. 1998. Consumer contributions to technology evaluation and transfer. *Technology and Disability* 9(3):103–118.

Lange B. 2000. The management of neoplastic disorders of haematopoiesis in children with Down's syndrome. *British Journal of Haematology* 110:512–524.

Lankasky K. 2004. A consumer's perspective on living with a disability: how change in function affects daily life. In: Kemp B, Mosqueda L, eds. *Aging with a Disability: What the Clinician Needs to Know.* Baltimore, MD: The Johns Hopkins University Press. Pp. 9–18.

LeBlanc A, Tonner MC, Harrington C. 2001. State Medicaid programs offering personal care services. *Health Care Financing Review* 22(4):155–173.

Leslie L, Rappo P, Abelson H, Jenkins RR, Sewall SR. 2000. Final report of the FOPE II pediatric generalists of the future workgroup. *Pediatrics* 106(5):1199–1223.

Lethbridge-Cejku M, Rose D. 2005. Summary Health Statistics for U.S. Adults, National Health Interview Survey, 2004. *Vital and Health Statistics* 10(228). [Online]. Available: http://www.cdc.gov/nchs/data/series/sr_10/sr10_228.pdf [accessed April 27, 2007].

Levi R, Hultling C, Sieger A. 1995. The Stockholm Spinal Cord Injury Study. 2. Associations between clinical patient characteristics and post-acute medical problems. *Paraplegia* 33(10):585–594.

Levine S. 2005. Suit wins changes for disabled at hospital: D.C. facility faces up to $2 million in modifications to ensure equal care. *The Washington Post*, November 3, p. B09.

Levy CE, Chow JW, Tillman MD, Hanson C, Donohue T, Mann WC. 2004. Variable-ratio pushrim-activated power-assist wheelchair eases wheeling over a variety of terrains for elders. *Archives of Physical Medicine & Rehabilitation* 85(1):104–112.

Lichtenstein R, Thomas JW. 1987. Including a measure of health status in Medicare's health maintenance organization capitation formula: reliability issues. *Medical Care* 25(2):100–110.

Light DW. 1992. The practice and ethics of risk-rated health insurance. *The Journal of the American Medical Association* 267(18):2503–2508.

Lilja M, Bergh A, Johansson L, Nygard L. 2003. Attitudes towards rehabilitation needs and support from assistive technology and the social environment among elderly people with disability. *Occupational Therapy International* 10(1):75–93.

Lindgren CL, Oermann MH. 1993. Effects of an educational intervention on students' attitudes toward the disabled. *Journal of Nursing Education* 32(3):121–126.

Ling G. 2005. Keeping a pact. *DARPATech.* August 9–11 Issue, pp. 56–58. [Online]. Available: http://www.arpa.mil/darpatech2005/presentations/dso/ling.pdf [accessed April 27, 2007].

Litvak S, Kennedy J. 1991. *Policy Issues Affecting the Medicaid Personal Care Services Optional Benefit.* World Institute on Disability. [Online]. Available: http://aspe.hhs.gov/daltcp/reports/optnales.htm [accessed April 27, 2007].

Loftis CW, Salinsky E. 2006. *Medicare and Mental Health: The Fundamentals.* National Health Policy Forum Background Paper. Washington, DC: The George Washington University. [Online]. Available: http://www.nhpf.org/pdfs_bp/BP_Mcare&MentalHlth_11-27-06.pdf [accessed April 27, 2007].

Long S, Coughlin T. 2004–2005. Access to care for disabled children under Medicaid. *Health Care Financing Review* 26(2):89–102.

Lopez-Soto E, Sheldon JR, eds. 2002. *Benefits Management for Working People with Disabilities: An Advocate's Manual.* Buffalo, NY: Neighborhood Legal Services, Inc.

Lopez-Soto E, Sheldon JR. 2005. *Policy and Practice Brief: Medicaid and Persons with Disabilities; A Focus on Eligibility, Covered Services, and Program Structure.* Ithaca, NY: Employment and Disability Institute Collection, Cornell University. [Online]. Available: http://digitalcommons.ilr.cornell.edu/cgi/viewcontent.cgi?article=1059&context=edicollect [accessed April 27, 2007].

Loprest P, Maag E. 2001. *Barriers to and Supports for Work Among Adults with Disabilities: Results from the NHIS-D.* Washington, DC: The Urban Institute. [Online]. Available: http://www.urban.org/UploadedPDF/adultswithdisabilities.pdf [accessed April 27, 2007].

Loprest P, Wittenburg D. 2005. *Choices, Challenges, and Options: Child SSI Recipients Preparing for the Transition to Adult Life.* The Urban Institute. [Online]. Available: http://www.urban.org/UploadedPDF/411168_ChildSSIRecipients.pdf [accessed April 27, 2007].

Lotstein DS, McPherson M, Strickland B, Newacheck PW. 2005. Transition planning for youth with special health care needs: results from the National Survey of Children with Special Health Care Needs. *Pediatrics* 115(6):1562–1568.

LSU (Louisiana State University). 2006. *Statistical Summary America's Major Wars.* The United States Civil War Center, Civil War Collections & the Civil War Book Review. Hill Memorial Library, LSU. [Online]. Available: http://www.cwc.lsu.edu/cwc/other/stats/warcost.htm [accessed April 27, 2007].

Lubitz J, Cai L, Kramarow, Lentzner H. 2003. Health, life expectancy, and health care spending among the elderly. *New England Journal of Medicine* 349(11):1048–1055.

Luft H. 1987. *Health Maintenance Organizations: Dimensions of Performance.* New Brunswick, NJ: Transaction Books. (Originally published by New York: Wiley, 1981.)

Luft H, Miller R. 1988. Patient selection in a competitive health system. *Health Affairs (Millwood)* 7(3):97–119.

Luke A, Roizen NJ, Sutton M, Schoeller DA. 1994. Energy expenditure in children with Down syndrome correcting metabolic rate for movement. *Pediatrics* 125(5 Pt 1):829–838.

Lunney J, Lynn J, Foley D, Lipson S, Guralnik J. 2003. Patterns of functional decline at the end of life. *The Journal of the American Medical Association* 289:2387–2392.

Luscombe B. 2003. This bold house: easy-grip handles, flat thresholds, and adjustable-height vanities are just the beginning in the world's most accessible house. *AARP The Magazine* September–October Issue. [Online]. Available: http://www.aarpmagazine.org/lifestyle/Articles/a2003-08-28-bold_house.html [accessed April 27, 2007].

Maag E, Wittengurg D. 2003. *Real Trends or Measurement Problems? Disability and Employment Trends from the Survey of Income and Program Participation.* [Online]. Available: http://www.urban.org/UploadedPDF/410635_Real_or_Measurement.pdf [accessed April 27, 2007].

MacIntyre D. 1962. *Voluntary Health Insurance and Rate Making.* Ithaca, NY: Cornell University Press.

Magrab P, Millar HEC. 1989. *Surgeon General's Conference: Growing up and Getting Medical Care: Youth with Special Health Care Needs: A Summary of Conference Proceedings.* Washington, DC: Georgetown University Child Development Center.

Mann C. 2005. *The New TennCare Waiver Proposal: What Is the Impact on Children?* Georgetown University Health Policy Institute. [Online]. Available: http://ihcrp.georgetown.edu/pdfs/tenncareandchildren.pdf [accessed April 27, 2007].

Mann C, Guyer J. 2005. *House Budget Bill Would Eliminate All Current Federal Medicaid Benefit Standards for Six Million Children and Other Vulnerable People.* Georgetown University Health Policy Institute. [Online]. Available: http://www.cbpp.org/11-10-05health3.pdf [accessed April 27, 2007].

Mann W, Ottenbacher K, Fraas L, Tomita M, Granger C. 1999. Effectiveness of assistive technology and environmental interventions in maintaining independence and reducing home care costs for the frail elderly. *Archives of Family Medicine* 8(3):210–217.

Manton KG, Gu X. 2001. Changes in the prevalence of chronic disability in the United States black and non-black population above age 65 from 1982 to 1999. *Proceedings of the National Academy of Sciences USA* 98(11):6354–6359.

Manton KG, Stallard E. 1992. Analysis of underwriting factors for AAPCC (adjusted average per capita cost). *Health Care Financing Review* 14(1):117–132.

Manton KG, Corder LS, Stallard E. 1993. Estimates of change in chronic disability and institutional incidence and prevalence rates in the U.S. elderly population from the 1982, 1984, and 1989 National Long Term Care Survey. *Journals of Gerontology* 48(4):153–166.

Manton KG, Corder LS, Stallard E. 1997. Chronic disability trends in elderly United States populations: 1982–1984. *Proceedings of the National Academy of Sciences USA* 94:2593–2598.

Manton KG, Gu X, Lamb VL. 2006. Change in chronic disability from 1982 to 2004/2005 as measured by long-term changes in function and health in the U.S. elderly population. *Proceedings of the National Academy of Sciences USA* 103(48):18374–18379. [Online]. Available: http://www.pnas.org/cgi/reprint/103/48/18374 [accessed March 29, 2007].

Marge M. 1988. Health promotion for persons with disabilities: moving beyond rehabilitation. *American Journal of Health Promotion* 2(4):29–35.

Marge M. 1990. Testimony to the Institute of Medicine Committee on Health Objectives for the Year 2000. Quoted in *Healthy People 2000: Citizens Chart the Course*. Washington, DC: National Academy Press. P. 64.

Marge M, ed. 1998. *Healthy People 2010 Disability Objectives: Private Sector and Consumer Perspectives*. Proceedings and Recommendations of a Conference, Alexandria, VA, April 20. New York: American Association on Health and Disability. [Online]. Available: http://www.cdc.gov/ncbddd/dh/publications/hpmarge.htm [accessed April 27, 2007].

Marge M. 1999. Defining a prevention agenda for secondary conditions. In: Simeonsson R, McDevitt E, eds. *Issues in Disability & Health: The Role of Secondary Conditions and Quality of Life*. Chapel Hill: University of North Carolina.

Markus A, Rosenbaum S, Cyprien S. 2004. *SCHIP-Enrolled Children with Special Health Care Needs: An Assessment of Coordination Efforts Between State SCHIP and Title V Programs*. Kaiser Commission on Medicaid and the Uninsured. [Online]. Available: http://www.kff.org/medicaid/loader.cfm?url=/commonspot/security/getfile.cfm&PageID=31921.

Markwalder A. 2005. *A Call to Action: A Guide for Managed Care Plans Serving Californians with Disabilities*. Oakland, CA: Disability Rights Activists. [Online]. Available: http://www.dralegal.org/downloads/pubs/call_to_action.pdf [accessed April 27, 2007].

Marmor T. 1973. *The Politics of Medicare*. Chicago, IL: Aldine Publishing Company. (Reprint; originally published by Routledge & Kegan Paul, Ltd.)

Marshall VW, Mueller MM. 2002. *Rethinking Social Policy for an Aging Workforce and Society. Insights from the Life Course*. Ottawa, Ontario, Canada: Canadian Policy Research Network.

Martin KE, Rogal DL, Arnold SB. 2004. *Health-Based Risk Assessment: Risk Adjusted Payments and Beyond*. Washington, DC: Health Care Financing and Organization. [Online]. Available: http://www.hcfo.net/pdf/riskadjustment.pdf [accessed April 27, 2007].

Masoro EJ. 1999. *Challenges of Biological Aging*. New York: Springer Publishing Co.

Mathews TJ. 2006. *Trends in Spina Bifida and Anencephalus in the United States, 1991–2003*. Hyattsville, MD: National Center for Health Statistics. [Online]. Available: http://www.cdc.gov/nchs/products/pubs/pubd/hestats/spine_anen.htm [accessed April 27, 2007].

Mathiowetz N. 2001. Methodological issues in the measurement of persons with disabilities. *Research in Social Science and Disability* 2:125–144.

Mathis J. 2004. *The ADA's Application to Insurance Coverage*. Washington, DC: Brazelon Center for Mental Health Law. [Online]. Available: http://www.bazelon.org/issues/disabilityrights/resources/insurance.htm [accessed April 27, 2007].

Mayer ML, Skinner AC, Slifkin RT. 2004. Unmet need for routine and specialty care: data from the National Survey of Children with Special Health Care Needs. *Pediatrics* 113(2):e109–e115. [Online]. Available: http://pediatrics.aappublications.org/cgi/content/abstract/113/2/e109 [accessed March 16, 2007].

Maynard FM, Julius M, Kirsch N, Lampman R, Peterson C, Tate D, Waring W, Werner R. 1991. *The Late Effects of Polio: A Model for Identification and Assessment of Preventable Secondary Conditions.* Ann Arbor: Post-Polio Research and Training Program, Department of Physical Medicine and Rehabilitation, University of Michigan.

McConachie H, Colver AF, Forsyth RJ, Jarvis SN, Parkinson KN. 2006. Participation of disabled children: how should it be characterized and measured? *Disability and Rehabilitations* 28(18):1157–1164.

McDonagh JE. 2000. Child-adult interface: the adolescent challenge. *Nephrology, Dialysis, Transplantation* 15:1761–1765.

McDonagh JE. 2006. *Growing up Ready for Emerging Adulthood: An Evidence Base for Professionals Involved in Transitional Care for Young People with No Chronic Illness and/or Disabilities.* [Online]. Available: http://217.35.77.12/archive/england/papers/health/pdfs/04137428.pdf [accessed April 27, 2007].

McDonagh JE, Kelly DA. 2003. Transitioning care of the pediatric recipient to adult caregivers. *Pediatric Clinics of North America* 50(6):1561–1583.

McInerny TK, Cull WL, Yudkowsky BK. 2005. Physician reimbursement levels and adherence to AAP well-visit and immunization recommendations. *Pediatrics* 115(4):833–838.

McManus M. 2001. *Private Health Insurance Coverage of Hearing Services for Children.* Maternal and Child Health Policy Research Center. [Online]. Available: http://www. infanthearing.org/financing/docs/Private%20Health%20Insurance%20for%20Children s%20Hearing%20Services.pdf [accessed April 27, 2007].

McManus M, Kohrt A, Bradley J, Walsh L. 2003. *Medical Home Crosswalk to Reimbursement.* [Online]. Available: http://www.medicalhomeinfo.org/tools/Coding/Crosswalk%20-%20Final.doc.

McMenamin TM, Hale TW, Kruse D, Kim H. 2005. *Designing Questions to Identify People with Disabilities in Labor Force Surveys: The Effort to Measure the Employment Level of Adults with Disabilities in the CPS.* Washington, DC: Bureau of Labor Statistics. [Online]. Available: http://www.bls.gov/ore/pdf/st050190.pdf [accessed April 27, 2007].

McMenamin TM, Miller SA, Polivka AE. 2006. *Discussion and Presentation of the Disability Test Results from the Current Population Survey.* Bureau of Labor Statistics Working Paper No. 396. [Online]. Available: http://www.bls.gov/ore/pdf/ec060080.pdf [accessed April 27, 2007].

McNeil JM. 1997. Americans with Disabilities; 1994–95. *Current Population Reports*, Report No. P70-61. Washington, DC: U.S. Government Printing Office. [Online]. Available: Available: http://www.census.gov/prod/3/97pubs/p70-61.pdf [accessed April 27, 2007].

McNeil JM. 2001. Americans with Disabilities: 1997. *Current Population Reports*, Report No. P70-73. Washington, DC: U.S. Government Printing Office. [Online]. Available: http://www.census.gov/prod/2001pubs/p70-73.pdf [accessed April 27, 2007].

McPherson M, Arango P, Fox H, Lauver C, McManus M, Newacheck PW, Perrin J. 1998. A new definition of children with special health care needs. *Pediatrics* 102(1 Pt 1): 137–139.

McPherson M, Weissman G, Strickland BB, van Dyck PC, Blumberg SJ, Newacheck PW. 2004. Implementing community-based systems of services for children and youths with special health care needs: how well are we doing? *Pediatrics* 113(5 Suppl):1538–1544.

McQuaid EL, Kopel SJ, Klein RB, Fritz GK. 2003. Medication adherence in pediatric asthma: reasoning, responsibility, and behavior. *Journal of Pediatric Psychology* 28(5):323–333.

Meaney MJ, Szyf M. 2005. Environmental programming of stress responses through DNA methylation: life at the interface between dynamic environment and a fixed genome. *Dialogues in Clinical Neuroscience* 7(2):103–123.

Medicare Rights Center. 2006. *Medicare HMOs: Denials.* [Online]. Available: http://www. medicarerights.org/casesmhdenials.html [accessed April 27, 2007].

MedPac (Medicare Payment Advisory Commission). 2004. Section 3D: Home Health Services. In: *Report to Congress: Medicare Payment Policy*. Washington, DC: Medicare Payment Advisory Commission. [Online]. Available: http://www.medpac.gov/publications%5Cco ngressional_reports%5CMar04_Ch3D.pdf [accessed April 27, 2007].

MedPac. 2005a. Medicare Advantage payment areas and risk adjustment. In: *Report to the Congress: Issues in a Modernized Medicare Program*. Washington, DC: Medicare Payment Advisory Commission. Pp. 41–55. [Online]. Available: http://www.medpac.gov/ publications%5Ccongressional_reports%5CJune05_ch2.pdf [accessed April 27, 2007].

MedPac. 2005b. *Medicare Payment Policy—Report to Congress*. Washington, DC: Medicare Payment Advisory Commission [Online]. Available: http://www.medpac.gov/publications/ congressional_reports/Mar05_EntireReport.pdf [accessed April 27, 2007].

MedPac. 2006. *Medicare Advantage Benchmarks and Payments Compared with Average Medicare Fee-for-Service Spending*. Washington, DC: Medicare Payment Advisory Commission. [Online]. Available: http://www.medpac.gov/publications/other_reports/ MedPAC_briefs_MA_relative_payment.pdf [accessed April 27, 2007].

Mehrotra A, Epstein AM, Rosenthal MB. 2006a. Do integrated medical groups provide higher-quality medical care than individual practice associations? *Annals of Internal Medicine* 145(11):826–833.

Mehrotra A, Grier S, Dudley RA. 2006b. The relationship between health plan advertising and market incentives: evidence of risk-selective behavior. *Health Affairs (Millwood)* 25(3):759–765.

Mele N, Archer J, Pusch BD. 2005. Access to breast cancer screening services for women with disabilities. *Journal of Obstetric, Gynecologic, and Neonatal Nursing* 34(4):453–464.

Melgar T, Brands C, Sharma N. 2005. Health care transition. *Pediatrics* 15(5):1449–1450.

Mendelsohn S. 2006. *Using State Insurance Laws to Advance the Cause of Assistive Technology*. United Cerebral Palsy, Health and Wellness. [Online]. Available: http://www. ucp.org/ucp_channeldoc.cfm/1/16/11431/11431-11431/1058/1/16/11431/11431-11431/ 1058?PrintFriendly=Yes [accessed April 27, 2007].

Mendelsohn S. 2007. Role of tax law in the development and use of accessible medical instrumentation. In: Winters JM, Story MF, eds. *Medical Instrumentation: Accessibility and Usability Considerations*. Boca Raton, FL: CRC Press. Pp. 59–80.

Merlis M. 2005. *Fundamentals of Underwriting in the Nongroup Health Insurance Market: Access to Coverage and Options for Reform*. National Health Policy Forum Background Paper. Washington, DC: The George Washington University. [Online]. Available: http:// www.nhpf.org/pdfs_bp/BP_Underwriting_04-13-05.pdf [accessed April 27, 2007].

Miles K. 2004. Transition from pediatric to adult services: experiences of HIV-positive adolescents. *AIDS Care* 16(3):305–314.

Miller K, DeMaio T. 2006. *Report of Cognitive Research and Proposed American Community Survey Disability Questions*. Study Series *(Survey Methodology No. 2006-6)*. [Online]. Available: http://www.census.gov/srd/papers/pdf/ssm2006-06.pdf [accessed April 27, 2007].

Mitchell JB, Khatutsky G, Swigonski NL. 2001. Impact of the Oregon Health Plan on children with special health care needs. *Pediatrics* 107(4):736–743.

Mo B, Lindbaek M, Harris S, Rasmussen K. 2004. Social hearing measured with the Performance Inventory for Profound and Severe Loss: a comparison between adult multichannel cochlear implant patients and users of acoustical hearing aids. *International Journal of Audiology* 43(10):572–578.

Mokdad AH, Ford ES, Bowman BA, Nelson DE, Engelgau MM, Vinicor F, Marks JS. 2000. Diabetes trends in the U.S.: 1990–1998. *Diabetes Care* 23(9):1278–1283.

Moon S, Shin J. 2006. The effect of the Americans with Disabilities Act on economic well-being of men with disabilities. *Health Policy* 76(3):266–276.

Moore JD, Smith DG. 2005–2006. Legislating Medicaid: considering Medicaid and its origins. *Health Care Financing Review* 27(2):45–52.

Morera C, Manrique M, Ramos A, Garcia-Ibanez L, Cavalle L, Huarte A, Castillo C, Estrada E. 2005. Advantages of binaural hearing provided through bimodal stimulation via a cochlear implant and a conventional hearing aid: a 6-month comparative study. *Acta Oto-Laryngologica* 125(6):596–606.

Morgan RO, Virnig BA, DeVito CA, Persily NA. 1997. The Medicare-HMO revolving door—the healthy go in and the sick go out. *New England Journal of Medicine* 337(3): 169–175.

Msall ME, Avery RC, Tremont MR, Lima JC, Rogers ML, Hogan DP. 2003. Functional disability and school activity limitations in 41,300 school-age children: relationship to medical impairments. *Pediatrics* 111(3):348–353.

Mueller J, principal investigator. 2000. *Oxo International Becomes a Universal Design Icon.* The Center for Universal Design, North Carolina State University. [Online]. Available: http://www.design.ncsu.edu/cud/projserv_ps/projects/case_studies/oxo.htm [accessed April 27, 2007].

Murphy H, Higgins E. 1994. *An Investigation of the Compensatory Effectiveness of Assistive Technology on Postsecondary Students with Learning Disabilities. Final Report.* California State University. [Online]. Available: http://eric.ed.gov/ERICDocs/data/ericdocs2/content_storage_01/0000000b/80/23/ae/c8.pdf [accessed April 27, 2007].

Murphy KP, Bliss PM. 2004. Aging with cerebral palsy. In: Winters JM, Story MF, eds. *Medical Instrumentation: Accessibility and Usability Considerations.* Boca Raton, FL: CRC Press. Pp. 196–212.

Murphy KP, Molnar GE, Lankasky K. 1995. Medical and functional status of adults with cerebral palsy. *Developmental Medicine and Child Neurology* 37(12):1075–1084.

Murray N. 2003. *Historical Overview of Disability Policy.* [Online]. Available: http://www.wheelchairnet.org/WCN_Living/Docs/Historicaloverview.html [accessed April 27, 2007].

Murugappan G. 2006. *DARPA Aims to Revolutionize Prosthetics Within Four Years.* The Johns Hopkins University News-Letter. [Online]. Available: http://www.jhunewsletter.com/media/storage/paper932/news/2006/11/16/Features/Darpa.Aims.To.Revolutionize.Prosthetics.Within.Four.Years-2468572.shtml?norewrite200612081307&sourcedomain=www.jhunewsletter.com [accessed April 27, 2007].

NAC/AARP (National Alliance for Caregiving/AARP). 1997. *Family Caregiving in the U.S.: Findings from a National Survey.* Washington, DC: NAC and AARP.

NAC/AARP. 2004. *Caregiving in the U.S.* [Online]. Available: http://www.caregiving.org/data/04finalreport.pdf [accessed April 27, 2007].

Nageswaran S, Roth MS, Kluttz-Hile CE, Farel A. 2006. Medical homes for children with special healthcare needs in North Carolina. *North Carolina Medical Journal* 67(2):103–109.

Nagi SZ. 1965. Some conceptual issues in disability and rehabilitation. In: Sussman M, ed. *Sociology and Rehabilitation.* Washington, DC: American Sociological Association.

Nagi SZ. 1991. Disability concepts revisited: implications for prevention. In: Pope A, Tarlov A, eds. *Disability in America: Toward a National Agenda for Prevention.* Washington, DC: National Academy Press. Pp. 309–327.

NAHU (National Association of Health Insurance Underwriters). 2005. *Analysis of State-Level Health Insurance Market Reforms.* [Online]. Available: http://www.nahu.org/legislative/market_reform/revised_markets_paper.pdf [accessed April 27, 2007].

NARIC (National Rehabilitation Information Center). 2006a. Assistive technology outcomes. *RehabWire—News from the National Rehabilitation Information Center.* 8(1):unpaged. [Online]. Available: http://www.naric.com/public/RehabWire/060201.cfm [accessed April 27, 2007].

NARIC. 2006b. Search page for "Rehabilitation Engineering Research Centers." [Online]. Available: http://www.naric.com/research/pd/results.cfm?type=type&display=brief&criteria=Rehabilitation%20Engineering%20Research%20Centers%20(RERCs) [accessed April 27, 2007].

NARIC. 2006c. Search page for "Rehabilitation Research and Training Center." [Online]. Available: http://www.naric.com/research/results.cfm?search=1&type=all&criteria=Rehabilitation%20Research%20and%20Training%20Center&phrase=yes&startrow=1 [accessed April 27, 2007].

NASBO (National Association of State Budget Officers). 2006. *The Fiscal Survey of States.* [Online]. Available: http://www.nasbo.org/Publications/PDFs/FiscalSurveyJune06.pdf [accessed April 27, 2007].

NASPGHAN (North American Society for Pediatric Gastroenterology, Hepatology and Nutrition.) 2002. Transition of the patient with inflammatory bowel disease from pediatric to adult care. *Journal of Pediatric Gastroenterology and Nutrition* 34:245–248.

National Emphysema Treatment Trial Research Group. 2003. Cost Effectiveness of Lung-Volume–Reduction Surgery for Patients with Severe Emphysema. *New England Journal of Medicine* 348(21):2092–2102.

National Spinal Cord Injury Statistical Center. 2006. *Spinal Cord Injury: Facts and Figures at a Glance.* University of Alabama at Birmingham. [Online]. Available: http://images.main. uab.edu/spinalcord/pdffiles/Facts06.pdf [accessed April 27, 2007].

National Task Force on Technology & Disability. 2004. *Within Our Reach: Findings and Recommendations of the National Task Force on Technology & Disability.* Jackson, MI: Colonial Press.

NCBDDD (National Center on Birth Defects and Developmental Disabilities). 2005. *Folic Acid: PHS Recommendations.* Atlanta, GA: Centers for Disease Control and Prevention. [Online]. Available: http://www.cdc.gov/ncbddd/folicacid/health_recomm.htm [accessed April 27, 2007].

NCCDPHP (National Center for Chronic Disease Prevention and Health Promotion). 2006. *Technical Information and Data: 2005 Summary Data Quality Report.* Atlanta, GA: Centers for Disease Control and Prevention. [Online]. Available: http://www.cdc.gov/ brfss/technical_infodata/2005QualityReport.htm [accessed April 27, 2007].

NCCSDO (National Co-Ordinating Centre for NHS Service Delivery and Organization). 2002. *The Transition from Child to Adult Health and Social Care.* [Online]. Available: http://www.sdo.lshtm.ac.uk/files/adhoc/11-briefing-paper.pdf [accessed April 27, 2007].

NCD (National Council on Disability). 2000a. *Back to School on Civil Rights.* [Online]. Available: http://www.ncd.gov/newsroom/publications/2000/backtoschool_1.htm [accessed April 27, 2007].

NCD. 2000b. *Federal Policy Barriers to Assistive Technology.* [Online]. Available: http://www. ncd.gov/newsroom/publications/2000/assisttechnology.htm [accessed April 27, 2007].

NCD. 2000c. *Promises to Keep: A Decade of Federal Enforcement of the Americans with Disabilities Act.* [Online]. Available: http://www.ncd.gov/newsroom/publications/2000/ promises_1.htm [accessed April 27, 2007].

NCD. 2001. *The Accessible Future.* Washington, DC: National Council on Disability. [Online]. Available: http://www.ncd.gov/newsroom/publications/2001/accessiblefuture.htm [accessed April 27, 2007].

NCD. 2004a. *Design for Inclusion: Creating a New Marketplace—Industry White Paper.* [Online]. Available: http://www.ncd.gov/newsroom/publications/2004/inclusion_whitepaper. htm [accessed April 27, 2007].

NCD. 2004b. *Position Paper: Improving Federal Disability Data.* [Online]. Available: http://www.ncd.gov/newsroom/publications/2004/improvedata.htm [accessed April 27, 2007].

NCD. 2005. *The State of the 21st Century Long-Term Services and Supports: Financing and Systems Reform for Americans with Disabilities.* [Online]. Available: http://www.ncd.gov/newsroom/publications/2005/longterm_services.doc [accessed April 27, 2007].

NCD. 2006. *Over the Horizon: Potential Impact of Emerging Trends in Information and Communication Technology on Disability Policy and Practice.* [Online]. Available: http://www.ncd.gov/newsroom/publications/2006/pdf/emerging_trends.pdf [accessed April 27, 2007].

NCEH (National Center for Environmental Health). 2004. *Children's Blood Lead Levels in the United States.* [Online]. Available: http://www.CDC.gov/nceh/Lead/research/kidsBLL.htm [accessed April 27, 2007].

NCHS (National Center for Health Statistics). 2005a. *Health, United States, 2005.* Hyattsville, MD: NCHS. [Online]. Available: http://www.cdc.gov/nchs/data/hus/hus05.pdf [accessed April 27, 2007].

NCHS. 2005b. *National Health and Nutrition Examination Survey, 2005–2006: Let's Improve our Health.* [Online]. Available: http://www.cdc.gov/nchs/data/nhanes/OverviewBrochureEnglish_May05.pdf [accessed April 27, 2007].

NCHS. 2005c. *Prevalence of Overweight Among Children and Adolescents: United States, 1999–2002.* [Online]. Available: http://www.cdc.gov/nchs/products/pubs/pubd/hestats/overwght99.htm [accessed April 27, 2007].

NCHS. 2006a. *1994 National Health Interview Survey on Disability, Phase I and Phase II (Survey Goals and Objectives).* [Online]. Available: http://www.cdc.gov/nchs/about/major/nhis_dis/nhisddes.htm [accessed April 27, 2007].

NCHS. 2006b. *Health Measures in the New 1997 Redesigned National Health Interview Survey (NHIS).* [Online]. Available: http://www.cdc.gov/nchs/about/major/nhis/hisdesgn.htm [accessed April 27, 2007].

NCHS. 2007. Difficulty Performing Activities of Daily Living, by Age, Residence, Sex, Race and Ethnicity: Medicare Beneficiaries from the Medicare Current Beneficiary Survey, 1992-2004. *Trends in Health and Aging* http://209.217.72.34/aging/TableViewer/tableView.aspx?ReportId=362 [accessed April 27, 2007].

NCLD (National Center for Learning Disabilities). 2006. *IDEA Parent Guide—A Comprehensive Guide to Your Rights and Responsibilities Under the Individuals with Disabilities Education Act (IDEA 2004).* [Online]. Available: http://www.ncld.org/images/stories/downloads/parent_center/idea2004parentguide.pdf [accessed April 27, 2007].

NCMRR (National Center for Medical Rehabilitation Research). 2001. *Cooperative Multicenter Traumatic Brain Injury Clinical Trials Network.* [Online]. Available: http://grants.nih.gov/grants/guide/rfa-files/RFA-HD-01-007.html [accessed April 27, 2007].

NCMRR. 2002. *Summary Minutes of the National Advisory Board on Medical Rehabilitation Research Meeting,* Bethesda, MD, May 2–3. [Online]. Available: http://www.nichd.nih.gov/about/overview/advisory/nmrrab/minutes/2002may.cfm [accessed April 27, 2007].

NCMRR. 2006. *Report to the NACHID (National Advisory Child Health and Human Development) Council, January 2006.* [Online]. Available: http://www.nichd.nih.gov/publications/pubs/upload/ncmrr_report_online_2006.pdf [accessed April 27, 2007].

NCSET (National Center on Secondary Education and Transition). 2005. *Key Provisions on Transition: IDEA 1997 Compared to H.R. 1350 (IDEA 2004).* [Online]. Available: http://ncset.org/publications/related/ideatransition.asp [accessed April 27, 2007].

NCSL (National Conference of State Legislators). 2007. *2007 Bills on Universal Health Care Coverage Legislatures Fill in the Gaps.* [Online]. Available: http://www.ncsl.org/programs/health/universalhealth2007.htm [accessed April 27, 2007].

Nelson C, Higman S, Sia C, McFarlane E, Duggan A. 2005. Medical homes for at-risk children: parental reports of clinician-parent relationships, anticipatory guidance, and behavior changes. *Pediatrics* 115(1):48–56.

Neumann PJ, Rosen AB, Weinstein MC. 2005. Medicare and cost-effectiveness analysis. *New England Journal of Medicine* 353(14):1516–1522.

Newacheck PW, Halfon N. 2000. Prevalence, impact, and trends in childhood disability due to asthma. *Archives of Pediatrics & Adolescent Medicine* 154(3):287–293.

Newacheck PW, Budetti PP, McManus P. 1984. Trends in childhood disability. *American Journal of Public Health* 74(3):232–236.

Newacheck PW, Budetti PP, Halfon N. 1986. Trends in activity-limiting chronic conditions among children. *American Journal of Public Health* 76(2):178–184.

Newacheck P, Strickland B, Shonkoffs J, Perrin J, McPherson M, McManus M, Lauver C, et al. 1998. An epidemiologic profile of children with special health care needs. *Pediatrics* 102(1):117–123.

Newhouse JP. 1992. Medical care costs: how much welfare loss? *Journal of Economic Perspective* 6(3):3–21.

Newhouse JP. 1993. *Free for All? Lessons from the RAND Health Insurance Project.* Cambridge, MA: Harvard University Press.

Newhouse JP, Manning WG, Keeler EB, Sloss EM. 1989. Adjusting capitation rates using objective health measures and prior utilization. *Health Care Financing Review* 10(3):41–54.

New Mobility Magazine. 2006. *Reeve's Chair Lands in Chop Shop.* July. [Online]. Available: http://www.newmobility.com/review_article.cfm?id=1174&action=browse [accessed April 27, 2007].

Newschaffer CJ. 2006. Investigating diagnostic substitution and autism prevalence trends. *Pediatrics* 117(4):1436–1437.

Newschaffer CJ, Falb MD, Gurney JG. 2005. National autism prevalence trends from United States special education data. *Pediatrics* 115(3):e277–e282.

NHATP (New Hampshire Assistive Technology Partnership). 2001. *Assistive Technology Funding Manual: A Guide to Assistive Technology Funding Sources.* [Online]. Available: http://72.14.209.104/u/unhsites?q=cache:jRvi5OyAxesJ:iod.unh.edu/publications/pdf/manual-AT-Funding.pdf+Assistive+Technology+Funding+Manual:+A+Guide+to+Assistive+Technology+Funding+Sources&hl=en&ct=clnk&cd=1&gl=us&ie=UTF-8 [accessed April 27, 2007].

NHLBI (National Heart, Lung, and Blood Institute). 1996. *Data Fact Sheet: Congestive Heart Failure in the United States: A New Epidemic.* Bethesda, MD: U.S. Department of Health and Human Services.

NIA (National Institute on Aging). 2004. *Factbook 2004: National Institute on Aging Intramural Research Program.* [Online]. Available: http://www.grc.nia.nih.gov/branches/osd/factbook2004.pdf [accessed April 27, 2007].

NICHD (National Institute of Child Health and Human Development). 1993. *Research Plan for the National Center for Medical Rehabilitation Research.* NIH Publication No. 93-3509. [Online]. Available: http://www.nichd.nih.gov/about/ncmrr/plan.pdf [accessed April 27, 2007].

NICHQ (National Initiative for Children's Healthcare Quality). 2005. *Spread the Medical Home Concept. Comprehensive Final Report.* [Online]. Available: http://www.medicalhomeinfo.org/model/downloads/LC/MHLC_2_Final_Report_Final.doc [accessed April 27, 2007].

NIDRR (National Institute on Disability and Rehabilitation Research). 2005. *NIDRR's Support of Capacity Building in Rehabilitation Research.* [Online]. Available: http://www.foundationforpmr.org/summit/NIDRR Support of Capacity Building.doc [accessed April 27, 2007].

NIDRR. 2006. Department of Education: National Institute on Disability and Rehabilitation Research—Notice of Final Long-Range Plan for Fiscal Years 2005–2009. *Federal Register* 71(31):8166–8200. [Online]. Available: http://www.ed.gov/legislation/FedRegister/other/2006-1/021506d.pdf [accessed April 27, 2007].

NIH (National Institutes of Health). 1993. *Research Plan for the National Center for Medical Rehabilitation Research.* Public Health Service, NIH Publication No. 93-3509. [Online]. Available: http://www.nichd.nih.gov/publications/pubs/upload/NCMRR_Research_Plan_1993.pdf [accessed April 27, 2007].

NIH. 2006a. *Estimates of Funding for Various Diseases, Conditions, Research Areas.* [Online]. Available: http://www.nih.gov/news/fundingresearchareas.htm [accessed April 27, 2007].

NIH. 2006b. *Types of Grant Programs.* [Online]. Available: http://grants.nih.gov/grants/funding/funding_program.htm [accessed April 27, 2007].

NIH. Undated. *What is PROMIS? Primary Goals of PROMIS.* [Online]. Available: http://www.nihpromis.org/what_is_promise/goals.asp [accessed April 27, 2007].

NLM (National Library of Medicine). 2006. *Technology Transfer.* [Online]. Available: http://ghr.nlm.nih.gov/ghr/glossary/technologytransfer [accessed April 27, 2007].

Nordenfelt L. 2003. Action theory, disability and ICF. *Disability and Rehabilitation* 25(18):1075–1079.

Norvell DC, Czerniecki JM, Reiber GE, Maynard C, Pecoraro JA, Weiss NS. 2005. The prevalence of knee pain and symptomatic knee osteoarthritis among veteran traumatic amputees and nonamputees. *Archives of Physical Medicine & Rehabilitation* 86(3):487–493.

Nosek MA, Howland CA. 1997. Breast and cervical cancer screening among women with physical disabilities. *Archives of Physical Medicine & Rehabilitation* 78(12 Suppl 5): S39–S44.

Nosek MA, Hughes RB, Petersen NJ, Taylor HB, Robinson-Whelen S, Byrne M, Morgan R. 2006. Secondary conditions in a community-based sample of women with physical disabilities over a 1-year period. *Archives of Physical Medicine & Rehabilitation* 87(3):320–327.

Novak M. 2001. *Working on Accessible Web Content Guidelines and Designing More Usable Documents.* Trace Center, University of Wisconsin—Madison. [Online]. Available: http://trace.wisc.edu/docs/navtools2001/index.html [accessed April 27, 2007].

NRC (National Research Council). 1976. *Science and Technology in the Service of the Physically Handicapped.* Washington, DC: National Academy of Sciences.

NRC/IOM (Institute of Medicine). 2003. *Enhancing the Vitality of the National Institutes of Health: Organizational Change to Make New Challenges.* Washington, DC: The National Academies Press.

NRC/IOM. 2004. *Children's Health, the Nation's Wealth: Assessing and Improving Child Health.* Washington, DC: The National Academies Press.

NSF (National Science Foundation). 2001. *NSF Congressional Highlight: Summary of NSF Appropriation for FY 02.* [Online]. Available: http://www.nsf.gov/about/congress/107/highlights/cu01_1127.jsp [accessed April 27, 2007].

NSF. 2005. *Biomedical Engineering/Research to Aid Persons with Disabilities (BME/RAPD).* [Online]. Available: http://www.nsf.gov/eng/bes/biomedidetail.jsp#RAPDHomeCare.

NTFTD (National Task Force on Technology and Disability). 2004. *NTFTD Within Our Reach Report: Table of Contents.* Draft Report. [Online]. Available: http://www.ntftd.org/report/tableofcontents.htm [accessed April 27, 2007].

NTIA/ESA (National Telecommunications and Information Administration/Economics and Statistics Administration). 2002. Computer and Internet use among people with disabilities. In: *A Nation Online: How Americans Are Expanding Their Use of the Internet.* [Online]. Available: http://www.ntia.doc.gov/ntiahome/dn/html/Chapter7.htm [accessed April 27, 2007].

Nyman JA. 2005. *Health Insurance Theory: The Case of the Missing Welfare Gain.* [Online]. Available: http://www.aria.org/rts/proceedings/2005/Nyman%20-%20Vanishing.pdf [accessed April 27, 2007].

O'Brien G. 2001. Adult outcome of childhood learning disability. *Developmental Medicine and Child Neurology* 43(9):634–638.

Oeffinger KC, Mertens AC, Sklar CA, Kawashima T, Hudson MM, Meadows AT, Friedman DL, Marina N, Hobbie W, et al. 2006. Chronic health conditions in adult survivors of childhood cancer. *New England Journal of Medicine* 355(15):1572–1582.

Oermann MH, Lindgren CL. 1995. An educational program's effects on students' attitudes toward people with disabilities: a 1-year follow-up. *Rehabilitation Nursing* 20(1):6–10.

Ogden C, Carroll M, Curtin L, McDowell M, Tabak C, Flegal K. 2006. Prevalence of overweight and obesity in the United States, 1999–2004. *The Journal of the American Medical Association* 295(13):1549–1555.

Ogonowski J, Kronk R, Rice C, Feldman H. 2004. Inter-rater reliability in assigning ICF codes to children with disabilities. *Disability and Rehabilitation* 26(6):353–361.

Ohio Department of Health. 1995a. *Standards of Care & Outcome Measures for Children with Cerebral Palsy.* The Committee on Children with Disabilities of the Bureau for Children with Medical Handicaps and Ohio Chapter, American Academy of Pediatrics. [Online]. Available: http://www.odh.ohio.gov/ASSETS/F5782B7A9C974CD8BC9C524BCC468A49/palsy.pdf [accessed April 27, 2007].

Ohio Department of Health. 1995b. *Standards of Care & Outcome Measures for Children with Chronic Pulmonary Disease.* The Pulmonary Standards Committee of the Bureau for Children with Medical Handicaps. [Online]. Available: http://www.odh.ohio.gov/ASSETS/AAF1BCCB7A5C40888ADA3FD51501F672/pulmonary.pdf [accessed April 27, 2007].

Ohio Department of Health. 1995c. *Standards of Care & Outcome Measures for Children with Craniofacial Deformities.* The Craniofacial Standards Committee of the Bureau for Children with Medical Handicaps. [Online]. Available: http://www.odh.ohio.gov/ASSETS/3799ACED0D4749D881B0B6DA4D1BA322/cranio.pdf [accessed April 27, 2007].

Ohio Department of Health. 1995d. *Standards of Care & Outcome Measures for Children with Myelodysplasia.* The Myelodysplasia Standards Committee of the Bureau for Children with Medical Handicaps. [Online]. Available: http://www.odh.ohio.gov/ASSETS/2914BC5B47314DF9836088DA4551E9F9/bifida.pdf [accessed April 27, 2007].

Okochi J, Utsunomiya S, Takahashi T. 2005. Health measurement using the ICF: test-retest reliability study of ICF codes and qualifiers in geriatric care. *Health and Quality of Life Outcomes* 3:46. [Online]. Available: http://www.pubmedcentral.org/picrender.fcgi?artid=1199614&blobtype=pdf [accessed April 27, 2007].

Olenik LM, Laskin JJ, Burnham R, Wheeler GD, Steadward RD. 1995. Efficacy of rowing, backward wheeling and isolated scapular retractor exercise as remedial strength activities for wheelchair users: application of electromyography. *Paraplegia* 33(3):148–152.

Olin G, Dougherty DD. 2006. *Characteristics and Medical Expenses of Adults 18- to 64-Years Old with Functional Limitations, Combined Years 1997–2002.* Agency for Healthcare Research and Quality Working Paper No. 06002. [Online]. Available: http://www.meps.ahrq.gov/mepsweb/data_files/publications/workingpapers/wp_06002.pdf#xml=http://207.188.212.220/cgi-bin/texis/webinator/search/pdfhi.txt?query=Working+Paper+No.+06002&pr=MEPSPUBS&prox=page&rorder=500&rprox=500&rdfreq=500&rwfreq=500&rlead=500&sufs=0&order=r&cq=&id=459ca6313b [accessed April 27, 2007].

Olsen DG, Swigonski NL. 2004. Transition to adulthood: the important role of the pediatrician. *Pediatrics* 113(3):159–162.

Olson LM, Tang SS, Newacheck PW. 2005. Children in the United States with discontinuous health insurance coverage. *New England Journal of Medicine* 353(4):382–391.

OMB (Office of Management and Budget). 2004. *Department of Veterans Affairs PART Assessments.* Program Assessment Rating Tool (PART). Pp. 38–48. [Online]. Available: http://www.whitehouse.gov/omb/budget/fy2005/pma/va.pdf [accessed April 27, 2007].

OMB. 2005. *Department of Veterans Affairs PART Assessments.* Program Assessment Rating Tool (PART). [Online]. Available: http://www.whitehouse.gov/omb/budget/fy2006/pma/va.pdf [accessed April 27, 2007].

OTA (Office of Technology Assessment). 1982. Technology and its appropriate application. In: *Technology and Handicapped People.* Washington, DC: U.S. Government Printing Office. [Online]. Available: http://www.wws.princeton.edu/ota/disk3/1982/8229/822907.pdf [accessed April 27, 2007].

OTA. 1985. Technologies, functional impairment and long-term care. In: *Technology and Aging in America.* Washington, DC: U.S. Government Printing Office. [Online]. Available: http://www.wws.princeton.edu/ota/disk2/1985/8529/852909.pdf [accessed April 27, 2007].

Packer TL, Iwasiw C, Theben J, Sheveleva P, Metrofanova N. 2000. Attitudes to disability of Russian occupational therapy and nursing students. *International Journal of Rehabilitation Research* 23(1):39–47.

PAFP (Pennsylvania Academy of Family Physicians). 2006. *Medical Management Series: Home Improvement.* [Online]. Available: http://www.kff.org/medicare/upload/Understanding-the-Health-Care-Needs-and-Experiences-of-People-with-Disabilities-Findings-from-a-2003-Survey.pdf [accessed April 27, 2007].

PAI (Protection and Advocacy). 2002. *Accessing Assistive Technology.* [Online] Available: http://www.pai-ca.org/pubs/533201.htm [accessed April 27, 2007].

Palfrey JS, Sofis LA, Davidson EJ, Liu J, Freeman L, Ganz ML. 2004. The Pediatric Alliance for Coordinated Care: evaluation of a medical home model. *Pediatrics* 113(5):1507–1516.

Palsbo SE, Kailes JI. 2006. Disability-competent health systems. *Disability Studies Quarterly* 26(2). [Online]. Available: http://chhs.gmu.edu/ccid/pdf/DisabilityCompetentHealthSystems.pdf [accessed April 27, 2007].

Palsbo SE, Post R. 2003. Financial risk reduction for people with disabilities in Medicaid programs. *Manage Care Quarterly.* 11(2):1–7.

Pandya S. 2005. *Caregiving in the United States.* AARP Public Policy Institute Fact Sheet, Washington, DC. [Online]. Available: http://assets.aarp.org/rgcenter/il/fs111_caregiving.pdf [accessed April 27, 2007].

Pastor PN, Reuben CE. 2005. Racial and ethnic differences in ADHD and LD in young school-age children: parental reports in the National Health Interview Survey. *Public Health Reports* 120(4):383–392.

Patel V, Pauly M. 2002. Guaranteed renewability and the problem of risk variation in individual health insurance markets. *Health Affairs, Web Exclusive* (August 28):280–289. [Online]. Available: http://content.healthaffairs.org/cgi/reprint/hlthaff.w2.280v1 [accessed April 27, 2007].

Patrick DL, Erickson P. 1993. *Health Status and Health Policy: Quality of Life in Health Care Evaluation and Resource Allocation.* New York: Oxford University Press.

Perenboom RJ, Chorus AM. 2003. Measuring participation according to the International Classification of Functioning, Disability and Health (ICF). *Disability and Rehabilitation* 25(11–12):577–587.

Perkins J, Youdelman M, National Health Law Program. 2004. *Defining "Medical Necessity" in State Medicaid Programs.* [Online]. Available: www.healthlaw.org/library.cfm?fa=download&resourceID=62045&appView=folder&print [accessed April 27, 2007].

Perlin J. 2006. *Hearing on VA Research: Investing Today to Guide Tomorrow's Treatment.* Statement of Jonathan Perlin on the VA Medical and Prosthetic Research Program before the Senate Committee on Veteran's Affairs, April 27. [Online]. Available:http://veterans. senate.gov/index.cfm?FuseAction=Hearings.CurrentHearings&rID=591&hID=196 [accessed April 27, 2007].

Perlin J, Kolodner R, Roswell R. 2004. The Veterans Health Administration: quality, value, accountability, and information as transforming strategies for patient-centered care. *American Journal of Managed Care* 10(11):828–836. [Online]. Available: http://www1. va.gov/cprsdemo/docs/AJMCnovPrt2Perlin828to836.pdf [accessed April 27, 2007].

Perrin JM. 2002. Health services research for children with disabilities. *Milbank Quarterly* 80:303–324.

Perrin JM, Boudreau AA. 2006. Reducing deficits and the health of children, youth, and families. *Ambulatory Pediatrics* 6(4):185–186.

Perrin JM, Shayne MW, Bloom SR. 1993. *Home and Community Care for Chronically Ill Children.* New York: Oxford University Press.

Perrin JM, Kuhlthau K, McLaughlin TJ, Ettner SL, Gortmaker SL. 1999. Changing patterns of conditions among children receiving SSI disability benefits. *Archives of Pediatrics & Adolescent Medicine* 153(1):80–84.

Perry J. 2004. Aging with poliomyelitis. In: Kemp B, Mosqueda L, eds. *Aging with a Disability: What the Clinician Needs to Know.* Baltimore, MD: The Johns Hopkins University Press. Pp. 175–195.

Peters CP. 2005. *Children with Special Health Care Needs: Minding the Gaps.* National Health Policy Forum Background Paper. Washington, DC: The George Washington University. [Online]. Available: http://www.nhpf.org/pdfs_bp/BP_CSHCN_06-27-05.pdf [accessed April 27, 2007].

Peters CP. 2006. *EPSDT: Medicaid's Critical but Controversial Benefits Program for Children.* National Health Policy Forum Background Paper. Washington, DC: The George Washington University. [Online]. Available: http://www.nhpf.org/pdfs_ib/IB819_EPSDT_11-20-06.pdf [accessed April 27, 2007].

Pettersson I, Berndtsson I, Appelros P, Ahlstrom G. 2005. Lifeworld perspectives on assistive devices: lived experiences of spouses of persons with stroke. *Scandinavian Journal of Occupational Therapy* 12(4):159–169.

Pfizer Pharmaceutical Company. 2003. *Utilization of Veterans Affairs Medical Care Services by United States Veterans.* [Online]. Available: http://www.pfizer.com/pfizer/download/ health/pubs_facts_veterans.pdf#search=%22%22length%20of%20stay%22%20veteran s%20hospitals%20pfizer%22 [accessed April 27, 2007].

Pham HH, Simonson L, Elnicki DM, Fried LP, Goroll AH, Bass EB. 2004. Training U.S. medical students to care for the chronically ill. *Academic Medicine* 79(1):32–40.

Phelps, CE. 2003. *Health Economics*, 3rd ed. Reading, MS: Addison-Wesley Press.

Phillips B, Zhao H. 1993. Predictors of assistive technology abandonment. *Assistive Technology* 5(1):36–45.

Physical Disabilities Branch. Undated. *About Us.* Bethesda, MD: National Institutes of Health. [Online]. Available: http://pdb.cc.nih.gov/aboutus/ [accessed April 27, 2007].

Pilotto A, Franceschi M, Leandro G, Paris F, Niro V, Longo MG, D'Ambrosio LP, Andriulli A, Di Mario F. 2003. The risk of upper gastrointestinal bleeding in elderly users of aspirin and other non-steroidal anti-inflammatory drugs: the role of gastroprotective drug. *Aging Clinical and Experimental Research* 15(6):494–499.

Pirkl J. 1994. *Transgenerational Design.* New York: Van Nostrand Reinhold.

Platts-Mills T. 2005. Asthma severity and prevalence: an ongoing interaction between exposure, hygiene, and lifestyle. *PLoS (Public Library of Science) Medicine* 2(2):122–126.

Plewis I, Calderwood L, Hawkes D. 2004. *National Child Development Study and 1970 British Cohort Study Technical Report: Changes in the NCDS and BCS70 Populations and Samples Over Time*. Centre for Longitudinal Studies, Institute of Education, University of London. [Online]. Available: http://www.cls.ioe.ac.uk/core/documents/download.asp?id=209&log_stat=1 [accessed April 27, 2007].

Pope GC, Ellis RP, Ash AS, Ayanian JZ, Bates DW, Burstin H, Iezzoni LI, Marcantonio E, Wu B. 2000. *Diagnostic Cost Group Hierarchical Condition Category Models for Medicare Risk Adjustment*. Final Report to the Health Care Financing Administration, U.S. Department of Health and Human Services. [Online]. Available: http://www.cms.hhs.gov/Reports/downloads/pope_2000_2.pdf [accessed April 27, 2007].

Pope GC, Kautter J, Ellis RP, Ash AS, Ayanian JZ, Iezzoni LI, Ingber MJ, Levy JM, Robst J. 2004. Risk adjustment of the Medicare capitation payments using the CMS-HCC model. *Health Care Financing Review* 25(4):119–141.

Population Reference Bureau. 2005. *Record Number of Women in the U.S. Labor Force*. [Online]. Available: http://www.prb.org/Articles/2001/RecordNumberofWomenintheUSLaborForce.aspx [accessed April 27, 2007].

Preston S. 2005. Deadweight?—the influence of obesity on longevity. *New England Journal of Medicine* 352(11):1135–1137.

Priest D, Hull A. 2007a. Soldiers face neglect, frustration at army's top medical facility. *The Washington Post*, February 18, A01.

Priest D, Hull A. 2007b. Hospital investigates former aid chief. *The Washington Post*, February 20, A01.

Prouty R, Lakin KC, Coucouvanis K, Anderson L. 2005. Progress toward a national objective of Healthy People 2010: "reduce to zero the number of children 17 years and younger living in congregate care." *Mental Retardation* 43(6):456–460.

Pueschel SM, Scola FH, Pezzullo JC. 1992. A longitudinal study of atlanto-dens relationships in asymptomatic individuals with Down syndrome. *Pediatrics* 89(6):1194–1198.

Quality of Life Technology Center. 2006. *Research Foundations*. [Online]. Available: http://www.qolt.org/Research/index.html [accessed April 27, 2007].

Rainville J, Bagnall D, Phalen L. 1995. Health care providers' attitudes and beliefs about functional impairments and chronic back pain. *The Clinical Journal of Pain* 11(4):287–295.

Ralston E, Zazove P, Gorenflo D. 1996. Physicians' attitudes and beliefs about deaf patients. *The Journal of the American Board of Family Practice* 9(3):167–173.

Ramirez A, Farmer G, Grant D, Papachristou T. 2005. Disability and preventive cancer screening: results from the 2001 California Health Interview Study. *American Journal of Public Health* 95(11):2057–2064.

Ramlow J, Alexander M, LaPorte R, Kaufman C, Kueller L. 1992. Epidemiology of the post-polio syndrome. *American Journal of Epidemiology* 136(7):769–786.

Rasch JD. 2006. *World Wide Web Review Guide for the CRC Examination: Legislative History of the American State-Federal Vocational Rehabilitation Program*. [Online]. Available: http://luna.cas.usf.edu/~rasch/leg.html [accessed April 27, 2007].

Ravesloot CH, Seekins T, Walsh J. 1997. A structural analysis of secondary conditions experienced by people with physical disabilities. *Rehabilitation Psychology* 42(1):3–16.

Ravesloot CH, Seekins T, Cahill T, Lindren S, Nary DE, White G. 2006. Health promotion for people with disabilities: development and evaluation of the Living Well with a Disability program. *Health Education Research Advance Access* 2006 Oct 10. [Epub ahead of print.]

Reester H, Missmar R, Tumlinson A. 2004. *Recent Growth in Medicaid Home and Community-Based Services.* Kaiser Commission on Medicaid and the Uninsured. [Online]. Available: http://www.kff.org/medicaid/upload/Recent-Growth-in-Medicaid-Home-and-Community-Based-Service-Waivers-PDF.pdf [accessed April 27, 2007].

Rehabilitation Engineering Research Center on Technology Transfer (University of Buffalo). Undated. *Public Policy Project: Federal Legislation.* [Online]. Available: http://cosmos.buffalo.edu/t2rerc/research/public-policy/legislation.htm [accessed April 27, 2007].

Reid GJ, Irvine MJ, McCrindle BW, Sananes R, Ritvo PG, Siu SC, Webb GD. 2004. Prevalence and correlates of successful transfer from pediatric to adult health care among a cohort of young adults with complex congenital heart defects. *Pediatrics* 113(3 Pt 1):197–205.

Reilly JJ, Armstrong J, Dorosty AR, Emmett PM, Ness A, Rogers I, Steer C, Sheriff A. 2005. Early life risk factors for obesity in childhood: cohort study. *British Medical Journal* 330(7504):1357–1359.

Reilly T. 2003. Transition from care: status and outcomes of youth who age out of foster care. *Child Welfare* 82:727–746.

Reis J, Breslin M, Iezzoni L, Kirschner K. 2004. *It Takes More Than Ramps to Solve the Crisis of Healthcare for People with Disabilities.* Chicago: Rehabilitation Institute of Chicago. [Online]. Available: http://www.ric.org/community/RIC_whitepaperfinal82704.pdf [accessed April 27, 2007].

Reiss J, Gibson R. 2006. Health care transition of adolescents and young adults with disabilities and special health care needs: new perspectives. In: Field MJ, Jette AM, Martin L, eds. *Workshop on Disability in America: A New Look.* Washington, DC: The National Academies Press. Pp. 166–184.

RESNA (Rehabilitation Engineering and Assistive Technology Society of North America). 2002. *RESNA Technical Assistance Project Small Group Meeting on "Establishing a Dialog on Assistive Technology and Private Health Insurance."* Meeting Summary, Hartford, CT, May 17. [Online]. Available: http://www.resna.org/taproject/library/statestrategies.html [accessed April 27, 2007].

RESNA. 2003. *Progress and Outcomes: A Report on the State Assistive Technology Act Projects, 2000-2001.* [Online]. Available:http://www.resna.org/taproject/library/accomplish/Policy_Final.pdf [accessed April 27, 2007].

RESNA. 2005. *Letter to Drs. Hughes, Brennen, Oleck, and Norris [Medical Directors for the Durable Medical Equipment Regional Carriers] from the Board of Directors of RESNA in response to the [September 14, 2005] request for comments on the Power Mobility Device Draft Local Coverage Determination.* [Online]. Available: http://www.resna.org/RESNA's%20Response%20To%20The%20Request%20For%20Comments%20On%20The%20Power%20Mobility%20Device%20Draft%20Local%20Coverage%20Determination%20.doc [accessed April 27, 2007].

RESNA. 2006. *Letter to Secretary Leavitt and Dr. McClellan of the US Department of Health and Human Services.* September 12. [Online]. Available: http://www.resna.org/GovernAffairs/CMS-power%20wc%20LCD%209-11-06.pdf [accessed April 27, 2007].

Resnick MD, Bearman PS, Blum RW, Bauman KE, Harris KM, Jones J, Tabor J, Beuhring T, Sieving RE, Shew M, et al. 1997. Protecting adolescents from harm. Findings from the National Longitudinal Study on Adolescent Health. *The Journal of the American Medical Association* 278(10):823–832.

Reswick J. 2002. How and when did the rehabilitation engineering center program come into being? *Journal of Rehabilitation Research and Development* 39(6):11–16.

Reynolds SL, Crimmins EM, Saito Y. 1999. Cohort differences in disability and disease presence. *Gerontologist* 38(5):578–590.

Riemer-Reiss ML, Wacker RR. 2000. Factors associated with assistive technology discontinuance among individuals with disabilities. *Journal of Rehabilitation* 66(3):44–50.

Riley GF. 2004. The cost of eliminating the 24-month Medicare waiting period for Social Security disabled-worker beneficiaries. *Medical Care* 42(4):387–394.

Rimmer JH, Shenoy SS. 2006. Impact of exercise on targeted secondary conditions. In: Field MJ, Jette AM, Martin L, eds. *Workshop on Disability in America: A New Look.* Washington, DC: The National Academies Press. Pp. 205–221.

Robinson J. 2002. Renewed emphasis on consumer cost sharing in health insurance benefit design. *Health Affairs, Web Exclusive* (March 20):139–154. [Online]. Available: http://content.healthaffairs.org/cgi/content/abstract/hlthaff.w2.139v1 [accessed April 27, 2007].

Robitaille S. 2001. Santa's assistive little helpers: children with special needs need special toys, so here's a quick guide to some neat and nifty gift ideas for disabled youngsters. *Business Week Online.* [Online]. Available: http://www.businessweek.com/bwdaily/dnflash/dec2001/nf20011212_5346.htm [accessed April 27, 2007].

Roelands M, Van Oost P, Buysse A, Depoorter A. 2002. Awareness among community-dwelling elderly of assistive devices for mobility and self-care and attitudes towards their use. *Social Science & Medicine* 54(9):1441–1451.

Roizen NJ, Patterson D. 2003. Down's syndrome. *Lancet* 361(9365):1281–1289.

Roizen NJ, Mets MB, Blondis TA. 1994. Ophthalmic disorders in children with Down syndrome. *Developmental Medicine and Child Neurology* 36(7):594–600.

Rona RJ, Gulliford MC, Chinn S. 1993. Effects of prematurity and intrauterine growth on respiratory health and lung function in childhood. *British Medical Journal* 306(6881):817–820.

Rose KA. 1999. A survey of the accessibility of chiropractic clinics to the disabled. *Journal of Manipulative and Physiological Therapeutics* 22(8):523–529.

Rosen DS, Blum RW, Britto M, Sawyer SM, Siegel DM. 2003. Transition to adult health care for adolescents and young adults with chronic conditions. Position paper of the Society for Adolescent Medicine. *Journal of Adolescent Health* 33(4):309–311.

Rosenbaum S. 2006. *Defined-Contribution Plans and Limited-Benefit Arrangements: Implications for Medicaid Beneficiaries.* Washington, DC: The George Washington University Medical Center. [Online]. Available: http://www.gwumc.edu/sphhs/healthpolicy/chsrp/downloads/Rosenbaum_AHIP_FNL_091306.pdf [accessed April 27, 2007].

Rosenbaum S, Stewart A, Sonosky C. 2002. *Negotiating the New Health System Fourth Edition Medicaid Managed Care General Service Agreements.* [Online]. Available: http://www.gwumc.edu/sphhs/healthpolicy/nnhs4/GSA/ [accessed April 27, 2007].

Rosenbaum S, Mauery R, Shin P, Hidalgo J. 2005. *National Security and U.S. Child Health Policy: The Origins and Continuing Role of Medicaid and EPSDT.* School of Public Health and Health Services, The George Washington University. [Online]. Available: www.gwumc.edu/sphhs/healthpolicy/chsrp/downloads/mil_prep042605.pdf [accessed April 27, 2007].

Rosenkranz J. 2005. *Utilization of Aid & Attendance/Homebound Pension by Veterans and Their Survivors to Access Long-Term Care in the Home, Respite Care & Prescription Medicine Coverage.* Report of Findings: 2005 White House Conference on Aging. [Online]. Available: http://www.whcoa.gov/about/policy/meetings/Schmeiding/Rosenkranz.pdf [accessed April 27, 2007].

Rosenthal M. 2005. *Testimony Presented to the House Subcommittee on Employer-Employee Relations Hearing on Examining Pay-for-Performance Measures and Other Trends in Employer-Sponsored Health Care.* May 17. [Online]. Available: http://www.cmwf.org/usr_doc/Rosenthal_testimony_05-17-2005.pdf [accessed April 27, 2007].

Ruff R. 2006. VA research and development. Presentation to the Committee on Disability in America, Institute of Medicine, Washington, DC, January 9.

Russell JN, Hendershot GE, LeClere F, Howie J, Adler M. 1997. *Trends and Differential Use of Assistive Technology Devices: United States, 1994.* Washington, DC: U.S. Department of Health and Human Services. [Online]. Available: http://www.cdc.gov/nchs/data/ad/ad292.pdf [accessed April 27, 2007].

Rust KL, Smith RO. 2005. Assistive technology in the measurement of rehabilitation and health outcomes. *American Journal of Physical Medicine & Rehabilitation* 84(10):780–793; quiz 794–796.

RWJF (The Robert Wood Johnson Foundation). 2004. *Foundation Aims at Taking Consumer-Directed Service Model for Medicaid to National Level.* RWJF News Release. [Online]. Available: http://www.rwjf.org/newsroom/newsreleasesdetail.jsp?id=10139 [accessed April 27, 2007].

RWJF. 2006. *The State of Kids' Coverage.* [Online]. Available: http://coveringkidsandfamilies.org/press/docs/2006StateofKidsCoverage.pdf [accessed April 27, 2007].

Sakai T, Yamada H, Nakamura T, Nanamori K, Kawasaki Y, Hanaoka N, Nakamura E, Uchida K, Goel VK, Vishnubhotla L, et al. 2006. Lumbar spinal disorders in patients with athetoid cerebral palsy; a clinical and biomechanical study. *Spine* 31(3):E66-E70.

Salmi J, Huupponen T, Oksa H, Oksala H, Koivula T, Raita P. 1986. Metabolic control in adolescent insulin-dependent diabetics referred from pediatric to adult clinic. *Annals of Clinical Research* 18(2):84–87.

Sanchez J, Byfield G, Brown TT, LaFavor K, Murphy D, Laud P. 2000. Perceived accessibility versus actual physical accessibility of healthcare facilities. *Rehabilitation Nursing* 25(1):6–9.

Sanford J. 1996. *A Review of Technical Requirements for Ramps: Final Report.* Architectural and Transportation Barriers Compliance Board. [Online]. Available: http://www.access-board.gov/research/Ramps/report.htm [accessed April 27, 2007].

Sanford J, Bruce C. 2006. *The Physical Environment as an Independent Measure: A Framework for Understanding the Role of Environmental Attributes in Activity and Performance Outcomes.* Presented at the Living in Our Environment, the Promise of the ICF Conference, Vancouver, British Columbia, Canada, June 5–7. [Online]. Available: http://www.icfconference.com/New%20Presentations/Tuesday%20(York%20Room)/1030-1200%20-%20Environmental%20Factors/Jon%20A.%20Sanford%20-%20Environmental%20Factors.pdf [accessed April 27, 2007].

Sardell A, Johnson K. 1998. The politics of EPSDT policy in the 1990s: policy entrepreneurs, political streams, and children's health benefits. *Milbank Quarterly* 76(2):175–205.

SBA (U.S. Small Business Administration). 2001. *SBIR and STTR Programs and Awards.* [Online]. Available: http://www.sba.gov/sbir/indexsbir-sttr.html [accessed April 27, 2007].

Scal P. 2002. Transition for youth with chronic conditions: primary care physicians' approaches. *Pediatrics* 110(6 Pt2):1315–1321.

Scal P, Ireland M. 2005. Addressing transition to adult health care for adolescents with special health care needs. *Pediatrics* 115(6):1607–1612.

Scal P, Evans T, Blozis S, Okinow N, Blum R. 1999. Trends in transition from pediatric to adult health care services for young adults with chronic conditions. *Adolescent Health* 24(4):259–264.

Scherer MJ. 2005. *Living in the State of Stuck: How Technology Impacts the Lives of People with Disabilities, Fourth Edition.* Cambridge, MA: Brookline Books.

Schidlow DV, Fiel SB. 1990. Life beyond pediatrics. Transition of chronically ill adolescents from pediatric to adult health care systems. *Medical Clinics of North America* 74(5):1113–1120.

Schiller JS, Adams PF, Coriaty Nelson Z. 2005. Summary health statistics for the U.S. population: National Health Interview Survey, 2003. National Center for Health Statistics. *Vital and Health Statistics* 10(224). [Online]. Available: http://www.cdc.gov/nchs/data/series/sr_10/sr10_224.pdf [accessed April 27, 2007].

Schmeler MR, Bundy A, Petro T, Stonfer MJ. 2003. Cost and quality outcome of a power wheelchair leasing program for persons with terminal disease. In: *Proceedings of the 19th International Seating Symposium*, Orlando, FL. Pp. 187–188.

Schmidt L. 2004. *Effects of Welfare Reform on the Supplemental Security Income (SSI) Program*. National Poverty Center: Policy Brief No. 4. [Online]. Available: http://www.npc. umich.edu/publications/policy_briefs/brief4/brief4.pdf [accessed April 27, 2007].

Schneider A, Elias R, Garfield R, Rousseau D, Wachino V. 2002. Appendix 1: Medicaid Legislative History, 1965–2000. In: *The Medicaid Resource Book*. The Kaiser Commission on Medicaid and the Uninsured. [Online]. Available: http://www.kff.org/medicaid/loader. cfm?url=/commonspot/security/getfile.cfm&PageID=14255 [accessed April 27, 2007].

Schoeni RF, Freedman VA, Wallace R. 2001. Persistent, consistent, widespread, and robust? Another look at recent trends in old-age disability. *The Journals of Gerontology, Series B: Psychological Sciences and Social Sciences* 56(4):S206–S218.

Schoeni RF, Martin L, Andreski P, Freedman VA. 2005. Persistent and growing socioeconomic disparities in disability among the elderly: 1982–2002. *American Journal of Public Health* 95(11):2065–2070.

Schoeni RF, Freedman VA, Martin LG. In press. Socioeconomic and demographic disparities in trends in old-age disability. In: Cutler DM, Wise DA, eds. *Health in Older Ages: The Causes and Consequences of Declining Disability Among the Elderly*. Chicago, IL: The University of Chicago Press. [Online]. Available: http://www.nber.org/books/disability/ index.html [accessed April 27, 2007].

Schulz R, Noelker LS, Rockwood K, Sprott R, eds. 2006. *The Encyclopedia of Aging*, 4th ed. (two-volume set). New York: Springer Publishing Co.

Schuntermann MF. 2005. The implementation of the International Classification of Functioning, Disability and Health in Germany: experiences and problems. *International Journal of Rehabilitation Medicine* 28(2):93–102.

Schupf N, Winsten S, Patel B, Pang D, Ferin M, Zigman WB, Silverman W, Mayeux R. 2006. Bioavailable estradiol and age at onset of Alzheimer's disease in postmenopausal women with Down syndrome. *Neuroscience Letters* 406(3):298–302.

Schwartz L, Engel JM, Jensen MP. 1999. Pain in persons with cerebral palsy. *Archives of Physical Medicine & Rehabilitation* 80(10):1243–1246.

Schwemberger JG, Mosby JE, Doa MJ, Jacobs DE, Ashley PJ, Brody DJ, Brown MJ. 2005. Blood lead levels—United States, 1999–2002. *Morbidity and Mortality Weekly Report* 54(20):513–516. [Online]. Available: http://www.cdc.gov/mmwr/preview/mmwrhtml/ mm5420a5.htm [accessed April 27, 2007].

Sears MR, Greene JM, Willan AR, Taylor DR, Flannery EM, Cowan JO, Herbison GP, Poulton R. 2002. Long-term relation between breastfeeding and development of atopy and asthma in children and young adults: a longitudinal study. *Lancet* 360:901–907.

Seekins T, Clay J, Ravesloot C. 1994. A descriptive study of secondary conditions reported by a population of adults with physical disabilities served by three independent living centers in a rural state. *Journal of Rehabilitation* 60(2):47–51.

Seekins T, Traci M, Bainbridge D, Humphries K, Cunningham N, Brod R, Sherman J. 2006. Promoting health and preventing secondary conditions among adults with developmental disabilities. In: Field MJ, Jette AM, Martin L, eds. *Workshop on Disability in America: A New Look*. Washington, DC: The National Academies Press. Pp. 251–264.

Seelman KD. 2007. Technology for full citizenship: challenges for the research community. In: Winters JM, Story MF, eds. *Medical Instrumentation: Accessibility and Usability Considerations*. Boca Raton, FL: CRC Press. Pp. 307–319.

Seidman DS, Laor A, Gale R, Stevenson DK, Denon YL. 1991. Is low birthweight a risk factor for asthma during adolescence? *Archives of Disease in Childhood* 66:584–587.

Seigel WM, Golden NH, Gough JW, Lashley MS, Sacker IM. 1990. Depression, self-esteem, and life events in adolescents with chronic disease. *Journal of Adolescent Health Care* 11:501–504.

Seigle NS. 2001. The father of invention. *People with Disabilities* 11(2) (unpaged). New Jersey Council on Developmental Disabilities. [Online]. Available: http://www.njddc. org/pwd11-2/pwd11-2-2.htm [accessed April 27, 2007].

Seltzer MM, Heller T, Krauss MW. 2004. Introduction to the Special Issue on Aging. *American Journal of Mental Retardation* 109(2):81–82.

Shaheen S. 1997. The beginnings of chronic airflow obstruction. *British Medical Journal* 53(1):58–70.

Shattuck PT. 2006. The contribution of diagnostic substitution to the growing administrative prevalence of autism in US special education. Pediatrics 117(4):1028–1037.

Shaw KL, Southwood TR, McDonagh JE. 2005. Growing up and moving on in rheumatology: transitional care and quality of life in a multicentre cohort of adolescents with juvenile idiopathic arthritis. *Rheumatology (Oxford)* 44(6):806–812.

Shaw KL, Southwood TR, McDonagh JE. 2006. Growing up and moving in rheumatology: parents as proxies of adolescents with juvenile idiopathic. *Arthritis and Rheumatism* 55(2):189–198.

Shekelle PG, Maglione M, Morton SC. 2003. *Preponderance of Evidence: What to Do About Ephedra*. RAND Organization. [Online]. Available: http://www.rand.org/publications/ randreview/issues/spring2003/evidence.html [accessed April 27, 2007].

Short A, Mays G, Mittler J. 2003. Disease Management: A Leap of Faith to Lower-Cost, Higher-Quality Health Care. *Issue brief (Center for Studying Health System Change)* Oct;(69):1–4.

Shumway-Cook A, Patla AE, Stewart A, Ferrucci L, Ciol M, Guralnik J. 2002. Environmental demands associated with community mobility in older adults with and without mobility disabilities. *Physical Therapy* 82(7):670–681.

Shumway-Cook A, Patla A, Stewart A, Ferrucci L, Ciol MA, Guralnik J. 2003. Environmental components of mobility disability in community-living older persons. *Journal of the American Geriatrics Society* 51(3):393–398.

Sie IH, Waters RL, Adkins RH, Gellman H. 1992. Upper extremity pain in the postrehabilitation spinal cord injured patient. *Archives of Physical Medicine & Rehabilitation* 73(1):44–48.

Simeonsson RJ. 2006. Defining and classifying disability in children. In: Field MJ, Jette AM, Martin L, eds. *Workshop on Disability in America: A New Look*. Washington, DC: The National Academies Press. Pp. 67–87.

Simeonsson RJ, McDevitt L, eds. 2002. *Issues in Disability and Health: The Role of Secondary Conditions and Quality of Life*. Chapel Hill: University of North Carolina Press.

Simeonsson RJ, Leonardi M, Lollar D, Bjorck-Akesson E, Hollenweger J, Martinuzzi A. 2003. Applying the International Classification of Functioning, Disability, and Health (ICF) to measure childhood disability. *Disability and Rehabilitation* 25(11–12):602–610.

Simmons T, O'Neill G. 2001. *Households and Families:2000. Census 2000 Brief.* [Online]. Available: http://www.census.gov/prod/2001pubs/c2kbr01-8.pdf [accessed April 27, 2007].

Smeltzer S. 2006. Preventive health screening for breast and cervical cancer and osteoporosis in women with physical disabilities. *Family & Community Health* 29:35S–43S.

Smith C, Cowan C, Heffler S, Catlin A, The National Health Accounts Team. 2006. National health spending in 2004: recent slowdown led by prescription drug spending. *Health Affairs (Millwood)* 25(1):186–196. [Online]. Available: http://content.healthaffairs.org/ cgi/reprint/25/1/186 [accessed April 27, 2007].

Smith D. 2001. Health care management of adults with Down syndrome. *American Family Physicians* 64(6):1031–1038, 1039–1040.

Smith G, O'Keeffe J, Carpenter L, Doty P, Kennedy G, Burwell B, Mollica R, Williams L. 2000. *Understanding Medicaid Home and Community Services: A Primer.* Center for Health Policy Reseach, The George Washington University. [Online]. Available: http://aspe.hhs.gov/daltcp/reports/primer.htm [accessed April 27, 2007].

Smith JM. 2002. Foster care children with disabilities. *Journal of Health & Social Policy* 16(1–2):81–92.

Smith RO, Rust KL, Lauer A, Boodey E. 2005. *Technical Report—History of Assistive Technology Outcomes (Version 1.0).* University of Wisconsin–Milwaukee. [Online]. Available: http://www.r2d2.uwm.edu/atoms/archive/technicalreports/fieldscans/tr-fs-history.html [accessed April 27, 2007].

Snyder SL. 2006. About the encyclopedia covers: visualizing variation. In: Albrecht GL, ed. *Encyclopedia of Disability,* Vol. 1. Thousand Oaks, CA: Sage Publications. Pp. xx–xxv.

Solberg LI, Brekke ML, Fazio CJ, Fowles J, Jacobsen DN, Kottke TE, Mosser G, O'Connor PJ, Ohnsorg KA, Rolnick SJ. 2000. Lessons from experienced guideline implementers: attend to many factors and use multiple strategies. *Joint Commission Journal on Quality Improvement* 26(4):171–188.

Solomon J. 2006. *The Illusion of Choice: Vulnerable Medicaid Beneficiaries Being Placed in Scaled-Back "Benchmark" Benefit Packages.* Washington, DC: Center on Budget and Policy Priorities. [Online]. Available: http://www.cbpp.org/9-14-06health.pdf [accessed April 27, 2007].

Somers HM, Somers AR. 1961. *Doctors, Patients, and Health Insurance.* Washington, DC: The Brookings Institution.

Sonn U, Davegardh H, Lindskog AC, Steen B. 1996. The use and effectiveness of assistive devices in an elderly urban population. *Aging (Milano)* 8(3):176–183.

Sophocles A. 2003. *Coding on the Basis of Time for Physician Services.* Family Practice Management, American Academy of Family Physicians. [Online]. Available: http://www.pafp.com/MMS/coding/medical-home-coding-for-time.pdf [accessed April 27, 2007].

Southall DP, Stebbens VA, Mirza R, Lang MH, Croft CB, Shinebourne EA. 1987. Upper airway obstruction with hypoxaemia and sleep disruption in Down syndrome. *Developmental Medicine and Child Neurology* 29(6):734–742.

Spector SA, Gordon PL, Feuerstein IM, Sivakumar K, Hurley BF, Dalakas MC. 1996. Strength gains without muscle injury after strength training in patients with post-polio muscular atrophy. *Muscle & Nerve* 19(10):1282–1290.

Spengler R, Wagner R. 2005. *Developing the New CDC Research Agenda.* Office of Public Health Research, Centers for Disease Control and Prevention. [Online]. Available: http://www.academyhealth.org/2005/pdf/spenglerr.pdf [accessed April 27, 2007].

Spillman BC. 2004. Changes in elderly disability rates and the implications for health care utilization and cost. *Milbank Quarterly* 82(1):157–194.

Spillman BC, Black KJ. 2005a. *Staying the Course: Trends in Family Caregiving.* The Urban Institute. [Online]. Available: http://assets.aarp.org/rgcenter/il/2005_17_caregiving.pdf [accessed April 27, 2007].

Spillman BC, Black KJ. 2005b. *The Size of the Long-Term Care Population in Residential Care: A Review of Estimates and Methodology.* Health Policy Center, The Urban Institute. [Online]. Available: http://aspe.hhs.gov/daltcp/reports/ltcpopsz.pdf [accessed April 27, 2007].

Spillman BC, Black KJ. 2006. *The Size and Characteristics of the Residential Care Population: Evidence from Three National Surveys.* Contract No. HHS-100-03-0010. Washington, DC: Office of the Assistant Secretary for Planning and Evaluation, U.S. Department of Health and Human Services.

SSA (Social Security Administration). 2003a. *Historical Background and Development of Social Security*. [Online]. Available: http://www.ssa.gov/history/briefhistory3.html [accessed April 27, 2007].

SSA. 2003b. *Ticket to Work and Work Incentives*. Annual Report to the President and Congress. [Online]. Available: http://www.ssa.gov/work/panel/whats_new/ssadmin24ahtml. doc [accessed April 27, 2007].

SSA. 2005a. *A Brief History*. [Online]. Available: http://ssa.gov/history/pdf/2005pamphlet.pdf [accessed April 27, 2007].

SSA. 2005b. *Find Your Retirement Age*. [Online]. Available: http://www.ssa.gov/retirechartred. htm [accessed April 27, 2007].

SSA. 2006a. *Children Receiving SSI, 2005*. Office of Policy. [Online]. Available: http://www.ssa. gov/policy/docs/statcomps/ssi_children/2005/summary.html [accessed April 27, 2007].

SSA. 2006b. *Information on the Ticket to Work Program for Youth*. [Online]. Available: http://www.ssa.gov/work/Ticket/Ticket_Info_Youth.html [accessed April 27, 2007].

SSA. 2006c. Projected future course for SSA disability programs. In: *Trends in the Social Security and Supplemental Security Income Disability Programs*. SSA Publication No. 13-11831. Washington, DC: SSA. [Online]. Available: http://www.ssa.gov/policy/docs/ chartbooks/disability_trends/sect06.pdf [accessed April 27, 2007].

SSA. 2006d. *Social Security Administration Strategic Plan for FY 2006–FY 2011*. [Online]. Available: http://www.ssa.gov/strategicplan2006.pdf [accessed April 27, 2007].

SSA. 2006e. *Social Security Beneficiary Statistics*. [Online]. Available: http://www.socialsecurity. gov/OACT/STATS/OASDIbenies.html [accessed April 27, 2007].

SSA. 2007a. *Benefits for Children with Disabilities*. SSA Publication No. 05-10026. [Online]. Available: http://www.ssa.gov/pubs/10026.pdf [accessed April 27, 2007].

SSA. 2007b. *Fact Sheet: Social Security*. [Online]. Available: http://www.ssa.gov/pressoffice/ factsheets/basicfact-alt.pdf [accessed April 27, 2007].

SSAB (Social Security Advisory Board). 2006. *A Disability System for the 21st Century*. [Online]. Available: http://www.ssab.gov/documents/disability-system-21st.pdf [accessed April 27, 2007].

Stapleton DC, Burkhauser RV eds. 2003. *The Decline in Employment of People with Disabilities: A Policy Puzzle*. Kalamazoo, MI: W.E. Upjohn Institute for Employment Research.

Starr P. 1982. *The Social Transformation of American Medicine*. New York: Basic Books, Inc.

Stebbens VA, Dennis J, Samuels MP, Croft CB, Southall DP. 1991. Sleep related upper airway obstruction in a cohort with Downs's syndrome. *Archives of Disease in Child* 66(11):1333–1338.

Stein REK. 2006. Trends in disability in early life. In: Field MJ, Jette AM, Martin L, eds. *Workshop on Disability in America: A New Look*. Washington, DC: The National Academies Press. Pp. 143–156.

Stein REK, Silver EJ. 2002. Comparing different definitions of chronic conditions in a national data set. *Ambulatory Pediatrics* 2(1):63–70.

Steinfeld E, Danford S. 2006. *Universal Design and the ICF*. Presented at the Living in Our Environment, the Promise of the ICF Conference: Vancouver, British Columbia, Canada, June 4–5. [Online]. Available: http://www.icfconference.com/New%20Presentations/ICF %20Presentation%20Notes.pdf [accessed April 27, 2007].

Steinmetz E. 2006. Americans with disabilities: 2002. *Current Population Reports*, U.S. Census Bureau. [Online]. Available: http://www.sipp.census.gov/sipp/p70s/p70-107.pdf [accessed April 27, 2007].

Stern SM. 2003. Counting people with disabilities: how survey methodology influences estimates in census 2000 and the census 2000 Supplemental Survey. Presented at the Annual Conference of the American Statistical Association, San Francisco, CA, August 3-7.

Stern SM. 2006. *American Community Survey as a Source of Disability Data*. Presentation for the ISDS State of the Art Conference: Developing Improved Disability Data, July 12. [Online]. Available: www.icdr.us/disabilitydata/Day1_SessI/S_Stern.ppt [accessed April 27, 2007].

Stern SM, Brault M. 2005. *Disability Data from the American Community Survey: A Brief Examination of the Effects of a Question Redesign in 2003*. [Online]. Available: http://www.census.gov/hhes/www/disability/ACS_disability.pdf [accessed April 27, 2007].

Stevens DP, Holland GJ, Kizer KW. 2001. Results of a nationwide Veterans Affairs initiative to align graduate medical education and patient care. *The Journal of the American Medical Association* 286(9):1061–1066.

Stoddard S, Jans L, Ripple J, Kraus L. 1998. *Chartbook on Work and Disability in the United States, 1998*. An InfoUse Report. Washington, DC: U.S. National Institute on Disability and Rehabilitation Research. [Online]. Available: http://www.infouse.com/disabilitydata/workdisability/ [accessed April 27, 2007].

Story M, Mueller J, Mace R. 1998. *The Universal Deign File*. Raleigh, NC: The Center for Universal Design.

Story M, Mueller J, Montoya-Weiss M. 2003. *Evaluating the Universal Design Performance of Products*. The Center for Universal Design. [Online]. Available: http://www.design.ncsu.edu/cud/pubs_p/pudperformproduct.htm [accessed April 27, 2007].

Strauss D, Ojdana K, Shavelle R, Rosenbloom L. 2004. Decline in function and life expectancy of older persons with cerebral palsy. *NeuroRehabilitation* 19(1):69–78.

Strickland B, McPherson M, Weissman G, van Dyck P, Huang Z, Newacheck P. 2004. Access to the medical home: results of the National Survey of Children with Special Health Care Needs. Supplement Article. *Pediatrics* 113(5):1485–1492.

Strongin R. 2001. *Medicare Coverage: Lessons from the Past, Questions for the Future*. National Health Policy Forum Background Paper. Washington, DC: The George Washington University. [Online]. Available: http://www.nhpf.org/pdfs_bp/BP_MedicareCoverage_8-01.pdf [accessed April 27, 2007].

Stuck AE, Walthert JM, Nikolaus T, Bula CJ, Hohmann C, Beck JC. 1999. Risk factors for functional status decline in community-living elderly people: a systematic literature review. *Social Science & Medicine* 48(4):445–469.

Stuck AE, Egger M, Hammer A, Minder C, Beck J. 2002. Home visits to prevent nursing home admission and functional decline in elderly people: systematic review and meta-regression analysis. *The Journal of the American Medical Association* 287(8):1022–1028.

Sturm R, Ringel JS, Andreyeva T. 2004. Increasing obesity rates and disability trends. *Health Affairs (Millwood)* 23(2):199–205.

Summer L, Ihara E. 2005. *The Medicaid Personal Care Services Benefit: Practices in States That Offer the Optional State Plan Benefit*. Georgetown University Health Policy Institute. [Online]. Available: http://assets.aarp.org/rgcenter/health/2005_11_medicaid.pdf [accessed April 27, 2007].

Summer L, Mann C. 2006. *Instability of Public Health Insurance Coverage for Children and Their Families: Causes, Consequences, and Remedies*. The Commonwealth Fund Publication No. 935. Washington, DC: Georgetown University Health Policy Institute. [Online]. Available: http://www.cmwf.org/usr_doc/Summer_instabilitypubhltinschildren_935.pdf [accessed April 27, 2007].

Super N. 2002. *Medigap: Prevalence, Premiums, and Opportunities for Reform*. National Health Policy Forum Background Paper. Washington, DC: The George Washington University. [Online]. Available: http://www.nhpf.org/pdfs_ib/IB782_Medigap_9-9-02.pdf [accessed April 27, 2007].

Szilagyi PG, Shenkman E, Brach C, LaClair BJ, Swigonski N, Dick A, Shone LP, Schaffer VA, Col JF, Eckert G, et al. 2003. Children with special health care needs enrolled in the State Children's Health Insurance Program (SCHIP): patient characteristics and health care needs. *Pediatrics* 112(6):e508–e520.

Taggard DA, Menezes AH, Ryken TC. 2000. Treatment of Down syndrome-associated craniovertebral junction abnormalities. *Journal of Neurosurgery* 93(2 Suppl):205–213.

Tai Q, Kirshblum S, Chen B, Millis S, Johnston M, DeLisa JA. 2002. Gabapentin in the treatment of neuropathic pain after spinal cord injury: a prospective, randomized, double-blind, crossover trial. *Journal of Spinal Cord Medicine* 25(2):100–105.

Tamblyn R, Laprise R, Hanley J, Abrahamowicz M, Scott S, Mayo N, Hurley J, Grad R, Latimer E, Perreault R, et al. 2001. Adverse events associated with prescription drug cost-sharing among poor and elderly persons. *The Journal of the American Medical Association* 285(4):421–429.

Tanenbaum SJ, Hurley RE. 1995. Disability and the managed care frenzy: a cautionary note. *Health Affairs (Millwood)* 14(4):213–219.

Tang SS, Yudkowsky BK, Davis JC. 2003. Medicaid participation by private and safety net pediatricians, 1993 and 2000. *Pediatrics* 112(2):368–372.

TATRC (Telemedicine & Advanced Technology Research Center). 2006. *FY07 EMEDD Advanced Medical Technology Initiative.* [Online]. Available: http://www.tatrc.org/ [accessed April 27, 2007].

Taugher M. 2004. *Focus Groups on Assistive Technology Use and Outcomes: A Consumer Perspective.* University of Wisconsin—Milwaukee. [Online]. Available: http://www.r2d2.uwm.edu/atoms/archive/technicalreports/tr-consumerfg.pdf [accessed April 27, 2007].

Taylor DH, Hoenig H. 2004. The effect of equipment usage and residual task difficulty on use of personal assistance, days in bed, and nursing home placement. *Journal of the American Geriatric Society* 52(1):72–79.

Tedeschi B. 2006. Do the Rights of the Disabled Extend to the Blind on the Web? *The New York Times,* November 6, C6.

Teitelbaum J, Kurtz J, Rosenbaum S, The George Washington University Medical Center. 2005. *Definitions of "Disability": Current Federal Standards and Implications of Reform for Medicaid Coverage.* Funded by the Center for Health Care Strategies, Inc. [Online]. Available: http://www.chcs.org/usr_doc/Disability_Def_Policy_Brief_FINAL_062105.pdf [accessed April 27, 2007].

Telfair J, Alexander LR, Loosier PS, Alleman-Valez PL, Simmons J. 2004. Providers' perspectives and beliefs regarding transition to adult care for adolescents with sickle cell disease. *Journal of Health Care for the Poor and Underserved* 15(3):443–461.

Tennessee Department of Finance and Administration. 2006. *TennCare Medicaid.* [Online]. Available: http://tennessee.gov/sos/rules/1200/1200-13/1200-13-13.pdf [accessed April 27, 2007].

Tervo RC, Azuma S, Palmer G, Redinius P. 2002. Medical students' attitudes toward persons with disability: a comparative study. *Archives of Physical Medicine & Rehabilitation* 83:1537–1542.

Tervo RC, Symons F, Stout J, Novacheck T. 2006. Parental report of pain and associated limitations in ambulatory children with cerebral palsy. *Archives of Physical Medicine & Rehabilitation* 87(7):928–934.

Thomas PW. 2005. *"75% Rule" Will Force People with Disabilities into Nursing Homes.* Washington, DC: American Association of People with Disabilities. [Online]. Available: http://www.aapd-dc.org/News/health/rule75.html [accessed April 27, 2007].

Thorin E, Yovanoff P, Irvin L. 1996. Dilemmas faced by families during their young adults' transitions to adulthood: a brief report. *Mental Retardation* 34(2):117–128.

Thorkildsen R. 1994. *Research Synthesis on Quality and Availability of Assistive Technology Devices.* Technical Report No. 7. Eugene, OR: National Center to Improve the Tools of Education and the College of Education. [Online]. Available: http://idea.uoregon.edu/~ncite/documents/techrep/tech07.pdf [accessed April 27, 2007].

Thyberg I, Hass UA, Nordenskiold U, Skogh T. 2004. Survey of the use and effect of assistive devices in patients with early rheumatoid arthritis: a two-year follow-up of women and men. *Arthritis & Rheumatism* 51(3):413–421.

Thyen U, Terres NM, Yazdgerdi SR, Perrin JM. 1998. Impact of long-term care of children assisted by technology on maternal health. *Journal of Developmental & Behavioral Pediatrics* 19:273–282.

Tinker A, McCreadie C, Stuchbury R, Turner-Smith A, Cowan D, Bialokoz A, Lansley P, Bright K, Flanagan S, Goodacre K, et al. 2004. *Introducing Assistive Technology into the Existing Homes of Older People: Feasibility, Acceptability, Costs and Outcomes.* Institute of Gerontology, King's College London. [Online]. Available: http://www.kcl.ac.uk/kis/schools/life_sciences/health/gerontology/pdf/reki.pdf [accessed April 27, 2007].

To TP, Lim TC, Hill ST, Frauman AG, Cooper N, Kirsa SW, Brown DJ. 2002. Gabapentin for neuropathic pain following spinal cord injury. *Spinal Cord* 40(6):282–285.

Tobias J, Vanderheiden G. 1998. *Why Companies Might Adopt Universal Design: An Initial Report from the Universal Design Research Project.* Proceedings of the 21st RESNA Annual Conference, Minneapolis, MN, June 26–30. Arlington, VA: Rehabilitation Engineering & Assistive Technology Society of North America. Pp. 349–351.

Toder E, Thompson LH, Favreault M, Johnson RW, Perese K, Ratcliffe C, Smith KE, Uccello CE, Waidmann T, Berk J, et al. 2002. *Modeling Income in the near Term: Revised Projections of Retirement Income Through 2020 for the 1931–1960 Birth Cohorts, Final Report.* Washington, DC: The Urban Institute. [Online]. Available: http://www.urban.org/url.cfm?ID=410609 [accessed April 27, 2007].

Towner E, Dowswell T. 2002. Community-based childhood injury prevention interventions: what works? *Health Promotion International* 17(3):273–284.

Treischmann RB. 1987. *Aging with a disability.* New York: Demos Publications.

Trefler E, Fitzgerald SG, Hobson DA, Bursick T, Joseph R. 2004. Outcomes of wheelchair systems intervention with residents of long-term care facilities. *Assistive Technology* 16(1):18–27.

Trude S. 2003. *Patient Cost Sharing: How Much Is Too Much?* Center for Studying Health System Change, Issue Brief No. 72. [Online]. Available: http://www.hschange.org/CONTENT/630/ [accessed April 27, 2007].

Tuffrey C, Pearce A. 2003. Transition from pediatric to adult medical services for young people with chronic neurological problems. *Journal of Neurology, Neurosurgery and Psychiatry* 74:1011–1013.

Tunis SR. 2005. A clinical research strategy to support shared decision making. *Health Affairs (Millwood)* 24(1):180–184.

Turk MA. 2006. Secondary conditions and disability. In: Field MJ, Jette AM, Martin L, eds. *Workshop on Disability in America: A New Look.* Washington, DC: The National Academies Press. Pp. 185–193.

Turk MA, Weber RJ, Pavin M, Geremski CA, Brown C. 1995. Medical secondary conditions among adults with cerebral palsy. *Archives of Physical Medicine & Rehabilitation* 76:1055.

Turk MA, Weber RJ, Pavin M, Geremski CA, Segore S. 1996. Pain complaints in adults with cerebral palsy. *Archives of Physical Medicine & Rehabilitation* 77:940.

Turk MA, Geremski CA, Rosenbaum PF, Weber RJ. 1997a. The health status of women with cerebral palsy. *Archives of Physical Medicine & Rehabilitation* 78(12 Suppl 5):S10–S17.

Turk MA, Geremski CA, Rosenbaum PF. 1997b. *Secondary Conditions of Adults with Cerebral Palsy: Final Report.* Syracuse: State University of New York Health Science Center at Syracuse.

Turk MA, Scandale J, Rosenbaum PF, Weber RJ. 2001. The health of women with cerebral palsy. *Physical Medicine & Rehabilitation* 12(1):153–168.

UCP (United Cerebral Palsy). 2006. *Durable Medical Equipment Used Outside the Home Should Be Covered by Medicare Part B.* Washington, DC: UCP National. [Online]. Available: http://www.ucp.org/ucp_generaldoc.cfm/1/8/11210/11210-11210/2301 [accessed April 27, 2007].

USCCR (U.S. Commission on Civil Rights). 2002. *U.S. Commission on Civil Rights Recommendations for the Reauthorization of the Individuals with Disabilities Education Act.* [Online]. Available: http://www.usccr.gov/pubs/idea/recs.htm [accessed April 27, 2007].

U.S. Census Bureau. 2004. *Table 2a. Projected Population of the United States, by Age and Sex: 2000–2050.* [Online]. Available: http://www.census.gov/ipc/www/usinterimproj/natprojtab02a.pdf [accessed April 27, 2007].

U.S. Census Bureau. 2005a. *2004 American Community Survey.* [Online]. Available: http://factfinder.census.gov/servlet/DatasetMainPageServlet?_program=ACS&_submenuId=&_lang=en&_ts= [accessed April 27, 2007].

U.S. Census Bureau. 2005b. Percent childless and births per 1,000 women in the last year: selected years, 1976–2004. *Current Population Survey, 1976–2004.* [Online]. Available: http://www.census.gov/population/socdemo/fertility/tabH1.csv [accessed April 27, 2007].

U.S. Census Bureau. 2006a. *Overview of the Survey of Income and Program Participation (SIPP).* [Online]. Available: http://www.sipp.census.gov/sipp/overview.html [accessed April 27, 2007].

U.S. Census Bureau. 2006b. *Reengineering the SIPP: The New Dynamics of Economic Well-Being System.* Paper prepared for a meeting of the Census Advisory Committee of Professional Associations, Suitland, MD, October 27. [Online]. Available: www.sipp.census.gov/sipp/DEWS/Reengineering%20the%20SIPP_September%2027.doc [accessed April 27, 2007].

U.S. Department of Commerce. 2006. *Annual Report on Technology Transfer: Approach and Plans, FY 2005 Activities and Achievements.* Supplemental Report. [Online]. Available: http://www.technology.gov/reports/TechTrans/FY2005.pdf [accessed April 27, 2007].

U.S. Department of Education. 2000. *To Assure the Free Appropriate Public Education of All Children with Disabilities.* Twenty-Second Annual Report to Congress on the Implementation of the Individuals with Disabilities Education Act. [Online]. Available: http://www.ed.gov/about/reports/annual/osep/2000/preface.pdf [accessed April 27, 2007].

U.S. Department of Education. 2005. *Twenty-Five Years of Progress in Educating Children with the Disabilities through IDEA.* [Online]. Available:http://www.ed.gov/policy/speced/leg/idea/history.html [accessed April 27, 2007].

U.S. Department of Education. 2006a. Assistance to states for the education of children with disabilities and preschool grants for children with disabilities; final rule. *Federal Register* 71(156):46540–46845.

U.S. Department of Education. 2006b. *Centers for Independent Living.* [Online]. Available: http://www.ed.gov/programs/cil/index.html [accessed April 27, 2007].

U.S. Department of Education. 2006c. *Twenty-Sixth Annual Report to Congress on the Implementation of the Individuals with Disabilities Education Act,* Vols. 1 and 2. Washington, DC: Office of Special Education and Rehabilitation Services. [Online]. Available: http://www.ed.gov/about/reports/annual/osep/2004/index.html [accessed April 27, 2007].

U.S. Department of Justice. 1995. *The Americans with Disabilities Act: Checklist for Readily Achievable Barrier Removal.* [Online]. Available: http://www.justice.gov/crt/ada/racheck. pdf#search=%22%22readily%20achievable%22%20ADA%22 [accessed April 27, 2007].

U.S. Department of Justice. 2000a. *Enforcing the ADA: Looking Back on a Decade of Progress.* [Online]. Available: http://www.usdoj.gov/crt/ada/pubs/10thrpt.htm#anchor60011 [accessed April 27, 2007].

U.S. Department of Justice. 2000b. *Information Technology and People with Disabilities: The Current State of Federal Accessibility.* Presented by the Attorney General to the President of the United States, April. [Online]. Available: http://www.usdoj.gov/crt/508/report/content.htm [accessed April 27, 2007].

U.S. Department of Justice. 2001. *Background and Questions and Answers: October 26, 2001 DOJ Clarifying Memorandum Regarding Limited English Proficiency and Executive Order 13166.* [Online]. Available: http://www.usdoj.gov/crt/cor/lep/Oct26BackgroundQ&A. htm [accessed April 27, 2007].

U.S. Department of Justice. 2002a. *Commonly Asked Questions and Answers Regarding Executive Order 13166.* [Online]. Available: http://www.usdoj.gov/crt/cor/Pubs/lepqapr. htm [accessed April 27, 2007].

U.S. Department of Justice. 2002b (last revised). *Delivering on the Promise: Self-Evaluation to Promote Community Living for People with Disabilities.* Report to the President on Executive Order 13217. [Online]. Available: http://www.hhs.gov/newfreedom/final/dojfull. html [accessed April 27].

U.S. Department of Justice. 2004. *Enforcing the ADA: A Status Report from the Department of Justice.* [Online]. Available: http://www.usdoj.gov/crt/ada/julsep04.htm [accessed April 27, 2007].

U.S. Department of Justice. 2005a. *Advanced Notice on Proposed Rulemaking: Nondiscrimination on the Basis of Disability in State and Local Government Services and Nondiscrimination on the Basis of Disability by Public Accommodations and in Commercial Facilities.* [Online]. Available: http://www.usdoj.gov/crt/ada/anprm04.htm [accessed April 27, 2007].

U.S. Department of Justice. 2005b. *Hospital Guarantees Equal Access to Medical Services. Disability Rights Online News.* [Online]. Available: http://www.justice.gov/crt/ada/newsltr1005scrn.pdf [accessed April 27, 2007].

U.S. Department of Justice. 2005c. *Settlement Agreement between the United States of America and Greater Southeast Community Hospital.* U.S. Department of Justice Complaint No. 202-16-123. [Online]. Available: http://www.ada.gov/secommhosp.htm [accessed April 27, 2007].

U.S. Department of Justice. 2005d. *Settlement Agreement between the United States of America and Valley Radiologists Medical Group, Inc.* U.S. Department of Justice Complaint No. 202-11-136. [Online]. Available: http://www.usdoj.gov/crt/ada/vri.htm [accessed April 27, 2007].

U.S. Department of Justice. 2005e. *Settlement Agreement Among the United States of America, Plaintiffs Equal Rights Center, Dennis Christopher Butler, Rosemary Ciotti, George Aguehounde, and Marsha Johnson and Washington Hospital Center.* U.S. Department of Justice Complaint No. 202-16-120. [Online]. Available: http://www.usdoj.gov/crt/ada/whc.htm [accessed April 27, 2007].

U.S. Department of Justice. 2006a. *ADA Business Brief: Communicating with People Who Are Deaf or Hard of Hearing in Hospital Settings.* Civil Rights Division, U.S. Department of Justice. [Online]. Available: http://www.usdoj.gov/crt/ada/hospcombr.htm [accessed April 27, 2007].

U.S. Department of Justice. 2006b. *Privacy Impact Assessments: Official Guidance.* [Online]. Available: http://www.usdoj.gov/pclo/pia_manual.pdf [accessed April 27, 2007].

U.S. Department of Labor. 2004a. *The Health Insurance Portability and Accountability Act (HIPAA)*. [Online]. Available: http://www.dol.gov/ebsa/newsroom/fshipaa.html [accessed April 27, 2007].

U.S. Department of Labor. 2004b. *Ticket to Work and Work Incentive Improvement Act*. [Online]. Available: http://www.dol.gov/odep/pubs/ek00/ticket.htm [accessed April 27, 2007].

U.S. Department of Labor. 2007. *FAQs About COBRA Continuation Health Coverage*. [Online]. Available: http://www.dol.gov/ebsa/faqs/faq_consumer_cobra.html [accessed April 27, 2007].

U.S. House of Representatives, Committee on Science. 1998. *Unlocking our Future: Toward a New National Science Policy*. September 1998. [Online]. Available: http://www.access.gpo.gov/congress/house/science/cp105-b/science105b.pdf [accessed April 27, 2007].

U.S. House of Representatives, Committee on Ways and Means. 1971. *Report on H.R. 1, the Social Security Amendments of 1972*. House Report 92-231, 92nd Congress, 1st session. Washington, DC: U.S. Government Printing Office.

U.S. House of Representatives, Committee on Ways and Means. 1974. *The Development of the Disability Program Under Old-Age Survivors Insurance, 1935–1974*. Social Security Online, Legislative Histories. [Online]. Available: http://ssa.gov/history/pdf/dibreport.pdf [accessed April 27, 2007].

U.S. House of Representatives, Committee on Ways and Means. 2003. Section 10—Title XX Social Services Block Grant Program: Overview, Allocation Formula, and Funding. [Online]. Available: http://waysandmeans.house.gov/media/pdf/greenbook2003/Section10.pdf [accessed April 27, 2007].

U.S. Public Health Service. 1979. *Healthy People: The Surgeon General's Report on Health Promotion and Disease Prevention*. Washington, DC: U.S. Government Printing Office. [Online]. Available: http://profiles.nlm.nih.gov/NN/B/B/G/K/_/nnbbgk.pdf [accessed April 27, 2007].

U.S. Public Health Service. 2001. *The Surgeon General's Call to Action to Prevent and Decrease Overweight and Obesity*. Rockville, MD: Office of the Surgeon General, U.S. Department of Health and Human Services. [Online]. Available: http://www.surgeongeneral.gov/topics/obesity/calltoaction/CalltoAction.pdf [accessed April 27, 2007].

U.S. Public Health Service. 2005. *The Surgeon General's Call to Action to Improve the Health and Wellness of Persons with Disabilities*. Rockville, MD: Office of the Surgeon General, U.S. Department of Health and Human Services. [Online]. Available: http://www.surgeongeneral.gov/library/disabilities/calltoaction/calltoaction.pdf [accessed April 27, 2007].

U.S. Senate, Committee on Appropriations. 2001. *Report on Departments of Labor, Health and Human Services, and Education, and Related Agencies Appropriation Bill, 2002 (to accompany S 1536)*. [Online]. Available: http://thomas.loc.gov/cgi-bin/cpquery/T?&report=sr084&dbname=107& [accessed April 27, 2007].

U.S. Senate, Committee on Appropriations. 2004. *Departments of Labor, Health and Human Services, and Education, and Related Agencies Appropriation Bill, 2005*. [Online]. Available: http://frwebgate.access.gpo.gov/cgi-bin/getdoc.cgi?dbname=108_cong_reports&docid=f:sr345.108.pdf [accessed April 27, 2007].

U.S. Senate, Committee on Finance. 2004. *Hearings: Strategies to Improve Access to Medicaid Home and Community Based Services*. April 7. [Online]. Available: http://finance.senate.gov/sitepages/hearing040704.htm [accessed April 27, 2007].

VA (U.S. Department of Veterans Affairs). 2004. *VA Research Currents* 4(10):1–4. [Online]. Available: http://www.research.va.gov/resources/pubs/docs/va_research_currents_october_04.pdf [accessed April 27, 2007].

VA. 2006a. *Barrier Free Design Guide: A Supplement to the Uniform Federal Accessibility Standards*. [Online]. Available: http://www.va.gov/facmgt/standard/dguide/barrfree.doc [accessed April 27, 2007].

VA. 2006b. *Rehabilitation Research and Development Service*. [Online]. Available: http://www.research.va.gov/programs/rrd.cfm [accessed April 27, 2007].

VA. 2006c. *Secretary Nicholson: VA Reaches Out to Veterans and Spouses—"Aid and Attendance" an Under-Used Benefit*. Office of Public Affairs News Release, December 19. [Online]. Available: http://www1.va.gov/opa/pressrel/pressrelease.cfm?id=1265 [accessed April 27, 2007].

Valet RS, Kutny DF, Hickson GB, Cooper WO. 2004. Family reports of care denials for children enrolled in TennCare. *Pediatrics* 114(1):e37–e42.

Vanderheiden G. 2002. Interaction for diverse users. In: Jacko J, Sears A, eds. *Human-Computer Interaction Handbook*. Mahwah, NJ: Lawrence Erlbaum Associates, Inc.

Vanderheiden G, Tobias J. 2000. *Universal Design of Consumer Products: Current Industry Practice and Perceptions*. Proceedings of the XIVth Triennial Congress of the International Ergonomics Association and 44th Annual Meeting of the Human Factors and Ergonomics Society, San Diego, CA, July 30–August 4.

Van Dyck PC, Kogan MD, McPherson MG, Weissmna GR, Newacheck PW. 2004. Prevalence and characteristics of children with special health care needs. *Archives of Pediatrics & Adolescent Medicine* 158(9):884–890.

Vanelli M, Caronna S, Adinolfi B, Chiari G, Gugliotta M, Arsenio L. 2004. Effectiveness of an uninterrupted procedure to transfer adolescents with type 1 diabetes from the pediatric to the adult clinic held in the same hospital: eight-year experience with the Parma protocol. *Diabetes, Nutrition, and Metabolism* 17(5):304–308.

Van Houtven C, Domino M. 2005. Home and community-based waivers for disabled adults: program versus selection effects. *Inquiry* 42(1):43–59.

Vascellaro JE. 2006. Web sites improve service for blind people: Google, AOL, Yahoo retool pages boosting compatibility with screen-reading aids. *The Wall Street Journal*, July 20, D1.

Veehof M, Taal E, Rasker J, Lohmann J, Van de Laar M. 2006. Possession of assistive devices is related to improved psychological well-being in patients with rheumatic conditions. *Journal of Rheumatology* 33(8):1679–1683.

Verbrugge LM, Jette AM. 1994. The disablement process. *Social Science & Medicine* 38(1):1–14.

Verbrugge LM, Sevak P. 2002. Use, type, and efficacy of assistance for disability. *The Journals of Gerontology, Series B: Psychological Sciences and Social Sciences* 57(6):S366–S379.

Verbrugge LM, Yang LS. 2002. Aging with disability and disability with aging. *Journal of Disability Policy Studies* 12(4):253–267.

Verbrugge LM, Yang LS, Juarez L. 2004. Severity, timing, and structure of disability. *Social and Preventive Medicine* 49(2):110–121.

Verdier JM. 2006. *Medicare Advantage Rate Setting and Risk Adjustment: A Primer for States Considering Contracting with Medicare Advantage Special Needs Plans to Cover Medicaid Benefits*, Center for Health Care Strategies. [Online]. Available: http://www.chcs.org/usr_doc/Medicare_Advantage_State_Primer.pdf [accessed April 27, 2007].

Verdeir JM, Au M. 2006. *Medicare Advantage Special Needs Plans Site Visits*. Washington, DC: Mathematica Policy Research, Inc. [Online]. Available: http://www.medpac.gov/publications/contractor_reports/Jun06_MA_SNP.pdf#search=%22cms%20medicare%20%22special%20needs%20plans%22%22 [accessed April 27, 2007].

Verville R, DeLisa JA. 2003. Evolution of National Institutes of Health options for rehabilitation research. *American Journal of Physical Rehabilitation and Development* 82:565–579.

Verza R, Carvalho ML, Battaglia MA, Uccelli MM. 2006. An interdisciplinary approach to evaluating the need for assistive technology reduces equipment abandonment. *Multiple Sclerosis* 12(1):88–93.

Vettleson U. 2006. *Summary of the Deficit Reduction Act of 2006.* Dorsey & Whitney LLP. [Online]. Available: http://www.dorsey.com/news/news_detail.aspx?id=216965503 [accessed April 27, 2007].

Vladeck B. 2002. *Round Pegs and Square Holes: Medicare and Chronic Care.* Prepared for the Study on Medicare and Chronic Care in the 21st Century, National Academy of Social Insurance, April. [Online]. Available: http://www.nasi.org/usr_doc/round_pegs_and_square_holes.doc [accessed April 27, 2007].

W3C (World Wide Web Consortium). 2006. *WCAG 2.0 Quick Reference: A Summary of All WCAG 2.0 Requirements (success criteria) and Techniques Sufficient to Meet Them.* Draft document. [Online]. Available: http://www.w3.org/WAI/WCAG20/quickref/ [accessed April 27, 2007].

Wadsworth ME, Kuh DJ. 1997. Childhood influences on adult health: a review of recent work from the British 1946 national birth cohort study, the MRC National Survey of Health and Development. *Pediatric and Perinatal Epidemiology* 11(1):2–20.

Wagner EH, Austin BT, Davis C, Hindmarsh M, Schaefer J, Bonomi A. 2001. Improving chronic illness care: translating evidence into action. *Health Affairs (Millwood)* 20(6):64–78.

Wagner M, Newman L, Cameto R, Garza N, Levine P. 2005. *After High School: A First Look at the PostSchool Experiences of Youth with Disabilities.* A report from the National Longitudinal Transitional Study 2. [Online]. Available:http://www.nlts2.org/reports/2005_04/nlts2_report_2005_04_complete.pdf [accessed April 27, 2007].

Waidmann TA, Liu K. 2000. Disability trends among elderly persons and implications for the future. *The Journals of Gerontology, Series B: Psychological Sciences and Social Sciences* 55(5):S298–S307.

Waldrop J, Stern S. 2003. *Disability Status: 2000. Census 2000 Brief.* [Online]. Available: http://www.census.gov/prod/2003pubs/c2kbr-17.pdf [accessed April 27, 2007].

Walsh EG, Nason A, Moore A, Khatutsky G, Caswell C. 2003. *Pilot Test of the Medicare Health Survey for PACE and EverCare.* Waltham, MA: RTI International. [Online]. Available: http://www.rti.org/pubs/PilotTestPACE.pdf [accessed April 27, 2007].

Wang Q. 2005. *Disability and American Families: 2000.* U.S. 2000 Special Report. [Online]. Available: http://www.census.gov/prod/2005pubs/censr-23.pdf [accessed April 27, 2007].

Warms CA, Turner JA, Marshall HM, Cardenas DD. 2002. Treatments for chronic pain associated with spinal cord injuries: many are tried, few are helpful. *Clinical Journal of Pain* 18(3):154–163.

Wechsler H. 2004. *HHS Efforts to Combat the Obesity Epidemic Among Children and Adolescents.* Testimony before the U.S. House of Representtatives, Committee on Energy and Commerce, Subcommittee on Oversight and Investigations, June 16. [Online]. Available: http://www.hhs.gov/asl/testify/t040616.html [accessed April 27, 2007].

Weisel-Jones S. 2005. Transition to Independence: Preparing Children with Special Health Care Needs for Adulthood. *Children's Hospitals Today*, Winter 2005. [Online]. Available: http://www.childrenshospitals.net/AM/Template.cfm?Section=Home&TEMPLATE=/CM/ContentDisplay.cfm&CONTENTID=17104 [accessed April 27, 2007].

Welch P, Palames C. 1995. A brief history of disability rights legislation in the United States. In: Welch P, ed. *Strategies for Teaching Universal Design.* Boston, MA: Adaptive Environments Center.

Werner EE. 1997. Vulnerable but invincible: high-risk children from birth to adulthood. *Acta Paediatrica Supplement* 422:103–105.

Wessner CW. 2006. *The Small Business Innovation Research Program.* Testimony of Charles W. Wessner before the Small Business and Entrepreneurship Committee. U.S. Senate, July 12. [Online]. Available: http://www7.nationalacademies.org/ocga/testimony/Small_Business_Innovation_Research_Program.asp [accessed April 27, 2007].

West J. 1994. *Federal Implementation of the Americans with Disabilities Act, 1991–1994.* New York: Millbank Memorial Fund.

Westwood A, Henley L, Willcox P. 1999. Transition from pediatric to adult care for persons with cystic fibrosis: patient and parent perspectives. *Journal of Pediatrics and Child Health* 35(5):442–445.

While A, Forbes A, Ullman R, Lewis S, Mathes L, Griffiths P. 2004. Good practices which address continuity during transition from child to adult care: synthesis of the evidence. *Child Care Health and Development* 30:439–452.

White MJ, Olson RS. 1998. Attitudes toward people with disabilities: a comparison of rehabilitation nurses, occupational therapists, and physical therapists. *Rehabilitation Nursing* 23(3):126–131.

White PH. 2002. Access to health care: health insurance considerations for young adults with special health care needs/disabilities. *Pediatrics* 110(6 Pt 2):1328–1335.

Whiteneck G. 2006. Conceptual models of disability: past, present, and future. In: Field MJ, Jette AM, Martin L, eds. *Disability in America: A New Look.* Washington, DC: The National Academies Press. Pp. 50–66.

Whittaker J. 2005. *Social Security Disability Insurance (SSDI) and Medicare: The 24-Month Waiting Period for SSDI Beneficiaries Under Age 65.* Congressional Research Service Report for Congress. [Online]. Available: http://digital.library.unt.edu/govdocs/crs/data/2005/upl-meta-crs-7749/RS22195_2005Jul14.pdf [accessed April 27, 2007].

WHO (World Health Organization). 1980. *International Classification of Impairments, Disabilities, and Handicaps: A Manual of Classification Relating to the Consequences of Disease.* Geneva, Switzerland: WHO.

WHO. 1995. *Field Trial: WHOQOL-100. The 100 Questions with Response Scales.* Geneva, Switzerland: WHO. [Online]. Available: http://www.who.int/evidence/assessment-instruments/qol/documents/WHOQOL-100.pdf [accessed April 27, 2007].

WHO. 1999. *Annotated Bibliography of the WHO Quality of Life Assessment Instrument— WHOQOL (DRAFT).* Geneva, Switzerland: WHO. [Online]. Available: http://depts.washington.edu/yqol/docs/WHOQOL_Bibliography.pdf [accessed April 27, 2007].

WHO. 2001. *International Classification of Functioning, Disability and Health ICF.* Geneva, Switzerland: WHO.

WHO. 2006. *International Statistical Classification of Diseases and Related Health Problems 10th Revision (Version for 2007).* [Online]. Available: http://www.who.int/classifications/apps/icd/icd10online/ [accessed April 27, 2007].

WHOQOL (WHO Quality of Life Assessment Instrument) Group. 1993. Study protocol for the World Health Organization project to develop a quality of life assessment instrument. *Quality of Life Research* 2(2):153–159.

Wiklund ME. 2007. Human Factors Standards for Medical Devices Promote Accessibility. In: Winters J, Story M, eds. *Medical Instrumentation: Accessibility and Usability Considerations.* Boca Raton, FL: CRC Publishing. Pp. 225–232.

Wilber N, Mitra M, Walker DK, Allen D, Meyers AR, Tupper P. 2002. Disability as a public health issue: findings and reflections from the Massachusetts survey of secondary conditions. *Milbank Quarterly* 80(2):393–421.

Williams B, Dulio A, Claypool H, Perry MJ, Cooper BS. 2004. *Waiting for Medicare: Experiences of Uninsured People with Disabilities in the Two-Year Waiting Period for Medicare.* The Commonwealth Fund Publication No. 786. [Online]. Available: http://www.cmwf.org/usr_doc/786_Williams_waiting_for_Medicare.pdf [accessed April 27, 2007].

Williams CH, Fuchs BC. 2004. *Expanding the Individual Health Insurance Market: Lessons from the State Reforms of the 1990's.* The Synthesis Project, Policy Brief No. 4. The Robert Wood Johnson Foundation. [Online]. Available: http://www.rwjf.org/publications/synthesis/reports_and_briefs/pdf/no4_policybrief.pdf#search=%22%22health%20insurance%22%20%22guaranteed%20renewal%22%22 [accessed April 27, 2007].

Wilson-Costello D, Friedman H, Minich N, Fanaroff AA, Hack M. 2005. Improved survival rates with increased neurodevelopmental disability for extremely low birth weight infants in the 1990s. *Pediatrics* 115(4):997–1003.

Winters JM, Story MF, eds. 2007a. *Medical Instrumentation: Accessibility and Usability Considerations.* Boca Raton, FL: CRC Press.

Winters JM, Story MF. 2007b. Report of the Workshop on Accessible Interfaces for Medical Instrumentation: draft guidelines and future directions. In: Winters JM, Story MF, eds. *Medical Instrumentation: Accessibility and Usability Considerations.* Boca Raton, FL: CRC Press. Pp. 419–448.

Winters JM, Story MF, Barnekow K, Kailes JI, Premo B, Schweir E, Danturthi S, Winters JM. 2007. Results of a national survey on accessibility of medical instrumentation for consumers. In: Winters JM, Story MF, eds. *Medical Instrumentation Accessibility and Usability Considerations.* Boca Raton, FL: CRC Press. Pp. 13–28.

Wolf DA, Hunt K, Knickman J. 2005. Perspectives on the recent decline in disability at older ages. *Milbank Quarterly* 83 (3):365–395.

Wolff JL, Agree EM, Kasper JD. 2005. Canes, walkers and wheelchairs: what does Medicare pay for and who benefits? *Health Affairs (Millwood)* 24(4):1140–1149.

Wood WM, Karvonen M, Test DW, Browder D, Algozzine. 2004. Promoting student self-determination skills in IEP planning. *Teaching Exceptional Children* 36(3):8-16. [Online]. Available: http://www.transitiontocollege.net/percpubs/SelfDeterminationArticle.pdf [accessed April 27, 2007].

Wright C, Parkinson K, Drewett R. 2006. How does maternal and child feeding behavior relate to weight gain and failure to thrive? Data from a prospective birth cohort. *Pediatrics* 117(4):1262–1269.

Xiang H, Stallones L, Chen G, Hostetler SG, Kelleher K. 2005. Nonfatal injuries among US children with disabling conditions. *American Journal of Public Health* 95(11):1970–1975.

Yezierksi R. 1996. Pain following spinal cord injury: the clinical problem and experimental studies. *Pain* 68(2-3):185–194.

Young K. 2006. Groups fighting wheelchair limit: Medicare plans $5,300 max, stair-climbing iBot costs $26,100. *Chicago Sun-Times*, July 19. [Online]. Available: http://www.findarticles.com/p/articles/mi_qn4155/is_20060719/ai_n16541498 [accessed March 15, 2007].

Zaslavsky AM, Buntin MJ. 2002. Using survey measures to assess risk selection among Medicare managed care plans. *Inquiry* 39(2):138–151.

Zimmerman B, Schwalberg R, Gallagher J, Harkins M, Sines E. 2000. *Title V Roles in Coordinating Care for Children with Special Health Care Needs.* Health Resources and Services Administration, U.S. Department of Health and Human Services. [Online]. Available: http://www.jhsph.edu/WCHPC/Publications/cshcn-final.pdf [accessed April 27, 2007].

A

Study Activities

In late 2004, at the request of the Centers for Disease Control and Prevention (CDC), the Institute of Medicine (IOM) began a study to review progress and developments since the publication of the IOM's 1991 report *Disability in America* and its 1997 report *Enabling America*. The study was to identify continuing gaps in disability science and propose steps to strengthen the evidence base for public and private actions to reduce the impact of disability and related conditions on individuals and society in the United States. The assessment of principles and scientific evidence for disability policies and services was to take international perspectives and models into account. (Discussions with CDC clarified that this assessment should focus primarily on international efforts to develop a conceptual framework and classification scheme for disability.)

The study's statement of task identified several specific topics for consideration, including

- methodological and policy issues related to the definition, measurement, and monitoring (surveillance) of disability and health over time;

- trends in the amount, types, and causes of disability;
- aging with disability and secondary health conditions;
- transitions from child/adolescent to adult services and community participation;
- role of assistive technologies and physical environments in increasing participation in society (e.g., through employment, community-based living) of people with disabilities;
- selected questions related to the financing of health care services, including payment for assistive technologies and risk adjustment of managed care and provider payments; and
- directions for research.

For administrative reasons, the study began with a limited set of tasks and the charge to conduct an invitational workshop and prepare a workshop summary report that did not include conclusions and recommendations. In planning the workshop, which was held in August 2005, one objective was to develop information that would be useful in the second phase of the project, which would result in a report with conclusions and recommendations. As discussions about the study progressed, CDC enlisted support for the second phase of the study from the National Institute on Disability and Rehabilitation Research (Department of Education) and the National Center for Medical Rehabilitation Research (National Institutes of Health).

To oversee the workshop phase of the study, the IOM appointed a 10-member committee. The table of contents for the resulting workshop report is included in Appendix B. The IOM added four additional committee members as part of the study's second phase.

The study committee met five times between August 2005 and September 2006. In addition to the August 2005 workshop, which provided background on the first four topics, the committee conducted two public meetings and commissioned five background papers (which appear as appendixes to the report). The agendas of the workshop and other public meetings are included below. The committee submitted its report for review under procedures of the National Research Council in December 2006, and the report was released in April 2007.

INSTITUTE OF MEDICINE
WORKSHOP ON DISABILITY IN AMERICA: AN UPDATE
Keck Center of the National Academies
August 1, 2005

8:30   Welcomes and Introductions

Alan Jette, Ph.D., Chair
Institute of Medicine Committee on Disability in America

Jose Cordero, M.D.
Director, National Center on Birth Defects and Development
Centers for Disease Control and Prevention

Steven James Tingus, M.S.
Director, National Institute on Disability and Rehabilitation
    Research

Michael Weinrich, M.D.
National Center for Medical Rehabilitation Research

8:45   **Disability Concepts, Models, and Measures**

Issues and Questions Involving Adults
    Gale Whiteneck, Ph.D.
    Director of Research
    Craig Hospital

Issues and Questions Involving Children and Adolescents
    Rune Simeonsson, Ph.D.
    Professor of Education
    University of North Carolina

Research on Environmental Factors
    Julie Keysor, Ph.D.
    Assistant Professor of Physical Therapy
    Boston University Sargent College of Health and
    Rehabilitation Sciences

Discussion

10:20   **Break**

10:45   **Trends in Disability**

Trends in Disability in Late Life
    Vicki Freedman, Ph.D.
    Professor of Health Systems and Policy
    School of Public Health
    University of Medicine and Dentistry of New Jersey

Trends in Disability in Midlife
   Jay Bhattacharya, Ph.D.
   Assistant Professor of Medicine
   Center for Primary Care and Outcomes Research
   Stanford University

Trends in Disability in Early Life
   Ruth E. K. Stein, M.D.
   Professor of Pediatrics
   Albert Einstein College of Medicine/Children's Hospital at
   Montefiore

Discussion

Noon   Lunch

1:00   Aspects of Disability Across the Life Span

Risk Factors for Disability in Late Life
   Jack Guralnik, M.D., Ph.D.
   Chief, Epidemiology and Demography Section
   National Institute on Aging

Transitions for Adolescents with Disabilities
   John G. Reiss, Ph.D.
   Chief, Division of Policy and Program Affairs
   Institute for Child Health Policy
   University of Florida College of Medicine

Discussion

**2:00   Secondary Health Conditions: Concepts, Data, and Examples
         (Part I)**

Overview
   Margaret A. Turk, M.D.
   Professor of Physical Medicine and Rehabilitation
   State University of New York Upstate Medical University

Secondary Health Conditions and Aging with Disability:
   Consumer Perspective
   June Kailes, M.S.W.
   Disability Policy Consultant

Effects of Exercise on Specific Secondary Conditions
   James H. Rimmer, Ph.D.
   Director, Center on Health Promotion Research for Persons
   with Disabilities
   University of Illinois at Chicago

Discussion

3:30   **Break**

3:50   **Secondary Health Conditions (Part II)**

Secondary Conditions with Spinal Cord Injury
   William A. Bauman, M.D.
   Professor of Medicine and Rehabilitation Medicine
   Mount Sinai School of Medicine

Depression as a Secondary Condition in Adults with Disability
   Bryan Kemp, Ph.D.
   Professor of Medicine and Psychology
   University of California, Irvine

Preventing the Progression of Secondary Conditions with
   Developmental Disabilities
   Tom Seekins, Ph.D.
   Director
   University of Montana Rural Institute
   Discussion

Adjourn

* * * * *

INSTITUTE OF MEDICINE
COMMITTEE ON DISABILITY IN AMERICA: A NEW LOOK

Keck Center of the National Academies
October 5, 2005, Open Session

8:30   **Welcomes and Introductions**

8:45   **Discussion with Study Sponsors**

Mark Swanson, M.D.
Team Leader, Disability and Health Team
National Center on Birth Defects and Development
Centers for Disease Control and Prevention

Steven James Tingus, M.S.
Director, National Institute on Disability and Rehabilitation
   Research

Michael Weinrich, M.D.
Director, National Center on Medical Rehabilitation Research

10:45   Adjourn open session

*****

INSTITUTE OF MEDICINE
COMMITTEE ON DISABILITY IN AMERICA: A NEW LOOK
Keck Center of the National Academies
January 9, 2006

10:30   Welcome and Introductions

U.S. Department of Justice
Irene Bowen, J.D.
Deputy Chief, Disability Rights Section, Civil Rights Division

Veterans Health Administration
Robert Ruff, M.D., Ph.D.
Acting Director, Rehabilitation Research & Development Services

U.S. Department of Health and Human Services
Margaret Giannini, M.D.
Director, Office on Disability

Noon   Lunch

1:00   Welcome and Introductions

American Association of People with Disabilities
    Andrew J. Imparto
    President and CEO

National Alliance for Caregiving
    Gail Gibson Hunt
    President and CEO

National Coalition for Assistive and Rehabilitation Technology
    Rita Hestak
    President

1:45   American Foundation for the Blind
        Mark Richert
        Director of Public Policy

        Paralyzed Veterans of America
        Fred Cowell
        Health Policy Analyst

        United Cerebral Palsy
        Stephen Bennett
        President and CEO

2:30   Break

3:00   American Academy of Pediatrics
        Paul H. Lipkin, M.D.
        Chairperson, AAP Council on Children with Disabilities

        American Academy of Physical Medicine and Rehabilitation
        Steve Gnatz, M.D., M.H.A.
        President

        American Physical Therapy Association
        Ken Harwood, P.T., Ph.D.
        Director, Division of Practice and Research

        Rehabilitation Engineering and Assistive Technology Society of North America
        Rory A. Cooper, Ph.D.
        President

Adjourn

The following organizations provided written statements: AARP Public Policy Institute, American Spinal Injury Association, and American Association on Mental Retardation.

B

Table of Contents for
Workshop on Disability in America: A New Look (2006)

Based on a Workshop of the Committee on
Disability in America: A New Look
Marilyn J. Field, Alan M. Jette, and Linda Martin, *Editors*
Board on Health Sciences Policy, Institute of Medicine
The National Academies Press, 2006
(Report available at www.nap.edu/catalog/11579.html.)

CONTENTS

Secondary Health Conditions: Part II, 29
References, 36

(List of tables, boxes, and figures is omitted.)

C

Risk Adjustment of Insurance Premiums in the United States and Implications for People with Disabilities

*David J. Knutson**

This paper provides an update on the current status of formal methods of risk adjustment of payments to health plans and an assessment of the implications of these methods for people with disabilities. The paper examines the development, implementation, and impact of risk adjustment methods intended for use by multiple purchasers and payers in the United States. Purchasers and payers include, in particular, public programs, such as Medicare and Medicaid, as well as large and small employer-sponsored group plans and individual insurance plans.

The paper also evaluates the strengths and weaknesses of various risk adjustment methods, emphasizing their adequacy in setting payment for health plans that enroll people with disabilities. Emerging issues and trends related to improving risk assessment methods and their impact on improved access to financing and health care for disabled people are also explored.

*Director of Health Systems Studies, Park Nicollet Institute for Research and Education, Minneapolis, Minnesota.

394

Iezzoni's *Risk Adjustment for Measuring Health Care Outcomes*, the foundation reference on risk adjustment, provides a comprehensive introduction to the concepts and techniques of risk adjustment as a generic tool (Iezzoni, 2003). This paper focuses on one particular purpose of risk adjustment: setting payments for health plans. Risk adjustment is a tool that can be used to improve the fairness of payment by accounting for enrollees' health when capitated reimbursement levels are set. Improving the fairness of payment is achieved by removing or diminishing economic incentives for avoiding people who might generate high costs because of their underlying health status. Improved risk adjustment methods help reduce information asymmetry among stakeholders and support transparency for managing and regulating risk pools to achieve equitable and efficient health care financing policy objectives.

For this application of risk adjustment, the risk is the medical expenditure level and the time frames involved with typical insurance or managed care contracts, which are usually 12 months. The risk adjustment methods addressed here focus on the use of risk factors to predict or explain individual or group variations in medical expenditures for a 12-month period.

INSURANCE PROGRAMS FOR PEOPLE WITH DISABILITIES

Medicare and Medicaid programs fund a large proportion of health care for people with disabilities. The financing mechanism is primarily fee for service; however, both Medicare and state Medicaid programs are attempting to expand managed care for people with disabilities. The Medicare Advantage program, authorized by the Medicare Modernization Act of 2003, continues Medicare's 1985 authority to contract with managed care plans. The legislation also authorized, through December 2008, new special needs plans (SNPs) that can disproportionately or exclusively enroll Medicare beneficiaries with special needs: institutionalized individuals, individuals dually eligible for Medicaid and Medicare, and individuals with high-cost chronic diseases.

The vast majority of SNP proposals received through the end of 2005 were for beneficiaries dually eligible for Medicaid and Medicare. Most SNPs chose to enroll exclusively populations with special needs instead of a greater percentage of individuals with special needs in a traditional plan. To date, more than 400 SNPs have been approved. Of these 37 are for institutionalized individuals, 13 are for individuals with chronic diseases, and the remainder is for individuals dually eligible for Medicaid and Medicare. These plans will compete with traditional Medicare Advantage plans, and their capitation payments will be based on the same risk adjustment method used by typical Medicare Advantage plans.

SNPs that selectively or exclusively enroll high-risk or disabled beneficiaries want the most accurate risk adjustment methodology possible to be used so that they will be assured of adequate funding. Unfortunately, as will be described here, even the best risk adjustment methods in use today significantly underestimate the actual cost of health care for individuals with major chronic illnesses and disabilities.

When the Medicare managed care program began in the mid-1980s, the demographic methods used for the risk adjustment of payments were not very accurate in allocating capitation payments on the basis of the relative needs of the beneficiary. The Centers for Medicare and Medicaid Services (CMS) has now adopted a state-of-the-art diagnosis-based risk adjuster for Medicare managed care plan payment, has added a frailty adjuster (a population sample, survey-based, functional status risk factor) to improve payment accuracy for specific demonstration programs for disabled people, and is considering using this functional status risk factor for all Medicare Advantage plans.

For many years state Medicaid programs, through federal waiver authorizations, have contracted with managed care plans to provide health care coverage for Medicaid beneficiaries. In nearly every case, managed care plans have been paid a risk-adjusted capitation. The major risk adjustment concern for the coverage of disabled populations covered by Medicaid, as it is for coverage by Medicare Advantage, is the accuracy of the methods used to adjust the payments to health plans on the basis of risk and its economic impact on health plans that enroll people with disabilities. As discussed below, many states do not use state-of-the-art risk adjustment methods.

Medicaid demonstration projects that serve individuals dually eligible for Medicare and Medicaid must contract with Medicare SNPs by 2008 if they wish to integrate Medicare and Medicaid payments. From the standpoint of the accuracy of risk-based payment rates, there may be less concern for the Medicaid side of managed care financing for people dually eligible for Medicaid and Medicare now that the implementation of Medicare Part D (coverage of prescription drugs) has shifted a major cost item from Medicaid to Medicare. For managed care programs financed exclusively by the Medicaid program, the level of concern for implementing the most accurate form of risk adjustment is even greater than it is for Medicare.

The central issue of risk adjustment and its implications for people with disabilities are relevant to most purchasers who offer more than one health plan to their beneficiaries and who provide the primary coverage for medical care. In other words, wherever risk selection occurs, the need for risk adjustment becomes critical to provide adequate capitation payments on behalf of people with high-cost conditions, including disabilities that require costly medical care.

MEDICAL COSTS AND POPULATIONS

Medical costs are highly skewed in any population. A relatively small proportion of the population (15 to 20 percent) accounts for two-thirds or more of the total health care expenditures for the entire population. Another way to characterize the skew is that about 80 percent of the population typically has medical costs below the mean per capita medical cost for the population. With no risk adjustment, a capitation payment system would pay far too much for 80 percent of the population and significantly underpay for the 20 percent whose costs are above the mean. If enrollment were randomly distributed across the population, the over- and underpayments would average to the right amount.

This skewed cost distribution is found in the general population and also in insurance programs exclusively for people with disabilities, even though the average cost per capita varies substantially between the two populations. A skewed distribution is also found in the Medicaid population. Ireys and colleagues (1997) found that in a pediatric Medicaid population, the medical costs for beneficiaries with selected chronic illnesses ranged from 10 to 29 times the mean for all children in the population. Specific examples include cardiopulmonary disease, the costs for which were 10 times greater than the mean for all children; cystic fibrosis, the costs for which were 14 times greater; chronic respiratory disease, the costs for which were 20 times greater; muscular dystrophy, the costs for which were 17 times; and, spina bifida, the costs for which were 11 times greater.

When one considers the distribution of medical costs for people with disabilities, the relationship between functional status and diagnosis becomes complex. Whereas the average cost for populations with disabilities is higher than that for the general population, the risk distribution is similar to that for the general population. For example, for Medicare beneficiaries over age 65 years enrolled in a Medicare Advantage health plan, CMS currently includes a risk factor indicator of whether a Medicare beneficiary was originally eligible for Medicare because of a disability. The average cost for this "ever disabled" population over age 65 years is nearly 50 percent higher than for the Medicare population over age 65 years as a whole. However, not all people with disabilities have medical costs that are greater. The specific diagnoses must be taken into account. Most of the difference in cost between a population with disabilities and a general population is explained by the type and the number of diagnoses recorded. Functional status, which may be considered a more direct measure of disability, in fact, adds only a modest improvement in the ability of current risk adjustment models to predict medical costs.

Kronick and colleagues (1995) reported that for a number of state Medicaid programs designed exclusively for people with disabilities (noninstitutionalized individuals and individuals not dually eligible for Medicaid and Medicare), 30 percent of the people with disabilities had no diagnosis of a chronic illness and their medical costs were similar to those for the general population. However, those with major chronic conditions had medical costs that were many times greater. For example, individuals with a diagnosis of multiple sclerosis had costs eight times greater than those with no diagnosis of a chronic disease. (The analysis included prescription drug costs.) Individuals with cardiovascular disease had costs 10 times greater than for those with no chronic disease, and those with quadriplegia had costs ranging from 3 to 34 times greater than for those with no chronic disease. This range also demonstrates that what would seem to be a direct risk factor (i.e., disability status), without reference to the presence of a chronic health condition, can fail to capture the high degrees of variability in health status and health care costs among people with disabilities. Pope and colleagues (2004) identified five conditions that predict higher medical costs (ranging from $2,200 to $9,700 in additional payments) for the disabled population over age 65 years enrolled in Medicare (over 12 percent of all beneficiaries). The conditions include some blood diseases, chemical dependency and related psychoses, and opportunistic infections.

Certain constellations of chronic illness diagnoses may serve as indicators of disability. These diagnosis-related risk factors are used by risk assessment models currently in the vanguard of methods for adjusting health plan payment. Most models rely exclusively on claims data—namely, data on diagnoses rather than functional status—and therefore the adequacy of the performance of risk adjustment methods for people with disabilities will be similar to the adequacy of their performance for populations with any high-cost chronic condition.

RISK SEGMENTATION IN INSURANCE MARKETS AND THE NEED FOR HEALTH-BASED RISK ADJUSTMENT

The need for health care can be influenced by disease, functional status, and socioeconomic factors. Risk selection is defined as the set of processes leading to the selective enrollment of individuals in health plans, which produces risk segmentation. Risk segmentation results from the uneven enrollment of higher- or lower-risk individuals across competing health plans or physician practices, so that some groups attract a disproportionate enrollment of higher-risk individuals. Segmentation is a problem if the payment system does not adjust payment on the basis of enrollee risk.

Risk selection occurs primarily when consumers have a choice of insurance plans or a choice of whether and when to buy health insurance. When individuals can choose among competing insurance plans, those who expect to use a lot of health care services will tend to be attracted to the more generous health plans, even when the premium is higher; and individuals with no chronic health care needs will be more likely to choose the lowest-cost plan, even if the benefits are relatively sparse or restrictive. The health plan characteristics that produce this selective attractiveness include benefit design (e.g., coverage of home health care services or mental health services), cost-sharing requirements (e.g., deductibles or co-payments when services are used), and ease of access to specialized services (e.g., no requirements for prior review for the use of specialized services or no requirement to use preferred specialty providers in the provider network) (Batavia and DeJong, 2001). Studies have found evidence of risk selection in a number of settings, including the benefit program for federal employees.

It is conventional wisdom that plans avoid being the only plan in a particular market with an academic medical center in its network, the best mental health benefits, open access to specialists, or richer prescription drug benefits (Knutson and Wrightson, 2002; Kronick et al., 1996). Each of these features is expected to attract those who use health care services more often. The magnitude and effects of risk selection in health insurance have been debated for many years. Although it is undeniable that risk selection occurs, the primary debates are related to its effects and to the means of addressing related problems, primarily those concerning efficiency and equity. Many debates are limited to issues within the bailiwick of particular disciplines. Economists discuss the efficiency and asymmetry of information. For actuaries, advising clients on detecting and avoiding adverse selection is a primary issue. Without summarizing each discipline's own take on the topic, it is apparent, to those who consider social and health policy, that risk selection in insurance markets generates a high potential for inequity for individuals with chronic and disabling conditions, whose future health care costs will be significantly and predictably higher than those for the general population (Batavia and DeJong, 2001; Kronick et al., 2000).

Therefore, in a market in which health plans compete for individual enrollees and payments to plans are not adjusted to reflect the risk of the enrollees, those plans that attract the healthiest enrollees will generally be more profitable and plans that consistently attract less healthy individuals may not be able to survive. Risk adjustment of payments to health plans is intended to protect individuals from this dynamic.

Medicare Example

Individuals become eligible for Medicare when they reach the age of 65 years or 29 months after they qualify for Social Security Disability Insurance benefits. In traditional Medicare, acute-care services are paid for on a fee-for-service basis, unless the beneficiary chooses to enroll in one of a number of Medicare Advantage plans. These plans operate as insurance

TABLE C-1 Distribution of Difference
Between HMO and Fee-for-Service Mean
Risk Factors for Medicare Beneficiaries in
428 U.S. Counties

Percent Difference	Frequency (No. of Counties)
–25.7 to –22.5	8
>–22.5 to –17.5	63
>–17.5 to –12.5	178
>–12.5 to –7.5	133
>–7.5 to –2.5	34
>–2.5 to +2.5	11
>+2.5 to +7.5	1

SOURCE: Greenwald et al. (2000).

plans and receive a monthly premium (capitated payment) for each beneficiary enrolled. Between 1985 and 2000, the premium was based on the
U.S. average per capita cost for beneficiaries, for whom the risk is adjusted
by age, gender, institutional status, medical enrollment status, and county
of residence.

Most studies have found that, in comparison with the established fee-
for-service system, the managed care plans enrolled healthier individuals.
Although earlier studies—which used limited methods and measures to
assess the risk presented by beneficiaries—found little or no risk selection
(Eggers and Prihoda, 1982; Hill et al., 2002), later studies, including those
that used more direct and accurate risk assessment methods, found strong
evidence of positive selection between Medicare health plans and traditional
Medicare fee-for-service plans.

For example, Lubitz and colleagues (1985) found that 106 of the 108
health plans studied experienced favorable selection. More recent studies
have further reinforced the findings of positive selection (Greenwald, 2000;
Greenwald et al., 2000; Zaslavsky and Buntin, 2002). A study by CMS, using the best available version of a claims-based risk assessment tool, found
that the relative risk (compared with that for the traditional fee-for-service
Medicare population) was "favorable" for all but three plans. Their enrollees ranged from approximately 3 percent to 15 percent favorable selection.
Table C-1 presents the average risk for the beneficiaries of a health maintenance organization (HMO) compared with the risk for fee-for-service plan
beneficiaries in the same counties.

Because the premium rates were normalized on the basis of the rates for
the Medicare fee-for-service population and because the demographic risk
adjustment methods in use during the early years of the Medicare managed
care program were poor predictors of risk ($r2$ = 1 to 3 percent), plans were

significantly overpaid compared with the payments expected from budget assumptions. This prompted CMS to introduce a risk adjuster that was based on health data rather than or in addition to demographic data.

The health plan industry resisted the transition for a number of reasons. What was clear was that the vast majority of plans in the program at that time, once CMS used a more accurate risk adjustment, would see their payments reduced (Blumenthal et al., 2005; Weissman et al., 2005).

How did the risk selection dynamic involve Medicare beneficiaries with disabilities? Disabled beneficiaries under age 65 years were eligible for both managed care and the traditional fee-for-service program. Actual enrollment distributions between managed care and the traditional fee-for-service program were similar by age group, but the population over age 65 years originally eligible for Medicare because of a disability was, on average, less prevalent in managed care plans than in fee-for-service plans, although the difference was not large. Although the beneficiary risk levels were much lower for Medicare managed care plans than for the fee-for-service Medicare program, for the vast majority of managed care plans, the prevalence of those enrolled who were eligible for Medicare because of a disability did not differ from that for the fee-for-service program (Greenwald et al., 2000). One explanation for this apparent inconsistency is that the plans attracted the least costly segment of those with disabilities, just as they had with the general Medicare population.

Outside the Medicare program, the Risk Adjustment Impact Study (RAIS) (which was funded by the Robert Wood Johnson Foundation) also found evidence of risk selection. The study found that relative risk scores across competing plans in one state Medicaid program ranged from 0.70 to 1.36. Significant selection bias was found in all programs or markets studied. Had the plans' payment rates been determined by using traditional demographic risk adjusters rather than the more accurate adjustment method actually used, the plan with the highest risk group of enrollees would have been seriously underpaid and the other plans would have been overpaid. Table C-2 presents the findings of selection bias across competing plans from RAIS.

Relevance for Large and Small Employers

Large employer-sponsored health insurance programs offering employees a choice of health plans also introduce the opportunity for risk selection. In their plan designs and in their marketing to employers and to their employees, plans strategically position themselves to avoid a disproportionate share of high-risk enrollees. In response, employers and consultants have devised a number of mechanisms that employers can use to reduce the opportunities for and effects of risk selection.

TABLE C-2 Percent Relative Risk Difference Between High- and Low-Risk Participating Health Plans

	Percent Difference in Relative Risk		
Program	Year 1	Year 2	Year 3
Medicaid waiver programs			
State 1—disabled population	46	66	37
State 2—disabled population	36	27	21
State 3—disabled population	24	28	30
State 4 —TANF	13	9	NA[a]
State Employee Health Benefit Program	22	26	27
Provider groups (capitated commercial)	43	100	100

[a]NA = not available.

SOURCE: Knutson (2003).

Keenan and colleagues (2001) also found that only a handful of large employers adopted HBRA between 1998 and 2000. Some economists have commented on the continuing low demand for formal risk adjustment among large employers (Glazer and McGuire, 2000). Many have also expressed the view that formal risk adjustment, such as that used by Medicare and many state Medicaid programs, may not be needed in the employer insurance market. Others suggest that employers may deliberately use the risk selection dynamic to get rid of options with more generous benefits. That is, they let adverse selection operate to price these plans out of existence.

Some employers self-fund their employees' health care and, through the Employee Retirement Income Security Act, avoid most insurance regulations. Selection issues are less important for these employer plans, unless a self-funded product is offered along with an insured plan. In that case, the issues become similar to those associated with offering more than one insured plan. Specifically, the employer may overpay if the insured plan attracts lower-risk enrollees than the self-insured plan.

Small employers face a particularly difficult set of issues. They are too small to bear the risk of self-insurance and so must purchase products that offer full insurance. Their premiums are determined through a risk evaluation of each employee and dependent by using either past insurance claims information from various sources or questionnaires, or both. A small-group plan is a product offered to a group usually without individual exclusions; that is, the plan usually cannot refuse to insure a given employee within an employee group; however, unlike large-group plans, the rates for small groups are based on the individually projected risk for each covered individual. The group is either accepted or denied by the health plan. (Some states sponsor high-risk pools that accept individuals who have been denied coverage in the market). The total premium for the group is usually the sum of the individual rates for each covered individual in the group. Thus, a very-high-cost employee or dependent can have a major impact on the total premium or on even whether the employer receives an offer of coverage.

Various strategies have been used to create small-employer insurance purchasing groups or pools both to spread the risk across a larger population and to reduce administrative costs. Such pools, many of which have used a form of risk adjustment, have been difficult to maintain. They have been vulnerable to "cherry picking" by health plans, which happens when those plans selectively offer their own small-group products to low-risk employers and attract them out of the larger risk pool. The small-group pools usually welcome all employers, but individual health plans can choose the small groups to which they will offer insurance. In some cases, an insurer will offer its health benefit product to businesses that are also participating in the small-group pool at a rate lower than that of the same product offered by the pool because the pool's risk may be higher than that of a given employer. This process removes the lower risk employers from the employer pool, thus forcing the pool to raise prices. This selection dynamic often leads to a "death spiral" during which the lower-risk employers increasingly abandon the pool and premiums for the remaining members increase until a sustainable risk pool no longer exists. One major example of such a situation was the demise of PacAdvantage, a small-group insurance pool in California.

Consumer-Driven Plans

In addition, with the advent of so-called consumer-driven products, such as health savings accounts or health reimbursement accounts, combined with health plans with high deductibles, employers are reducing their financial contribution for health insurance and shifting more of the cost of care to employees, primarily by increasing the deductible thresholds for standard benefit programs

When products with high deductibles and health savings accounts are offered to employees along with traditional products with richer benefits, the risk selection opportunity appears to be raised substantially. In making these changes, employers are usually not taking into account the differences in their employees' health care needs and other circumstances. Studies show some indication that individuals with higher incomes disproportionately selected these less expensive, less rich health plans (Parente et al., 2004). In their longitudinal study of consumer-driven health plans, Parente and colleagues did not detect significant adverse selection or utilization cost differences, but they were quick to point out that the consumer-driven health plan experience is in the early phase and that more research is needed.

One can see that risk selection for employers is ultimately determined by the combination of whom they employ and of the differences in the generosity of the health insurance benefits that they offer their employees. If an employer manages to hire and retain only healthy employees, risk selection is less of a problem. Risk selection is also less of a problem if an employer offers only one plan, although an employer who has more employees with health problems will pay more for insurance (other things being equal) than an employer with few such employees. Concerns about discrimination in the hiring and retention of employees (for example, by the use of health plan data to target employees for layoffs) enter the domain of the Americans with Disabilities Act.

The RAIS study, in addition to surveys of purchasers and health plans, included a survey of all U.S. members of the health section of the Society of Actuaries (SOA) to evaluate the implementation and impact of formal health-based risk adjustment (HBRA) methods that were based primarily on diagnoses (Knutson, 2003).The actuary survey included actuaries who consulted with purchasers and those who worked for or consulted with insurers. It found that actuaries reported that they believed that the use of formal risk adjustment is far less important for employers than for Medicaid or Medicare managed care programs. However, actuarial consultants have reported that the rate of use of these tools is growing as consultants use them to evaluate health plan performance and advise employers on health plan selection and oversight.

Non-Group Insurance

Small employers are dropping health insurance as fringe benefits at the same time that non-group-insurance options are, once again, being considered as a way of extending insurance to those who are not eligible for either public or employer-based insurance. Health plans competing in this market are particularly vulnerable to risk selection problems, for example, when people wait until they develop health problems to buy insurance. As described below, health plans have created a variety of mechanisms to protect themselves.

What happens in this individual insurance market to people with a greater need for health care? Hadley and Reschovsky (2003) reported that the probability of purchasing non-group insurance was 50 percent lower for people in fair to poor health and that premiums were 43 to 50 percent higher for this group than for beneficiaries in excellent health. In some cases, no insurer will cover the former group of individuals, and in other cases, the premium will be unaffordable.

Preventing and Managing Risk Selection

Purchasers and policymakers have devised a number of tools and strategies to try to prevent selection or to mitigate the problems it creates. For example, a study by Palsbo and Post (2003) reported on strategies that state Medicaid programs employ with competing managed care plans that serve Medicaid beneficiaries. These include the use of risk corridors, risk pools, stop-loss reinsurance, and risk classification (risk adjustment). The authors reported that only 12 of the states studied used the same type of state-of-the-art risk adjuster that CMS uses for the Medicare Advantage program. Since publication of the study, however, state policymakers appear to be showing renewed interest in implementing health-based payment for managed care plans.

In addition to risk management strategies, purchasers rely on regulation of health plan rate setting and enrollment to reduce or manage selection in the small group and individual market. Still, most health economists conclude that the best means of addressing risk selection is appropriate risk adjustment.

The views of actuaries on health-based risk adjustment are also informative. Actuaries assess risk and advise on premiums on behalf of purchasers or health plans. The RAIS actuary survey reported that actuaries judged that HBRA reduced the financial impact of selection bias on health plans. Based on a scale of 0 (no financial problem) to 10 (extremely serious financial problem), the rating dropped from 6.8 without HBRA to 3.5 with HBRA.

Half of all actuary respondents thought that the profession would establish a HBRA-related standard of actuarial practice within 5 years. Those with HBRA experience were more likely to believe this (54 percent) than those without HBRA experience (43 percent). More than two-thirds of the actuary respondents (76 percent with direct HBRA experience, 56 percent without experience) thought that HBRA has advanced the actuarial field, and over half (67 percent with experience, 46 percent without experience) thought that more purchasers should implement HBRA. Actuaries with and without HBRA experience now widely believe that HBRA is a useful tool and that it will become a standard of practice.

The RAIS survey of U.S. actuaries included a series of questions about the need for purchaser implementation of HBRA. The actuaries were also asked to imagine that they were advising large employers offering a choice of plans, including Medicaid managed care programs for the disabled, and then indicate how strongly they would advocate the implementation of HBRA for determining payments to health plans or for determining adjustments to employee premium contributions in defined-contribution plans. Sixty-six percent reported that they would "very or somewhat strongly" recommend the use of HBRA for the Medicaid programs, with 21 percent "not sure." Forty-two percent would "very or somewhat strongly" recommend HBRA for large employers, with 16 percent "not sure." Thirty-six percent would "very or somewhat strongly" recommend HBRA for employers adjusting employee premium contributions, with 19 percent "not sure."

The actuary responses were also analyzed for the subset of respondents employed by prominent health plans. Seventy-four percent of actuaries employed by health plans and 40 percent of consultant actuaries would "very or somewhat strongly" recommend the implementation of HBRA in Medicaid programs for the disabled, with 16 and 13 percent, respectively, "not sure," whereas only 45 percent of actuaries employed by health plans and 47 percent of managed care consulting actuaries would "very or somewhat strongly" recommend the implementation of HBRA for determining payments to plans to a large employer, with 14 and 7 percent, respectively, "not sure." Thirty-six percent of actuaries employed by managed care organizations and 45 percent of managed care consulting actuaries would "very or somewhat strongly" recommend to a large employer the implementation of HBRA for determining adjustments to employee premium contributions.

LESSONS FROM PURCHASERS WHO HAVE IMPLEMENTED HBRA FOR HEALTH PLAN PAYMENT

What can we learn from the experience of those purchasers who have implemented HBRA for payment? The earlier-cited RAIS study included Medicare Advantage, six state Medicaid programs, a small-employer-group pool, and two state employee benefit programs. The following key findings are highlighted: All purchasers indicated that HBRA had contributed to fairer payments, that HBRA was needed, and that the implementation of HBRA had been worth the effort. All purchasers have had to address health plan resistance to the risk adjustment of their payments, and as one would expect, the resistance came primarily from plans whose members presented a lower-than-average risk.

The survey of participating health plans found that one-third of the plans received increased payments under HBRA, one-third received decreased payments, and one-third received the same payments. The plans were evenly distributed when they were asked if HBRA had a strong positive or a strong negative financial impact on product viability. The plans expressed concern about data issues, such as the quality of the data and the cost of data collection, the financial viability of the product, the financial effects of selection bias without HBRA, and the effort required to implement risk adjustment compared with the benefit. The nature of these concerns generally reflected whether a plan's revenue had increased, decreased, or remained the same. A significant minority (31 percent) reported that HBRA enabled program participation by some health plans that financially could not have done so without HBRA. A similar number (28 percent) reported that HBRA had caused some low-risk plans to drop the product. Overall, however, the responses of health plans that have experienced payment based on HBRA are positive—even for plans that experienced negative financial results. Health plans reported that HBRA

- was more accurate than traditional methods of rate setting (87 percent),
- produced a fairer payment system (81 percent),
- did not require the collection of unnecessary and costly data (77 percent),
- significantly reduced concern about the negative financial impact of adverse selection (decreased concern by two-thirds), and
- should be part of public health policy for plan payment (79 percent).

Many health plans reported that they used HBRA internally, mostly for provider profiling (46 percent) and product management (66 percent).

The researchers reported that state officials and administrators believed that the process improved the efficiency of the payment programs and gave health plans more incentive to focus on providing quality care as opposed to selection strategies. In February 2002, CMS, in conjunction with the Center for Health Program Development and Management at the University of Maryland—Baltimore Campus distributed a questionnaire to CMS regional offices to assess states' experiences with HBRA. The questionnaire was distributed to the 40 states that had comprehensive Medicaid managed care programs or primary care case management programs that were not currently using HBRA. Of the 35 states that responded, 28 states (80 percent) reported that they were interested in learning more about risk adjustment, and 23 states (67 percent) reported that they had considered using risk adjustment for their Medicaid programs.

CMS has withstood significant plan resistance to changes in risk-adjustment methods, but it did make some compromises. For example, CMS implemented the Selected Significant Condition risk adjustment model in 2004. CMS is also using this new risk adjustment method in the financing formulas for most of the recent demonstration projects that it has initiated in the traditional Medicare program and in rate setting for its managed care program.

The author is not aware of surveys that have explored the views or experiences of employees or health plan members related to risk adjustment as such, and as far as the author knows, public and private purchasers who use the method do not mention its use in materials provided to employees or plan members. This presumably reflects, among other concerns, the complexity of the methods and the circumstances that prompt their use.

ADEQUACY OF CAPITATION PAYMENT FOR PEOPLE WITH DISABILITIES

A perfect risk adjuster would pay a capitated payment to health plans that exactly fits the actual cost along the entire cost distribution for the population. In other words, there should be no systemic bias; there should be only random error based on sample size. Achieving this would, in principle, make health plan managers less anxious about the risk of enrollees. In fact, such a perfect fit might very well lead managers to desire high-cost enrollees if they could enroll a stable actuarial number because these enrollees would bring much higher revenues per capita; they may also present plans with a greater opportunity to achieve profits by improving efficiency at the health care services level. The incentive for health plans to support selective enrollment strategies is directly related to the extent to which the rate-setting method, with market regulations held constant, overpays for healthy enrollees and underpays for high-cost enrollees. The bigger the gap between paid amounts and actual costs, the more the health plan will be rewarded for focusing on avoiding these high-cost enrollees rather than seeking better ways to provide care for them.

HBRA methods that use direct indicators of disease burden and health status are growing in use. They are much better predictors than traditional demographic methods and have far fewer perverse incentives (e.g., to increase spending in order to increase payments) than rates based on the prior expenditures of an individual or group. However, they as yet may not produce adequate payments to remove plan concern with adverse selection for people with disabilities who have high-cost chronic conditions.

Achieving Payment Accuracy for Populations with Disabilities

For the general population, the predictability of medical expenditures at the individual enrollee level historically has been assumed to be about 6 to 15 percent of the observed variation (Newhouse et al., 1989). Using prior utilization information for Medicaid beneficiaries with disabilities in six states, Kronick and colleagues (2000) produced predictions that ranged from 29 to 51 percent. It is both the large proportion of the total cost accounted for by these beneficiaries and the consistency of health care over time that produces this predictability.

Risk adjustment is important for populations with disabilities (1) when such populations are enrolled in capitated health plans and (2) when the capitated health plan must compete in the mainstream insurance market. Current Medicare policy seems to be moving in this direction; that is, not only toward promoting managed care for people with disabilities, but also toward supporting SNPs that would compete with traditional managed care plans in the mainstream Medicare Advantage market. This trend will expose the limits of even the best risk adjustment methods currently in practical use.

The problem is partly with the current state of the art of risk adjustment. Although current claims and survey-based methods are a vast improvement over traditional rate-setting methods, they do not yet produce the perfect predictor described above. The problem also lies in a political and competitive environment dominated by traditional health plans that have historically enrolled less risky beneficiaries than the Medicare program in general and that have not supported the rapid implementation of improvements in risk adjustment. The SNPs that wish to focus on excelling in attributes that would attract people with chronic illnesses or people who are frail or disabled will want the most accurate risk adjuster possible, whereas medical assistance plans with healthier than average enrollees will receive less revenue with a better risk adjuster because the improved method will reduce overpayments for healthy beneficiaries.

During an examination of the progress of risk adjustment methods, one must be mindful that where risk selection already exists, and given the fact that the vast majority of the population (80 percent) has medical costs below the average per capita cost for the population as a whole, the funding allocation politics can be tricky. On a related theme, it is commonly found in competitive health plan markets that the majority of the plans have relatively positive risk compared with the risk for the pool as a whole, leaving only the one or two health plans with high-cost populations to advocate for better risk adjustment.

Predictive Accuracy of Risk Adjusters

Many evaluations of risk adjustment methods use individual enrollee-level statistical analysis to evaluate the overall predictive performance. Although this approach is valid and useful for the comparison of models, if one is concerned with the adequacy and fairness of health plan payment for people with disabilities, one must look directly at the predictive performance for people with disabilities. It is possible for the risk adjuster to perform materially better for the general population but remain problematic for people with disabilities. This kind of prediction performance evaluation is often represented by predictive ratios that compare predicted payments with actual expenditures for defined subpopulations within a risk pool. A predicted payment ratio of 1.00 is the most accurate. A ratio above that indicates overpayment and ratios below that indicate underpayment.

Evaluations of predictive ratios are of different types, each of which examines the extent to which a method overestimates and underestimates spending for different subpopulations. One approach segments the population by actual medical expenditure levels (by quintiles or deciles) and evaluates the predictive ratio for each segment. Another approach identifies subpopulations, using specific chronic conditions or functional status to evaluate predictive ratios. Finally, some studies create simulated health plans with various proportions of high-risk members (risk selection) and evaluate the predictive accuracy for the simulated plans. In some studies, actual enrollees in actual plans (not simulated) of policy interest have been studied directly (e.g., Program of All-Inclusive Care for the Elderly [PACE] programs). This paper includes findings from all types of evaluations.

Commonly Used Risk Factors Produce Different Levels of Payment Accuracy

Prior Utilization as a Risk Factor

An individual's prior utilization and related costs have historically been the most predictive of future costs. This has been the basis for what insurers call "experience rating."

Demographic Measures as Risk Factors

Analysts and purchasers have sought alternatives to simple prior utilization models because payments to health plans on the basis of members' past use of services creates a potential disincentive for plans to promote the prudent use of health care services. One approach relied on demographic variables, such as age, that are statistically associated with higher levels of use of services. The Medicare example of this approach was the Medicare average adjusted per capita cost (AAPCC). The AAPCC underpaid plans for people with major chronic conditions (who were in the upper quintile of cost) by 50 percent.

Health Status Measures as Risk Factors:
Diagnosis Codes and Functional Status

Early work to improve demographic-based methods focused on the use of diagnosis codes combined with age and gender and sometimes included additional risk factors, such as functional status. These early explorations represented a major advance in the field. Some studies found that functional status information alone predicted health care expenditures about half as well as diagnosis data alone. These studies also found that that functional status combined with diagnosis data only modestly improved the predictive performance compared with the predictive performance of models that used diagnosis data only (Fowles et al., 1996; Hornbrook and Goodman, 1996). Even for a Medicare population, functional status data do not add significantly to the overall predictive performance of the model on the basis of diagnosis data.

Diagnosis models included all inpatient diagnoses and the diagnoses for patients in ambulatory care settings and were implemented by a handful of public and private employers as well as some managed care programs and Medicare managed care from 1994 to 2000. The performance of the prominent risk adjusters was evaluated by SOA in 1995 and by other investigators (Dunn et al., 1995; Ellis et al., 1996; Fowles et al., 1996; Hwang et al., 2001; Ingber, 2000; Kronick et al., 1996, 2000).

With these methodological advances, the underprediction for the upper 20 percent and the overprediction for the low-risk beneficiaries were substantially reduced but not eliminated. In one example, Hwang and colleagues (2001) evaluated the performance of three prominent diagnosis-based risk adjustment methods for predicting the costs for chronic diseases for children enrolled in Medicaid. The diagnosis models significantly outperformed demographic methods overall for children with chronic health conditions. Nonetheless, these models still over-predicted 15 to 31 percent of the costs for children with no chronic conditions. When the percentage of children with chronic conditions reached 20 percent of the enrolled population, the payments to plans overall ranged from 92 to 105 percent of the actual costs. As the proportion of members with chronic disease rises beyond 20 percent, the plan underpayment worsened, dropping to between 84 and 95 percent of the actual costs. If the average cost per member per month (PMPM) for the overall risk pool were $200, with the best-performing diagnosis-based risk adjusters available, the loss per capita for a plan with a disproportionate share of children with chronic conditions would be $10 to $22 PMPM.

In 2001, SOA sponsored another comparison of the predictive performance of prominent diagnosis-based and prescription-based risk adjustment methods used as proxies for diagnosis, using claims and enrollment data from employers (Cumming et al., 2002). Prescription data-only models were found to perform almost as well as diagnosis-based models, and use of the combination of diagnosis and prescription data improved the performance of the model to a limited extent. That study also demonstrated underpayments for the highest-cost segments of the commercially insured population studied. Table C-3 summarizes the findings for commercially insured and Medicare populations.

TABLE C-3 Predictive Ratios for Alternative Risk Adjustment Models

| | Predictive Ratios[a] for the Following Quintiles of Actual Expenditures: | | | | |
| | First | | | | Fifth |
Model	(Lowest)	Second	Third	Fourth	(Highest)
Medicare (age/sex)[b]	2.66	1.93	1.37	0.95	0.44
Medicare (diagnoses)[b]	1.23	1.23	1.14	1.02	0.86
Commercial (SOA study, diagnosis model)[c]	8.26	6.04	2.94	1.73	0.53

[a]Predictive ratio = mean predicted cost divided by mean actual cost for subgroups, based on distribution of actual per capita expenditures.
[b]SOURCE: Pope et al. (2004).
[c]SOURCE: Cumming et al. (2002).

Many other studies have demonstrated the significant improvement in performance of health-based risk adjusters compared with the performance of previous methods. They have also consistently found a sufficient level of underprediction for the highest-cost segment of multiple populations, including those with disabilities, to raise continued concern about incentives for health plans to avoid high-risk individuals and to create barriers to access or services in mainstream insurance markets. Temkin-Greener and colleagues (2001) found that for a PACE population, the Medicare inpatient diagnosis-based risk adjustment method underpaid for any group from one to five limitations of activities of daily living with predictive ratios ranging from 0.90 to 0.62. Ettner and colleagues (2000) found that for an employer plan population, the diagnosis-based methods underpaid for psychiatric disabilities with predictive ratios of 0.83 to 0.85. Kronick and colleagues (2000) found that even for an exclusively disabled Medicaid population (non-dually eligible and noninstitutionalized), whereas demographic risk adjustment underpaid the upper quintile on the basis of prior costs with a predictive ratio of 0.37, a diagnosis-based model demonstrated substantial improvement but still had a predictive ratio of 0.71.

Ellis and colleagues (1996) concluded that for the Medicare population, a diagnosis-based group of models was a significant improvement over a demography-based model but continued to underpay, on the basis of prior costs, for the upper quintile of individuals. The predictive ratio for a demographic model was 0.48, whereas a model based only on diagnosis improved the accuracy to 0.85, and the addition of prior procedures and hospitalizations to the model left a 10 percent underprediction for individuals in the highest risk quintile.

Fowles and colleagues (1996) found that for a health plan with employer and Medicare enrollees, even a modest skewing of the distribution of high-cost enrollees simulating high-, medium-, and low-risk plans resulted in underpayments for the high-risk group by a per capita average of 4.5 percent for individuals under age 65 years and 6.7 percent for individuals over age 65 years when a diagnosis-based risk adjuster was used. Hwang and colleagues (2001) found that for a population of Medicaid children, use of a demographic risk adjuster underpredicted the costs for the upper quintile, with predictive ratios of 0.50, whereas a diagnosis-based model reduced the magnitude of underprediction to between 0.91 and 0.93 of actual costs.

Pope found that the use of a customized model for the Medicare managed care program based on diagnoses resulted in a large improvement in payments over those achieved by use of a previous demographic risk adjustment method. Nonetheless, it still resulted in underpayment for beneficiaries in the upper cost quintile. The predictive ratio for the demographic model was 0.44, and that for the diagnosis model was 0.85.

Mark and colleagues (2003) evaluated the predictive ratios for two diagnosis-based risk adjustment models and for one demographic model for a large employer-sponsored health plan. For the subpopulation of beneficiaries who had diagnoses of chronic conditions associated with a disability (measured by activities of daily living [ADLs]), the demographic model underpredicted costs by 50 percent. The two diagnosis-based models performed very well and provided 1.01 and 1.02 percent of the actual costs.

Thus, for these employers, it appears that the diagnosis risk adjusters significantly reduced the incentive for "cream skimming," a term that describes plan strategies designed to selectively attract lower-risk enrollees that produce profits.

Medicare Example

The advances in the Medicare risk adjustment method reflect the advances that have been achieved by using health status information in other sectors. In the mid-1980s, a prior hospitalization data-based model for Medicare HMO rate setting was demonstrated. This first demonstration of a diagnosis-based payment system for Medicare used principal inpatient diagnoses and some demographic data (the principal inpatient diagnostic cost group [PIP-DCG method) to replace the demographics-only-based model in use. The demonstration ran from 1986 to 1987 for a Medicare health plan in Minneapolis, Minnesota.

Compared with the AAPCC, the model based on the inpatient diagnosis reduced the underestimation of expenditures for beneficiaries in the top cost quintile from 50 percent to 12 to 15 percent. Temkin-Greener and colleagues (2001) found, however, that although the PIP-DCG model was a major improvement over the AAPCC, it underpredicted the overall costs for PACE programs by 38 percent. That is, it underpaid these plans, which had higher enrollments of individuals with chronic health conditions. For individuals with five limitations in ADLs, the underprediction was 62 percent.

In 2004, CMS introduced a selected condition diagnosis-based risk adjustment model (formally the hierarchical condition category model [the CMS-HCC model]) for health plan payments. This included diagnosis codes from ambulatory care settings and all of the inpatient codes. This selected condition-based model improved the overall payment prediction by about 25 percent, a major gain in overall performance. However, the underprediction for beneficiaries in the upper quintile of expenditures was 12 to 15 percent.

Table C-4 shows the payment accuracy for two capitation methods for Medicare populations in general and also for Medicare beneficiaries with functional disabilities, as measured by the number of ADLs.

In 2004, CMS implemented the selected conditions CMS-HCC model, which included up to 3,400 diagnoses from both ambulatory care and inpatient settings. This implementation was achieved despite health plan industry resistance to much of the plan ostensibly over concern with data burden and diagnosis-coding completeness. A compromise reduced the number of diagnosis codes but retained 90 percent of the predictive performance of a full diagnosis-based model. Another critical compromise eliminated the requirement that health plans submit procedure codes. This eliminated CMS's ability to calibrate the models with managed care data or to determine care patterns of managed care. Therefore, payment models for health plans will continue to be updated and calibrated on the basis of the data for the traditional Medicare fee-for-service program population, and the predictive performance will be somewhat lower than that which would be achieved if all diagnosis codes were included.

TABLE C-4 Medicare Predictive Ratios for Noninstitutional Beneficiaries by Functional Status, Pooled Data, 1991 to 1994

		Predictive Ratios for Noninstitutionalized Individuals with the Following Numbers of ADLs:				
Model	Total	All	0 ADL	1–2 ADLs	3–4 ADLs	5–6 ADLs
Demographic	1.00	1.00	1.36	0.81	0.63	0.46
CMS-HCC	1.00	0.97	1.18	0.87	0.76	0.64

SOURCE: Greenwald (2000).

To improve the predictive accuracy for frail elderly individuals and for individuals with major chronic conditions, CMS has also evaluated a frailty adjuster for medical assistance plans and for the PACE program using ADLs as risk factors. Kautter and Pope (2004) found that ADLs added an approximately 10 percent improvement in overall prediction when they were combined with diagnosis-based models.

IMPLEMENTATION FACTORS THAT CAN INFLUENCE THE ACCURACY OF RISK SCORES

In addition to the potential level of predictive performance of a risk assessment method, the success or usefulness of a risk assessment method also depends to a great extent on how the model is implemented. Implementation factors that affect the performance of a model include the extent to which the data required are readily available and adequate in quality, whether the chosen model fits the application, how the model was calibrated, and the time lag between diagnosis coding and payment adjustment.

Data Issues

From the perspective of the data used to assess risk, methods can be categorized by their reliance on demographics, prior expenditures, or health data, including self-reported health status. Methods that rely on demographic risk factors, such as age, gender, and program eligibility status, are easy to administer. Data can be collected from eligibility files. In addition, these measures are unrelated to the care process and therefore do not produce incentives to change treatment or coding to maximize the risk scores. Unfortunately, these methods have a poor predictive value at the individual or risk-skewed group level. As stated earlier, an individual's total prior medical expenditure is a reasonably good predictor of future expenditure. These data can easily be obtained from claims data. However, as noted earlier, the use of past spending to set payments does nothing to encourage the prudent use of health services.

Health status measures, such as diagnoses and prescriptions, are now predictors that are as good as prior use (Ash et al., 2000). They also provide useful medical management information. Plans must obtain diagnostic data from providers either on claims forms or through other means. Once diagnosis-based risk adjustment is introduced, changes in coding patterns are expected. For diagnosis-based methods, the main concern involves diagnoses in the ambulatory care setting. Historically, these codes have not been used as the basis for payment or rate setting. With the advent of HBRA, the result may be an underreporting of diagnoses and can result in underestimated risk-based payments.

Different health plans have different types of data problems. Staff model HMOs, which have historically had limited experience with fee-for-service billing, will have concerns about claims data completeness. Plans with information systems that truncate the number of diagnosis codes per record to less than three diagnoses per encounter may receive less risk credit than they deserve. Data may also be missing because of subcapitation or because of services that may be contracted or "carved" out to a specialty provider whose utilization data may not be integrated with the other claims or encounter data. For example, a common problem is missing mental health data for plans that carve out mental health services.

With HBRA, more complete diagnosis codes or more specific diagnoses can significantly increase the risk score. At the plan level, plans will attempt to capture and retain in their files all codes submitted by providers. At the provider level, when a risk adjustment system is calibrated or normalized on the basis of the existing coding patterns, coding practices may change in the directions of identifying more conditions that can be legitimately coded and providing more specific coding of the severity of conditions. Once a risk adjustment model is implemented, changes in coding practices that produce more complete and more specific coding create the appearance of a higher-risk population compared with the risk for the population used to calibrate the prediction model. The results inflate the total cost for that population. Purchasers will renormalize their models at regular intervals to prevent overpayment due to upcoding and other changes in coding practices.

A particular underreporting coding problem that is likely to disproportionately affect costs for people with disabilities and to result in underestimates is the lack of persistence of recording the diagnosis codes for major and often disability-related chronic conditions in the typical claims histories over time. For example, on the basis of Medicaid claims data from six states for people with disabilities, Kronick (2000) found that for more than 43 percent of those with the code for quadriplegia in Year 1, that important code was not carried over into Year 2, even though the individual had contact with the provider. The lack of year-to-year persistence was found for many major chronic conditions. The code for multiple sclerosis disappeared in Year 2 for 42 percent of individuals with that condition, and the code for ischemic heart disease disappeared for 67 percent of individuals.

Without the diagnosis recorded in the 12-month time frame of the typical risk assessment period applied in risk adjustment, the payment system assumes that no condition exists. Even if there is no direct link between a chronic condition and a high-cost treatment (e.g., quadriplegia), the often high-frequency occurrences of related acute conditions such as urinary tract infections do not get adequate value because, in a typical risk assessment model, without the strong signal (code) indicating the presence of the underlying major condition, these diagnoses of acute conditions do not predict future costs. The incentive for more complete coding produced by diagnosis-based risk adjustment has been shown to begin to alleviate the problem; but to the extent that it remains, it has a significant impact on the risk assessment for people with these major chronic conditions.

Plans with payments that have been adjusted by purchasers by using diagnosis-based risk adjusters, such as those participating in the Colorado and Maryland Medicaid programs, have, in many cases, made significant improvements in collecting the more complete data needed to set plan-level payments accurately.

For some purchasers, diagnosis data availability problems are such a concern that they substitute prediction models that are based on more easily obtained prescription data. Prescription data are timely, relatively accurate and complete for major drugs prescribed in the ambulatory care setting. In addition, these data do not need to be obtained from providers, eliminating a difficult data collection step. However, if prescribing is increased to raise a plan or provider's risk score, the incentives for efficiency may be poor. Prescription-based risk assessment models generally focus on drugs believed to be nondiscretionary. However, with off-label prescribing and to the extent that discretion remains in prescribing drugs for additional diseases or for less severe or marginal forms of the disease, caution should be exercised when prescription-based models are considered for provider payment applications.

Functional status and perceived health status information derived from surveys have also been evaluated for use as factors for risk adjustment. These studies have shown that significant nonrespondent underestimation bias can influence those results. Gaming or manipulation of surveys is also a concern.

Risk Adjustment Model Design Should Fit the Application

The risk adjustment methods may differ to some extent in the number of conditions that they incorporate. Some use almost all known diseases to assign risk scores. Others exclude minor, acute conditions, under the assumption that these conditions are not relevant to risk selection and do not represent significant per capita costs and that their inclusion may produce a clinically needless proliferation of these codes. If the user of risk adjustment wished to categorize all patients for an evaluation of how primary care providers are managing these frequent minor, acute conditions, for example, then the use of one of the methods that includes these conditions would be preferred.

Another difference is the assignment of disease measures to risk categories. This process may produce categories that are much too heterogeneous for a specific disease of interest. Some conditions are lumped with related, yet clinically quite distinct, diseases with similar costs. A disease such as diabetes, on the other hand, has its own category in most of these methods, and payment is affected by coding for diabetes more specifically. For other conditions, more detailed coding to describe severity will not change the assignment to a risk category, beyond that from the simple identification of the disease.

The approach to assigning individual risk scores also varies. Some methods are additive, with additional payment made for each additional disease category identified. For payment applications, some of these categories may be arranged in hierarchies of related conditions (e.g., pulmonary conditions), with payment made only for the highest-cost category in the hierarchy, the assumption being that the lower-cost categories in the hierarchy indicate complications related to the more significant condition. This approach avoids double counting. Other methods address this relatedness of conditions by assigning individuals to mutually exclusive risk categories derived by interacting all of the individual's conditions or by identifying the individual's dominant condition.

The methods have been designed to be as robust as possible to data problems while preserving predictive performance. The models typically require only one occurrence of the diagnosis or prescription in the assessment period to assign risk. The number of times that the same code appears is irrelevant. Discretionary or ill-defined indicators are often excluded or are assigned to risk categories to minimize gaming incentives. This means that data need not be perfectly complete and detailed to be adequate for risk adjustment.

Lag Issues

One concern for the implementation of payment adjustment is the lag between the date that the health problem was coded or that the prescription was ordered and the use of the information for payment adjustment. Lags reduce the accuracy of the payment in two ways: (1) the minimum length of the claims history required to produce a valid risk score will exclude some recently enrolled beneficiaries who do not meet the requirement, and (2) the longer the lag, the greater the loss of predictive power. It is more difficult to accurately predict events in the distant future than those in the proximate future. Lags occur in three ways, including (1) the length of the risk assessment time frame, (2) the time required for claims and enrollment data to be available to a plan or purchaser, and (3) the time required to implement the risk scoring.

A model that uses health data from a prior period to predict payments in a subsequent period will often require a minimum of 6 months of claims history to capture major chronic conditions and comorbidities; therefore, the model requires continuous enrollment throughout the assessment period. In addition, the model will require that the enrollee be enrolled each month in the payment period for the model to perform as well as it was designed to perform. A concurrent model uses health data from the same period to explain costs during that period. This so-called profiling model does not require a lengthy diagnosis history to assign a valid risk score to an enrollee. The prospective approach may not be critical for Medicare, which has a very stable enrollment, but it is relevant for some Medicaid and other programs, in which there is often high enrollment turnover and in which eligibility may terminate after weeks or months because individuals no longer meet the eligibility criteria.

Health plans will have unequal claims run-out periods (periods between the time that an expense is incurred and the time that the claim is processed). It is important to allow sufficient time for all the plans to reach a similar level of data collection completion; otherwise, payments will be biased. For diagnosis data, 4 months or more may be required to be adequate. (Prescription data may lag by only a month or less before they are available to a plan.)

It may require 2 months to receive updates of changes in the eligibility status of plan members from purchasers. For some large employers, the retroactive adjustment for new enrollment, enrollment status changes, or terminations may take even longer.

Purchasers can control how often and how fast they compute and assign risk scores. Combined with the usual claims run-out lag, the range can be from a minimum of 6 months up to a maximum of 24 months.

For individual-level prospective models, the enrollee must be continuously eligible for 6 to 12 months in the assessment period, 6 to 18 months in the claims delay period, and 1 to 12 months in the payment period for a health plan to be paid for the risk of that enrollee. This continuous enrollment requirement can remove up to 40 to 50 percent of any currently enrolled Medicaid population from the clinical condition risk assessment (e.g., all new enrollees), thus dramatically reducing the predictive performance of the total capitation system because the rates for enrollees generally must be based on the much poorer predictors of age and gender. Therefore, it is important to know to what extent the delay has reduced the performance of the model compared with its predictive performance from research studies, which often include no delay.

Model Calibration Issues

To determine that the costs for someone with a major chronic condition are some amount above the average for the population, the risk adjustment models must be normalized on the basis of some actual population.

It has been assumed that for the most valid payment, relative values could be achieved only by estimating the weights on the basis of the values for the actual insured population for which payments would be applied. Experience has taught that imported relative weights can be sufficiently valid and stable if they are estimated on the basis of a similar population, for example, Medicare, Medicaid, and commercial populations (with similar covered benefits). For some, however, it may be preferable to calculate weights on the basis of the user's population. This requires both a sufficiently large population and adequate data. Whether a user imports or calculates its own data, weights must be updated at regular intervals to account for changes in practice patterns, coding changes, and significant changes in benefit design. When one wishes the accuracy to be maximized for the highest-risk segment of the population, small numbers can present a problem in developing stable risk weights.

Although many of the diagnosis-based models are calibrated, of necessity, on the basis of fee-for-service data and although experience has taught that these weights are reasonably valid for managed care applications, there is a desire to move, when possible, to weights based on patient encounter data. There may be some gain in validity from encounter-based weights that reflects the clinical and coding practices of a managed care environment. The use of encounter data for the estimation of weights requires the highest standard for completeness. Although duplications of diagnoses can be tolerated in the risk assessment, duplications of charges could cause significant errors when proper weights are established. Another issue to be considered in the development of weights is how to apply charges to encounter data.

Current risk adjustment models do not directly capture the additional costs that would be incurred to reduce barriers for access to health care. For example, a number of investigators have found that risk models that have introduced factors associated with barriers to health care may predict a lower cost for an individual compared with that for another individual with an identical health status profile but no indicator of a barrier to access.

Typical risk adjustment models, like all traditional rate-setting models, establish payment levels on the basis of current practice patterns. If one wishes to provide incentives to improve the quality of care or to reduce existing barriers to access, features must be added to the payment models. Future research is needed to better integrate quality and disparity related incentive features into risk based payment models.

Implementation Environment

Another important consideration is the environmental context in which HBRA is being implemented. One such issue, especially for employees, is the concern with access to private information. A third party may need to collect and analyze the data. In addition, the payment model may require special calibration for the specific application or population. The model may also need to be updated frequently because the relationship between the risk measure and medical expenditures may change rapidly, for example, as prescribing patterns change and new drugs become available or as the availability of generic drugs reduces the costs for drugs that no longer are protected by patent.

Other factors may also need to be considered. If other major purchasers are using a particular approach, it may be less confusing to the market if the same approach is used. Finally, the cost of licensing and maintaining the software should be taken into account. Prices vary, and some in the public domain may require additional outside consultants for successful implementation.

CURRENT ISSUES AND TRENDS

For programs that want to excel or focus exclusively on health care for individuals with many health care needs, the remaining underpayment bias may still present a daunting financial barrier to provider accountability systems, such as tiered networks, competing in the mainstream insurance market. CMS, as was described above, is attempting to mainstream the financing for many demonstration projects and special programs, many of which serve people with disabilities.

A better understanding of both the underestimation bias and the prediction error associated with individuals with higher health care costs is needed. Rarely is this group addressed explicitly by risk adjustment models. The assumption is that plans will enroll enough of the overpaid (lower-cost) beneficiaries to balance out individuals with higher health care costs. Many times the rationale expressed is that, after all, "they are still insurance companies and the pooling of risk is their job." Here we confront the often implicit illogical application of insurance assumptions under conditions of chronic, and thus predictable, costs and the desire to finance adequate care by using a per capita budget to allow substitution (prevention) and fiscal restraint (not fee for service).

NEXT GENERATION

The widespread implementation of electronic medical records will provide a new source of clinical data that are feasibly obtainable, such as clinical, hematological, radiological, cognitive, psychological, and other laboratory test results. Such data are expected to improve the predictive performance of risk adjusters, especially in further refining the differentiation of the more severe and complex stages of a condition than the current diagnosis codes or coding practices allow. These studies are only now beginning. For example, Luft and Dudley (2004) have identified 100 verifiable, expensive, and predictable conditions that are good predictors, even from claims data, and that account for a large portion of overall medical expenditures. Also promising is that for many of the conditions, the residual unexplained risk due to limitations of diagnosis coding can be further refined by using the results of single diagnostic tests. This has not been considered feasible for insurance applications; however, with the promise of electronic medical records and the need for accuracy for expensive and deserving populations with the greatest needs, such as people with long-term disabilities, the opportunity may present itself to advance risk adjustment in a significant way. This access to new and richer data may also present the promising opportunity of incorporating quality measures with risk factors to begin the promise of building payment models that address both risk and quality differences.

Eventually, risk assessment will use more sophisticated modeling techniques that more closely fit the dynamics of enrollment length and pent-up demand; mechanisms of risk selection (Luft and Dudley, 2004); the behaviors of various health problems from a variable, relevant time frame or episode-of-illness perspective and from the perspective of a longer time frame; and financing models that support 3- to 5-year contracts or payment schemes to reduce the effects of externalities that exacerbate active risk selection and the inability to invest in preventive care.

So far, this paper has not addressed long-term care. The long-term care purchasers have developed a sophisticated case mix and risk assessment process to determine the need for institutional and long-term care and community services, as well as the level of care within a long-term care institution. Those who are working on the integration of Medicare and Medicaid for dually eligible individuals are confronting the remaining problems of risk adjusters described earlier in this paper and are increasingly interested in integrating acute-care risk adjustment with long-term care payments. Usually, a theoretically pure premium rate-setting process attempts to avoid the inclusion of setting of care or services because of a concern of reinforcing the overuse of health care services or constraining creative innovation. However, for some applications, such as health plan integration of long-term care with acute care, the inclusion of setting of care or prior utilization markers may improve the accuracy of the rates because the care delivery patterns are so different when a beneficiary is in an institution than in the community. This is in part because long-term care services may substitute for or prevent acute care utilization.

The integration problem remains, however, for people with long-term, significant chronic conditions when long-term care is a substitute for or prevents acute care utilization or vice versa. This problem is usually addressed by calibrating the risk adjustment models separately for populations who are dually eligible or who are in a long-term care facility or by adding an indicator to the risk model. The problem becomes especially difficult when an overlap in the coverage of services exists between both payers and the payers disagree over how many health care services are needed. This has been a major problem for mental health services, which do require a licensed physician and are, to some extent, covered by both Medicare and Medicaid and for which, under managed care plans, utilization controls place limits on mental health services that are more restrictive. The variation in mental health costs for the Medicaid-covered portion for dually eligible mental health services is greater than that for other health problems, many of which are driven by Medicare coverage policy. Now that prescription costs for the dually eligible are Medicare's responsibility, states may experience the need to coordinate Medicaid coverage around a complex set of formularies for Part D. Under these circumstances the coordination of benefits makes risk adjustment and the rate setting that it supports particularly difficult.

CONCLUSIONS

The use of the best risk adjustment methods for multiple applications, including insurance plan payment, is now common practice. These tools not only produce more accurate allocations of resources than traditional actuarial methods and reduce the level of use of perverse incentives but also offer insights for managers and policy makers about who and what is producing real value, that is, cost-effectiveness, as performance is able to be better differentiated from risk.

The problem is that for individuals with the highest-cost medical needs, the current methods still underpredict expenditures to the extent that concerns about the effects of adverse selection remain, particularly for a plan that wishes to excel in care for those with significant long-term chronic conditions.

REFERENCES

Ash AS, Ellis RP, Pope GC, et al. Using diagnoses to describe populations and predict costs. *Health Care Financ Rev.* Spring 2000;21(3):7–28.

Batavia AI, DeJong G. Disability, chronic illness, and risk selection. *Arch Phys Med Rehab.* Apr 2001;82(4):546–552.

Blumenthal D, Weissman JS, Wachterman M, et al. The who, what, and why of risk adjustment: a technology on the cusp of adoption. *J Health Polit Policy Law.* Jun 2005; 30(3):453–473.

Cumming R, Knutson DJ, Cameron BA, Derrick B. *A Comparative Analysis of Claims-Based Methods of Health Risk Assessment for Commercial Populations.* Washington, DC: Society of Actuaries; May 24, 2002.

Dunn DL, Rosenblatt A, Taira DA, et al. *A Comparative Analysis of Methods of Health Risk Assessment.* Washington, DC: Society of Actuaries; December 21, 1995.

Eggers PW, Prihoda R. Pre-enrollment reimbursement patterns of Medicare beneficiaries enrolled in "at-risk" HMOs. *Health Care Financ Rev.* Sep 1982;4(1):55–73.

Ellis RP, Pope GC, Iezzoni L, et al. Diagnosis-based risk adjustment for Medicare capitation payments. *Health Care Financ Rev.* Spring 1996;17(3):101–128.

Ettner SL, Frank RG, Mark T, Smith MW. Risk adjustment of capitation payments to behavioral health care carve-outs: how well do existing methodologies account for psychiatric disability? *Health Care Manag Sci.* Feb 2000;3(2):159–169.

Fowles JB, Weiner JP, Knutson D, Fowler E, Tucker AM, Ireland M. Taking health status into account when setting capitation rates: a comparison of risk-adjustment methods. *JAMA.* Oct 23–30 1996;276(16):1316–1321.

Glazer J, McGuire TG. Optimal risk adjustments in markets with adverse selection: an application to managed care. *Am Econ Rev.* 2000;90:1055.

Greenwald LM. Medicare risk-adjusted capitation payments: from research to implementation. *Health Care Financ Rev.* Spring 2000;21(3):1–5.

Greenwald LM, Levy JM, Ingber MJ. Favorable selection in the Medicare+Choice program: new evidence. *Health Care Financ Rev.* Spring 2000;21(3):127–134.

Hadley J, Reschovsky JD. Health and the cost of nongroup insurance. *Inquiry.* Fall 2003; 40(3):235–253.

Hill SC, Thornton C, Trenholm C, Wooldridge J. Risk selection among SSI enrollees in TennCare. *Inquiry.* Summer 2002;39(2):152–167.

Hornbrook MC, Goodman MJ. Chronic disease, functional health status, and demographics: a multi-dimensional approach to risk adjustment. *Health Serv Res.* Aug 1996; 31(3):283–307.

Hwang W, Ireys HT, Anderson GF. Comparison of risk adjusters for Medicaid-enrolled children with and without chronic health conditions. *Ambul Pediatr.* Jul–Aug 2001; 1(4):217–224.

Iezzoni LI. *Risk Adjustment for Measuring Health Care Outcomes,* 3rd ed. Chicago, IL: Health Administration Press; 2003.

Ingber MJ. Implementation of risk adjustment for Medicare. *Health Care Financ Rev.* Spring 2000;21(3):119–126.

Ireys HT, Anderson GF, Shaffer TJ, Neff JM. Expenditures for care of children with chronic illnesses enrolled in the Washington State Medicaid program, fiscal year 1993. *Pediatrics.* Aug 1997;100(2 Pt 1):197–204.

Kautter J, Pope GC. CMS frailty adjustment model. *Health Care Financ Rev.* Winter 2004; 26(2):1–19.

Keenan PS, Buntin MJ, McGuire TG, Newhouse JP. The prevalence of formal risk adjustment in health plan purchasing. *Inquiry.* 2001;38:245–259.

Knutson D. Health-based risk adjustment: payment and other innovative uses. Unpublished manuscript. Presented at Robert Wood Johnson HCFO and Kaiser Permanente IHP May 23, 2003 Invitational Meeting. 2003:1–12.

Knutson D, Wrightson W. The Buyer's Health Care Action Group's pricing and payment system. In: *Financial Strategy for Managed Care Organizations: Rate Setting, Risk Adjustment and Competitive Advantage.* Chicago, IL: Health Administration Press; 2002:227-238.

Kronick R, Zhou Z, Dreyfus T. Making risk adjustment work for everyone. *Inquiry.* Spring 1995;32(1):41–55.

Kronick R, Dreyfus T, Lee L, Zhou Z. Diagnostic risk adjustment for Medicaid: the disability payment system. *Health Care Financ Rev.* Spring 1996;17(3):7–33.

Kronick R, Gilmer T, Dreyfus T, Lee L. Improving health-based payment for Medicaid beneficiaries: CDPS. *Health Care Financ Rev.* Spring 2000;21(3):29–64.

Lubitz J, Beebe J, Riley G. Improving the Medicare HMO payment formula to deal with biased selection. *Adv Health Econ Health Serv Res.* 1985;6:101–126.

Luft HS, Dudley RA. Assessing risk-adjustment approaches under non-random selection. *Inquiry.* Summer 2004;41(2):203–217.

Mark TL, Ozminkowski RJ, Kirk A, Ettner SL, Drabek J. Risk adjustment for people with chronic conditions in private sector health plans. *Med Decis Making.* Sep–Oct 2003; 23(5):397–405.

Newhouse JP, Manning WG, Keeler EB, Sloss EM. Adjusting capitation rates using objective health measures and prior utilization. *Health Care Financ Rev.* Spring 1989; 10(3):41–54.

Palsbo SE, Post R. Financial risk reduction for people with disabilities in Medicaid programs. *Manag Care Q* 2003;11:1–7.

Parente ST, Feldman R, Christianson JB. Employee choice of consumer-driven health insurance in a multiplan, multiproduct setting. *Health Serv Res.* Aug 2004;39(4 Pt 2): 1091–1112.

Pope GC, Kautter J, Ellis RP, et al. Risk adjustment of Medicare capitation payments using the CMS-HCC model. *Health Care Financ Rev* 2004;25:119–141.

Temkin-Greener H, Meiners MR, Gruenberg L. PACE and the Medicare+Choice risk-adjusted payment model. *Inquiry.* Spring 2001;38(1):60–72.

Weissman JS, Wachterman M, Blumenthal D. When methods meet politics: how risk adjustment became part of Medicare managed care. *J Health Polit Policy Law.* Jun 2005; 30(3):475–504.

Zaslavsky AM, Buntin MJ. Using survey measures to assess risk selection among Medicare managed care plans. *Inquiry.* Summer 2002;39(2):138–151.

D

The Americans with Disabilities Act in a Health Care Context

*Sara Rosenbaum**

INTRODUCTION

This paper examines the Americans with Disabilities Act (ADA)[1] in the context of health care. Encompassed in this analysis are issues related to health care access, coverage, and financing. The interaction of the ADA with employment laws governing the health care workforce is considered separately (see Appendix E). This analysis also assumes the presence of legal disputes involving "qualified" persons with "disabilities," as the term is used under the ADA, since the question of who is "qualified" would consume an entire legal analysis in its own right.[2]

Any legal analysis involving health care can be daunting, because it entails an examination of the notoriously complicated interaction between law and the health care system. When the focus is on the relationship between civil rights and health care financing, the juncture can be particularly rocky because of the inherent contradictions between health care financing laws on the one hand and the law of civil rights on the other. At their core, the web of laws that together comprise the law of health care financing rests heavily on the law of insurance, which in turn emphasizes the legality

---

*Harold and Jane Hirsh Professor of Health Law and Policy and Chair, Department of Health Policy, The George Washington University School of Public Health and Health Services.

[1]42 U.S.C. §12101 et seq.
[2]For an overview of legal developments in this area in the 16 years since the ADA's enactment, see National Council on Disability, *Righting the ADA* (Washington, D.C.: NCD, 2004). Available at http://www.ncd.gov/newsroom/publications/2004/publications.htm (accessed July 22, 2006).

of exclusion and risk avoidance. In contrast, civil rights laws enacted to protect persons with disabilities are fundamentally intended to advance the societal embrace of individuals whose health status can carry the potential for a greater consumption of resources. Legal disputes involving the allocation of resources within particular covered populations inevitably operate as a flashpoint for this deep, underlying policy tension.

The fundamental purpose of the ADA is to achieve the integration of persons with disabilities into all facets of society, including health care.[3] At the same time, the complex and intricate web of federal and state laws that govern public and private health care and health care financing are embedded in the principles of markets[4] and federalism; these principles in turn vest health system players—physicians, hospitals, public programs, employers, and health insurers—with substantial discretion regarding health care undertakings and health care finance. Reconciling the ADA's aspirational goals and specific legal provisions with the U.S. health care system's market orientation[5] is a daunting task, particularly when the regulatory focus is on whom health care professionals must serve or what health insurance programs must cover and pay for.

The analysis that follows underscores the complexity of this topic. Part II describes the ADA's basic provisions. Part III considers the ADA in the context of health care access, while Part IV explores the ADA and the law of health care financing. The paper concludes with a discussion of options for ensuring access to the civil rights protections conferred under law.

The principal conclusions drawn from this review can be summarized as follows:

• First, when the claim by a qualified individual with a disability is understood to be one that involves discrimination in the provision of health care—that is, failing to offer health services in an accessible manner—courts are likely to view the dispute as one that falls within the ADA's remedial scope. That is, assuming that a plaintiff can show conduct considered discriminatory under the ADA and that a defendant cannot prove an affirmative defense—that is, cannot bring its conduct within a legally permissible exception to the rule of nondiscriminatory conduct—the ADA provides a

---

[3] 42 U.S.C. §12101, defining the term "public accommodation" to include health care services.

[4] For an exhaustive discussion to date of the use of law to advance health care markets, see U.S. Department of Justice and Federal Trade Commission, *Improving Health Care: A Dose of Competition*. Available at http://www.ftc.gov/reports/healthcare/040723healthcarerpt.pdf (accessed November 23, 2006).

[5] *A Dose of Competition*, supra. For a legal comparison of national health policies here and abroad, see Timothy Stoltzfus Jost, *Disentitlement* (New York: Oxford University Press, 2003).

remedy. In situations involving accessible care, therefore, the major social challenge is how to create remedies that foster accessibility without placing an undue burden on the program.

• Second, when the claim is one that involves discrimination in the design of health insurance coverage so as to inherently limit the flow of resources to persons whose disabilities create greater health needs, plaintiffs inevitably lose, since any changes would inevitably require an expansion or restructuring of coverage design itself, a remedy that courts view as beyond the remedial limits of the ADA. For example, courts will not order insurers to add coverage for wheelchairs or expand or redesign formulary limits.

• Third, plaintiffs can prevail, however, if they can show that the discrimination occurs not as part of plan design but as a result of discriminatory choices in how the plan is administered and can also show that the remedy they seek does not involve a "fundamental alteration," that is, a change in the design of the plan itself. For example, courts may be willing to classify as discriminatory an insurer's refusal to pay for covered physical therapy for a child with cerebral palsy if it turns out that the denial is based on claims reviewer's unfounded opinion that children with cerebral palsy cannot improve.[6]

• Fourth, where health care financing cases are concerned, it can be difficult to predict when an ADA claim will be viewed by courts involving remediable discriminatory administration or nonremediable discriminatory design. The same facts may give rise to different judicial approaches to resolving this tension between coverage design and coverage administration, especially when the focus is on whether a claim should be paid. In these cases, it can be unclear as to whether a service is covered but withheld from particular individuals or whether the insurer's position is that the claim is for an uncovered service.

AN OVERVIEW OF THE ADA

Termed a "quiet revolution"[7] and "a celebration of the uniquely American notion that all of our citizens can contribute to society if we provide

---

[6]See, e.g., *Bedrick v. Travelers Insurance Co.* (93 F. 3d 149 (4th Cir, 1996)), in which such a dispute was won on the grounds of arbitrary and unfair administration of an Employee Retirement Income Security Act health benefit plan. This type of fact pattern might also give rise to a remediable ADA claim.

[7]Statement of Senator Tom Harkin honoring the 15th anniversary of the ADA, *Cong. Rec.* S. 8804 (July 25, 2005). Available at http://thomas.loc.gov/cgi-bin/query/D?r109:4:./temp/ ~r1092WcqGT (accessed November 23, 2006).

them with the tools and opportunities they need,"[8] the ADA established a "clear and comprehensive national mandate for the elimination of discrimination against people with disabilities."[9] The Act provides broad protections in the areas of employment, public services, public accommodations, and services operated by private entities and in the areas of transportation and telecommunications.

The ADA is a complex legislative structure and a cobbling together of a series of separate legislative measures reported by various congressional committees with jurisdiction over the range of subject areas addressed by the Act. The end result is a civil rights statute of broad applicability, particularly compared with laws that prohibit discrimination on the basis of race and national origin, which are discussed further below.

Persons protected under the ADA are "qualified individuals with a disability."[10] A disability under the terms of the Act is a physical or mental impairment that substantially limits one or more major life activities or a record of having such an impairment or being perceived by others as having such an impairment.[11] Qualified persons with disabilities are persons who can perform the essential functions of employment[12] with or without accommodation or who meet the essential eligibility requirements for the receipt of services or the participation in programs or activities provided by a public entity.[13]

Several titles of the ADA are directly relevant to this analysis. (Only Title IV, which relates to telecommunications, is not directly related to health care.) Title I prohibits discrimination in employment. It defines employment to include "employee compensation . . . and other terms, conditions, and privileges of employment."[14] As such, terms would include employer-sponsored health insurance. Four separate federal agencies—the Equal Opportunity Employment Commission, the U.S. Department of Transportation, the Federal Communications Commission, and the U.S. Department of Justice—enforce the legislation's employment provisions.[15]

Title II prohibits the denial of benefits or exclusionary conduct under programs and services operated by public entities. In so doing, Title II

---

[8]Statement of Senator John Kyl honoring the 15th anniversary of the ADA, *Cong. Rec.* S. 8771 (July 25, 2006). Available at http://thomas.loc.gov/cgi-bin/query/F?r109:8:./temp/ ~r1092WcqGT:e29790 (accessed November 23, 2006).

[9]Id.

[10]42 U.S.C. §12102(2).

[11]Id.

[12]42 U.S.C. §12111-12117.

[13]42 U.S.C. §12131(2).

[14]42 U.S.C. §12112(a).

[15]U.S. Department of Labor, *Disability Resources: the ADA.* Available at http://www.dol.gov/dol/topic/disability/ada.htm (accessed November 23, 2006).

incorporates and extends the reach of earlier law, Section 504 of the Rehabilitation Act of 1973,[16] by encompassing public entities generally, including not only executive agencies but the legislative and judicial branches of state and local governments[17] and their instrumentalities,[18] regardless of the direct presence of federal funds.[19] Title II sets not only a nondiscrimination standard but also an "equality of opportunity" requirement in publicly operated settings.[20] This equal opportunity obligation can require a more rigorous modification of services than might otherwise be the case; for example, it may require public clinic mental health counselors to be able to communicate in American Sign Language (ASL) rather than the lower standard of requiring mental health counselors without such language skills to be accompanied by translators.[21]

As with Title I, an array of federal agencies[22] has the power to investigate and enforce the law, including the U.S. Department of Justice and the U.S. Department of Health and Human Services, in the case of both publicly operated and federally supported health care services.[23] Although the sweep of ADA Title II reaches all public entities, as with other aspects of the ADA, there is limited specific interpretive guidance on the applicable rules for public entities that may or may not receive federal funds.

Title III, which is, in some respects, the most far-reaching ADA title in a health care context, prohibits discrimination by wholly private enterprises that are considered places of public accommodation.[24] In a dramatic departure from earlier civil rights laws prohibiting discrimination on the basis of race or national origin, Title III classifies private health care services as

---

[16]29 U.S.C. §794(a).

[17]U.S. Department of Justice, *Non-Discrimination on the Basis of Disability in State and Local Governments.* Available at http://www.usdoj.gov/crt/ada/reg2.html (accessed November 23, 2006).

[18]42 U.S.C. §12131(1).

[19]*Tugg v. Towey* 861 F. Supp. 1201, 1205 (S.D. Fl., 1994); *Tennessee v. Lane* 504 U.S. 514 (2004) §794(a).

[20]28 C.F.R. §35.130(b)(1)(i-iii).

[21]Id.

[22]See U.S. Department of Justice, *ADA Investigative Agencies.* Available at http://www.usdoj.gov/crt/ada/investag.htm (accessed November 23, 2006).

[23]U.S. Department of Health and Human Services, Office of Civil Rights, *Your Rights Under the Americans with Disabilities Act.* Available at http://www.hhs.gov/ocr/ada.html (accessed November 23, 2006). In its final rules implementing Title II, the U.S. Department of Justice notes under "Compliance Procedures" that Congress expected that activity-relevant federal agencies (in the case of health services, the U.S. Department of Health and Human Services) would interpret and enforce standards in the case of public health facilities. Available at http://www.usdoj.gov/crt/ada/reg2.html (accessed November 23, 2006).

[24]42 U.S.C. §12182.

a public accommodation and without regard to whether service providers are considered recipients of federal financing.[25]

The fifth and final title covers a number of topics, the most relevant of which for this analysis appears in a section labeled "Construction."[26] This provision, which has come to be known as the "insurance safe harbor," provides as follows:

(c) Insurance

Subchapters I through III of this chapter and title IV of this Act shall not be construed to prohibit or restrict—

(1) an insurer, hospital or medical service company, health maintenance organization, or any agent, or entity that administers benefit plans, or similar organizations from underwriting risks, classifying risks, or administering such risks that are based on or not inconsistent with State law; or

(2) a person or organization covered by this chapter from establishing, sponsoring, observing or administering the terms of a bona fide benefit plan that are based on underwriting risks, classifying risks, or administering such risks that are based on or not inconsistent with State law; or

(3) a person or organization covered by this chapter from establishing, sponsoring, observing or administering the terms of a bona fide benefit plan that is not subject to State laws that regulate insurance.

Paragraphs (1), (2), and (3) shall not be used as a subterfuge to evade the purposes of . . . this chapter.

The ADA is remedial; that is, the law requires entities covered by the Act to make "reasonable modifications" in activities, programs, and services in the case of qualified individuals with disabilities. Covered entities under both Titles II and III are given certain affirmative defenses, the most prominent of which is a claim that a requested change in fact constitutes a "fundamental alteration"[27] rather than a reasonable modification; the concept of fundamental alteration is understood as a change that affects the basic character of the activity, good, or service.[28] Additional affirmative defenses allowed under the law are that the plaintiff poses a "direct threat"[29] or that the requested change represents an "undue burden." In a few areas, the law is anticipatory only, in recognition of the need for some level of

---

[25]42 U.S.C. §12181(7). For a general discussion of the unique nature of this provision in relation to earlier laws, see Joel Teitelbaum and Sara Rosenbaum, "Medical care as a public accommodation: moving the discussion to race," 29 *Am. J. Law Med.* 381 (2003).

[26]42 U.S.C. §12201.

[27]See *PGA Tour v. Martin*, 532 U.S. 661 (2001) (Title III) and *Olmstead v. L.C.* 527 U.S. 581 (1999).

[28]*PGA v. Martin* 532 U.S. 682–683.

[29]*Bragdon v. Abbott* 526 U.S. 1131 (1999).

restraint in the implementation of standards. For example, different and more stringent rules on accessibility apply to new construction compared with rules that apply to the removal of barriers in existing facilities.[30]

Individuals may enforce the ADA privately through litigation to redress a violation of rights guaranteed under law. With respect to government enforcement of the various titles of the ADA, responsibility cuts across various agencies. The U.S. Department of Justice acts as the principle source of regulatory standards[31] and formal enforcement actions, with interpretive guidance and investigatory powers vested in other federal agencies responsible for the program within their spheres of expertise. Thus, for example, the U.S. Department of Health and Human Services has the authority to interpret the health care-specific meaning of Title II's broad regulatory standards[32] and to investigate complaints.[33] The U.S. Department of Justice retains enforcement authority over health care entities, which under ADA Title III are places of public accommodation; the regulations specify no formal role for other federal agencies.[34]

Investigation by federal agencies can result in the filing of enforcement complaints by the U.S. Department of Justice on behalf of affected individuals and the federal government itself. These complaints can result in settlements or proceed to full trial. Agency settlements, when they are finally reached, are publicly available and may have important implications for similar covered entities.[35]

Judicial decisions involving private or government enforcement efforts tend to be viewed as carrying greater weight, since under the United States Constitution it is the judicial branch of government that has the ultimate authority to determine what the law means.[36] It is not infrequent to find that courts give only limited weight to the rulings of federal agencies.[37]

---

[30]28 C.F.R. §§35.150–151 (public facilities); 28 C.F.R. §36.401–402 (public accommodations).

[31]All ADA regulations can be viewed at http://www.usdoj.gov/crt/ada/adahom1.htm (accessed November 23, 2006).

[32]See U.S. Department of Health and Human Services, Office of Civil Rights, *Civil Rights on the Basis of Disability*. Available at http://www.hhs.gov/ocr/discrimdisab.html#rights (accessed November 23, 2006).

[33]U.S. Department of Health and Human Services, Office of Civil Rights, *How to File a Discrimination Complaint with the Office for Civil Rights*. Available at http://www.hhs.gov/ocr/discrimhowtofile.html (accessed November 23, 2006).

[34]28 C.F.R. §36.501.

[35]U.S. Department of Justice, *Enforcing the ADA: A Status Report from the Justice Department*. Available at http://www.usdoj.gov/crt/ada/statrpt.htm (accessed November 23, 2006).

[36]*Marbury v, Madison*, 1 Cranch 137 (1803).

[37]*Doe v. Mutual of Omaha Ins. Co.*, 179 F. 3d 557 (7th Cir., 1999); rehearing and suggestion for rehearing en banc denied (Aug 03, 1999); cert. den. *Doe v. Mutual of Omaha Ins. Co.*, 528 U.S. 1106 (2000) (limited or no weight was given to the Equal Employment Opportunity Commission interpretation of insurance "safe harbor" in an ADA enforcement case involving allegations of discrimination by a health insurer).

THE ADA AND ACCESS TO HEALTH CARE

Physical Access to Health Care Services

The essential starting point for understanding the significance of the ADA in a health care context is the common law, the basic set of judicially fashioned legal principles that form the foundation of the American legal system.[38] As part of common law, health care professionals and institutions were considered to have no legal duty of care. As private enterprises, they were not considered places of public accommodation in the nature of inns and common carriers; as a result, and regardless of the threat posed, they had no legal obligation either to undertake care[39] or to refrain from discriminatory practices in the selection of their customers.[40]

During the latter half of the 20th century, the "no-duty" principle was legislatively abrogated (i.e., set aside or modified) in certain respects, most notably in state laws related to hospital emergency care and, ultimately, in the case of federal law governing the conduct of hospitals, specifically, the Hospital Survey and Construction Act of 1946 (the Hill Burton Act) and the Emergency Treatment and Labor Act.[41] Earlier, Title VI the Civil Rights Act of 1964 had established a nondiscrimination principle in the case of health care services furnished by private providers receiving federal funds, with a non-statutory exception in the case of private physicians receiving payments under Medicare Part B only.[42] At the same time, Title II of the 1964 Act, which prohibited discrimination by public accommodations, used a definition of public accommodation that did not reach health care

---

[38]Oliver Wendell Holmes, Jr., *The Common Law*, 1881. Available online at http://www.law. harvard.edu/library/collections/special/online-collections/common_law/Contents.php (accessed January 4, 2007).

[39]Many people confuse the concept of a "Good Samaritan" with the no-duty principle. A Good Samaritan is one who undertakes care and who then is held to a lesser duty of care in consideration of his or her good act. The undertaking itself is totally voluntary, however.

[40]Rand Rosenblatt, Sylvia Law, and Sara Rosenbaum, *Law and the American Health Care System* (New York: Foundation Press, 1997; 2001-2002 Supplement), Ch. 1, The impact of U.S. law on medicine as a profession; Sara Rosenbaum, "The impact of United States law on medicine as a profession," *JAMA* 289:1546–1556 (2003).

[41]Rand Rosenblatt, Sylvia Law, and Sara Rosenbaum, *Law and the American Health Care System* (New York: Foundation Press, 1997), Ch. 1, The impact of U.S. law on medicine as a profession.

[42]For a history of how Medicare-participating physicians gained a (nonstatutory) exception from Title VI, see David Barton Smith, *Health Care Divided* (Ann Arbor: University of Michigan Press, 1999). Current legal interpretation of physicians' Part B exemption limits the exemption to physicians participating in "traditional" Medicare, that is, Medicare Part B direct fee-for-service payments only. See, e.g., U.S. Department of Health and Human Services, Office of Civil Rights, *Guidance to Federal Financial Assistance Recipients Regarding Title VI Prohibition Against National Origin Discrimination Affecting Limited English Proficient Persons*. Available at http://www.hhs.gov/ocr/lep/revisedlep.html (accessed November 23, 2006).

services. Most hospitals did, however, receive some form of federal funds (e.g., payments for serving Medicare beneficiaries) and were thereby prohibited from discriminating on the basis of race or national origin.

The ADA fundamentally expanded on this abrogation of the common law by explicitly classifying health care services as a public accommodation. No legislative history accompanies this significant expansion of the concept of "place of public accommodation." Indeed, discussions by the author with persons involved in the drafting of Title III suggests that, perhaps in a sign of the times, by 1990 it simply did not occur to anyone (including the American Medical Association, which supported the law) that health care (which figured prominently in the minds of disability advocates as an example of discrimination and was so identified in the Preamble to the statute)[43] was anything other than a place of public accommodation.

Although it is most frequently cited as the case that established asymptomatic human immunodeficiency virus (HIV) infection as a disability, the U.S. Supreme Court's decision in *Bragdon v. Abbott*[44] is equally powerful for its holding that confirmed that private health care providers are places of public accommodation for the purposes of ADA enforcement. They are thus are prohibited from engaging in conduct considered discriminatory.[45]

Title III of the Act classifies a broad array of conduct as discriminatory: subjecting individuals, either directly or "through contractual arrangements" to a "denial of the opportunity to participate in or benefit from" the goods and services of public accommodations; affording individuals an opportunity to participate that is "not equal" to that afforded other individuals; or to provide qualified individuals with goods, services, or accommodations "different or separate from" that afforded other individuals unless separate or different services are necessary to provide individuals with goods, services, or accommodations as effective as that provided to others.[46]

Importantly, Title III requires only that discriminatory conduct be shown in effect, not as a matter of intent, prohibiting administrative methods that "have the effect of discriminating on the basis of disability" or that perpetuate discrimination.[47] Beyond its general prohibitions, Title III sets forth a detailed list of prohibited activities (many of which transfer easily to health care settings), as well as a series of affirmative defenses that place the burden of proof squarely on a health care facility. For example, it is con-

---

[43]42 U.S.C. §12101(a)(3).

[44]524 U.S. 624 (1999).

[45]Rand Rosenblatt, Sylvia Law, and Sara Rosenbaum, *Law and the American Health Care System* (New York: Foundation Press, 1997), Ch. 1, The impact of U.S. law on medicine as a profession.

[46]42 U.S.C. §12182.

[47]Id.

sidered discriminatory to impose eligibility criteria that would screen out individuals with disabilities (e.g., refusing to provide mental health services to persons who are infected with HIV or who are deaf) unless a facility can show that the criteria are necessary for the provision of the services being offered.[48] Likewise, it would be discriminatory to fail to make "reasonable modifications in policies, practices and procedures" when such modifications are "necessary to afford" services to individuals with disabilities (e.g., offering patient education materials in braille) unless a health care provider can demonstrate that making such modifications would "fundamentally alter" the nature of the service.[49] It also would be discriminatory for a health care facility to fail to treat an individual "in the most integrated setting appropriate to the needs of the individual."[50] It would also be a violation of the Act to "take such steps as may be necessary to ensure" that qualified individuals with disabilities are not "excluded, denied services, segregated or otherwise treated differently than other individuals because of the absence of auxiliary aids and services," unless the facility can demonstrate that such steps would "fundamentally alter" the nature of the service or would "result in an undue burden."[51]

Title III also provides, however, that "nothing . . . shall require an entity to permit an individual to participate" in offered services where the individual "poses a direct threat to the health or safety of others."[52] The term "direct threat" means "a significant risk to the health or safety of others that cannot be eliminated by a modification of policies, practices, or procedures or by the provision of auxiliary aids or services."[53]

Interpretive guidance issued by the U.S. Architectural and Transportation Compliance Board (the "Access Board") sets forth guidelines for the construction and alteration of all facilities and buildings falling within Titles II and III of the ADA, thereby covering both public and private health care facilities.[54] The guidelines specifically discuss the accessibility of medical care facilities, defined as facilities "in which people receive physical or medical treatment or care and where persons may need assistance in responding to an emergency and where the period of stay may exceed 24 hours".[55]

Whether the office of a private health care professional constitutes a

---

[48]42 U.S.C. §12182(b)(1)(A)(i).
[49]42 U.S.C. 12182(b)(A)(ii).
[50]42 U.S.C. §12182(b)(2)(B).
[51]42 U.S.C. 12182(b)(A)(iii).
[52]42 U.S.C. 12182(b)(3).
[53]42 U.S.C. §12182.
[54]Access Board, *ADA Accessibility Guidelines for Buildings and Facilities*. Available at http://www.access-board.gov/adaag/html/adaag.htm (accessed November 23, 2006).
[55]Id.

place of public accommodation governed by the ADA's nondiscrimination and "most integrated setting" provisions was tested in *Bragdon v. Abbott*,[56] which involved the refusal of a dentist to fill a cavity of a person with asymptomatic HIV in his office. In essence, the defendant was charged with administering his dental practice in a discriminatory fashion, and his intent to discriminate was irrelevant. Bragdon's defense was that the patient posed a direct threat, which in turn eliminated his duty of care. The U.S. Supreme Court's decision contains a valuable discussion of the conditions under which health care providers can succeed on a "direct threat" defense.

During the trial, Bragdon attempted to challenge the evidentiary value of universal precautions guidelines of the Centers for Disease Control and Prevention (CDC), which set forth a series of steps that, if adopted by health professionals, would eliminate any "significant" risk associated with the treatment of persons with HIV. Defendant's arguments failed; on appeal, the Court of Appeals treated the CDC guidelines as conclusive evidence of insignificant risk, thereby denying Bragdon the right to mount a "direct threat" defense at all. The Court ruled, however, that although the CDC guidelines carried weight, they were not conclusive and could be challenged for their reliability,[57] leaving the door open to future "direct threat" defenses by public accommodations, even where government guidelines specify the procedures for eliminating a threat. (When the case was remanded for further proceedings on the direct threat defense, Bragdon was unable to prove the existence of a threat or to overcome the presumption of an insignificant threat created by the CDC guidelines).

The ADA defense that a proposed reasonable modification in fact creates an "undue burden" on a defendant is also common in a health care context. The concept of an "undue burden" is a requested modification that poses "significant difficulty or expense."[58] In health care, where the cost of the service is high to begin with and the importance of effective communication is great, the case law suggests some skepticism on the part of courts regarding the claim when the issue is interpreters, although the courts have a greater willingness to consider the defense when removal of architectural barriers in existing construction is the issue.

For example, in *Majocha v. Turner*,[59] the refusal of a pediatric practice to furnish an ASL interpreter during a consultative visit was held actionable, after the practice not only refused to secure translation services but went so far as to send plaintiffs a letter advising them that they were refusing

---

[56] 524 U.S. 624 (1999).

[57] The U.S. Supreme Court remanded the case for further proceedings on the direct threat question, and Bragdon was unable to show evidence to lead the trial court to reject the guidelines.

[58] *Davis v. Flexman* 109 F. Supp 2d 776 (S. D. Oh., 1999).

[59] 166 F. Supp. 2d 316 (W.D. Pa., 2001).

service altogether. The family persisted in its request for an ASL interpreter. Noting that federal guidelines on auxiliary aids specifically recognized the importance of effective communication in a health care context, the ruling of Court of Appeals in this case underscored the high bar faced by health care providers that seek to challenge requested reasonable accommodations under "undue burden" theory.

In contrast, *Mannick v. Kaiser Foundation Health Plan*[60] illustrates the type of factual pattern that can result in an undue burden finding. In *Mannick*, a patient with advanced multiple sclerosis, hospitalized for days in a patient room whose bathroom facilities were not wheelchair accessible, brought suit, alleging a violation of Title III. The hospital in question was an older one, and the issue was the extent to which the defendant, under the less restrictive "readily achievable" standard governing the modification of older facilities, was required to make its patient rooms wheelchair accessible. Noting that "readily achievable in the context of existing and non-modernized construction" meant "easily achievable without much difficulty or expense," the court concluded that cost is a key consideration, as is the nondiscriminatory nature of a defendant's efforts to overcome the problems posed by architectural barriers. In this case, the hospital was able to show that bed baths in lieu of showers, as well as bedside commodes, are techniques used for disabled and nondisabled patients alike.

In sum, Title III of the ADA reaches private health care settings and represents a sweeping and detailed prohibition against discrimination in health care. Because the statute reaches both direct and contractual arrangements, the law applies not only directly to medical care settings but also to corporate health care systems, such as health maintenance organizations, preferred provider organizations, and other managed care entities that arrange for covered services through participating provider networks.[61] Although Title III offers certain affirmative defenses, including fundamental alteration, direct threat, and undue burden, the burden of proof lies with the health care entity.

A recent review of Title III discrimination in health care settings documents the breadth of ADA enforcement actions—initiated by both private parties and government agencies—involving health care providers.[62] The review found that between 1994 and 2003, the U.S. Department of Justice, which has legal enforcement authority under Title III, reported more than 114 health care-related cases involving facility accessibility, accessibility of

---

[60] WL 1626909 (N.D. Ca., 2006).

[61] *Woolfolk v. Duncan*, 872 F. Supp. 1381 (E.D. Pa., 1995).

[62] Judy Panko Reis, Mary Lou Breslin, Lisa Iezzoni, and Kristi Kirschner, *It Takes More Than Ramps to Solve the Crisis of Healthcare for People with Disabilities* (Chicago: Rehabilitation Institute of Chicago, 2004).

equipment, effective communication, and denial of services. The review found actions across numerous health care settings, both office- and institution-based settings. Only a small number involved the denial of care to persons with HIV. Physical barriers affecting people with limited mobility and ineffective communication techniques for people with hearing or vision loss dominated the cases.[63]

A recent settlement by the U.S. Department of Justice and plaintiffs with the Washington Hospital Center similarly shows the breadth of claims that can arise against public accommodations and the nature of remedies that are considered by enforcement agencies to fall within the scope of their powers. The settlement, filed in the fall of 2005, involved an investigation into all phases of hospital operations. The hospital agreed to renovate patient rooms, create new accessible patient rooms, develop and implement barrier removal plans, purchase accessible equipment, review hospital policies and train staff, and appoint an ADA compliance officer.[64]

The Access Board focuses on architectural barriers that arise in the "design, construction, and alteration" of buildings and facilities.[65] The specific obligations of hospital and health care clinics and facilities to adapt their health care services to the needs of patients through the use of specialized equipment and supplies (e.g., appropriate exam tables or modified diagnostic equipment, such as mammography machines suitable for use with patients in wheelchairs) would appear to be precisely the type of interpretive guideline that could be developed by the Office for Civil Rights of the U.S. Department of Health and Human Services, much as that office has developed similar applied guidance governing the provision of translation and interpreter services for persons with limited English proficiency. No such detailed applications of the broad guidelines appear to exist. Additionally, because ADA compliance is a condition of participation in Medicare and Medicaid, the Centers for Medicare and Medicaid Services also would have the authority to establish minimum accessibility standards as a condition of participation in both programs. In general, federal agencies such as the Office of Civil Rights of the U.S. Department of Health and Human Services and the Centers on Medicare and Medicaid Services have been remarkably inactive in using their legal powers either to directly interpret and enforce civil rights laws or to establish conditions of participation in

---

[63]Id., p. 15.

[64]http://www.usdoj.gov/crt/ada/whc.htm (Accessed March 3, 2007)

[65]Access Board, *ADA Accessibility Guidelines for Buildings and Facilities*, §1, Purpose. Available at http://www.access-board.gov/adaag/html/adaag.htm (accessed November 23, 2006).

federal programs that are aimed at the achievement of the broad goals of civil rights legislation.[66]

More Subtle Forms of Discrimination

The fact that physical and hearing access should dominate the U.S. Department of Justice complaint process is not surprising and should not be taken as a sign that perhaps more subtle forms of discrimination aimed at avoiding certain patients does not exist. Overt physical and communication barriers are the most visible forms of discrimination, as are architectural barriers and the failure to promote the accessibility of services through the use of specialized equipment. However, health care entities can engage in other, more subtle forms of discrimination, such as the refusal to serve "disruptive" patients or members of Medicaid managed care plans.[67] Neither the U.S. Department of Justice nor the Office for Civil Rights at the U.S. Department of Health and Human Services maintains written interpretive guidelines related to services to qualified persons with mental disabilities by public facilities or places of public accommodation.

The Interaction Between ADA Violations and Medical Malpractice

In the United States, the failure of health care professionals and institutions to adhere to reasonable standards of health care practice constitutes the basis of liability for medical negligence. Because the ADA reaches conduct that denies equality of opportunity, presumably, medical injuries resulting from a health care provider's failure to make reasonable modifications in accordance with applicable federal requirements could serve as evidence regarding the unreasonableness of the provider's conduct in relation to the professional standard of care, the legal concept against which liability is measured. Thus, for example, the failure of a provider to adapt a health care setting to the needs of patients with physical or hearing disabilities could constitute evidence not only of an ADA violation but also of a violation of state medical liability law.

Although the potential for this type of legal parallelism is mostly speculative, one recent case illustrates how the failure to make reasonable modifications in health care services can lead to medical injury actionable

---

[66]Sara Rosenbaum and Joel Teitelbaum, "Civil rights enforcement in the modern health care system: reinvigorating the role of the federal government in the aftermath of *Alexander v Sandoval*," *Yale J. Health Policy Law Ethics* 3:215–252 (2003).

[67]Sara Rosenbaum, Peter Shin, Marcie Zakheim, et al., *Negotiating the New Health System: A Nationwide Study of Medicaid Managed Behavioral Health Care Contracts*, Vols. 1-2 (Washington, DC: Center for Health Policy Research, The George Washington University Medical Center, 1997).

under state law, as well as federal legal violations. In *Abernathy v. Valley Medical Center*,[68] the hearing impaired patient, who suffered from severe abdominal pain, was unable to receive appropriate emergency care at the defendant hospital because of inadequate accommodations in the form of written notes and a nurse who knew "some" sign language. The court concluded that the claim fell well within the legal standards governing the obligations of hospitals; because medical injury was alleged, the case might have as plausibly been brought as a negligence case. Because the nexus between ADA compliance and the quality of care can be readily seen in the case of medical injury disputes arising from the failure to make reasonable modifications, it is possible to understand ADA compliance as an aspect of health care services risk management.[69]

ADA AND HEALTH CARE COVERAGE AND FINANCING

Overview

As noted earlier, ADA challenges involving health care coverage and financing can be classified into two basic categories: one involving health plan administration and the other involving the underlying design of the health benefit plan or health insurance coverage agreement in question. The first category of challenges encompasses situations in which the allegation is essentially that a plan administrator (e.g., a private health insurer, a self-insuring employer, or a Medicaid agency or its managed care contractor) is implementing the design of its service coverage in a discriminatory fashion. For example, if a plan covers physical therapy services as a broad class of benefit, an administrator's decision to deny coverage in the case of a plan participant with an underlying disability could be held to be discriminatory, since the remedy—excluding unfounded opinion from the interpretation of the meaning of a plan—is a reasonable modification of health plan operations.

The second type of challenge is one in which the content of the coverage itself includes an embedded exclusion. Imagine a benefit plan in which physical therapy is covered, but the terms of the contract limit the coverage to therapy needed to restore the previous range of motion. In such a situation, the plan's very terms discriminate against persons who may need the therapy to attain but not restore lost motion; the content builds discrimination directly into its terms. The former limitation may be actionable under the ADA; the latter is not, because courts have held that to remediate

---

[68]2006 WL 1515600 (W.D. Wash., 2006).
[69]See discussion of the ADA in a quality context in *It Takes More Than Ramps*, op. cit., pp. 1–11.

such limitations involves a fundamental alteration in the terms of coverage themselves.

Crucial to the outcome of insurance cases therefore is whether the courts view the conduct of the insurer or the benefit plan to be one involving design (i.e., the content of insurance) or administration. The preponderance of cases raising discriminatory administration claims appear to involve challenges to state Medicaid administration, presumably because of the disproportionate reliance on Medicaid by persons who are qualified individuals with disabilities. The most important/well-known case of this kind is *Olmsted v. L.C.*, which is considered further below.

Insurance discrimination cases are heavily evidence driven and turn on how courts interpret and apply the ADA and other disability statutes (such as Section 504 of the Rehabilitation Act of 1973) to what they perceive to be the critical facts of the case. Furthermore, because cases are fact driven and depend for their outcome on the application of complex legal standards to equally complex factual situations, the judicial outcome is highly variable. Case law is replete with both winners and losers the outcomes of whose cases were not predicted by observers before the decision.[70]

A basic aspect of insurance design is the definition of medical necessity used in the terms of coverage. In the example given above involving the discriminatory denial of physical therapy, the plan might use a general definition of medical necessity (i.e., care is medically necessary if the evidence shows that furnishing the benefit is consistent with appropriate standards of professional practice). The definition has two meanings; the first meaning is coverage in relation to the overall design of the plan (no coverage for services that are not considered professionally appropriate, such as surgery undertaken for purely cosmetic purposes). The second type involves the application of a medical necessity definition to a specific situation in which a patient seeks an indisputably covered benefit. To return to the physical therapy example, an insurer's informal conclusion that therapy is not medically necessary because persons with disabilities cannot improve is informal, is not compelled by the design of coverage, and does not rest on informed medical judgment.

In fact, both types of medical necessity decisions can involve questions of medical fact and judgment. For example, if an insurer categorically excludes facial reconstruction surgery as cosmetic and therefore not medically necessary, this is not the end of the story potentially. The factual question, which insurance laws would permit on appeal, is whether the procedure

---

[70]Sara Rosenbaum and Joel Teitelbaum, *Olmstead at Five: Assessing the Impact* (Washington, DC: Kaiser Commission on Medicaid and the Uninsured). Available at http://www.kff.org/medicaid/7105a.cfm (accessed July 23, 2006), reviewing post-Olmstead cases decided through spring 2004.

sought by the patient is one whose underlying medical facts would cause a reasonable decision maker to classify the surgery as medical in nature rather than cosmetic. On the other hand, if the coverage agreement specifically excludes breast reconstruction following a mastectomy, there is no appealable issue if the event leading to the reconstruction request is a mastectomy.

In sum, certain types of medical necessity decisions involve purely legal interpretations related to the content of coverage. Appealable cases are those that rest on factual questions to be resolved by a decision maker.

Olmstead and Discriminatory Allocation of Resources Within an Established Plan Design

A signature case in the field of discrimination in the administration of insurance is *Olmstead v L.C.*[71] In *Olmstead*, plaintiffs mounted an ADA Title II claim of discriminatory administration of a public health care financing program. The fact that the public financing scheme involved Medicaid added a critical dimension to the case, since the defendant, the administrator of the public program, could present a theory of the case stating that what plaintiffs sought was more coverage, not fairer administration of existing coverage. The U.S. Supreme Court rejected this view, finding instead that the case involved the discriminatory administration of Georgia's Medicaid program. Nonetheless, once it turned to the remedial question—how to remedy the discriminatory practice of failing to make the state's community benefit coverage accessible to plaintiffs—the Court was forced to confront the problem of coverage design.

The *Olmstead* decision is best known for its eloquent central holding that medically unjustifiable institutionalization constitutes discrimination under Title II of the ADA. In this regard the decision serves as a reminder that even public insurance programs are subject to ADA scrutiny. At the same time, the effort on the part of the *Olmstead* court to parse the remedy so as to avoid the fundamental alteration problems inherent in altering benefit design has led to years of judicial involvement in dozens of similar cases, many of which have had unsatisfactory conclusions from the plaintiffs' viewpoint.

The facts of *Olmstead* are relatively well known. Two Georgia women, who were both qualified individuals with disabilities, received public funding for long-term institutional care but were unable to get the state Medicaid program to cover long-term personal care and other services provided in the community, even though the women's own treating physicians deter-

---

[71]527 U.S. 581 (1999). Note that that the *Olmstead* and *Bragdon* cases occurred in the same term of the U.S. Supreme Court, a not unusual tendency on the part of the Court to take a related series of cases in order to explore the dimensions of a particular body of law.

mined that institutional care was not medically justifiable. The state Medicaid plan covered more than 2000 "home and community based services slots" under a special federal law permitting states to extend home coverage to persons at risk for institutional placement, but the legislature had funded only a fraction of the federally approved services. Federal law permits states to cap the number of placements funded under the state plan, and states are also allowed to limit their request to a certain number of "slots." The trial record showed that Georgia had some 2,100 federally approved slots but funded the state share of the costs at a level sufficient to support only about 700 placements.

Beyond its "unjustifiable institutionalization" holding, the U.S. Supreme Court was then forced to confront a more basic fact: a state Medicaid program that, even if it is properly administered, covered less than the full amount of the community services needed (federal Medicaid law permits states to place a fixed, aggregated cap on the home- and community-based services that they will finance, and while Medicaid spending on community services has increased significantly,[72] coverage is still less than demand). The Court refused to order the state to spend more than its plan specified to ensure appropriate financing of community services up to the level of need,[73] precisely because such a step would have constituted a fundamental alteration of the state's scheme for financing health care for persons with mental disabilities. Instead, the Court set a "reasonable pace" standard, which in practice has operated as a judicial instruction to slowly reallocate spending priorities within an existing benefit design:[74]

> To maintain a range of facilities and to administer services with an even hand, the State must have more leeway than the courts below understood the fundamental-alteration defense to allow. If, for example, the State were to demonstrate that it had a comprehensive, effectively working plan for placing qualified persons with mental disabilities in less restrictive settings, and a waiting list that moved

---

[72]Heidi Reester, Raad Missmar, and Anne Tumlinson, *Recent Growth in Medicaid Home and Community Based Services* (Washington, DC: Kaiser Commission on Medicaid and the Uninsured). Available at http://www.kff.org/medicaid/upload/Recent-Growth-in-Medicaid-Home-and-Community-Based-Service-Waivers-PDF.pdf (accessed November 23, 2006).

[73]The Court of Appeals would have had the state furnish community services to all persons for whom institutional care was unnecessary, so long as the annual per-capita cost of community care was less than the institutional cost. This remedy could have, however, resulted in greater expenditures if persons in need of institutional care moved in to take the place of those living in the community so that the total population of people receiving long-term-care services grew.

[74]Critical to the U.S. Supreme Court's decision was the notion that the entire 2,100 home- and community-based care slots were part of the coverage scheme but were going unused because of discriminatory underfunding of community placements and deliberate overfinancing of institutional care.

at a reasonable pace not controlled by the State's endeavors to keep its institutions fully populated, the reasonable-modifications standard would be met.[75]

Within the context of the ADA, the U.S. Supreme Court arguably did what it could to avoid breaching the limits imposed by the fundamental alteration defense. At the same time, the ambiguous balancing framework set out in its decision has triggered years of challenges by plaintiffs attempting to push states harder to rebalance their spending. Cases have involved both classes of plaintiffs and individual plaintiffs, and the decisions have created a jumble of winners and losers.

In some of the cases, plaintiffs have prevailed because they have convinced the courts that the issue is a state's failure to make an adequate effort to fairly allocate its resources within its existing benefit design. In other cases, plaintiffs have lost because the courts perceive the dispute as one involving demands for more—or faster—community coverage, thereby tipping the case into the realm of fundamental alteration.[76]

A recent decision by the U.S. Court of Appeals in *The ARC v. Braddock*[77] illustrates the difficulties encountered in the *Olmstead* litigation. *The ARC* involved a class challenge to Washington State's investment in community services. The court opened its decision by noting that once again it was navigating "the murky waters between two statutory bodies: the ADA and the Medicaid Act."[78] That action posed the following specific question: whether a state violates the ADA when it limits the number of people that can participate in a Medicaid waiver program providing disabled persons with alternatives to institutionalization."[79]

The specifics of the case focused on Washington State's 10,000-person limit on Medicaid home and community care slots. The U.S. Court of Appeals noted that federal Medicaid law specifically contemplates a cap on slots as a state plan option. The court then proceeded to offer a lengthy and thoughtful explanation that attempted to distinguish between factual situations that raise the issue of unlawful discrimination and those that exhibit compliance with the "reasonable pace" standard. The court noted that *Olmstead* did not force the U.S. Supreme Court to consider lifting the waiver cap because the state had never allocated funds to the slots that were already part of its state plan. The Court of Appeals also noted that in an

---

[75] 527 U.S. 605–606.

[76] *Olmstead at Five*, op. cit.

[77] 427 F. 3d 615 (9th Cir., 2005).

[78] 427 F. 3d 617.

[79] Id.

earlier decision, Townsend v. Quasim,[80] the issue was the improper administration of benefit design when the state forced medically needy individuals into nursing facilities while extending community services to categorically needy persons and was thereby discriminatory on its face. The present case, however, like an earlier case in the same circuit, *Sanchez v. Johnson*,[81] involved the very size of the waiver program. The plaintiffs, in essence, were asking for more services than the state presently covered; and therefore, the court rejected the claim, concluding that the state's deinstitutionalization plan was acceptable in light of the facts surrounding its effort to retool its Medicaid program to more heavily emphasize community-based care. In neither *Sanchez* nor the present case did the mere existence of a cap violate *Olmstead*; instead, the issue was the size of the state's program and the pace at which the state was moving to raise the cap on community coverage. The court's discussion of the facts underscores the tipping point in *Olmstead* cases when challenges to administration become challenges to design:

> Plaintiffs acknowledge that the state's HCBS [home and community-based services] program is capped at 9,977 disabled persons, and the program is operating at capacity. Yet they argue the program is not large enough. . . . The record reflects that Washington's commitment to deinstitutionalization is as "genuine, comprehensive and reasonable" as the state's commitment in Washington's HCBS program is substantial in size, providing integrated care to nearly 10,000 Medicaid-eligible disabled persons in the state. The waiver program is full, and there is a waiting list that admits new participants when slots open up. Unlike in *Townsend*, all Medicaid-eligible disabled persons will have an opportunity to participate in the program once space becomes available, based solely on their mental-health needs and position on the waiting list.

> Further, the size of Washington's HCBS program increased at the state's request from 1,227 slots in 1983 . . . to 9,977 slots beginning in 1998. The annual state budget for community-based disability programs such as HCBS more than doubled from $167 million in fiscal year 1994, to $350 million in fiscal year 2001, despite significant cutbacks or minimal budget growth for many state agencies. During the same period, the budget

---

[80]*Townsend*, discussed in *Olmstead at Five*, involved a challenge to the institutionalization of a man whose monthly income rose by literally a few dollars, but enough to place him just above the cutoff for categorically needy Medicaid coverage and into the realm of the medically needy "spend-down" program. Washington State covered community services for categorically needy persons only, and he was forced to give up his 17-year community residential placement and to enter a nursing home. Despite the fact that institutional versus community services were part of the state's benefit design for Medicaid, the court held that the case involved discriminatory administration of long-term-care assistance and ordered relief. In short, the court flipped a design case into the administration classification.

[81]416 F. 3d 103 (9th Cir., 2005) involving a challenge to the size of California's community care program.

for institutional programs remained constant, while the institutionalized population declined by 20%. Today, the statewide institutionalized population is less than 1,000. . . . We do not hold that the forced expansion of a state's Medicaid waiver program can *never* be a reasonable modification required by the ADA. What we do hold is that, in this case, Washington has demonstrated it has a "comprehensive, effectively working plan," and that its commitment to deinstitutionalization is "genuine, comprehensive and reasonable." [82]

The Ninth Circuit Court thus looked at the rate of growth over time in terms of both funds and services and compared that rate of growth to those of other human services during the same time period. While the court left the door open to future reconsideration, it appears that the pace of investment would have to slow considerably before the Court might be persuaded.

Another helpful exploration of how the balancing test is approached from an evidentiary perspective can be found in *Martin v. Taft*,[83] a case involving a class action by 12,000 persons who alleged that the state was, effectively, doing nothing to help them move into community settings. Plaintiffs sought an order establishing a 5-year remedial time frame. In ordering a trial on the issue of reasonable pace, the court also set out what each side would have to prove.

> The initial burden of demonstrating that a reasonable accommodation is available rests with plaintiffs. Once the plaintiff meets the burden of demonstrating this element, along with the other prima facie elements, the burden then shifts to the State to show that the requested accommodation is not reasonable.[84]

The court went on to note that plaintiffs erred in relying on *Olmstead* for the proposition that waiting lists moving at a reasonable pace constituted the sole means by which defendants could prove the reasonableness of their efforts and resist a faster pace as a fundamental alteration.

> The presence or absence of an existing state plan and a waiting list that moves at a reasonable pace does nothing whatsoever to answer whether, in the first instance, a reasonable modification is available. . . . In addition, as *Olmstead* requires a far more involved inquiry than cost per individual; it directs the Court to consider all of the demands on the State's mental health budget, as well as the State's legitimate interest in maintaining a broad range of services to address the different needs of individuals. . . . [D]efendants must do far more than make *arguments* such as that defendants are not motivated by the desire to keep institutions

---

[82]427 F. 3d 618–621.
[83]222 F. Supp. 940 (S.D. Ohio, 2005).
[84]2222 F. Supp. 2d 986–990.

full. . . . [T]hey must *demonstrate* that making the modifications would fundamentally alter the nature of the existing community-based service program. Failure to carry this burden could result in the entry of judgment in favor of plaintiffs.

In other words, the court rejected the notion that movement toward community services was the only plausible defense and invited defendants to show that other state needs (such the medical need to maintain treatment services) prevented further investment in community services. The trial court went so far as to argue that a state could show that it satisfied the *Olmstead* test even in the absence of any plan or further reasonably paced movement by proving that it already was reasonably accommodating the need for community care, based on the current expenditure of resources. The court then set out the criteria by which it would judge defendants' "fundamental alteration" defense at trial:

1. The resources available to the State; 2. The State's responsibility to care for and treat a large and diverse population of persons with mental disabilities, including those who will require services in an institutional setting; [and] 3. Whether the relief plaintiffs seek would be inequitable given the above considerations.[85]

Other Discriminatory Administration Challenges

In a non-*Olmstead* context, several other Title II discriminatory administration claims have met with success. For example, in *Rodde v. Bonta*[86] the court upheld an injunction against the closure of the Rancho Los Amigos National Rehabilitation Center in Los Angeles County, California, which was part of the county's hospital system. The basis for the injunction against the closure was the county's inability to demonstrate that it had equally appropriate and physically accessible services elsewhere in the system for plaintiffs, all of whom were patients with serious and long-term medical conditions. In effect, the county had made no reasonable accommodation for patients with disabilities prior to instituting a closure plan, thus creating a legal result similar to that for the *Washington Hospital Center* case (which focused on physical and communications accessibility) settlement discussed above.

In addition, a 2003 decision by the U.S. Court of Appeals for the Second Circuit found a violation of the ADA in the manner in which New York City was administering its public programs for persons with HIV and AIDS. As in *Olmstead* case, the court examined the burdens placed upon the plaintiffs in their efforts to secure services used by other populations,

---

[85]222 F. Supp. 2d 986–990.
[86]357 F. 3d 988 (9th Cir., 2004).

with and without disabilities, dependent on public services. The case centered on patient support services that were designed to assist plaintiffs—all persons experiencing AIDS and HIV-related illnesses and in weakened conditions—navigate the welfare system but that, in fact, were never furnished. As in *Olmstead*, the services covered under the New York City plan were available on paper only and were never funded or furnished. In this case, the missing services were patient support and enabling services that made health care accessible and effective.

Challenges to Coverage Design

There are very few cases in which the challenge is directly against coverage design, but the few that do exist underscore that modifying the design of an insurance plan is considered a fundamental alteration. The basic case in the field is *Alexander v. Choate*,[87] a 20-year-old U.S. Supreme Court decision that arose under Section 504 of the Rehabilitation Act of 1973, the predecessor to ADA Title II. Once again, the case involved Medicaid, but this time the challenge was to Tennessee's 14-day annual limit on inpatient hospital care. The essence of the claim was that the 14-day hospital inpatient coverage limit left persons with disabilities with insufficient coverage in light of their greater health care needs. Plaintiffs offered numerous alternatives, specifically, the adoption of a diagnosis-related group-style, per-case limit that varied by diagnosis or condition, recognized length-of-stay "outlier" cases, and averaged payment across more and less expensive patients. In plaintiffs' view, such an alternative, which would have allowed variability linked to underlying condition (e.g., lower payments for less complex cases and higher payments for more resource-intensive cases), would have had a less harsh impact on persons with disabilities. In essence, plaintiffs' theory of the case was that the issue at hand was the means of administering hospital inpatient payments. The appellate court agreed that plaintiffs had made out a prima facie claim and that the burden of proof shifted to states as defendant to offer alternatives or explain why alternatives would be unreasonable. The state appealed.

After ruling that discriminatory intent was not necessary to make out a Section 504 claim, Justice Thurgood Marshall, writing for a unanimous U.S. Supreme Court, made clear that in the Court's view, the claim amounted to a challenge to benefit design, that is, a direct attack on the content of coverage, as well as a request for individually tailored coverage, rather than a case to address discriminatory plan administration. Section 504, the Court held, required only that persons with handicaps (the predecessor term for disabilities) be given meaningful access "to the benefit that

---

[87]469 U.S. 287 (1985).

the [program] offers."[88] Rejecting arguments that the "benefit offered" in this case was inpatient hospital care and that limits on the benefit therefore were a matter of plan administration, the court characterized the 14-day benefit as an embedded aspect of the plan's coverage design itself. The question thus became simply whether all persons, regardless of disability, had equal access to the coverage:

> To the extent respondents further suggest that their greater need for prolonged inpatient care means that, to provide meaningful access to Medicaid services, Tennessee must single out the handicapped for *more* than 14 days of coverage, the suggestion is simply unsound. At base, such a suggestion must rest on the notion that the benefit provided through state Medicaid programs is the amorphous objective of "adequate health care." But Medicaid programs do not guarantee that each recipient will receive that level of health care precisely tailored to his or her particular needs. Instead, the benefit provided through Medicaid is a particular package of health care services, such as 14 days of inpatient coverage. That package of services has the general aim of assuring that individuals will receive necessary medical care, but the benefit provided remains the individual services offered—not "adequate health care."[89]

In essence, the U.S. Supreme Court rejected the effort to equate coverage with adequacy of care and assumed that the equality of treatment standard was met under Section 504 as long as all persons, regardless of handicap, had equal access to whatever coverage was available. It rejected any notion that Section 504 somehow altered the discretion of state Medicaid programs, acting under federal Medicaid law, over matters of benefit design:

> Respondents argue that the inclusion of any annual durational limitation on inpatient coverage in a state Medicaid plan violates § 504. The thrust of this challenge is that all annual durational limitations discriminate against the handicapped because (1) the effect of such limitations falls most heavily on the handicapped and because (2) this harm could be avoided by the choice of other Medicaid plans that would meet the State's budgetary constraints without disproportionately disadvantaging the handicapped. [Section] 504 does not require the changes respondents seek. In enacting the Rehabilitation Act and in subsequent amendments, Congress did focus on several substantive areas—employment, education, and the elimination of physical barriers to access—in which it considered the societal and personal costs of refusals to provide meaningful access to the handicapped to be particularly high. But nothing in the pre- or post-1973 legislative

---

[88]469 U.S. 720.
[89]469 U.S. 721.

discussion of § 504 suggests that Congress desired to make major inroads on the States' longstanding discretion to choose the proper mix of amount, scope, and duration limitations on services covered by state Medicaid.[90]

Later cases considering the same issues—the legality of restrictive benefit design under civil rights law applicable to persons with disabilities—reached the identical conclusion. As noted, by their very nature, the *Olmstead* cases raise questions of benefit design, at least from the viewpoint of defendants, and the cases show the tension that arises as courts struggle with the challenge of how to characterize the claims presented and fashion a remedy.

Perhaps the most significant example of the rejection of benefit design challenges in an ADA context is *Doe v. Mutual of Omaha*,[91] which eliminated any notion that the ADA could be used to challenge benefit design limits. The case opened with this startling introduction:

> Mutual of Omaha appeals from a judgment that the AIDS caps in two of its health insurance policies violate the public accommodations provision of the Americans with Disabilities Act. One policy limits lifetime benefits for AIDS or AIDS-related conditions (ARC) to $25,000, the other limits them to $100,000, while for other conditions the limit in both policies is $1 million. Mutual of Omaha has stipulated that it "has not shown and cannot show that its AIDS Caps are or ever have been consistent with sound actuarial principles, actual or reasonably anticipated experience, bona fide risk classification, or state law." It also concedes that AIDS is a disabling condition within the meaning of the Americans with Disabilities Act.[92]

With this introduction, Judge Richard Posner, one of the nation's most influential jurists and a prominent proponent of markets, proceeded to demolish the argument that the ADA somehow altered the market freedoms enjoyed by insurers, much as Justice Marshall had disposed of any notion that Section 504 in some way altered the basic rules of state Medicaid discretion over coverage design (within federal limits). In an opinion notable for the strength of its tone, the *Mutual of Omaha* case made clear that Title III reaches the physical aspects (such as whether the offices of insurers are physically available), as well as the sale of insurance products to persons with disabilities, but does not reach content.

The majority decision went on to dismiss the very presence of an insurance "safe harbor" as evidence of congressional intent to reach the content

---

[90]469 U.S. 723.
[91]179 F 3d 557 reh.den. (1999); cert. den. *Doe v Mutual of Omaha Ins. Co.* 528 U.S. 1106 (2000).
[92]137 F. 3d 558.

of coverage, despite the fact that the safe harbor on its face sets the standard for distinguishing between lawfully structured product design and design that is not lawful:

> The plaintiffs argue . . . that the insurance exemption has no function if section 302(a) does not regulate the content of insurance policies, and so we should infer that the section does regulate that content. But . . . the industry may have obtained the rule of construction in section 501(c) just to backstop its argument that [Title III] regulates only access and not content. . . . Or it may have worried about being sued . . . for refusing to sell an insurance policy to a disabled person. . . . For Mutual of Omaha to take the position that people with AIDS are so unhealthy that it won't sell them health insurance would be a prima facie violation of [Title III]. But the insurance company just might be able to steer into the safe harbor provided by section 501(c), provided it didn't run afoul of the "subterfuge" limitation, as it would do if, for example, it had adopted the AIDS caps to deter people who know they are HIV positive from buying the policies at all.[93]

SUMMARY

This review suggests that the ADA has made a significant contribution in the realm of physical access to care among persons with disabilities, removing many of the grounds on which a private health care provider or health care system might refuse to accept persons with disabilities into care. The ADA has also had a notable impact on the extent to which public and private health insurers can be held accountable for discriminatory administration. However, once a dispute is understood as being centered on the question of coverage design and content—meaning the amount of benefits, the range of benefits, and the definitions used to allocate benefits—the ADA ceases to offer a remedy, since any modification of coverage design itself arguably becomes a fundamental alteration.

One aspect of this analysis bears further reflection, namely, the notable absence of health care-specific guidelines for use in services and coverage. Such guidelines, even if they are not actively enforced by federal investigators, can serve an immensely useful process in guiding health care service providers and insurers on questions of corporate compliance, a major focus of all health care entities in the modern world. Neither the U.S. Department of Justice nor the U.S. Department of Health and Human Services appears to have used its considerable authority to develop comprehensive guidance tailored to the health care industry that might delineate the stan-

---

[93]137 F. 3d 560.

dards of compliance expected under public programs and public health care accommodations.

The need for such guidance ranges from a clear explanation regarding the meaning of the broad federal rules within health care facilities to an explanation of the types of health benefit administration practices that could be considered discriminatory. While the Access Board sets standards for the modification and construction of facilities, these standards do not speak to internal equipment and operations that play an equal role in access, nor is there language guidance for health services providers in an ADA context that is comparable to the guidance that applies to persons with limited English proficiency. Robust ADA guidance regarding public and private insurance and employee health plan administration is also lacking. At what point do certain practices become discriminatory methods of administration? When would medical necessity decision making, for example, lose its "design" characteristics and become the arbitrary denial of coverage to persons with disabilities? When might the refusal to pay a claim cease being a limitation on coverage and be transformed into the discriminatory withholding of covered benefits because of the patient's disability? The cases—as well as the complexity of health care itself—suggest a need for carefully developed guidelines that help health care corporations understand the meaning of the ADA in both health care and coverage decision making and payment.

ACKNOWLEDGMENT

The author thanks Nancy Lopez for research assistance.

E

The Employment Discrimination Provisions of the Americans with Disabilities Act: Implementation and Impact

Kathryn Moss and Scott Burris*

INTRODUCTION

Signing the Americans with Disabilities Act (ADA) in 1990, President George H. W. Bush described it as an "historic new civil rights Act. . . . the world's first comprehensive declaration of equality for people with disabilities" (National Council on Disability, 2004b, p. 30). Others called it "a watershed in the history of disability rights, . . . the most far-reaching legislation ever enacted against discrimination of people with disabilities" (U.S. Congress, Office of Technology Assessment, 1994). A substantial body of disability law—including the Rehabilitation Act of 1973, the Education for All Handicapped Children Act of 1975 (now known as the Individuals with Disabilities Education Act), the Fair Housing Amendments Act of 1988, and numerous state antidiscrimination disability statutes—was already in place, but the ADA seemed to promise a dramatic change in the place of people with disabilities in American society. The ADA was broader in scope than existing federal laws, prohibiting discrimination not just in employment and public programs but also in public accommodations. It covered private employers and service providers and not just public and publicly funded ones (Miller, 1998). The ADA emerged from Congress with bipartisan support, carrying an explicit promise to people with disabilities of "equality of opportunity, full participation, independent living, and economic self sufficiency." The statute would, it was predicted, significantly af-

*K. Moss, Cecil G. Sheps Center for Health Services Research, University of North Carolina at Chapel Hill. S. Burris, James E. Beasley School of Law, Temple University.

fect "not just persons with disabilities and persons charged with respecting and enforcing human rights, but virtually every segment of our society—*all* Americans" (Gostin and Beyer, 1993. p. xiii).

Measuring the impact of a major civil rights statute is difficult (Donahue and Heckman, 1991). Impact depends upon the complex process of implementation by courts, enforcement agencies, and employers (Blumrosen, 1993; Edelman and Suchman, 1997). "Impact" can take a variety of forms, from increases in wages and employment rates to significant changes in social or organizational norms. The causal role of a civil rights statute is difficult to disaggregate from other social and economic factors, such as labor market conditions generally and government interventions on a number of interrelated fronts (Heckman, 1990). In the case of the ADA's employment provisions, assessment is further complicated by differences between the population defined as disabled in data sources that monitor the employment and economic status of the U.S. population and the narrower group of people whose employment rights are actually protected by the law (Blanck et al., 2003; Burris and Moss, 2000; Kruse and Schur, 2003; Schwochau and Blanck, 2000).

The evidence suggests that the employment effects of the ADA have been, at best, mixed. Many studies find a decline in employment rates among the disabled, a decline which some have attributed to the ADA. Some find that the abysmally low wages of people with disabilities have not changed with the enactment of the ADA and may even have declined. Negative employer attitudes toward the disabled persist. The courts have interpreted the statute narrowly, and enforcement has been flawed. Yet there are also indications that the ADA has helped people with disabilities. Tens of thousands of individuals with disabilities have directly benefited by filing claims under the law. Organizations have adopted new employment practices and policies, and many people with disabilities have gained new leverage in pursuing their career goals. There is evidence that the segment of the disabled population actually protected by the employment provisions of the statute has seen an improvement in employment rates.

This paper summarizes what is known about the effects of the ADA's employment rules. It reviews how the law has been operationalized and how the employment experiences of people with disabilities have changed since its passage. It begins with a brief overview of the ADA's provisions. The next part reviews the evidence for three kinds of effects of the ADA: impact on wages and employment rates, changes in employer attitudes and practices, and the law's empowering effect for people with disabilities. We then turn to a review of how the implementation of the law by courts and administrative agencies and countervailing social welfare policies complicate the assessment of the statute's effectiveness.

THE ADA AND ITS EMPLOYMENT
PROVISIONS: A BRIEF OVERVIEW

The ADA prohibits discrimination against individuals with disabilities (Americans with Disabilities Act of 1990). It is based on and supplements the 1973 Rehabilitation Act and other earlier laws (Feldblum, 2000). The ADA has five sections, referred to in the law as "Titles." Title I contains its employment provisions; the other titles deal with matters that include state and local government services and access to public accommodations.

The ADA's definition of "disability" is a crucial factor in the effort to understand its effects. In general, people are considered disabled for the purposes of the ADA if they satisfy at least one of three criteria: they have "a physical or mental impairment that substantially limits one or more of the major life activities," they have "a record of such an impairment," or they are "regarded as having such an impairment." Title I prohibits employment discrimination only against "qualified individuals with disabilities." A qualified individual with a disability is one who meets the skill, experience, education, and other job-related requirements of a position and who can perform the essential functions of the job under the same conditions as any other worker or with what is known as a "reasonable accommodation" to the disability. "Reasonable accommodations" are defined in Title I as changes to the work environment or process that allow a person with a disability to enjoy equal employment opportunity; they include making facilities accessible, restructuring jobs, modifying work schedules, reassigning the worker to a more suitable position if one is available, and modifying equipment or devices. An accommodation is not considered reasonable if it creates an undue burden for the employer. "Undue burden" includes financial hardship, but also accommodations that are disruptive or that would change the nature or operation of a business.

Title I applies to all employers with 15 or more employees, both private and public, as well as to employment agencies, labor organizations, and joint labor-management committees. It prohibits discrimination against qualified individuals with a disability in any aspect of employment. The prohibition embraces discrimination in job application procedures, hiring, firing, advancement, compensation, fringe benefits, and job training. Inquiries about the existence, nature, or severity of a disability before an individual is hired are prohibited, although an employer may require a medical examination after a job offer has been made if it is required of all new employees, is job related, and is consistent with business necessity.

The enforcement of the ADA differs from title to title (Parry, 1998). Under Title I, individuals who believe that they have been subject to employment discrimination because of a disability may file an administrative charge with the U.S. Equal Employment Opportunity Commission (EEOC) or an equivalent state or local human rights agency. Later, they may file a lawsuit, but only after they have received a "right-to-sue letter" from the agency. Federal law provides that winning plaintiffs can recover attorney's fees from the defendant but offers no guarantee that legal services will be provided or paid for in the prosecution of the suit.

MEASURING THE EFFECTS OF TITLE I

Congress intended the elimination of disability-based employment discrimination to increase the ability of people with disabilities to participate in the labor market on the same basis as others. We consider here several indicators that may be used to measure Title I's success: (1) employment rates and wage disparities, (2) employer attitudes and practices, and (3) "empowerment" effects among people with disabilities themselves.

Employment Rates and Wage Disparities

The results of studies both on what happened to the wage and employment rates of people with disabilities in the decade following the passage of the ADA and whether the ADA was the cause of the various changes that they identified differ (Hotchkiss, 2003). There is consensus that the employment rate declined in the 1990s for people reporting that they had conditions that limit their ability to work, but whether this trend extended to wages or to people more likely to be protected by Title I is still debated. Disagreement starts with whether the most commonly used data sets properly define disability and also extends to more arcane points of study methodology. Analysis is complicated by the changing judicial interpretation of "disability" over time and the fact that in many states people with disabilities had substantial protection from discrimination even before the ADA was passed. These issues are fully discussed elsewhere (Blanck et al., 2003; Kruse and Schur, 2003; Stapleton and Burkhauser, 2003). In this section, we briefly summarize the findings and most significant methodological issues.

Most studies of employment rates use one of three nationally representative data sets: the Current Population Survey (CPS), the National Health Interview Survey, and the Survey of Income and Program Participation (SIPP), all of which define "disability" primarily in terms of a self-reported health condition that limits or entirely prevents an individual from working. The researchers analyzing these data generally agree that the rate of employment for working-aged adults with disabilities declined during the 1990s, not only absolutely but also relative to the rate for those without disabilities (Acemoglu and Angrist, 2001; Burkhauser et al., 2003; DeLeire, 2000; Houtenville and Burkhauser, 2004; Kruse and Schur, 2003; Moon and Shin, 2006; Stapleton and Burkhauser, 2003).

Fewer studies have looked at changes in wages over time. DeLeire analyzed SIPP data for men between 1986 and 1995 and found no significant declines (DeLeire, 2000). Acemogolu and Angrist, using similar methods, analyzed CPS data for men and women between the ages of 21 and 58 years over the same time period and reached the same conclusion (Acemoglu and Angrist, 2001). Moon and Shin, using SIPP data for men between 1990 and 1992, found that the logarithm of the real wages of people with disabilities had declined relative to those of men without disabilities (Moon and Shin, 2006).

Title I's definition of disability excludes people who cannot work (or who require more than a "reasonable" accommodation to do so), and it covers people who have no serious impairment or work limitations but are mistakenly treated as if they had. Thus the employment rate of people with serious work limitations is a flawed indicator of the statute's effect on those whom it was designed to help. A set of questions on the SIPP about functional and activity limitations that do not prevent work allowed Kruse and Schur to investigate changes in a segment of the disabled population that more closely approximates that covered by Title I (Kruse and Schur, 2003). They found that employment rates did decrease in the 1990s for individuals reporting a work disability but that employment rates actually increased for those with functional and activity limitations that do not prevent work (Kruse and Schur, 2003). Disagreement about the validity of studies based on a work-limitation definition of disability persists, even as the Bureau of Labor Statistics works to craft a new definition more compatible with the ADA for use in the CPS (Burkhauser et al., 2002; McMenamin et al., 2006; National Council on Disability, 2004a).

Researchers have tested many explanations for the employment outcomes that they found. They have studied the importance of demographic factors and education (Houtenville and Daly, 2003), changes in the nature of work or in the job market (Stapleton et al., 2003), the changing size and composition of the disabled population (Kaye, 2003), changes in the costs of health care and modes of health care financing (Goodman and Waidmann, 2003; Hill et al., 2003; Yelowitz, 1998), and expansions of the Social Security Disability Income (SSDI) and Supplemental Security Income (SSI) programs, including both lowering of the eligibility requirements and increases in benefits for some recipients (Burkhauser et al., 2001; Houtenville and Burkhauser, 2004). Reviewing these data, two leading researchers concluded that SSDI and SSI expansion had played a more significant role than any other factor, including the ADA (Stapleton and Burkhauser, 2003).

Table E-1 lists the studies that have focused on the effect of the ADA on employment among people with disabilities. Most used the work-limitation definition of disability and depended primarily on the temporal associa-

458

THE FUTURE OF DISABILITY IN AMERICA

TABLE E-1 Studies of the Effect of the ADA on Employment Rates and Wages

Study	Data Source	Time Period	Study Population	Definition of Disability
DeLeire (2000)	SIPP	1986–1995	Men ages 18–64 years with and without disabilities	Work limitation
Acemoglu and Angrist (2001)	CPS	1986–1995	Men and women ages 21–58 years with and without disabilities	Work limitation
Kruse and Schur (2003)	SIPP	1990–1994	Men and women ages 21–58	Classification was based on 14 different SIPP disability measures representing three dimensions: activity limitations, receipt of disability income, and reported ability to work
Beegle and Stock (2003)	U.S. Census	1970, 1980, and 1990	Men and women ages 18–64 years with and without disabilities	Work limitation
Houtenville and Burkhauser (2004)	CPS	1986–1995	Men and women ages 21–58 years with and without disabilities	Work limitation
Jolls and Prescott (2004)	CPS	1988–1998	Men and women ages 21–58 years	Work limitation
Moon and Shin (2006)	SIPP	1990–1992	Men ages 20–62 years with and without disabilities	Classification was based on responses concerning use of a wheelchair or long-term use of a cane, crutches, or a walker; activity limitations; reporting one or more disability conditions; and receiving federal benefits based on an inability to work.

tion between the date of passage (1990) or the effective date (1992) of the ADA's Title I and employment changes to prove causation. Using both simple pre-post and year-by-year analyses, Moon and Shin (2006), DeLeire (2000), and Acemogolu and Angrist (2001) all found robust declines in employment rates: Moon and Shin on the order of 6 percent and DeLeire of 7 percent. Acemoglu and Angrist reported sharp drops in annual weeks of employment for men with disabilities aged 21 to 58 years and women with disabilities under age 40 years. Moon and Shin also found a decline in the logarithm of the real wages of men with disabilities of 5.3 percent relative to that of men without disabilities, although it was significant only at the 0.1 level. Econometric modeling led both DeLeire and Acemoglu and Angrist to attribute the declines specifically to the reasonable accommodation requirement of Title I; Acemoglu and Angrist thought that the reduction in the rates of employment among disabled individuals also reflected employers' expectation of increased lawsuit costs.

The use of a different definition of disability and different time periods leads to different results. Kruse and Schur used 14 different measures of disability from the SIPP that represented permutations along three dimensions (activity limitations, receipt of disability income, and reported ability to work) to facilitate comparisons between people more and less likely to be covered by the ADA (Kruse and Schur, 2003). They found that the subgroup of people most likely to be covered by Title I saw an improvement in employment rates, while for others employment declined.

Houtenville and Burkhauser (2004) replicated the study of Acemoglu and Angrist (2001), testing the sensitivities of different definitions of disability, as well as the effects of different periods of time. They confirmed that the employment rate for people with a work limitation did indeed decline when the rate was measured by the annual number of weeks that an individual worked during one calendar year. The use of a 2-year time period, however, suggested that employment began to decline in the mid-1980s and actually sharply improved in 1992 for some age-sex categories. They concluded that there was "little evidence of a negative effect of the ADA on the population with longer term disabilities and some evidence of a positive effect of the ADA" (Houtenville and Burkhauser, 2004, p. 7).

All the studies that have attempted to test the impact of the ADA by temporal association with national trends in employment and wages suffer from the same flaw: many states had laws against discrimination on the basis of disability before the ADA came into effect, so we cannot assume that the implementation of Title I represented a change in the rules for all employers and workers. Two studies specified state-law variables that made it possible to compare the rates of employment and wages for people with disabilities in states with and without various ADA-like disability protections at the same points in time.

Beegle and Stock compared state-level employment conditions for people with disabilities at three points, in 1970, 1980, and 1990. Because all three times were before the time of the implementation of the ADA, it should be understood that the study used similar state laws as a proxy for the federal statute (Beegle and Stock, 2003). They found that disability discrimination laws were associated with lower relative earnings among disabled individuals and with slightly lower rates of relative labor force participation rates among disabled individuals. However, once they controlled for differential time trends in employment among disabled and nondisabled individuals, there was no systematic negative relationship between the laws and the relative employment rates of disabled individuals. Of course, this also suggests that there was no substantial *positive* impact of state disability discrimination laws.

Jolls and Prescott studied states with three different legal conditions between 1990 and 1993: states with no protections comparable to the ADA, in which the ADA would represent an entirely new influence; "protection without accommodation" states, whose law prohibited employment discrimination against people with disabilities but did not require reasonable accommodation; and "ADA-like" states, whose protections for the employment rights of people with disabilities both prohibited discrimination and required reasonable accommodation (Jolls and Prescott, 2004). They found that employment rates for disabled individuals began to decline in 1993 relative to pre-ADA levels in all three categories of states. The extent to which the ADA was new law made no significant difference, making it difficult as a general matter to attribute the declines to employers' reaction to new legal requirements.

The design of the study of Jolls and Prescott (2004) allowed them to test the effects of specific ADA mandates. They found that the employment rates of individuals with disabilities fell 10 percent in the early days of the ADA in "protection without accommodation" states compared with that in states that already had full "ADA-like" statutes, indicating that the reasonable accommodation requirement had an independent negative effect on employment. Yet they also found little or no differences between pre- and post-ADA employment rates among people with disabilities in states that had had no protection before, indicating that the ADA did not have a significant impact in states where it brought entirely new mandates. Considering other important confounding variables—including the size of the employer covered, differences between states in eligibility for disability benefits and the amounts of disability benefits, states' economic environments, and preexisting state group-specific trends in employment rates among disabled individuals—Jolls and Prescott concluded that apart from a short-term effect of the new reasonable accommodation requirement, there was no link between the ADA and the employment declines experienced by people with disabilities starting in 1993 and continuing forward (Jolls and Prescott, 2004).

Employer Practices and Attitudes

The ADA requires employers to eliminate discriminatory practices and promote equal opportunity by making reasonable accommodations for workers with disabilities. We can assess the impact of the ADA on employment by asking what employers have done to comply with the law and whether there is evidence that the attitudes of employers to people with disabilities have improved. Existing data show a high level of awareness of the law and substantial compliance activity. They do not shed much light on the sincerity or the effectiveness of employer efforts and suggest that negative attitudes toward disabled people persist.

At the time of enactment, many employers were uninformed about the ADA and had significant concerns about the costs that it was going to impose. This seems to have changed rather quickly. More durable has been the negative attitudes about people with disabilities, especially those with certain types of disabilities (Bruyere et al., 2006; Greenwood and Johnson, 1987). Employers feel more positively about people with physical or sensory disabilities than they do about people with psychiatric or cognitive disabilities (Baldwin, 1992; Scheid, 2005). There is less acceptance of people whose disabilities are perceived as having been caused by factors under their control than for "innocent" victims (for example, there is less acceptance of a person paralyzed in an accident caused by her own drinking than of a person paralyzed by the actions of a drunken stranger) (Bruyere et al., 2006; Hazer and Bedell, 2000; Mitchell and Kovera, 2006).

Given the poor empirical correlation between attitudes about disabled people and actual employer behavior (Bruyere et al., 2006), attitude studies may be more suggestive of the complexity of workplace decision making and the need for further research than conclusive about the employer response to the ADA. Organizations have historically made changes in policies, procedures, and organizational structures in response to a new national civil rights law (Edelman and Suchman, 1997). Organizational compliance actions create the environment in which managers make decisions about hiring, promotion, and accommodation. Perceptions of organizational adherence to the ADA have been found to be a better predictor of how managers put the ADA into practice than their personal attitudes about people with disabilities (Thakker and Solomon, 1999). Larger employers typically respond to antidiscrimination laws by creating policies and internal equal employment opportunity offices to help the organization draw the line between legal and illegal behavior and to minimize and resolve discrimination disputes. In a 1998 survey of human resource managers, 72 percent reported that their companies had formal procedures for requesting reasonable accommodations and presenting grievances (Bruyere, 2000). Employers too small to support a separate human resources or equal employment opportunity staff may respond to antidiscrimination law in less formal but still important ways (Barnes and Burke, 2006).

Aside from a number of small surveys, qualitative studies, and dissertations (Blackburn, 2003; Harlan and Robert, 1998; Unger, 1999), the best evidence on the organizational response to the ADA comes from a series of large probability surveys of human resources managers conducted by Bruyere and colleagues at Cornell University (Bruyere et al., 2006). General awareness of the law was high, with a large majority (80 to 90 percent) of both federal and private respondents reporting that they had received training in specific elements of the law, particularly reasonable accommodation and nondiscrimination in hiring (Bruyere, 2000).

Title I puts considerable emphasis on reasonable accommodation as an instrument for workplace inclusion, making the extent to which employers provide accommodations a good measure of compliance. Bruyere's surveys tracked 10 types of accommodations, including changes in accessibility, transportation, supervisory methods, and job requirements. The research found overall that most employers were making accommodations of all types, but there were important variations. As an employer, the federal government was substantially more likely to report the provision of accommodations of virtually every kind than private employers (Bruyere, 2000), and large employers reported a greater use of accommodations than smaller ones (Bruyere et al., 2006). The differences between federal and private employers and between small and large employers were largely accounted for by those that reported that they had never been asked for an accommodation but may also reflect a greater emphasis on compliance within the federal government. A lack of requests for accommodation could indicate an unsupportive environment, employee unfamiliarity with their rights, or the use of informal, undocumented accommodations in smaller workplaces. For all employers, physical accessibility, workplace or tool reconfiguration, and policy change accommodations were more common than changes in training, supervisory methods, or job structure (Bruyere, 2000).

Most federal government (95 percent) and private (82 percent) employers reported that they had made facilities more accessible. There were sharper differences in other areas. Government employers were twice as likely to report providing communication access to the hearing impaired (91 percent versus 43 percent) or visually impaired (77 percent versus 37 percent). Less than half of employers, federal or private, had provided flexible test-taking procedures or a scent-free environment, but most employers that did not provide these accommodations reported that no one had ever asked for them (Bruyere, 2000). A similar pattern and explanation emerged in studies comparing large and small private employers, with smaller employers consistently less likely to report various compliance activities (Bruyere et al., 2006).

The ADA requires a large number of changes in routine procedures that can also be used to mark employer compliance. Brueyere tracked 10 indicators in the hiring process, ranging from changing where recruiting was conducted to overcoming communication barriers with technology or interpreters and complying with restrictions on obtaining information about medical examinations and medical histories. As with the provision of reasonable accommodations after a disabled individual is hired, employers were much more likely to make what they reported to be "easy" changes, like ensuring physical accessibility in the interview site, than to take on communication barriers. Again, the federal government as an employer was much more likely to report providing these accommodations than private employers, apparently because private employers were less aware of how to overcome communication barriers.

A survey focusing on the private-sector use of adaptive information technologies found that less than half of the respondents reported that their organizations had experience in modifying a computer to make it accessible to an employee with a disability (Bruyere et al., 2005). Respondents employed by large organizations were more likely than those employed by small organizations to report familiarity with assistive technology and accessible web designs and to report that their organizations had made modifications to computers and adaptations to workstations. In general, however, there was a low level of familiarity with assistive technology. Almost half (46 percent) were familiar with screen magnifiers, approximately one-third were familiar with speech recognition software, about one-fourth were familiar with video captioning, about 20 percent were familiar with braille readers/displays, about 16 percent were familiar with screen readers, and only 13 percent were familiar with accessible web design.

These studies leave little doubt that employers are generally aware of the ADA and have taken steps to meet its requirements. They show that employers are making accommodations in hiring processes and in the workplace. The studies do not allow confident conclusions to be made about how well these measures are being implemented and the extent to which people with disabilities have benefited or perceived any benefits. Bruyere's respondents report that negative attitudes and a lack of information still stand as barriers to the hiring and retention of workers with disabilities and that smaller employers may need more help to understand and implement the law's requirements. More research is also recommended (Bruyere et al., 2006).

Empowerment Effects

The ADA could have a positive impact by empowering workers with more tools for achieving their goals or vindicating their rights. Filing an ADA complaint is one way in which people can use the law to defend their rights. More than 200,000 workers filed discrimination claims under ADA in the decade after the statute was passed (Moss et al., 2005), but research on how people "use" the law would predict that only a small minority of people with disabilities will invoke the ADA to deal with discrimination.

People often use a language of rights to define their social goals and position, and disadvantaged groups and their advocates often see the defining of rights as a policy solution to social problems. At the same time, research has consistently shown that Americans are loathe to sue (Felstiner et al., 1980-1981; Galanter, 1983) and that civil rights laws are among the least often invoked (Curran and Spalding, 1974; Engel and Munger, 2003). Research on the ADA suggests that people with disabilities conform to this pattern of law avoidance not simply because they are unaware of the law or are unable to get a lawyer but because filing a complaint implicates a variety of deep social and psychological issues (Engel and Munger, 2001; Moss et al., 2005; Studdert, 2002).

Just as organizations may comply with the law without active enforcement, individuals may "rely" on the law in their own strategies for daily living without formally invoking it (Burris and Moss, 2000). An important study by Engel and Munger explored this in the context of the ADA. Detailed life-history interviews with 60 people with a variety of disabilities found at least three ways in which the ADA was changing their lives, apart from litigation:

> First, rights can change the self-perceptions of individuals with disabilities, enabling them to envision more ambitious career paths by incorporating in their plans the reasonable accommodations and the nondiscriminatory treatment guaranteed by the ADA. . . . Second, ADA rights become active through cultural and discursive shifts even when rights do not directly transform an individual's self-perceptions. By becoming part of everyday speech, thought, and action, ADA rights affect the way others perceive individuals with disabilities as employees. . . . Third, ADA rights may become active through institutional transformations that are not directed at any particular individual. . . . [R]ights are sometimes implemented unilaterally by . . . employers, rather than through advocacy by the rights-bearers themselves (Engel and Munger, 2003, pp. 243–244).

While these "empowerment effects" are difficult to quantify, they must be seen as among the most important forms of impact that a civil rights law can have. Although the Engel and Munger study is qualitative, it offers intriguing suggestions that the ADA may be working through these mechanisms. Bruyere's work and some unpublished studies have found signs that people with disabilities are reluctant to ask for accommodations (Baldridge, 2002; Bruyere, 2000; Frank, 2004). Further research along these lines would be valuable.

RETHINKING THE "CAUSE" OF THE EFFECTIVENESS OF TITLE I

Relating changes in the employment situations of people with disabilities to Title I is not a straightforward matter. We can, however, reduce the uncertainty and guide reasonable inferences about cause and effect by clearly specifying how the ADA has been applied and identifying factors that might be confounding its intended effects. In this section we discuss several key factors: judicial interpretation of the statute's terms, how the law has been implemented in courts and administrative enforcement agencies, and the problem of countervailing social welfare policies.

Title I in the Courts: Narrowing the Protected Class

Title I did not purport to provide legal protection of employment opportunity to everyone with a disability but does provide legal protection of employment opportunity to those who meet its definition of a "qualified person with a disability." Many proponents of the ADA have argued that Congress intended the definition to be liberally applied, as it had been under the earlier Rehabilitation Act, so that even substantial accommodations would be deemed "reasonable" to encourage the inclusion of people with disabilities who have low levels of functioning and so that "impairment" and "major life activity" would be liberally construed to ensure that qualified people did not suffer employment discrimination simply because of prejudice, fear, or outdated stereotypes (Burgdorf, 1991, 1997; Feldblum, 2000). Over the last 15 years, however, the U.S. Supreme Court has led the federal courts in interpreting Title I narrowly (National Council on Disability, 2004b). We summarize the main rulings and then review the data on case outcomes.

Supreme Court Decisions: Narrowing the Protected Class

Membership in the protected class, a virtual nonissue under other discrimination statutes in which a plaintiff's status is obvious (for example, race or gender under Title VII of the Civil Rights Act of 1965 or age under the Age Discrimination in Employment Act), has been the single most litigated issue in ADA cases. Even under prior law, the status of a plaintiff as "disabled" was required to be determined in an "individualized inquiry," but as the ADA case law developed, the notion that disability determinations must be made on a case-by-case basis took on a decisive importance (Feldblum, 2000; *Albertson's, Inc. v. Kirkingburg*, 1999). Under this approach, a *person* is found to be disabled; conditions are not categorically disabilities. Thus it is not enough for the plaintiff to show that he or she has a condition, such as epilepsy or carpal tunnel syndrome, that as a general matter is plainly a disability. Rather, he or she must prove to the court exactly how this condition constitutes a substantial limitation of a major activity in his or her own life and yet does not prevent him or her from doing the job.

Many conditions—such as diabetes, hypertension, and depression—have been found to meet the definition of impairment under the law but are controllable through medication so that, at least most of the time, their effects on daily life are minimal. In a trio of important cases involving nearsightedness, hypertension, and monocular vision, the U.S. Supreme Court held that mitigating, or corrective, measures should be considered in determining whether an individual has a disability under the ADA (*Sutton v. United Airlines, Inc.*, 1999; *Murphy v. United Parcel Service*, 1999; *Albertson's, Inc. v. Kirkingburg*, 1999). Under this interpretation, an employer may discriminate against someone because he or she has, say, diabetes, but as long as the victim is successfully controlling the condition with medication he or she has no recourse under the ADA. Of course, if the employee is *not* controlling the condition, he or she not only suffers symptoms but may find him- or herself excluded from the ADA because he or she is too impaired to do the job even with a reasonable accommodation.

The U.S. Supreme Court also took a narrow view of the "regarded as" prong of the definition. In older cases under the Rehabilitation Act, the Supreme Court attributed this prong to Congress's concern with protecting the disabled against discrimination stemming not only from simple prejudice but also from "archaic attitudes and laws" and from "the fact that the American people are simply unfamiliar with and insensitive to the difficulties confront[ing] individuals with handicaps" (*School Board of Nassau County v. Arline*, 1987). In the *Sutton* and *Murphy* cases, however, the Court introduced what amounts to a rather difficult "intent" element into the inquiry. It required the employee to show not only that the employer regarded the employee as unable to do the job at issue because of disability but also that the employer has essentially thought out its decision in terms of the primary definition of disability. In *Sutton*, the court ruled against plaintiffs barred from serving as pilots for failing to meet vision requirements that they argued were more stringent than necessary:

> Petitioners have failed to allege adequately that their poor eyesight is regarded as an impairment that substantially limits them in the major life activity of working. They allege only that respondent regards their poor vision as precluding them from holding positions as a "global airline pilot." . . . Because the position of global airline pilot is a single job, this allegation does not support the claim that respondent regards petitioners as having a substantially limiting impairment (*Sutton v. United Airlines, Inc.*, 1999, pp. 492–493).

The mechanic involved in the *Murphy* case had been doing his job with excellent performance ratings for years but was fired because his hypertension barred him from getting the U.S. Department of Transportation truck-driver's license that his employer generally required mechanics to possess.

Murphy showed that he had not actually needed to drive in his work but failed to show that the employer "regarded him" as disabled because there was no evidence that the employer thought that he was too disabled to do any job other than the one that required the license. In both cases, people were fired because of impairments that the employer believed precluded them from doing the job that they had but were not protected by the ADA because they could not prove the employer thought about their fitness for a wide range of other, similar jobs.

The U.S. Supreme Court's rulings have restricted the definition in other significant ways. In *Toyota v. Williams*, there was no dispute that the plaintiff had suffered from carpal tunnel syndrome for many years; had changed job assignments several times because of it; and had trouble with basic manual tasks like gardening, dressing herself, and housework. In holding that her impairment did not substantially limit a major life activity, the Court ruled that "substantially" excluded "precludes impairments that interfere in only a minor way" with the activity and narrowed "major life activity" to mean one that is "of *central importance* to daily life" (*Toyota Motor Manufacturing of, Kentucky, Inc. v. Williams*, 2002, p. 197 [emphasis added]). Despite her undisputed impairment and the demonstrable limitations that it created, the plaintiff failed to qualify as disabled because "she could still brush her teeth, wash her face, bathe, tend her flower garden, fix breakfast, do laundry, and pick up around the house" (*Toyota Motor Manufacturing of Kentucky, Inc. v. Williams*, 2002, p. 202).

For many people with disabilities, medication, devices, adaptability, and sheer grit can mean that they are not in fact substantially limited in the activities of daily life. For them, the real barrier to participation in employment may be prejudice or stereotypes, meaning that when they suffer discrimination the only "major life activity" that their impairment has limited is work itself, and then only because of the attitudes or actions of others. Under prior law and in the early days of the ADA, "working" seemed to be well accepted as a major life activity, but in the *Sutton, Murphy*, and *Williams* cases, the U.S. Supreme Court cast serious doubt on this, suggesting that if the only activity impaired is working, the plaintiff will need to show that he or she is "unable to work in a broad class of jobs" (*Sutton v. United Airlines, Inc.*, 1999; *Murphy v. United Parcel Service*, 1999; *Toyota Motor Manufacturing of, Kentucky, Inc. v. Williams*, 2002). In the words of the National Council on Disability, "[t]here are extensive examples of situations in the case law in which plaintiffs have been fired, refused employment, or otherwise disadvantaged in the workplace because of their actual or perceived impairments but have been unable to bring ADA actions because they could not meet what one federal court of appeals called the 'weighty showing' of demonstrating that they would be precluded from a class or broad range of jobs" (National Council on Disability, 2004b).

Lower Court Decisions: Few Plaintiff Victories

The effect of narrowing U.S. Supreme Court and courts of appeals rulings can clearly be seen in the outcomes of reported ADA cases. A series of annual studies conducted by the editors of the *Mental and Physical Disability Law Reporter* has analyzed Title I final case decisions in federal courts (Allbright, 2001, 2002, 2003, 2004, 2005; Parry, 1998, 1999, 2000). The studies have highlighted how rarely plaintiffs secure a favorable court judgment or jury verdict in published ADA case decisions. Taking into account reversals on appeal, the plaintiff success rate in these cases ranged from just under 8 percent between 1992 and 1997 to as low as 3 percent from 2002 to 2004. Colker's study of published appellate decisions found that courts ruled in favor of defendants 94 percent of the time (Colker, 2001). Courts of appeals reversed prodefendant outcomes in trial courts only 21 percent of the time in Title I cases, whereas the rates were 26 to 48 percent in other types of cases that Colker reviewed. There was a similar gap in appellate reversals of trial court decisions in favor of plaintiffs: in ADA cases, plaintiff trial court victories were reversed 60 percent of the time, whereas the range was 33 to 52 percent in other kinds of cases. Only prisoners challenging their conditions of confinement were more likely than Title I plaintiffs to have a win reversal (69 percent) (Colker, 2001).

Case Outcomes Through Settlements: Benefits for Many Plaintiffs

While the studies of published Title I decisions demonstrate the impact of the narrow judicial interpretation of the law, reported case decisions are not a reliable indicator of overall outcomes, because most lawsuits are settled without a reported decision. Because settlements are voluntary, we presume that most of them entail some sort of payment or other benefit to the plaintiff. Moss and colleagues collected data from federal court files on a nationally representative sample of 4,114 lawsuits filed between 1993 and March 31, 2001, and linked the cases with administrative data obtained from the EEOC (Moss et al., 2005). Of the 3,624 federal court cases with identifiable outcomes, 2,219 (61 percent) were classified as settlements.[1] These findings are consistent with an earlier study of ADA cases in one judicial district (Rulli, 2000). The study confirmed that plaintiffs lose most cases that are decided by a judge on motions to dismiss or for summary judgment. Its finding that in ADA cases plaintiffs whose cases go to trial

---

[1]This included 1,397 cases (38.5 percent) in which the docket explicitly mentioned settlement and 822 (22 percent) in which settlement was inferred from the docket file information as a whole. Combining court rulings and settlements, the researchers found that up to 62 percent (n = 2,266) of the sample lawsuits may have brought some benefit to plaintiffs. For more details of the analysis, see the work of Moss et al. (2005).

do as well as plaintiffs in other civil rights cases supports the view that the narrow definition of disability is the main doctrinal factor driving the low success rate for plaintiffs.

The study of Moss et al. (2005) also indicated that the vast majority of people eligible to file a Title I lawsuit in federal court did not invoke this right. During the period covered by the study, 201,371 Title I charges filed with the EEOC or state or local fair employment practice agencies (FEPAs) were not resolved to the charging parties' satisfaction and were therefore eligible to be filed as lawsuits. The researchers estimated that only 27,725 lawsuits were actually filed, meaning that up to 87 percent of employment claims filed with state and federal agencies were abandoned without a resolution. The administrative process does serve a screening function, sparing the courts the labor of dealing with unsupported allegations, but the sheer volume of abandoned cases points to another important set of problems in the implementation of Title I, to which we turn next.

The Title I Enforcement System: Implementation Problems

Title I is enforced by the same agencies and under the same procedures as the nation's other employment discrimination laws. People who believe that they have been discriminated against in employment on the basis of a disability may file an administrative charge with the EEOC or a state or local FEPA that contracts with the EEOC, which initiates an administrative dispute resolution process. If the administrative process fails to produce a satisfactory result, the worker can file an ADA lawsuit in state or federal court. The effectiveness of this enforcement system has been weakened by chronic underfunding of the EEOC in the face of ever growing workloads (Moss et al., 2001).

The Administrative Charge Process

The EEOC has primary enforcement authority for Title I. It contracts with state and local FEPAs to help with receiving and investigating employment discrimination charges. In theory, each case is investigated by the agency to the point at which it is settled or it is determined that the charge is supported or not supported by "reasonable cause" to believe that discrimination has occurred. Individuals who want to get to court as quickly as possible can short-circuit the administrative process by asking for a "right to sue" letter. The EEOC can take unresolved cases to court itself, alone or in collaboration with a complainant's own attorney.

In fact, the EEOC has never been able to investigate all, or even most, complaints. It has had a backlog of cases since the earliest days, a backlog that by 1993, 1 year after Title I took effect, had reached 96,945 cases

(Moss et al., 2001; U.S. Government Accountability Office, 2005). Shortly after the ADA was enacted, the EEOC tried to deal with its backlog with a new system of intake triage. Based on the complainant's initial submission, new cases were separated into three categories: clearly meritorious (Category A) cases, clearly unsupported (Category C) cases, and cases whose merits could be determined only after further investigation (Category B). The agency made substantial progress in reducing case processing time, decreasing the inventory of charges awaiting resolution, focusing investigative resources onto cases it believed to be strong, increasing its rate of "reasonable cause" determinations, and increasing the monetary benefits received by charging parties. By September 2000, 149,123 charges had been filed and resolved with the EEOC under the ADA, with median benefits of $6,000 per closure.

The new system is efficient, but has never been validated for accuracy. The C categorization is probably the most reliable because it depends upon objective factors like whether the employer has enough workers to be covered by the ADA. About 25 percent of cases are classified as Category C and quickly dismissed. Categorization as a Category A case requires more of a "feel" for the facts that make for a strong case. About 17 percent of cases are put in Category A. The problem with Category B is that inclusion rests on the classifier's inability to assess the case's merits without further fact finding, and most cases (57 percent) are rated Category B. Because of insufficient staff resources, most Category B cases and even some Category A cases are never seriously investigated, so the fate of a complaint hangs on a subjective rating based on only the information that the complainant is able to articulate. Not surprisingly, good outcomes—settlements with benefits and reasonable cause findings—are highly correlated with the original classification decision. In spite of a very successful mediation program targeted at Category B cases (Moss et al., 2002), the majority of possibly meritorious ADA claims filed with the EEOC and FEPAs are never investigated or resolved.

Access to Legal Services

People do not need to retain an attorney to file a claim with the EEOC or a FEPA, nor does having an attorney during the administrative process raise the chances of resolving the case (Moss et al., 2001). The overall benefit rate for individuals with attorneys (17.2 percent) was nearly identical to the overall benefit rate for individuals without attorneys (17.1 percent). Having an attorney does have a significant effect on the size of monetary settlements. Median actual monetary benefits for individuals with attorneys were significantly higher ($19,750) than those for individuals without attorneys ($4,482). Median projected monetary benefits (mainly "front pay" or wage increases) were $19,500 for represented parties, whereas they were $16,200 for individuals without attorneys.

An inability to get legal help is probably one of the most important factors in the huge rate of claim abandonment between the administrative and judicial systems. People with attorneys during the EEOC/FEPA stage had significantly higher right-to-sue resolutions (31.4 percent) than individuals without attorneys (7.4 percent). Most (85 percent) Title I plaintiffs in federal court suits have attorneys, and those with attorneys had much better court results. The proportion of cases that were settled or decided for the plaintiff was about three times higher among plaintiffs who were represented by an attorney than among those representing themselves (68 versus 23 percent ($p < 0.0001$]) (Moss et al., 2005).

ADA Complainants with Psychiatric Disabilities

Among the most troubling findings of ADA implementation research has been a difference in experiences and outcomes for people with psychiatric disabilities. People with psychiatric disabilities were less likely than people with other disabilities to have a case classified as Category A by the EEOC and less likely than other to have a case resolved with benefits, even when categorization is controlled for (Moss et al., 2001; Ullman et al., 2001). They were slightly but significantly less likely to be referred by the EEOC to mediation, and employers were significantly less likely to agree to take part (Moss et al., 2002).

Once they were in court, people with psychiatric disabilities were significantly less likely than people with other disabilities to feel that they were "treated with respect," that the judge was "fair to both sides," and that they were satisfied overall with their experience of filing a lawsuit. These differences in perception corresponded to actual differences in the outcomes of the lawsuits filed by the two groups of plaintiffs. Plaintiffs with psychiatric disabilities were only half as likely as those with other disabilities to receive a settlement or favorable court decision, even when important cofactors, such as health status, education, and having a lawyer, were controlled for (Swanson et al., 2006). The data raise the possibility of "justice disparities" in the ADA enforcement system, that is, durable differences in outcomes between cases brought by people with psychiatric disabilities and those brought by people with other disabilities that are not attributable to differences in the legal and factual merits of the cases.

Countervailing Policies

For people whose disabilities are severe enough to place them on the margins of employability, the effects of Title I may be blunted by other elements of national disability policy. Expansion of eligibility for federal Social Security programs[2] made it easier for marginally employable people to get income and health benefits, a phenomenon that some believe was the main driver of the declining employment rates among the disabled in the 1990s (Stapleton and Burkhauser, 2003). Eligibility for these programs required leaving the workforce and proving that one was unable to engage in any substantial gainful activity. Historically, people receiving benefits under these programs encountered substantial disincentives to going back to work. Workers returning to low-wage or part-time work faced the prospect of earning less than they received in benefits. Because Medicare/Medicaid benefits were tied to social security disability eligibility, going back to work could also mean a gap in or total loss of health insurance (Stapleton et al., 2005). Court decisions under the ADA added another wrinkle: Defendants in discrimination cases may use an individual's application for or acceptance of disability benefits as evidence that the individual is not "otherwise qualified" to work and therefore not protected from discrimination (*Cleveland v. Policy Management Systems Corp.*, 1999).

The government has acted in recent years to reshape Social Security to encourage beneficiaries to return to work and assist them with doing so. Legislation has expanded eligibility to programs that allow people to work and still receive benefits for a time, that allow increased access to vocational rehabilitation programs, that give state Medicaid administrators greater leeway to cover people returning to work from disability, that defer medical eligibility reviews for people trying to return to work, and that have funded advocacy organizations to improve communication between individuals with disabilities and state agencies (Ticket to Work and Work Incentives Improvement Act of 1999). Research is under way to assess the implementation and outcomes of these initiatives.

CONCLUSIONS

Despite widespread perceptions (or assertions) that Title I has not "worked," the empirical picture is fuzzy and mixed. People with disabilities continue to have lower employment rates than other Americans, but whether this is because of or in spite of the ADA is not known. There is evidence that the law improved employment rates for the portion of the disabled population most clearly protected by Title I. Employers know about and are implementing the law but continue to have negative attitudes toward people with disabilities. There is no doubt that the ADA has been

---

[2]SSDI provides cash benefits and Medicare benefits for disabled workers. SSI is a needs-based program for adults and children ineligible for SSDI; it typically triggers eligibility for Medicaid (Social Security Advisory Board, 2006).

narrowly interpreted by courts and imperfectly enforced by administrative agencies and the judicial system.

In the face of these findings, it is useful to heed the reminder that "Legal protections from discriminatory practice are probably indispensable, but such guarantees cannot be the only strategy toward ending the discrimination and social exclusion faced by Americans with disabilities" (Scotch, 2000, p. 222). The ADA stands as a long-term commitment to integrating people with disabilities into the mainstream of American life. The agencies, courts, lawyers, and employers responsible for fulfilling the U.S. Congress's promise can do better and do more, but only in the context of a broader social change in attitudes about and behavior toward people with disabilities.

REFERENCES

Cases

Albertson's, Inc. v. Kirkingburg, 527 U.S. 555 (1999)
Cleveland v. Policy Management Systems Corp., 526 U.S. 795 (1999)
Murphy v. United Parcel Service, 527 U.S. 516 (1999)
School Board of Nassau County v. Arline, 480 U.S. 273 (1987)
Sutton v. United Airlines, Inc., 527 U.S. 471 (1999)
Toyota Motor Manufacturing, Kentucky, Inc. v. Williams, 534 U.S. 184 (2002)

Statutes, Regulations, and Legislative Materials

Age Discrimination in Employment Act, 29 U.S.C. §623 (2006)
Americans with Disabilities Act of 1990, 42 U.S.C. §§12101–12213 (2006)
Education for All Handicapped Children Act of 1975, P.L. 94-142, 89 Stat. 773 (Nov. 29, 1975) (now called the Individuals with Disabilities Education Act and codified at 20 U.S.C. §1400 et seq.)
Fair Housing Amendments Act of 1988, 42 U.S.C. §3613 et seq. (2006)
Rehabilitation Act of 1973, 29 U.S.C. §§791–794 (2006)
The Ticket to Work and Work Incentives Improvement Act of 1999, P.L. 106-170, 113 Stat 1860 (December 17, 1999)
Title VII of the Civil Rights Act of 1965, 42 U.S.C. §2000e-2(a) (2006)

Books, Articles, and Reports

Acemoglu, D., and J. D. Angrist. 2001. Consequences of Employment Protection? The Case of the Americans with Disabilities Act. *Journal of Political Economy* 109:915–957.
Allbright, A. 2001. 2000 Employment Decisions Under the ADA Title I—Survey Update. *Mental & Physical Disability Law Reporter* 25:508–510.
_____. 2002. 2001 Employment Decisions Under the ADA Title I—Survey Update. *Mental & Physical Disability Law Reporter.* May-Jun;26(3):394–398.
_____. 2003. 2002 Employment Decisions Under the ADA Title I—Survey Update. *Mental & Physical Disability Law Reporter* 27:387–389.

_____. 2004. Survey Update: 2003 Employer-Employee Wins Under ADA Title I. *Mental & Physical Disability Law Reporter* 28:319.

_____. 2005. 2004 Employment Decisions Under the ADA Title I—Survey Update. *Mental & Physical Disability Law Reporter* 29:513–516.

Baldridge, D.C. 2002. The Everyday ADA: The Influence of Requesters' Assessments on Decisions to Ask for Needed Accommodation. *Dissertation Abstracts International, Section A: Humanities and Social Sciences* 62:2807.

Baldwin, V.R. 1992. An Analysis of Subjective and Objective Indicators of Quality of Care in North Carolina Homes for the Aged. Ph.D. dissertation. Department of Health Policy and Administration, School of Public Health, University of North Carolina at Chapel Hill.

Barnes, J., and T.F. Burke. 2006. The Diffusion of Rights: From Rights on the Books to Organizational Rights Practices. *Law and Society Review* 40:493–524.

Beegle, K., and W.A. Stock. 2003. The Labor Market Effects of Disability Discrimination Laws. *Journal of Human Resources* 38:806–859.

Blackburn, R.D. 2003. Relationships Between Employers' Attitude Toward People with Disabilities, Awareness of ADA, and Willingness to Comply. *Dissertation Abstracts International, Section A: Humanities and Social Sciences* 63:2453.

Blanck, P., S. Schwochau, and C. Song. 2003. Is it Time to Declare the ADA a Failed Law? Pp. 301–337 in *The Decline in Employment of People with Disabilities: A Policy Puzzle*, edited by D. Stapleton and R. Burkhauser. Kalamazoo, MI: W.E. Upjohn Institute for Employment Research.

Blumrosen, A.W. 1993. *Modern Law: The Law Transmission System and Equal Employment Opportunity Commission*. Madison, WI: The University of Wisconsin Press.

Bruyere, S. 2000. *Disability Employment Policies and Practices in Private and Federal Sector Organizations*. Ithaca, NY: Cornell University, School of Industrial and Labor Relations Extension Division, Program on Employment and Disability.

Bruyere, S.M., W.A. Erickson, and S. VanLooy. 2005. Information Technology and the Workplace: Implications for Persons with Disabilities. *Disability Studies Quarterly* 25(2) [Online]. http://digitalcommons.ilr.cornell.edu/edicollect/98/ [accessed March 15, 2007).

Bruyere, S.M., W.A. Erickson, and S.A. Van Looy. 2006. The Impact of Business Size on Employer ADA Response. *Rehabilitation Counseling Bulletin* 49:194–206.

Burgdorf, R.L., Jr. 1991. The Americans with Disabilities Act: Analysis and Implications of a Second-Generation Civil Rights Statute. *Harvard Civil Rights/Civil Liberties Law Review* 26:413–522.

_____. 1997. "Substantially Limited" Protection from Disability Discrimination: The Special Treatment Model and Misconstructions of the Definition of Disability. *Villanova Law Review* 42:409–584.

Burkhauser, R.V., M.C. Daly, and A.J. Houtenville. 2001. How Working Age People with Disabilities Fared over the 1990s Business Cycle. In *Ensuring Health and Income Security for an Aging Workforce*, edited by P. Bardetti, R.V. Burkhauser, J. Gregory, and A. Hunt. Kalamazoo, MI: W.E. Upjohn Institute for Employment Research.

Burkhauser, R.V., M.C. Daly, A.J. Houtenville, and N. Nargis. 2002. Self-Reported Work-Limitation Data: What They Can and Cannot Tell Us. *Demography* 39:541–555.

Burkhauser, R.V., A. J. Houtenville, and D.C. Wittenburg. 2003. A User's Guide to Current Statistics on the Employment of People with Disabilities." Pp. 23–86 in *The Decline in Employment of People with Disabilities: A Policy Puzzle*, edited by D.C. Stapleton and R.V. Burkhauser. Kalamazoo, MI: W.E. Upjohn Institute for Employment Research.

Burris, S., and K. Moss. 2000. A Road Map for ADA Title I Research. Pp. 19–50 in *Employment, Disability, and the Americans with Disabilities Act: Issues in Law, Public Policy, and Research*, edited by P. D. Blanck. Evanston, IL: Northwestern University Press.

Colker, R. 2001. Winning and Losing Under the Americans with Disabilities Act. *Ohio State Law Journal* 62:239.

Curran, B.A., and F.O. Spalding. 1974. *The Legal Needs of the Public.* Chicago, IL: American Bar Foundation.

DeLeire, T. 2000. The Wage and Employment Effects of the Americans with Disabilities Act. *Journal of Human Resources* 35:693–715.

Donahue, J., and J. Heckman. 1991. Continuous vs. Episodic Change: The Impact of Civil Rights Policy on the Economic Status of Blacks. *Journal of Economic Literature* 29: 1603–1643.

Edelman, L., and M.C. Suchman. 1997. Legal Ambiguity and Symbolic Structures: Organizational Mediation of Civil Rights Law. *American Journal of Sociology* 97:1531–1576.

Engel, D., and F.W. Munger. 2001. Re-Interpreting the Effect of Rights: Career Narratives and the Americans with Disabilities Act. *Ohio State Law Journal* 62.:285-333.

Engel, D.M., and F.W. Munger. 2003. *Rights of Inclusion: Law and Identity in the Life Stories of Americans with Disabilities.* Chicago, IL: University of Chicago Press.

Feldblum, C. 2000. Definition of Disability Under Federal Anti-Discrimination Law: What Happened? Why? And What Can We Do About It?" *Berkeley Journal of Employment & Labor Law* 21:91–165.

Felstiner, W.L.F., R.L. Abel, and A. Sarat. 1980-1981. The Emergence and Transformation of Disputes: Naming, Blaming, Claiming. *Law and Society Review* 15:631–654.

Frank, J.J. 2004. The Avoidance of Help-Seeking: A Study of the Experiences of Persons with Severe Visual Impairment with the Americans with Disabilities Act (ADA) Accommodation Request Process for Print Access. *Dissertation Abstracts International, Section A: Humanities and Social Sciences* 64:4370.

Galanter, M. 1983. Reading The Landscape of Disputes: What We Know and Don't Know (and Think We Know) About Our Allegedly Contentious and Litigious Society. *U.C.L.A. Law Review* 31:18.

Goodman, N., and T. Waidmann. 2003. Is it Time to Declare the ADA a Failed Law? Pp. [339-368] in *Social Security Disability Insurance and the Recent Decline in the Employment Rate of People with Disabilities*, edited by D. Stapleton and R. Burkhauser. Kalamazoo, MI: W.E. Upjohn Institute for Employment Research.

Gostin, L.O., and H.A. Beyer. 1993. Preface. Pp. xiii in *Implementing the Americans with Disabilities Act: Rights and Responsibilities of All Americans*, edited by L. O. Gostin and H. A. Beyer. Baltimore, MD: P.H. Brookes Publishing Co.

Greenwood, R.J., and V.A. Johnson. 1987. Employer Perspectives on Workers with Disabilities. *Journal of Rehabilitation* 53:37–45.

Harlan, S.L., and P.M. Robert. 1998. The Social Construction of Disability in Organizations. *Work and Occupations* 25:397–435.

Hazer, J.T., and K.V. Bedell. 2000. Effects of Seeking Accommodation and Disability on Pre-employment Evaluations. *Journal of Applied Social Psychology* 30:1201–1223.

Heckman, J.J. 1990. The Central Role of the South in Accounting for the Economic Progress of Black Americans. *The American Economic Review* 80:242–246.

Hill, S.C., G.A. Livermore, and A.J. Houtenville. 2003. Rising Health Care Expenditures and the Employment of People with High-Cost Chronic Conditions. Pp. 181–215 in *The Decline in Employment of People with Disabilities: A Policy Puzzle*, edited by D.C. Stapleton and R.V. Burkhauser. Kalamazoo, MI: W.E. Upjohn Institute for Employment Research.

Hotchkiss, J. 2003. *The Labor Market Experience of Workers with Disabilities: The ADA and Beyond.* Kalamazoo, MI: W.E. Upjohn Institute for Employment Research.

Houtenville, A.J., and R.V. Burkhauser. 2004. *Did the Employment of People with Disabilities Decline in the 1990s, and was the ADA Responsible? A Replication and Robustness Check of Acemoglu and Angrist (2001).* Ithaca, NY: Cornell University Center for Economic Research on Employment Policy for Persons with Disabilities.

Houtenville, A.J., and M.C. Daly. 2003. Employment Declines Among People with Disabilities." Pp. 87–123 in *The Decline in Employment of People with Disabilities: A Policy Puzzle*, edited by D.C. Stapleton and R.V. Burkhauser. Kalamazoo, MI: W.E. Upjohn Institute for Employment Research.

Jolls, C., and J.J. Prescott. 2004. Disaggregating Employment Protection: The Case of Disability Discrimination. Working Paper 10740. http://www.nber.org/papers/w10740. Cambridge, MA: National Bureau of Economic Research.

Kaye, H.S. 2003. Employment and the Changing Disability Population." Pp. 217–258 in *The Decline in Employment of People with Disabilities: A Policy Puzzle*, edited by D.C. Stapleton and R.V. Burkhauser. Kalamazoo, MI: W.E. Upjohn Institute for Employment Research.

Kruse, D., and L. Schur. 2003. Employment of People with Disabilities Following the ADA. *Industrial Relations* 42:31–64.

McMenamin, T., S.M. Miller, and A.E. Polivka. 2006. Discussion and Presentation of the Disability Test Results from the Current Population Survey. Washington, DC: Bureau of Labor Statistics.

Miller, P.S. 1998. Genetic Discrimination in the Workplace. *Journal of Law, Medicine & Ethics* 26:178, 189–197.

Mitchell, T.L., and M.B. Kovera. 2006. The Effects of Attribution of Responsibility and Work History on Perceptions of Reasonable Accommodations. *Law and Human Behavior* 30:733.

Moon, S., and J. Shin. 2006. The Effect of the Americans with Disabilities Act on Economic Well-Being of Men with Disabilities. *Health Policy* 76:266–276.

Moss, K., S. Burris, M. Ullman, M.C. Johnsen, and J. Swanson. 2001. Unfunded Mandate: An Empirical Study of the Implementation of the Americans with Disabilities Act by the Equal Employment Opportunity Commission. *Kansas Law Review* 50:1–110.

Moss, K., J. Swanson, M. Ullman, and S. Burris. 2002. Mediation of Employment Discrimination Disputes Involving Persons with Psychiatric Disabilities. *Psychiatric Services* 53:988–994.

Moss, K., M. Ullman, J.W. Swanson, L.M. Ranney, and S. Burris. 2005. Prevalence and Outcomes of ADA Employment Discrimination Claims in the Federal Courts. *Mental & Physical Disability Law Reporter* 29:303–310.

National Council on Disability. 2004a. Improving Federal Disability Data. Position paper. National Council on Disability, Washington, DC., p. 30

_____. 2004b. Righting the ADA. National Council on Disability, Washington, DC.

Parry, J.W. 1998. Study Finds Employers Win Most ADA Title I Judicial and Administrative Complaints. *Mental & Physical Disability Law Reporter* 22:403–407.

_____. 1999. Trend: Employment Decisions Under ADA Title I—Survey Update. *Mental & Physical Disability Law Reporter* 23:294–298.

_____. 2000. 1999 Employment Decisions Under ADA Title I—Survey Update. *Mental & Physical Disability Law Reporter* 24:348–350.

Rulli, L. 2000. Employment Discrimination Litigation Under the ADA from the Perspective of the Poor: Can the Promise of Title I Be Fulfilled for Low-Income Workers in the Next Decade? *Temple Political & Civil Rights Law Review* 9:345–394.

Scheid, T.L. 2005. Stigma as a Barrier to Employment: Mental Disability and the Americans with Disabilities Act. *International Journal of Law and Psychiatry* 28:670–690.

Schwochau, S., and P.D. Blanck. 2000. The Economics of the Americans with Disabilities Act. Part III. Does the ADA Disable the Disabled? *Berkeley Journal of Employment and Labor Law* 21:271–313.

Scotch, R.K. 2000. "Models of Disability and the Americans with Disabilities Act." *Berkeley Journal Of Employment & Labor Law* 21:213–222.

Social Security Advisory Board. 2006. *A Disability System for the 21st Century.* Washington, DC: Social Security Advisory Board.

Stapleton, D.C., and R.V. Burkhauser. 2003. The Decline in Employment of People with Disabilities: A Policy Puzzle. Kalamazoo, MI: W.E. Upjohn Institute for Employment Research.

Stapleton, D.C., N. Goodman, and A.J. Houtenville. 2003. Have Changes in the Nature of Work or the Labor Market Reduced Employment Prospects of Workers with Disabilities? Pp. 125–179 in *The Decline in Employment of People with Disabilities: A Policy Puzzle,* edited by D.C. Stapleton and R.V. Burkhauser. Kalamazoo, MI: W.E. Upjohn Institute for Employment Research.

Stapleton, D.C., G.A. Livermore, B. O'Day, and A.J. Imparato. 2005. Dismantling the Poverty Trap: Disability Policy for the 21st Century. Rehabilitation Research and Training Center for Economic Research on Employment Policy for Persons with Disabilities, Cornell University, Ithaca, NY. Retrieved March 14, 2007 from http://digitalcommons.ilr.cornell.edu/edicollect/124.

Studdert, D. M. 2002. Charges of Human Immunodeficiency Virus Discrimination in the Workplace: The Americans with Disabilities Act in Action. *American Journal of Epidemiology* 156:219–229.

Swanson, J., S. Burris, K. Moss, M. Ullman, and L. Ranney. 2006. Justice Disparities: Does the ADA Enforcement System Treat People with Psychiatric Disabilities Fairly? *University of Maryland Law Review* 66:94–139.

Thakker, D., and P. Solomon. 1999. Factors Influencing Managers' Adherence to the Americans with Disabilities Act. *Administration and Policy in Mental Health* 26:213–219.

U.S. Congress, Office of Technology Assessment. 1994. *Psychiatric Disabilities, Employment, and the Americans with Disabilities Act.* Washington, DC: U.S. Government Printing Office.

U.S. Government Accountability Office. 2005. *Burgeoning Workload Calls for New Approaches.* Washington, DC: U.S. Government Accountability Office.

Ullman, M.D., M.C. Johnsen, K. Moss, and S. Burris. 2001. The EEOC Charge Priority Policy and Claimants with Psychiatric Disabilities. *Psychiatric Services* 52:644–649.

Unger, D.D. 1999. Workplace Supports: A View From Employers Who Have Hired Supported Employees. *Focus on Autism and Other Developmental Disabilities* 14:167–179.

Yelowitz, A.S. 1998. Why Did the SSI-Disabled Program Grow So Much? Disentangling the Effect of Medicaid. *Journal of Health Economics* 17:321–349.

F

Access to Telecommunications Technology by Americans with Disabilities: Key Laws and Policies

*Karen Peltz Strauss**

INTRODUCTION

The earliest federal disability laws enacted in the United States had little to do with ensuring access by people with disabilities to telecommunications technologies. These statutes placed far greater emphasis on providing access to the physical world than to the virtual world of telephone networks. For example, the Architectural Barriers Act of 1968 required federal buildings and facilities to be accessible to people with disabilities,[1] while the Rehabilitation Act of 1973 prohibited discrimination on the basis of disability in programs and activities that received federal funds.[2] The latter statute requires reasonable accommodations for qualified people with disabilities in federal employment (Section 501)[3]; by contractors who do business with the federal government (Section 503)[4]; and by federally assisted programs and activities, such as public schools, colleges and universities, police and fire departments, libraries, prisons, mass transit systems, and museums (Section 504).[5] These sections have been interpreted to require the auxiliary

---

*Principal, KPS Consulting.

[1]P.L. 90-480, 82 Stat. 718 (1968), codified at 42 U.S.C. §4151 et seq.

[2]P.L. 93-112, 87 Stat 390 (1973), codified at 29 U.S.C. §791 et seq.

[3]29 U.S.C. §791. See also 29 C.F.R. §1614.

[4]29 U.S.C. §793. See also 41 C.F.R. Part 60-741.

[5]29 U.S.C. §794. Each agency has its own rules governing the programs and activities funded or administered by that agency. The U.S. Department of Justice has guidelines to help implement and oversee compliance with this section. See 28 C.F.R. §§42.503; 42.511.

aids and services needed to ensure effective communication accommodations for people with disabilities, unless doing so would impose an undue hardship (significant difficulty or expense) on the operation of the covered entity.[6] Ways to achieve access include, but are not limited to, the use of assistive listening systems, hearing aid compatible (HAC) phones, sign language interpreters, amplifiers, captioning, television decoders, screen readers, and materials in braille.

Although a by-product of the Rehabilitation Act was the provision of some telephone access, the first real efforts to secure equal access to telecommunications services actually took place at the state level, through grassroots efforts to reduce telephone rates for teletypewriter (TTY) users.[7] At the time, all TTYs (also known as teletypewriters, text telephones, TDDs, or TTs) transmitted at a very slow speed of 60 words per minute. This paled in comparison to the 150 to 180 words per minute at which voice conversations were transmitted, resulting in large disparities between the costs of long-distance calls placed by TTY users and those placed by individuals who used conventional telephones. To compensate for the greater amount of time and toll charges required to complete a TTY call, local advocates launched efforts to secure service discounts from their state public service commissions. The first states to respond were New York, which approved a 25 percent discount for TTY toll charges in July 1977,[8] and Connecticut, which authorized a 75 percent reduction in TTY toll charges in December 1977.[9] By the end of the mid-1980s, all but three of the states offered such toll reductions.[10]

In the late 1970s and throughout the 1980s, disability advocates also lobbied their state legislatures, regulatory commissions, and local telephone

---

[6]To determine whether an undue hardship exists, the agency balances the cost and type of the accommodation against the budget, size, and nature of the agency. As noted below, this is the same test used to determine whether an access feature will result in an undue burden under the Americans with Disabilities Act or is readily achievable under Section 255 of the Communications Act.

[7]Karen Peltz Strauss, *A New Civil Right: Telecommunications Equality for Deaf and Hard of Hearing Americans* (Washington D.C.: Gallaudet University Press), 2006: 16.

[8]New York Public Service Commission Order 27205 (July 6, 1977).

[9]Connecticut Public Utilities Control Authority, Decision in Dkt. No. 77-0526, Application of Southern New England Telephone Company, and No. 77-0520, Petition of the Connecticut Office of Consumer Counsel Regarding Tariffs of the Southern New England Telephone Company Concerning Usage of Teletypewriter Units (December 16, 1977).

[10]Karen Peltz Strauss, "Television, Telephones, and TDDs . . . Access Is the Issue!" *Gallaudet Today* (Spring 1985): 17, 20. AT&T filed a federal tariff requesting reduction of all interstate TTY rates on August 21, 1981. See W. E. Albert, AT&T Administrator of Rates and Tariffs, letter to Secretary of the Federal Communications Commission, Transmittal 13822, August 21, 1981, referencing Tariff 263. This set the trend for AT&T's state affiliates, some of which volunteered to reduce their rates (e.g., Illinois and Massachusetts) and others of which were directed to do so by their state commissions (e.g., Arizona and Maine).

companies for affordable specialized customer premises equipment (SCPE), such as TTYs, amplifiers, light signalers, and artificial larynxes. Although conventional voice telephone users were able to lease telephones for only a few dollars a month, at the time, people with communication disabilities were forced to spend hundreds of dollars for their specialized equipment. In 1979, California and South Dakota became the first states to distribute free or low-cost TTYs to certified deaf and hard-of-hearing individuals.[11] Over the next several years, other states followed suit, and by the close of the 1980s, specialized devices were being distributed to thousands of individuals with communication disabilities in about half the states.[12]

These state equipment distribution programs varied considerably both in their eligibility criteria and in their methods of distribution. Some states offered cost-free leases, others provided low-interest loans or vouchers for equipment, and still others granted outright ownership of the adaptive equipment. In many states, these programs were mandated by law; others were the product of voluntary efforts by local telephone companies. Most of the programs were supported by small surcharges on the telephone bills of the states' telephone subscribers.

It was not until 1982 that the U.S. Congress first responded to the telecommunications needs of people with disabilities at the federal level, when it enacted the Telecommunications for the Disabled Act (TDA).[13] In that legislation, Congress relied on the Communications Act of 1934's universal service obligation to declare telephone access by people with hearing loss to be a priority in our nation's telecommunications policies. This obligation directs the Federal Communication Commission (FCC) to "make available, so far as possible to all the people of the United States . . . a rapid, efficient, nationwide, and worldwide wire and radio communication service with adequate facilities at reasonable charges."[14] Congress explained that the denial of telephone access to people with disabilities "would disserve the statutory goal of universal service [and] deprive many individuals of the opportunity to have gainful employment."[15] It further concluded that the "costs to society of such lost access, including impairment of the quality of life for disabled Americans, [would] far exceed [its] costs."[16]

---

[11]See e.g., Senate Bill 597, enacted as Chapter 1142, Statutes of 1979, and incorporated into California Pub. Util. Code §2881. The amount initially collected in California was 15 cents per subscriber; it was reduced to 3 cents after the collection of these charges created a surplus.

[12]Peltz Strauss, *A New Civil Right*: 26-27, 50-51; National Center for Law and the Deaf, "Summary of State TDD Distribution Programs and/or Dual Party Relay Programs" (March 1987, January 1988 editions), unpublished.

[13]P.L. 97-410, 94 Stat. 2043 (1982) codified at 47 U.S.C. §610, as amended (1988).

[14]47 U.S.C. §151.

[15]H. Rep. No. 888, 97th Cong., 2d Sess. 4 (1982).

[16]Id.

The TDA set the stage for a string of federal telecommunications laws requiring telephone and television access, many of which were similarly based on the FCC's obligation to provide universal service to the general public.[17] Through passage of the Hearing Aid Compatibility Act of 1988,[18] the Telecommunications Accessibility Enhancement Act,[19] Title IV of the Americans with Disabilities Act (ADA),[20] the Television Decoder Circuitry Act,[21] Sections 255 and 305 of the Telecommunications Act,[22] and Section 508 of the Rehabilitation Act,[23] Congress has consistently mandated that individuals with disabilities be included in the benefits of modern telecommunications, so that they can fully participate in employment, education, recreation, and other aspects of everyday life. These statutes have created mandates for hearing aid compatibility, telecommunications relay services, closed captioning, and other accessible telecommunications products and services in an effort to promote the independence, privacy, and productivity of the individuals for whom they have been enacted.

Federal mandates for accessibility have been a response to the failure of market forces to bring about much needed disability access features in telecommunications products and services. The reasons that markets have not worked well are several. They include the smaller market size of each disability group, the generally lower incomes of these groups, and the frequent need for people with disabilities to obtain expensive assistive technologies to get mainstream technologies to meet their needs.[24] Where market forces have failed, Congress has stepped in with regulatory mandates for telecommunications access, even where, in the same breath, it has deregulated other aspects of the telecommunications industry.

Congress has assigned the FCC the primary responsibility for implementing these various statutes, although collaborative consumer-industry forums have also played a significant role in helping to shape the nation's telecommunications policies. For example, the Telecommunications Access Advisory Committee (a federal advisory committee made up of telecommunications manufacturers and service providers, disability organizations, software developers, and assistive technology companies) worked with the Architectural Transportation Barriers Compliance Board (also known as the Access Board) from June through December 1996 to develop guidelines that formed the basis for the FCC's guidelines on Section 255, which re-

---

[17]Peltz Strauss, *A New Civil Right*: 34-35.
[18]P.L. No. 100-394, 102 Stat. 976 (1988), codified at 47 U.S.C. §610.
[19]P.L. No. 100-542, 102 Stat. 2721(1988), codified at 40 U.S.C. §762.
[20]P.L. No. 101-336, 104 Stat. 327 (1990), codified at 47 U.S.C. §225.
[21]P. L. No. 101-431, 104 Stat. 960 (1990), codified at 47 U.S.C. §§303(u); 330(b).
[22]P.L. No. 104-104, 110 Stat. 56 (1996), codified at 47 U.S.C. §§255; 713.
[23]P.L. 105-220, Title IV, §508(b), 112 Stat. 936 (1998), codified at 29 U.S.C. §794d.
[24]Peltz Strauss, *A New Civil Right*: 4.

quires all telecommunications products and services to be accessible. A few years later, the Electronic and Information Technology Advisory Committee, again operating under the aegis of the Access Board, reached consensus on guidelines for electronic and information technology access by federal agencies under Section 508. Similarly, an FCC-appointed negotiated rulemaking committee in 1995 produced recommendations for making wireline phones in most workplaces HAC under the TDA.

In addition to these regulatory activities, nongovernmental, standards-setting organizations have been called upon to define technical compliance with telecommunications access laws. The Electronics Industry Association (EIA) worked with captioning providers and television manufacturers to develop standards for the display of closed captions for both analog and digital television sets.[25] Similarly, since the mid-1990s, the Alliance for Telecommunications Industry Solutions has worked with telecommunications manufacturers and carriers and disability advocates to resolve technical issues associated with providing hearing aid and TTY access to wireless and cordless phone technologies. Finally, the Web Accessibility Initiative of the World Wide Web Consortium continues to coordinate discussion among disability and industry representatives, researchers, and governmental entities on solutions for making the Internet accessible to individuals with disabilities.[26]

FEDERAL LAWS

Telecommunications for the Disabled Act of 1982

Historical Background and Legislation

As noted above, the first federal law to specifically address telecommunications access was the TDA of 1982. This legislation was prompted by two major events that raised concerns about the future of telecommunications access for people with disabilities. The first was a decision by AT&T and other major telephone manufacturers to alter the internal composition of their telephones; the second was the divestiture of AT&T.

---

[25]EIA later changed its name to the Electronics Industry Alliance. The analog standard is contained at Television Receiver Performance Specification for Basic Closed Captioned Services, Draft Revision 6.0, EIA Standards Proposal, EIA/CEG Television Receiver Committee (R-4) (December 7, 1990), and was the basis for the FCC's analog captioning technical standards at 47 C.F.R. §15.119. The digital standard is contained at EIA-708-A, "Digital Television Closed Captioning" (November 23, 1998), revised at EIA-708-B, "Digital Television Closed Captioning" (December 1999), and was the basis for the FCC's digital captioning technical standards at 47 C.F.R. §15.122.

[26]See http://www.w3.org/WAI.

Hearing aid compatibility   There are two primary ways for a hearing aid to couple with telephones. One is through "acoustic coupling," which allows the hearing aid's microphones to pick up and amplify sounds from the phone's receiver. Because this method frequently does not create a tight seal between the hearing aid and the phone, individuals who use this coupling method can often hear distracting background noise and feedback that results when the hearing aid output is reflected off the handset and reamplified by the microphone. The second method, inductive coupling, allows the hearing aid user to turn off the microphone to eliminate that noise and feedback. Instead, the user's hearing aid has a small, coiled wire called a telecoil, or "T-coil," that receives the signal (i.e., telephone conversation) through a magnetic field in the telephone's handset. In the 1960s, most telephones in America were equipped with receivers that had sufficient magnetic field strength to couple with T-coil-equipped hearing aids.

In the 1970s, however, AT&T and GTE began increasing their reliance on lighter telephone handsets that used fewer expensive metallic materials and were more tamper resistant at payphones but that did not have magnetic fields strong enough to couple with hearing aid telecoils. As a consequence, hearing aid users with moderate to severe hearing loss began finding it harder to locate telephones that could inductively couple with their hearing aids. Efforts by people with disabilities to persuade the companies to switch back to the older HAC handsets achieved only moderate success.[27] Although the companies did eventually agree to install the new HAC receivers in all future payphones, to retrofit older payphone models, and to provide HAC telephones to individuals upon request, they continued producing the lighter, incompatible receivers and installing these in residences and businesses throughout the country.

When hearing aid users continued to complain about the many places where they could not access telephones, the companies created a portable telephone adapter that could convert the acoustic signals from any phone into magnetic signals to achieve inductive coupling. However, this solution was rejected by the hearing aid user community as being stigmatizing, costly, and cumbersome. Many of the affected individuals, especially senior citizens with limited dexterity, found it difficult to create the tight seal needed each time that the adapter had to be strapped onto the handset's receiver. More importantly, these consumers did not want to be treated differently from the general public; they insisted that it was their right to

---

[27]These efforts were largely spearheaded by a maverick group of senior citizens who called themselves the Organization for Use of the Telephone (OUT).

have *all* telephones universally compatible through inductive coupling with hearing aids.[28]

During the 1970s, as the number of telephones without inductive coupling proliferated throughout government agencies and private businesses, hearing aid advocates went to Congress to secure legislation that would require hearing aid compatibility on all telephones.[29] Ultimately, they were only partially successful. Rather than require universal compatibility, the TDA of 1982 created a new category of telephones—"essential telephones"—which would have to provide internal compatibility with hearing aids.[30] Included in this category were all phones that were coin operated, phones frequently needed for use by persons using hearing aids, and phones provided for emergency use. As a partial compromise for not requiring hearing aid compatibility on all phones, Congress also required all telephone packages to be conspicuously labeled so that consumers could easily locate HAC phones.[31]

Subsidies for SCPE   In addition to addressing the HAC issue, a second and equally important matter addressed in the TDA concerned the availability and affordability of the SCPE needed by people with disabilities to access the telephone network. This stemmed from concerns about a 1980 FCC ruling called the "Second Computer Inquiry," or "Computer II," which required local telephone companies to separate the provision of their telephone equipment from their regulated services to prevent the costs of producing telephone products from being subsidized with revenues from telephone services.[32] Although the goal of this ruling was to spur greater competition by new entrants into the telephone business, the new arrangement threatened to force people with disabilities to pay the full and sometimes exorbitant costs of SCPE. To prevent this from occurring, the TDA gave states the authority to allow their telephone companies to con-

---

[28]See, e.g., Statement of David Saks, OUT, Hearings on S. 604 and S. 2355 before the Subcommittee on Communications of the Senate Committee on Commerce, Science, and Transportation, 97th Cong., 2d Sess. (May 6, 1982): 27.

[29]During this period, several bills were introduced, although all failed to achieve passage. See, e.g., H.R. 5022, 96th Cong., 2d Sess. (1979); S. 2642, 96th Cong., 2d Sess. (1979); H.R. 375, 97th Cong, 1st Sess. (1981).

[30]P.L. 97-410, 94 Stat. 2043 (1982), codified at 47 U.S.C. §610, as amended (1988).

[31]47 U.S.C. §610(d). The House report explained that these labels had to explain "in a clear and understandable manner, whether and how persons with impaired hearing may use such equipment effectively." H. Rep. No. 888, 97th Cong., 2d Sess. 12 (1982).

[32]Second Computer Inquiry, 77 FCC 2d 384 (May 2, 1980), recon., 84 FCC 2d 50 (December 30, 1980), further recon., 88 FCC 2d 512 (1981), aff'd sub nom., *Computer and Communications Industry Assn v. FCC*, 693 F. 2d 198 (D.C. Cir. 1982), cert. den'd, 461 U.S. 938 (1983), aff'd on second further recon., FCC 84-190 (May 4, 1984), codified at 47 C.F.R. 64.702.

tinue subsidizing the costs of providing SCPE with the rates received from their general subscribers.[33] Congress explained that while deregulation of telecommunications equipment might ensure a competitive market for most ratepayers, this simply would not work for people with disabilities:

> For most ratepayers, deregulation may indeed ensure a competitive market in telephone sets and eliminate subsidies for such sets from local rates. For the disabled, however, the ban on cross-subsidization could mean unregulated price increases on the costly devices that are necessary for them to have access to the telephone network. Disabled persons who are unable to afford the full costs of this equipment will lose access to telephone service."[34]

FCC Regulations

FCC rules implementing the hearing aid provisions of the TDA established the magnetic field strength needed to achieve internal inductive coupling with telephones, set forth labeling requirements, and further defined which telephones were deemed to be "essential" under the TDA.[35] These phones fell into the following categories:

• *Telephones provided for emergency use*, including telephones in isolated locations (e.g., tunnels and elevators); telephones in confined settings (e.g., hospital rooms) needed to notify others about life-threatening or emergency situations, unless the individual had another alternative; and telephones installed with the explicit purpose of being able to contact public authorities in an emergency (e.g., call boxes that connected directly to emergency personnel);
• *Telephones frequently needed by people with hearing loss*, including telephones at the employee's workstation when needed to fulfill regular work duties; telephones in public buildings and businesses; credit card telephones; telephones in nursing homes, hospitals, and prisons where individuals could be confined; and telephones in at least 10 percent of rooms in hotels and motels; and
• *Coin-operated telephones*, including phones on public property or semipublic locations (e.g., drugstores, gas stations, and private clubs).

After passage of the TDA, the FCC modified its Computer II rule, clear-

---

[33]47 U.S.C. §610(g).
[34]H. Rep. No. 888 at 3-4.
[35]47 C.F.R. §68.316 contains the technical specifications for hearing aid compatibility, and 47 C.F.R. §68.112 defines essential telephones. This labeling requirement has since been removed from the *Code of Federal Regulations* because all newly manufactured phones are required to be HAC.

ing the way for continued cross-subsidization of the costs of SCPE, and for states to develop programs for the distribution of specialized equipment. The new rule, in effect to this day, states:

> Any communications common carrier may provide, under tariff, customer premises equipment (other than hearing aid compatible telephones as defined in part 68 of this chapter), needed by persons with hearing, speech, vision or mobility disabilities. Such equipment may be provided to persons with those disabilities or to associations or institutions that require such equipment regularly to communicate with persons with disabilities. Examples of such equipment include, but are not limited to, artificial larynxes, bone conductor receivers and TTs.[36]

Hearing Aid Compatibility Act of 1988

Historical Background and Legislation

During the years following passage of the TDA, the number of domestic and foreign manufacturers who began selling inexpensive and incompatible telephones in the United States significantly increased. Hearing aid users grew increasingly frustrated with the limited scope of the TDA's provisions as they watched millions of inaccessible handsets get installed in "nonessential" locations throughout the country. They returned to Congress to renew their attempts to secure passage of a HAC law that would enable them to use any telephone, regardless of where it was located.

Although it took an additional 6 years, Congress eventually responded with the Hearing Aid Compatibility Act of 1988, which required all wireline telephones manufactured or imported for use in the United States after August 16, 1989, to have an internal means of providing hearing aid compatibility.[37] Manufacturers of cordless telephones were given an additional 3 years to comply, though wireless phones were provisionally exempt pending further FCC review. Again, Congress relied on the FCC's universal service mandate to conclude that "advances in technology have made communication possible and it is time that hearing impaired persons are included in 'all the people:'"[38]

> No matter how broadly the FCC defines "essential," it is impossible to specify in advance all the telephones that a hearing aid user might need. Traveling salespeople, repairmen and women, doctors, and others who make house calls or work outside of an office, for instance, often use telephones that would not be classified as "essential.". . . Similarly, it is impos-

---

[36]47 C.F.R. §64.606(a).
[37]P.L. 100-394, 102 Stat. 976 (1988), codified at 47 U.S.C. §610.
[38]H. Rep. No. 674, 100th Cong., 2d Sess. 6 (1988), referring to 47 U.S.C. §151.

sible to predict beforehand when an emergency situation may arise. . . . In short, the situations in which a hearing aid user would need access to a telephone are innumerable.[39]

FCC Regulations

Although advocates were successful in finally securing a universal HAC law, a significant gap between the 1982 and the 1988 HAC statutes left consumers without the access that advocates had sought. Specifically, between the time that the 1982 Act was passed and the time that the 1988 Act went into effect, a huge number of incompatible phones were put into circulation, which left millions of hearing aid users with moderate to severe hearing loss without any means of using the telephone in hospitals, hotels, and many places of business. Hearing aid advocates spent the next several years trying to convince the FCC to expand its definition of HAC-required "essential telephone" locations to close this gap. This culminated in an FCC-led negotiated rulemaking that successfully produced a consensus among disability advocates, businesses, telephone manufacturers, and governmental agencies for a new schedule of deadlines that expanded the scope of existing HAC phones in workplaces, hotels and motels, and health care facilities.[40] In addition to inductive coupling, the new regulations (issued in 1996) created a new requirement for volume control on all wireline and cordless telephones manufactured in or imported into the United States after January 1, 2000.[41] Authority for this novel mandate was found in statements, contained in the legislative history of both the 1982 and 1988 Acts, confirming Congress's view that inductive coupling was only one of many ways of achieving hearing aid compatibility (volume control being another), as well as directives by Congress in both statutes encouraging the use of new technologies to achieve access.[42]

---

[39]S. Rep. No. 391, 100th Cong., 2d Sess. 3 (1988), citing to Testimony of Karen Peltz Strauss, Gallaudet University, before the Communications Subcommittee of the Senate Committee on Commerce, Science, and Transportation.

[40]*Access to Telecommunications Equipment and Services by Persons with Disabilities,* Report and Order, CC Dkt. No. 87-124, FCC 96-285, 11 FCC Rcd 8249 (July 3, 1996), amending 47 C.F.R. §68.112. See also 47 C.F.R. §68.4, containing the general requirements for handsets to be HAC under the 1988 Act.

[41]47 C.F.R. §68.6. The technical standards for volume control are contained at 47 C.F.R. §68.317. The FCC rejected arguments that competitive market forces would provide sufficient quantities of amplified telephones.

[42]For example, a finding in the 1988 Act "anticipated improvements in both telephone and hearing aid technologies." P.L. 100-394 §2. In addition, the House report stated that this Act did "not require induction as the sole method of telephone/hearing aid coupling. It is flexible and allows for other methods of compatibility." H. Rep. No. 674 at 12.

Wireless Telephones

Just as the struggle to obtain HAC wireline phones was reaching its final resolution, Americans began discovering the benefits of mobile telephones. The earliest wireless phones introduced in the United States relied on analog transmissions and did not pose a problem for hearing aid users. However, when digital wireless phones began to be deployed with increasing frequency in about the mid-1990s, it was discovered that these created electromagnetic interference that made their use with T-coil-equipped hearing aids very difficult. Digital wireless technologies produce pulsing signals as they send messages, which, when picked up by hearing aids, can cause buzzing or other high-pitched noises. Because the 1988 Act had exempted all wireless handsets from the hearing aid compatibility mandates, manufacturers were not engaging in efforts to eliminate this type of interference. Initial attempts to convince the wireless phone industry to resolve this problem produced few or no results, and in 1995, hearing aid advocates filed a petition with the FCC to lift the HAC exemption for these phones.

Although the FCC expressed serious concerns about the new accessibility barrier, the agency feared taking any regulatory action that would delay the rollout of wireless technologies in the United States. Instead, the FCC merely directed the wireless industry to work with consumers to resolve the new hearing aid compatibility problem on its own. But negotiations between the wireless industry and consumer advocates over the next 5 years failed to achieve a consensus on a solution for the mobile handset issue, and by the turn of the century, the precipitous decline in the availability of analog phones threatened to eliminate all wireless telephone access for these hearing aid wearers. By now, not only was more than 40 percent of the American public reliant on digital wireless telephone technologies, but these technologies promised far greater sound quality, versatility, and pricing than their analog predecessors. In 2000, consumers went back to the FCC to renew their request for a wireless hearing aid compatibility requirement.

Again, years went by without FCC action. Finally, during the summer of 2002, the FCC announced its intent to eliminate its "analog rule," a rule originally put into place in the early 1980s requiring all wireless carriers to provide analog service.[43] The FCC determined that the rule was no longer needed to foster competition and was now impeding innovation by forcing wireless carriers to operate in both the analog and digital modes. The FCC directed the wireless industry to gradually phase out these tech-

---

[43] *Year 2000 Biennial Regulatory Review—Amendment of Part 22 of the Commission's Rules to Modify or Eliminate Outdated Rules Affecting the Cellular Radiotelephone Service and other Commercial Mobile Radio Services*, Report and Order, WT Dkt No. 01-108, 17 FCC Rcd 18401 (September 24, 2002), Order on Reconsideration, FCC 04-22 (February 12, 2004).

nologies over a 5-year period (by February 18, 2008), during which time the industry would develop technical solutions for digital phone hearing aid compatibility. Failure to achieve access within this period would result in an extension of the analog rule for an unspecified period of time. The Commission explained that it was taking this action because market forces would not address the hearing aid problem:

> We find that, given the scarcity of digital devices that may be used with hearing aids, persons with hearing disabilities could be left without access to mobile telephony services in the event that the analog requirement is removed immediately and carriers are able to shut down their analog facilities. While we anticipate that market mechanisms will, for the most part, ensure access to digital services for most consumers . . . [t]he same economic incentives do not exist that would ensure that persons with hearing disabilities have adequate access to digital wireless service because they account for only a small percentage of mobile telephony users.[44]

While the FCC's new order created a powerful incentive for the wireless industry to achieve digital wireless accessibility within a specified time, the rapid decline in analog phones in retail establishments spurred advocates to continue pushing for an affirmative *mandate* for hearing aid compatibility. In July of 2003, consumers finally got their way in an FCC ruling that created a schedule for certain wireless phones to become HAC over the next several years (Box F-1)[45] This time, hearing aid compatibility was defined to include both inductive and acoustic coupling, as well as acceptable levels of interference.[46] By now, 88 percent of all wireless telephone subscribers used digital services.

As a guide to fulfilling the new requirements, companies were directed to comply with ANSI C63.19, a standard which had been devised by Standards Committee 63 on Electromagnetic Compatibility of the American

---

[44]Id. at ¶28, citing Reply Comments of the National Association of the Deaf.

[45]*Section 68.4(a) of the Commission's Rules Governing Hearing Aid-Compatible Telephones*, Report and Order, WT Dkt. 01-309, FCC 03-168, 18 FCC Rcd 16753 (released August 14, 2003), erratum, 18 FCC Rcd 18047 (2003), codified at 47 C.F.R. §20.19. On June 9, 2005, the FCC slightly modified the final rules, in response to a petition for reconsideration filed by the Cellular and Internet Telecommunications Association. *Section 68.4(a) of the Commission's Rules Governing Hearing Aid-Compatible Telephones*, Order on Reconsideration and Further Notice of Proposed Rulemaking, FCC 05-122, 18 FCC Rcd 11208 (June 21, 2005).

[46]The FCC relied on language in the legislative history of the 1988 HAC Act to expand the hearing aid compatibility requirement to acoustic coupling and reduced interference. The 1988 House report had stated: "The hearing aid bill will not freeze today's technology and inhibit future development. The bill only requires that telephones be compatible; it does not mandate any particular type of technology. Induction coupling and electromagnetic fields are not even mentioned. See H. Rep. No. 674 at 8. See also S. Rep. No. 391 at 2 ("Telephones may also be 'compatible' without a telecoil. Some telephones, for instance, contain internal amplifiers. . . . It is also possible that other means of 'compatibility' may be developed in the future.")

BOX F-1
Hearing Aid Compatibility Rules for Wireless Telephones
47 C.F.R. §20.19

Schedule of Deadlines

• By September 16, 2005, in order to achieve acoustic coupling without interference, every digital telephone manufacturer and carrier had to make available 2 handset models with reduced RF emissions for each air interface (CDMA, TDMA, GSM, iDEN).

• By September 16, 2005, each of the 5 largest digital wireless carriers (Verizon, T-Mobile, Cingular, Sprint, Nextel) had to make available, per air interface, either 4 handset models with reduced RF emissions or 25 percent of the total number of its handset models.

• By September 16, 2006, each of the 5 largest digital wireless carriers had to make available, per air interface, either 5 handset models with reduced RF emissions or 25 percent of the total number of its handset models.

• By September 16, 2006, in order to achieve inductive coupling, every digital manufacturer and carrier had to provide 2 handset models with telecoil coupling for each air interface.

• By February 18, 2008, 50 percent of all digital phones must have reduced RF emissions for acoustic coupling.

• After 2008, the FCC may review its regulations and determine whether it will require 100 percent acoustic coupling.

De Minimis Exemptions

• Digital manufacturers, carriers or service providers that offer 2 or fewer digital wireless handset models (on a per air interface basis) do not need to meet the wireless HAC mandates.

• Digital manufacturers or carriers that offer 3 digital wireless handset models must produce 1 compliant model.

Labeling

• Detailed information on the ASNI C63.19 rating system must be contained in a product manual.

• Conspicuous labeling of the phone's interference rating must appear on the outside of its box.

• Although the FCC does not have jurisdiction over hearing aid manufacturers, it encourages these companies to provide labeling on hearing aid immunity levels.

Reporting Requirements

The FCC requires wireless companies to regularly report on progress made to achieve HAC handsets, including their testing, standards setting activities, outreach activities, and the feasibility of achieving 100% HAC for all digital wireless phones after 5 years.

National Standards Institute (ANSI).[47] The standard assigns each hearing aid a rating for the level of immunity that it provides when used in both the microphone and telecoil modes. It also gives every wireless handset a rating for its magnetic signal strength, magnetic field emissions, and radio frequency emissions. Hearing aid users can then add together the ratings to determine how well each handset is expected to work with each hearing aid.

Cordless Telephones

Although most cordless wireline telephones have been HAC since their temporary exemption from the HAC Act expired in 1991, new concerns about the lack of compatibility in cordless phones that operate at a higher frequency—5.8 gigahertz (GHz)—have prompted a number of complaints to the FCC, as well as new efforts by telephone manufacturers, advocates, and Gallaudet University researchers to resolve this problem.

AMERICANS WITH DISABILITIES ACT

Historical Background and Legislation

As noted above, the Rehabilitation Act of 1973 prohibited discrimination on the basis of disability by programs that were federally operated, administered, or funded. However, until 1990, no federal law prohibited discrimination on the basis of disability by private retail establishments, private employers, and state and local governmental programs that did not receive federal aid. Originally patterned after the Civil Rights Act of 1964, the ADA closed this gap by prohibiting discrimination on the basis of disability in the private sector and by all local governments, whether or not they received federal financial assistance.[48] The goal of this omnibus statute was to promote the independence, productivity, and integration of all Americans with disabilities throughout society.[49] The Act is divided into five titles. Title IV, which focuses specifically on telecommunications, is discussed in detail below.

Title I, which covers private employers with 15 or more employees, employers in state and local governments, members of Congress, and others in the federal legislative branch, requires the provision of accessible

---

[47]The full title of ANSI C63.19 is the American National Standard for Methods of Measurement of Compatibility Between Wireless Communication Devices and Hearing Aids.

[48]P.L. 101-336, 104 Stat. 327 (1990), codified at §12101 et seq.

[49]The ADA was largely prompted by two reports prepared by the National Council on the Handicapped (later renamed the National Council on Disability): *Toward Independence*, released in 1986, and *On the Threshold of Independence*, released in 1988.

telecommunications and technologies when these are needed by qualified individuals with disabilities to perform the essential functions of a job; to apply for employment; or to enjoy other employee benefits and privileges, including training, social functions, and employee services.[50] Under Title II, state and local governments must provide effective communication to people with disabilities in their programs, services, and activities.[51] Entities covered under this title include, but are not limited to, social services, transportation, public education, libraries, judicial systems, and legislative proceedings. Title III similarly requires commercial facilities and places of public accommodation, including stores, hotels, movie theaters, restaurants, recreational facilities, and professional offices (e.g., the offices of lawyers, physicians, and accountants), to provide the auxiliary aids and services needed to ensure effective communication.[52] Accommodations or auxiliary aids and services that can be used to achieve effective communication under any of these titles include, but are not limited to, TTYs, telephone amplifiers, assistive listening devices, computer-aided transcription services, sign language interpreters, HAC telephones, captioning services and equipment, audio recordings, computer disks, large print, and materials in braille.[53] However, the entities covered under all three titles are required to provide such assistance only where doing so will not impose an undue burden upon their operations.[54]

In addition to the obligations described above, local governments that provide emergency telephone services must make those services directly accessible to callers using TTYs, so that these individuals need not rely on relay services or third parties to access 9-1-1 and other local emergency

---

[50]42 U.S.C. §12112 et seq.

[51]42 U.S.C. §12131 et seq. Title II guidelines on telecommunications access, issued by the U.S. Department of Justice, can be found at 28 C.F.R. §35.160-162.

[52]42 U.S.C. §12181 et seq. Title III guidelines on telecommunications access, again issued by the U.S. Department of Justice, are at 28 C.F.R. §36.303(c)—(e).

[53]Public accommodations that typically provide the opportunity to make telephone calls on "more than an incidental convenience basis" (e.g., hospitals and hotels), are specifically required to provide TTYs upon request. 28 C.F.R. §36.303(d)(1). According to the U.S. Department of Justice, TTY access must also be provided for security phones needed to enter public accommodations. 56 *Fed. Reg.* 35567 (July 26, 1991).

[54]Title I uses the term "undue hardship," but the factors used to assess this defense, found at 47 U.S.C. §12111(10), are nearly identical to those used for the undue burden standard under Titles II and III. Similarly, these factors are the same as those used for determining undue hardship under the Rehabilitation Act. They require balancing the cost and nature of the accommodation or aid with the financial resources of the facility and the impact of the accommodation or aid on its operations. See, e.g., 28 C.F.R. §36.104 (Title III).

authorities.[55] State and local governments also have a specific obligation to ensure that their websites are accessible to people with disabilities. Among other things, this requires ensuring that website materials are available in text versions so that persons who are blind or have vision disabilities can use talking screen readers to access that information.[56] The law on whether websites are covered under Title III, however, is less definitive. Although the U.S. Department of Justice has indicated that it does believe that Title III covers the websites of entities that are otherwise covered under the ADA,[57] two federal circuit courts have released opinions suggesting that the Act does not cover services provided in virtual space.[58] These opinions are in conflict with other federal court rulings that public accommodations cannot exclude people with disabilities from entering their facilities, whether their services are provided in physical or electronic space.[59]

In 1991, as required under the ADA, the Access Board released the ADA Accessibility Guidelines for Buildings and Facilities (ADAAG) that set forth technical specifications for making physical structures accessible.[60] A number of these guidelines directly pertain to telecommunications accessibility, including requirements to make a certain percentage of newly constructed or renovated hotel rooms TTY accessible and mandates for payphones in public places, such as covered malls, hospitals, convention centers, stadiums, and transportation depots, to be TTY accessible. The ADAAG also contains technical standards for equipping telephones with volume control features and hearing aid compatibility.[61]

---

[55]28 C.F.R. §35.162. The actual requirement to provide this access was contained in the legislative history of Title II at H. Rep. No. 485, Part 2, 101st Cong., 2d Sess., at 84–85 (May 15, 1990). Similar language was also inserted into the ADA Conference Report at Conf. Rep. No. 596, 101st Cong., 2d Sess., at 67–68 (July 12, 1990).

[56]More information about U.S. Department of Justice requirements to make local government websites accessible can be found at http://www.ada.gov/websites2.htm.

[57]Specifically, the U.S. Department of Justice submitted an amicus brief in *Hooks v. OK-Bridge, Inc.,* 232 F. 3d 208 (5th Cir. 2000), taking this position.

[58]*Chabner v. United of Omaha Life Insurance Company,* 225 F. 3d 1042 (9th Cir. 2000) (holding that an insurance office must be physically accessible but the provision of insurance policies to customers need not be equally accessible to people with disabilities); *Access Now, Inc. v. Southwest Airlines,* 385 F. 3d 1324 (11th Cir. 2004).

[59]*Doe v. Mutual of Omaha Insurance Comp.,* 179 F. 3d 557, 559 (7th Cir. 1999), cert. den'd, 120 S. Ct. 845 (2000) (ruling that the owner or operator of a store, website, or other facility that is open to the public, whether in physical or electronic space, cannot exclude individuals with disabilities nor treat them differently); *Carparts Distribution Center, Inc. v. Automotive Wholesaler's Association of New England, Inc.,* 37 F. 3d 12, 19 (ruling that public accommodations do not need to have physical structures to be covered by the ADA).

[60]36 C.F.R. Part 1191, Appendix A.

[61]Id. at §§4.1.3(17)(c); 10.3.1(12); 4.31.9.

Title IV—Telecommunications Relay Services

Background and Statutory Provisions

Prior to the 1960s, deaf individuals had virtually no way to communicate independently by telephone. This changed in 1968, when a deaf engineer named Robert Weitbrecht figured out a way to attach a telephone modem to outdated teletype machines that had been discarded by telecommunications companies and news services. Although Weitbrecht's invention enabled deaf people to send text directly over the telephone network to other individuals with these TTYs, a method was still needed to enable TTY users to make telephone calls to people who did not have one of these devices. Telecommunications relay services (TRS) were created for this purpose. To use a relay service, a TTY user calls a relay operator, also called a communications assistant (CA), and gives the CA the number of the person whom he or she wishes to call. After the CA connects the two parties, the caller types out his or her part of the conversation, which the CA then voices to the receiving party. When the hearing party responds, the CA types that part of the conversation back to the caller. The call continues in this fashion, with the CA reading everything that the caller types and typing back all responses.

The private and state relay services created in the 1970s and 1980s were underfunded and understaffed and generally placed limitations on the number and length of calls, operating hours, and even call content. Relay service quality was also inconsistent from state to state, with few standards for relay confidentiality or CA qualifications in grammar and spelling.[62] The vast majority of states also disallowed interstate calls, for fear of violating interstate boundaries. Title IV of the ADA was designed to eliminate the many barriers that confronted people who needed this service to communicate by telephone and create relay uniformity across the United States.[63] Once again, when enacting this provision, Congress relied on the Communications Act's universal service obligation.[64]

Under Title IV, telephone companies must provide relay services that enable people with hearing or speech disabilities to engage in telephone communication that is "functionally equivalent" to the conventional voice telephone communication enjoyed by people without these disabilities.[65] At a minimum, principles of functional equivalency require that

---

[62]See, for example, Bill White, "Dual Party Relays . . . How Far Will They Fly?" *Silent News*, May 1990 at 13.

[63]47 U.S.C. §225.

[64]47 U.S.C. §225(b)(1).

[65]47 U.S.C. §225(a)(3).

- TRS operate 24 hours every day;
- TRS users pay rates no greater than the rates paid for functionally equivalent voice communication services with respect to such factors as the duration of the call, the time of day, and the distance from the point of call origination to the point of its termination;
  - relay operators not refuse calls or limit the length of calls;
  - relay operators not disclose the content of any relayed conversation or keep records of the content of any conversation beyond the duration of the call; and
  - relay operators not intentionally alter a relayed conversation.[66]

Common carriers may fulfill their TRS responsibilities by providing these services individually, through designees, through a competitively selected vendor, or in concert with other carriers.[67] Congress also provided a mechanism for states to receive certification to operate relay programs on behalf of the carriers in their jurisdictions, so long as those states meet minimum relay standards set by the FCC and provide adequate procedures and remedies for enforcing these mandates.[68] At present, all 50 states plus the U.S. territories have relay certification.

FCC Regulations

Since 1991, the FCC has had an ongoing series of rulemaking proceedings to refine and update its TRS mandates.[69] Guiding these proceedings have been the overarching goals of achieving functionally equivalent telecommunications access and ensuring that TRS users are able to benefit from the most advanced relay technologies.[70] These proceedings have resulted in the availability of a host of relay services that can now meet diverse communication needs:

- **Text-to-speech relay services.** Text-to-speech relay services transmit conversations over the public switched telephone network (PSTN) between individuals who have TTYs or ASCII capability on their computers and voice telephone users. The CA converts everything that the text caller types into voice and the hearing person says into typed text. This service is mandated and must be provided 24 hours a day, 7 days a week.

---

[66]These various mandates are contained at 47 U.S.C. §225(d).

[67]47 U.S.C. §225(c).

[68]47 U.S.C. §225(f).

[69]These mandates are found at 47 C.F.R. §§64.604 and 64.605.

[70]The ADA explicitly directs the FCC to ensure that its Title IV rules encourage the use of existing technology and do not discourage or impair the development of improved technology. 47 U.S.C. §225(d)(2).

•   **Video relay services.** Video relay services (VRS), approved by the FCC in March of 2000,[71] use sign language interpreters, remotely accessed via a high-speed Internet connection, to voice everything that is signed by the deaf person and to sign back all voiced responses from the hearing party. These services allow native sign language users to converse naturally and to convey emotional content through the interpreter. Because they take place in real time, VRS can also facilitate conference calls and calls that have voice menu selections. In addition, because VRS are not text based, they are especially beneficial for children, senior citizens, and others who have difficulty typing. These services are not mandated, but providers who offer them must make them available 24 hours a day, 7 days a week.

•   **Speech-to-speech relay services.** Speech-to-speech relay services, approved in the FCC's March 2000 order, use specially trained CAs who can understand difficult-to-understand speech patterns. The CA listens to the caller and repeats what that person says to the called party. The individual with the speech disability can then hear the called party's responses without intervention from the CA. These services are mandated and must be provided 24 hours a day, 7 days a week.

•   **Internet protocol relay services.** Internet protocol (IP) relay services, approved by the FCC in April 2002,[72] allow a user to access text-based relay services via the Internet using a wired or wireless computer, personal digital assistant, web phone, or other IP-enabled device. This service is authorized, but not mandated.

•   **Captioned telephone relay services.** Captioned telephone relay services, approved by the FCC in August 2003,[73] enable users to simultaneously listen to and read the captions of what the hearing person involved in the call is saying. Unlike other forms of relay, callers may dial their parties directly and automatically get connected to the CA. Once the parties are connected, the CA revoices all conversation spoken by the hearing person. Voice recognition technology automatically transcribes these words from the CA's voice into text, which is then generated into captions and transmitted back to the caller, so that he or she can read what the hearing party is saying. At the same time, the person with hearing loss can use residual

---

[71]*Telecommunications Relay Services and Speech-to-Speech Services for Individuals with Hearing and Speech Disabilities*, Report and Order and Further Notice of Proposed Rulemaking, CC Dkt. No. 98-67, FCC 00-56, 15 FCC Rcd 5140 (March 6, 2000).

[72]*Provision of Improved Telecommunications Relay Services and Speech-to-Speech Services for Individuals with Hearing and Speech Disabilities*, Declaratory Ruling and Second Further Notice of Proposed Rulemaking, CC Dkt. No. 98-67, FCC 02-121, 17 FCC Rcd 7779 (April 22, 2002), Order on Reconsideration, FCC 03-46 (March 14, 2003).

[73]*Telecommunications Services and Speech-to-Speech Services for Individuals with Disabilities*, Declaratory Ruling, CC Dkt. No. 98-67, FCC 03-190, 18 FCC Rcd 16121 (August 1, 2003).

hearing to hear the hearing person's voice. Captioned telephone relay is very popular among older Americans who have lost their hearing because it closely mirrors the typical telephone experience. This service is authorized but not mandated.

• **Spanish relay services.** In its March 2000 order, the FCC established a mandate for common carriers to offer *interstate* relay services in Spanish. States can decide for themselves whether they wish to provide Spanish-language relay services for relay calls *within* their states.

• **Voice and hearing carryover.** The voice carryover (VCO) and hearing carryover (HCO) forms of TRS use CAs to convey messages for only one leg of each call. VCO is used by people who cannot hear but who can speak: the individual uses his or her own voice to talk directly to the called party and uses the CA only to type back responses. HCO allows a hearing individual with a speech disability to listen directly to the other party and to use the CA to speak what he or she types. VCO and HCO are mandated and must be provided 24 hours a day, 7 days a week.

• **Other mandated services.** In addition to the mandated services described above, the following relay services are mandated and must be provided 24 hours a day, 7 days a week: VCO to TTY, VCO to VCO, HCO to TTY, and HCO to HCO.

Other Relay Considerations

Confidentiality   The FCC has recognized that to achieve true functional equivalency to voice telephone calls, TRS providers must maintain the strict confidentiality of all relay calls. More specifically, the CA must act as a "transparent conduit relaying conversations without censorship or monitoring functions."

Speed of answer   The speed with which a relay call is answered is a prime indicator of the extent to which the service is functionally equivalent to voice telephone services. Because a relay service is intended to be a substitute for a voice telephone dial tone, the FCC requires that relay network facilities and CA staffing be sufficient so that under projected calling volumes, the probability of a busy response because of loop trunk congestion or CA unavailability is the functional equivalent of what a voice caller would experience when placing a call through the voice telephone network.[74]

Funding and cost recovery   The ADA provides that the costs incurred by intrastate TRS providers may be recovered from the subscribers to in-

---

[74]VRS are held to a different standard because these services are still relatively new and because there are a limited number of interpreters in the United States.

trastate services and that the costs attributable to interstate TRS may be recovered from the interstate jurisdiction. The two exceptions to this policy are expenses associated with the provision of VRS and IP relay. Because it is difficult to ascertain the geographic origination of these calls, their costs are recovered entirely from interstate subscribers. The National Exchange Carriers Administration collects contributions from all interstate and international telecommunications carriers, determines an appropriate rate of reimbursement, and dispenses funds to bona fide relay providers. States may decide for themselves how to fund their intrastate relay services.

Mandatory minimum standards   FCC rules set forth other mandatory minimum standards and technical requirements. These are summarized in Box F-2.

Future Issues

The major TRS-related issues currently under consideration by the FCC are described in the following sections.

VRS numbering   In July of 2000, the FCC released a ruling directing common carriers nationwide to allow all relay callers—deaf, hard-of-hearing, and hearing or speech disabled callers—to access relay services by dialing "7-1-1."[75] The goal was to make relay dialing fast, easy, and uncomplicated so that callers anywhere could be able to access these services. While 7-1-1 has been effective in facilitating relay access for PSTN-based calls, easy dialing remains a problem for VRS users. At present, when a hearing person tries to initiate a VRS call by dialing a provider's toll-free number, that person typically needs the IP address of the deaf VRS user's equipment to enable the interpreter to establish a video link with the person receiving the call. However, most residential IP addresses are dynamic; that is, they can change at any given time and are therefore very difficult to ascertain. To address this situation, some VRS providers use their own database of "proxy" or "alias" numbers, which allows VRS customers to have a constant "telephone number" that is automatically mapped to their dynamic IP address. Unfortunately, because these databases generally cannot be used from one provider to the next, deaf VRS users often have multiple telephone numbers or extensions (one for each VRS provider) to get calls from hearing people.

To remedy this situation, the FCC has opened a rulemaking proceeding

---

[75]*The Use of N11 Codes and Other Abbreviated Dialing Arrangements*, Second Report and Order, CC Dkt. No. 92-105, FCC 00-257 (August 9, 2000), codified at 47 C.F.R. §§64.601(1), 64.603.

requesting comment on the feasibility of establishing a single, open, and global database of proxy numbers that could be used by all service providers to allow hearing people to call any VRS user through any VRS provider without having to know every VRS users' current IP address.[76] This type of universal numbering would be neutral with respect to both the provider and the video equipment that the customer uses, just as are ordinary phone numbers.

Interoperability of VRS protocols   In a recent ruling, the FCC determined that all VRS consumers must be able to place VRS calls through the services of any VRS providers and that all VRS providers must be capable of receiving calls from and transmitting calls for any VRS consumer.[77] The order was prompted by the prior marketing practices of some VRS providers that had required consumers to use a single provider in exchange for free video equipment or broadband service. VRS users were able to access multiple VRS providers only by using multiple pieces of equipment or broadband connections, an arrangement that the FCC determined was both burdensome and inconsistent with notions of functional equivalency.

A related interoperability issue concerns the protocols used by VRS providers to transmit their calls over the Internet. Although the standard currently used for transmitting real-time voice and video over packet-based networks by most VRS providers is H.323, newer entrants to the VRS market are beginning to rely on Session Initiation Protocol (usually referred to as SIP) for this purpose. The FCC has opened a proceeding to determine whether it should adopt specific Internet protocols for VRS providers to prevent incompatible protocols from creating new barriers for VRS consumers.[78]

Emergency access   FCC rules require TRS providers to be capable of immediately and automatically transferring emergency 9-1-1 calls to an appropriate public safety answering point (PSAP) that can respond with fire, police, or medical attention.[79] An appropriate PSAP is defined as one that the caller would have reached by directly dialing 9-1-1 or that is capable of dispatching emergency services expeditiously. While PSTN-based TRS providers comply with this directive, it often takes longer to connect

---

[76]*Telecommunications Relay Services and Speech-to-Speech Services for Individuals with Hearing and Speech Disabilities, and the Americans with Disabilities Act of 1990*, Declaratory Ruling and Notice of Proposed Rulemaking, CG Dkt. No. 03-123, FCC 06-57 (May 9, 2006). Easy dialing access remains a problem for Internet-based text relay for the same reasons that it poses a problem for VRS.

[77]Id.

[78]Id. at ¶55.

[79]47 C.F.R. §§64.604(a)(4).

BOX F-2
TRS Mandatory Minimum Standards
47 C.F.R. §64.604 and §64.605

Technical Standards

- Mandated TRS and English VRS must be offered 24 hours a day, seven days a week.
- TRS providers must be capable of handling ASCII and Baudot formats, in any speed generally in use.
- TRS providers must answer 85% percent of all categories of TRS calls (except VRS) within 10 seconds by any method that enables the call to immediately be placed, and not put in a queue or on hold.
- Network facilities and CA staffing shall be sufficient so that under projected calling volume, the probability of a busy response due to loop trunk congestion or CA unavailability shall be functionally equivalent to what a voice caller would experience when placing a call through the voice telephone network.
- TRS providers must be capable of handling any type of call normally provided by common carriers except coin sent-paid calls, which are now exempt; the burden of proving the infeasibility of handling a particular type of call is on the carriers.
- TRS providers are prohibited from refusing single or sequential calls or limiting the length of relay calls.
- TRS providers must ensure user confidentiality and with the exception of STS calls, CAs may not keep records of the contents of any conversation. STS CAs may retain information from a call to facilitate the completion of consecutive calls.
- Relay conversations must be conducted in real time.
- TRS providers must be able to handle emergency (911) calls and relay them to the appropriate public safety answering point (PSAP). An appropriate PSAP is a PSAP that the caller would have reached through direct 911 dialing, or that is capable of dispatching emergency services expeditiously. The CA must pass along the caller's telephone number when a caller disconnects before being connected to emergency services. Waivers for this requirement are in place until 2008 for VRS and IP relay.
- TRS users may not be charged rates that are any greater than the rates paid for functionally equivalent voice communication services with respect to such factors as the duration of the call, the time of day, and the distance from the point of origination to the point of termination.
- TRS users must be given their choice of interexchange carrier for long distance calls to the same extent that voice telephone users are given this choice.
- TRS providers must have redundancy features that are functionally equivalent to the equipment in telephone central offices, including uninterruptible power for emergency use.
- TRS providers must give STS users the option of maintaining a list of names and telephone numbers used frequently by that individual.

Mandates Pertaining to Communication Assistants and VRS Interpreters

- CAs must have competent skills in typing, grammar, spelling, interpretation of typewritten ASL and familiarity with hearing and speech disability cultures, languages and etiquette.
- CAs must type at a minimum speed of 60 words per minute (Technological aids may be used to achieve this speed). Providers must give oral-to-type tests to verify this speed.

- CAs may not intentionally alter or disclose the content of a relayed conversation and must relay all conversations verbatim unless the user specifically requests summarization or requests interpretation of an ASL call. An STS CA may facilitate a call with the permission of the caller, so long as the CA does not interfere with the independence of the caller and the caller maintains control of the conversation.
- A CA answering or placing a call must stay with a TRS/VRS call for a minimum of 10 minutes and with an STS call for a minimum of 15 minutes to avoid disruptions to the call.
- TRS providers must undertake their best efforts to accommodate a user's request for a particular CA gender.
- VRS interpreters must be qualified, defined as able to interpret effectively, accurately, and impartially, both receptively and expressively, using any necessary specialized vocabulary.

Mandates Pertaining to Specific TRS or Telephone Features

TRS providers must be capable of handling

- answering machine and voice mail retrieval
- call release functionality
- speed dialing functionality
- three-way calling functionality
- pay-per-call calls
- interstate Spanish TRS calls

Interactive Voice Response Systems and Recorded Messages: CAs must use a hot key to inform TRS users when the incoming call is a recorded message or uses an interactive menu. TRS providers shall electronically capture recorded message and retain them for the length of the call. No additional charges may be imposed for additional calls needed to complete calls involving recordings or interactive messages.

Consumer Complaints

- Logs: Each state and interstate TRS provider must maintain a log of consumer complaints filed with the state or TRS provider, and must include in such logs the date each complaint was filed, the nature of each complaint, the date of resolution, and an explanation of the resolution. States and TRS providers shall submit summaries of these logs to the Commission each year.
- Contact persons: State TRS programs, interstate TRS providers, and TRS providers that have state contracts must provide the FCC with a contact person and/or office that handles TRS consumer information and TRS complaints. These are to be posted on the FCC's website: http://www.fcc.gov/cgb/dro/trs_contact_list.html.

Outreach

Common carriers have an obligation to ensure that individuals in their service areas, including people who are hard of hearing, speech disabled, senior citizens and members of the general population, are aware of the availability and use of all types of TRS. Ways to achieve this include publication of information in directories, billing inserts, and through directory assistance services. In addition, carriers providing telephone voice transmission services have an obligation to conduct ongoing education and outreach programs to publicize the availability of 711 TRS access in a manner "reasonably designed to reach the largest number of consumers possible."

emergency relay calls to appropriate 9-1-1 personnel than it takes to connect directly dialed voice 9-1-1 calls, because relay calls are routed through
the PSAPs' 10-digit administrative numbers rather than through the native
selective routing system. Thus, even where 9-1-1 relay access is provided,
many believe that this affords only second-class status to its users.

A more significant problem exists with respect to the handling of emergency calls made by VRS and Internet-based relay users. Although number
and location information for relay calls made over the PSTN can automatically be passed through to PSAPs, relay calls made over the Internet are
not linked to specific geographic locations and therefore cannot similarly
be automatically transferred. This limitation has led the FCC to waive the
requirement to handle emergency calls for VRS and text-based Internet relay service providers until 2008. On November 30, 2005, the FCC released
a notice of proposed rulemaking seeking comment on the best methods of
handling these emergency calls.[80] Among other things, the Commission is
seeking feedback on whether the solution for VRS and Internet-based relay
services should mirror the solution for voice over Internet protocol (VoIP)
services, which requires the customers of interconnected VoIP services to
register the physical location where they will be originating their calls so
that emergency authorities can be directed to the appropriate location.[81]

Telecommunications Accessibility Enhancement Act of 1988

Although the Architectural Barriers Act of 1968 required federal buildings to be accessible to people with disabilities, well into the 1980s most
federal government buildings did not have TTY devices. This left many
people with hearing loss without a means to contact federal governmental
agencies. To remedy this, in June 1986, the Access Board, in conjunction
with the U.S. Department of the Treasury and the Interagency Coordinating Council (ICC), announced the creation of a pilot federal relay service
that would relay calls between TTY users and governmental employees
who used conventional voice telephones.[82] When this service—initially
staffed with a single relay operator—quickly became overwhelmed with
calls, consumers approached Congress about expanding the federal relay
service and installing TTYs in all governmental offices. Although the latter
proposal was abandoned, in 1988, Congress passed the Telecommunica-

---

[80]*In the Matter of Telecommunications Relay Services and Speech-to-Speech Services for Individuals with Hearing and Speech Disabilities*, Notice of Proposed Rulemaking, CG Docket No. 03-123, FCC 05-196 (November 30, 2005).

[81]*In the Matter of IP-Enabled Services and E911Rrequirements for IP Enabled Service Providers*, First Report and Order and Notice of Proposed Rulemaking, WC Dkt. Nos. 04-36; 05-196, FCC 05-116 (June 3, 2005) (E911 Order).

[82]51 *Fed. Reg.* 23251 (June 26, 1986).

tions Accessibility Enhancement Act (TAEA), which created a new Federal Relay Service (FRS) that transferred the day-to-day relay operations from the Access Board to the General Services Administration (GSA).[83] By 1998, FRS evolved into a 24-hour-a-day, 7-day-a-week service, and by 2000, it had a staff of more than 100 operators who handled tens of thousands of inbound and outbound calls each month. The service now provides the full range of relay services that are available under the ADA.

In addition to its relay mandates, the TAEA directed GSA to work with the Access Board, the ICC, the FCC, and other federal agencies to take the actions needed to ensure that the federal telecommunications system is fully accessible to people with hearing and speech disabilities for communication with and within federal agencies and to promote research by federal agencies, state agencies, and private entities to "reduce the cost and improve the capabilities of telecommunications devices and systems that provide accessibility to hearing-impaired and speech-impaired individuals."[84] The Act also ordered the publication of a directory of the TTYs used in federal agencies,[85] required that each house of Congress establish a policy for its members to obtain TTYs,[86] and directed the federal government to adopt a TTY logo to signify the presence of TTY devices.[87]

Section 255 of the Telecommunications Act of 1996

Historical Background and Legislation

In the mid-to-late 1980s, the convergence of computer and telephone technologies, together with the introduction of new and innovative telecommunications services and equipment, prompted local telecommunications companies to seek federal legislative relief from many of the restrictions imposed upon them by the AT&T divestiture. When Congress started drafting legislation to ease some of these limitations, disability advocates took the opportunity to seek stronger safeguards for access to all telecommunications products and services by people with disabilities.

Up until this time, the only way for most people with disabilities to obtain telecommunications access was through reliance on specialized rather

---

[83]P.L. 100-542, 102 Stat. 2721(1988), codified at 40 U.S.C. §762a-d.

[84]40 U.S.C. §762b. Unfortunately, these provisions have not been enforced since the Act was passed.

[85]40 U.S.C. §762a(b)(5).

[86]40 U.S.C. §762d.

[87]40 U.S.C. §762a(b)(6). In July 1989, a contest held at Gallaudet University's Deaf Way Conference in Washington, D.C., resulted in the selection of a TTY logo created by a young deaf artist named Jennifer Hummel. The logo is now used to identify TTYs throughout governmental agencies and in many locations around the world.

than mainstream equipment. This approach created several problems. First, assistive devices were often expensive and hard to locate in retail establishments. Second, the technology associated with the specialized telecommunications equipment often lagged behind mainstream telecommunications technologies, which evolved at a very swift pace. Third, the access provided by the specialized equipment was generally slower, more complicated, or otherwise inferior to the access provided by mainstream equipment.

Also, people with disabilities did not want to continue having to "catch up" whenever new technologies were developed. Instead, they wanted their needs to be considered and access features to be built in *as* new products and services were being designed and developed. To this end, they asked Congress to incorporate principles of "universal design" into the Communications Act. This meant that they wanted telecommunications businesses to make their mainstream telecommunications products and services accessible to the widest range of individuals right "off the shelf," without the need for additional adaptation. When the Telecommunications Act of 1996 passed, Section 255 incorporated these principles of universal design for all telecommunications products and services. This section requires manufacturers of telecommunications equipment and customer premises equipment and providers of telecommunications services to design, develop, and fabricate their equipment and services so that they are accessible to and usable by individuals with disabilities, if accessibility and usability are readily achievable.[88] If accessibility and usability are not readily achievable, then a manufacturer or service provider must ensure that its equipment or service is compatible with peripheral devices or the SCPE that is commonly used by people with disabilities.

Determining whether something is readily achievable requires balancing the cost and nature of the access feature against the resources of the covered entity—much in the same way that an undue burden determination is made under the Rehabilitation Act or the ADA.[89] Not required are access features that are technically infeasible or that would so fundamentally alter the product that they would substantially reduce the functionality of the product, render some features inoperable, substantially and materially alter the shape, size, or weight of the product, or impede or deter the use of the product by other individuals.

A parallel obligation, contained in Section 251 of the Act, prohibits telecommunications carriers from installing network features, functions, or capabilities that do not comply with the Section 255 guidelines.[90] Section 251 requires that telecommunications carriers ensure that the configura-

---

[88]P.L. 104-104 (1996), 110 Stat. 56 (1996), codified at 47 U.S.C. §255.
[89]47 C.F.R. §§6.3(g).
[90]47 U.S.C. §251.

tion of their network architecture (i.e., hardware, software, and databases associated with the routing of telecommunications services) complies with the FCC's accessibility rules.

FCC Regulations

FCC rules on Section 255, effective since January 28, 2000, require telecommunications manufacturers and service providers to evaluate the accessibility, usability, and compatibility of equipment and services, as early and consistently as possible throughout their design, development, and fabrication. All basic and advanced telephone services including call waiting, speed dialing, call forwarding, computer-provided directory assistance, call monitoring, caller identification, call tracing and repeat dialing, interactive voice response systems, and voice menus are covered under the rules. In addition, under a ruling that came out in June 2007, services provided by interconnected voice-over Internet protocol providers are covered because of their functional similarity to traditional telephone services.[91]

The customer premises equipment covered by the rules includes all equipment used on an individual's premises to originate, route, or terminate telecommunications, as well as software integral to the operation of the telecommunications functions of the equipment, whether or not it is sold separately. Examples are wireline and wireless telephones, pagers, and fax machines.

Accessibility In determining whether a product is accessible, a manufacturer must evaluate the extent to which the product's various input, control, and mechanical functions, as well as its output, display, and control functions, are operable without vision, hearing, manual dexterity, speech, cognitive skills, and other functionalities.[92] All information needed to operate the product, including "text, static or dynamic images, icons, labels, sounds, or incidental operating cues," must also be made accessible to people with various types of disabilities.[93] Some of the access features that companies have already started to incorporate to meet the accessibility requirement include nibs or capital letters on keypads; vibrating features and volume control on telephones; jacks for TTYs; accessible telephone intercept mes-

---

[91]*Implementation of Section 255 and 251(a)(2) of the Communications Act of 1934, as Enacted by the Telecommunications Act of 1996, Access to Telecommunications Services, Telecommunications Equipment, and Customer Premises Equipment by Persons with Disabilities*, Report and Order and Further Notice of Inquiry, WT Dkt No. 96-198, FCC 99-181, 16 FCC Rcd 6417 (September 29, 1999), codified at 47 C.F.R. Parts 6 and 7.
[92]47 C.F.R. §6.3(a)(1).
[93]47 C.F.R. §6.3(a)(2).

sages; the ability to change the color, font, or lighting on keypads and screens; and the provision of speech output on cell phones.[94]

Usability   Telecommunications service providers and manufacturers must also evaluate whether their products and services are "usable by" individuals with disabilities.[95] This mandate requires functionally equivalent access to the full operation of and the documentation for the product, including instructions, product information, technical support hotlines and databases, customer support call centers, repair services, and billing departments. Among other things, companies must provide end-user product documentation in alternate formats (such as braille and large print) and access to services in alternate modes (TTY, e-mail, etc.) at no additional charge to the consumer requesting these accommodations.

The FCC has also stated that "usable by" requires manufacturers and service providers to include consumers with disabilities in market research projects, focus groups, pilot demonstrations, and product trials when a company otherwise engages in these activities. Similarly, companies must make reasonable efforts to validate unproven access solutions with people with disabilities or disability-related organizations.

Compatibility   The FCC's rules explain that the Section 255 requirement to make mainstream equipment compatible with peripheral devices applies to peripheral devices employed in connection with telecommunications equipment or customer premises equipment used to translate, enhance, or otherwise transform telecommunications into a form that is accessible to individuals with disabilities, such as TTYs, visual signaling devices, and amplifiers.[96] The requirement to achieve compatibility with SCPE covers equipment commonly used by individuals with disabilities to originate, route, or terminate telecommunications, such as direct-connect TTYs.[97] Assistive technology devices, such as hearing aids or eyeglasses, which have a broad application outside the telecommunications context, are not SCPE or peripheral equipment even if they are used in conjunction with telecommunications devices. In addition to its overall mandate to provide compatibility, FCC rules have four very specific requirements for telecommunications compatibility:

---

[94]The last accommodation was the product of a formal complaint under Section 255 against Verizon Wireless and Audiotext for their failure to make an accessible wireless phone for people who are blind or who have vision disabilities. The cell phone with speech output was produced after a settlement was reached between the parties.

[95]47 C.F.R. §6.3(k).

[96]47 C.F.R. §§6.3(b), (f).

[97]47 C.F.R. §§6.3(h).

- There must be external electronic access to all information and control mechanisms.
- There must be a connection point for external audio-processing devices.
- Products that have a function for voice communication shall provide a standard nonacoustic connection point for TTYs. Users must also be able to easily turn a microphone on and off to intermix speech with TTY (for VCO- and HCO-type functions).[98]
- Products shall support all cross-manufacturer nonproprietary standard signals used by TTYs.

Section 508 of the Rehabilitation Act of 1973

In the Workforce Investment Act of 1998, Congress strengthened the requirements of Section 508 of the Rehabilitation Act of 1973 to require all federal agencies to develop, procure, maintain, and use accessible electronic and information technologies, unless doing so would create an undue burden for the agency.[99] Access Board guidelines, released on December 21, 2000, have applied this mandate to telecommunications, computers, software applications, video and multimedia products and applications, and web-based intranet and Internet information and applications.[100] Among other things, the guidelines require federal agencies to maintain telecommunications products that provide hearing aid compatibility and amplification and that support TTY transmissions;[101] accessible caller identification devices for individuals who cannot see displays;[102] and TTY-compatible voice mail, auto-attendant, and interactive voice response telephone systems.[103]

---

[98]Because only VCO and not HCO was mentioned in the regulations, some companies have implemented the former feature but not the latter feature in their products.

[99]Rehabilitation Act Amendments of 1998, P.L. 105-220 §408(b), 112 Stat. 936 (1998), codified at 29 U.S.C. §794d.

[100]65 *Fed. Reg.* 80499-80528 (December 21, 2000), codified at 36 C.F.R. §1194 et seq. On April 25, 2001, GSA, the U.S. Department of Defense, and the National Aeronautics and Space Administration amended the Federal Acquisition Regulation to incorporate these standards. 66 *Fed. Reg.* 20894 et seq. (April 25, 2001), amending 48 C.F.R. Parts 2, 7, 10, 11, 12, 39.

[101]36 C.F.R. §1194.23(a) provides that "Telecommunications products or systems which provide a function allowing voice communication and which do not themselves provide a TTY functionality shall provide a standard non-acoustic connection point for TTYs. Microphones shall be capable of being turned on and off to allow the user to intermix speech with TTY use." In addition, Subsection (b) requires telecommunications products that include voice communication functionality to support all commonly used cross-manufacturer nonproprietary standard TTY signal protocols. Subsections (f) and (g) establish standards for telephone volume control for incoming and outgoing calls, while Subsections (h) and (i) cover hearing aid compatibility and access to wireless phones by hearing aid users.

[102]36 C.F.R. §1194.23(e).

[103]36 C.F.R. §1194.23(c) and (d).

The Access Board's standards also lay out various requirements for video and multimedia information to be captioned and video described, and for certain televisions, tuners, and computer equipment with television receivers to have built-in decoders for the receipt and display of closed captions and secondary audio program circuitry for the playback of video descriptions (narrative verbal descriptions inserted into the natural pauses of a video program to describe visual events that are not part of a program's audio track).[104] In addition, under the Section 508 guidelines, software applications and operating systems must be accessible,[105] as must information and documentation about the technologies used by the government, including user manuals, installation guides, and customer and technical support.

Television Decoder Circuitry Act

Historical Background and Legislation

Television programs began adding closed captioning to their programs in March 1980 when three networks—NBC, ABC, and PBS—entered into an agreement with the National Captioning Institute to provide 16 to 20 hours of captioned programming weekly. The agreement also provided for Sears to produce and sell stand-alone television decoders that would be capable of receiving and displaying closed captions.[106] Over the next decade, the number of programs containing captions jumped to about 200 programs per week, largely because of the millions of dollars in grants for closed captioning distributed by the U.S. Department of Education.[107] Despite the growth of this service, by the close of the decade, closed captioning faced a crisis. Less than 200,000 decoders had been purchased, far below the initial projections of 100,000 a year. With so small a viewing audience, television networks began questioning the wisdom of continuing to invest in this service.

The discrepancy between the possible market for decoders, which was

---

[104]36 C.F.R. §1194.24.

[105]36 C.F.R. §1194.21. In addition, products that transmit information or communication, shall "pass through cross-manufacturer, non-proprietary, industry-standard codes, translation protocols, formats or other information necessary to provide the information or communication in a usable format. Technologies which use encoding, signal compression, format transformation, or similar techniques shall not remove information needed for access or shall restore it upon delivery." 36 C.F.R. §1194.23(j).

[106]Sears offered two decoders; one was an "adapter unit" for $249 that connected to a television set, and the second was an "integrated TV receiver" that was built into a 19-inch color TV set and that sold for $500.

[107]"General Information About the Closed-Captioning Services," *nci for your information* [sic] (July 1987):3. These grants accounted for approximately one-third of the cost of providing captioning; the remaining two-thirds of the costs were picked up by television networks, producers, programmers, and advertisers.

estimated to be approximately 100 million people, and the number of these devices that had been purchased was attributed to a number of factors.[108] First, many people with hearing loss were simply unaware of the existence of decoders or where to purchase them. In addition, the complications involved in hooking up these devices to a television set, video cassette recorder, and cable box discouraged some consumers, especially senior citizens, from purchasing decoders. But the primary reason cited by consumers for not purchasing decoders was simply that there were not enough closed-captioned television programs to justify their cost. Although by that year the number of hours of programming with closed captioning totaled 390 per week, including nearly all prime-time programs on the major networks, a mere 90 of 1,400 local newscasts were closed captioned, and most daytime and basic cable programming was not captioned at all.[109]

The proponents of captioning believed that increasing the number of programs with captions would expand decoder purchases and audiences who used captioning, but an attempt to incorporate a requirement for television captioning in the ADA, which was then under consideration by the Congress, was rejected outright. Powerful lobbying by the motion picture and television industries made clear that the inclusion of such a mandate could kill the omnibus disability rights legislation.

A report released by the Commission on Education of the Deaf suggested a different solution.[110] It proposed that if all television sets were equipped internally with circuitry that decoded closed captions, the larger audiences that would be able to use this technology would create a strong incentive for the television industry to increase its captioned programming. More specifically, the new audiences would attract greater advertising revenues that could, in turn, help defray the costs of the networks' captioning investments. It was this reasoning that prompted consumers to push for the passage of legislation that would require captioning circuitry to be built into all new television sets. Advocates achieved success with the passage of the Television Decoder Circuitry Act of 1990, which required all televisions manufactured or imported into the United States with screens 13 inches or larger to be capable of displaying closed captions.[111]

---

[108]Many of these reasons were revealed in a survey conducted by the U.S. Department of Education in the spring of 1989. Renee Z. Sherman and Joel D. Sherman, *Analysis of Demand for Decoders of Television Captioning for Deaf and Hearing-Impaired Children and Adults* (Washington, D.C.: Pelavin Associates, June 1989).

[109]See, generally, S. Rep. No. 393, 101st Cong., 2d Sess. 2 (1990).

[110]Commission on Education of the Deaf, Frank Bowe, ed., *Toward Equality: Education of the Deaf* (Washington D.C.: Government Printing Office, 1988).

[111]P.L. 101-431, 104 Stat. 960 (1990), codified at 47 U.S.C. §§303(u), 330(b). The statute became effective on July 1, 1993. For an overview of the history behind and intent of this legislation, see Sy DuBow, "The Television Decoder Circuitry Act—TV For All," *Temple Law Review* 64, No. 2 (1991): 609; Peltz Strauss, *A New Civil Right*: 226-245.

FCC Regulations

In December 1990, the FCC issued standards that defined the size, font, color, placement, and intelligibility of the captions received and displayed by decoder circuitry in analog television sets.[112] Among other things, these required italicized or slanted standard characters, smooth scrolling of captions, upper- and lowercase letters, up to four lines of captions anywhere on the screen, a black background, and prominent labeling of captioning features with television receivers. A subsequent ruling by the FCC also made clear that when computers equipped with television circuitry are sold together with monitors that have viewable pictures measuring at least 13 inches, the computers must also be capable of receiving and displaying closed captions.[113]

In July 2000, the FCC updated its captioning specifications for *digital* television programming.[114] The new guidelines give viewers several new options, including the ability to choose among three caption sizes (standard, large, and small captions), eight fonts, eight background and foreground colors (white, black, red, green, blue, yellow, magenta, and cyan), various levels of background opacity (transparent, translucent, solid, and flashing), five character edges (none, raised, depressed, uniform, or drop shadowed), and up to six captioning services.[115] These standards apply to screens that measure 7.8 inches vertically, roughly the equivalent of a 13-inch diagonal analog screen. The mandates cover digital televisions that are sold with

---

[112]*Amendment of Part 15 of the Commission's Rules to Implement the Provisions of the Television Decoder Circuitry Act of 1990*, Report and Order, GEN Dkt. No. 91-1, FCC 91-119, 6 FCC Rcd 2419 (April 15, 1991), recon. granted in part, Memorandum Opinion and Order, 7 FCC Rcd 2279 (1992), codified at 47 C.F.R. §15.119. These performance and display standards are based on a report prepared by a task force of television set manufacturers, decoder circuitry manufacturers, and captioning agencies, working under the auspices of the Electronics Industries Association, later renamed the Electronics Industry Alliance. *Television Receiver Performance Specification for Basic Closed Captioned Services*, Draft Revision 6.0, EIA Standards Proposal, EIA/CEG Television Receiver Committee (R-4) (December 7, 1990).

[113]*Closed Captioning Requirements for Computer Systems Used as Television Receivers*, FCC Public Notice, DA 95-581 (March 22, 1995), 60 *Fed. Reg.* 16055 (March 29, 1995).

[114]Analog television pictures are comprised of 525 lines; line 21 is the last line of the television's "vertical blanking interval" before the television picture begins and is where closed captions are inserted. Because there is no vertical blanking interval in digital TVs, engineers had to find a different way for captions to be added to programs.

[115]*Closed Captioning Requirements for Digital Television Receivers*, Report and Order, ET Dkt. No. 99-254, MM Dkt. 95-176, FCC 00-259, 15 FCC Rcd 16788 (July 31, 2000), codified at 47 C.F.R. §15.122.

tuners, as well as all stand-alone digital television tuners and set-top boxes, whether or not these are sold with display screens over a certain size.[116]

Section 713 of the Communications Act of 1934: Closed-Captioning Mandates

Historical Background and Legislation

By the time that the Television Decoder Circuitry Act of 1990 became effective in July 1993, nearly 100 percent of all prime-time programming, children's programming, and national news programs on NBC, CBS, ABC, and PBS and most prime-time programming on Fox was shown with captions.[117] However, captioning on cable TV remained scarce, with approximately only 5 to 10 percent of all basic cable programs providing captioning. Concerned that the Decoder Act was not providing sufficient incentives for cable programmers to caption their programs, advocates returned to Congress. This time, they were successful in getting mandates for closed captioning of televised programming in Section 305 of the Telecommunications Act of 1996, which created a new Section 713 of the Communications Act.

Section 713 requires video programming first published or exhibited *after* the effective date of the FCC's regulations to be "fully accessible through the provision of closed captions."[118] The section also directs video programming providers or owners to "maximize the accessibility of video programming first published or exhibited prior to the effective date of such regulations through the provision of closed captions."[119] The statute allows the FCC to exempt certain programming from these requirements, where the provision of captioning is economically burdensome, is inconsistent with contracts in effect at the time that the 1996 Act was enacted, or would result in an undue burden for the video programming provider or program owner.[120]

A separate provision contained in Section 713, which directed the FCC to commence an inquiry on the provision of video descriptions, prompted

---

[116]The FCC reasoned that separately purchased digital tuners would most likely be used with screens measuring at least 7.8 vertical inches and that the ability to control the size, color, and font of captions meant that viewers would be able to discern captions on small screens. Id. at ¶47.

[117]"Closed Captioned Programming Currently Available," Fact Sheet, The Caption Center (June 1993).

[118]47 U.S.C. §713(b)(1).

[119]47 U.S.C. §713(b)(2).

[120]47 U.S.C. §713(d). The last exemption is granted only upon individual petitions filed with the FCC. The Act does not draw a distinction between the "economically burdensome" and "undue burden" standards, other than to provide that the former is used for categorical exemptions and the latter is used for exemptions upon request.

the agency to also promulgate, in 2000, regulations requiring video descriptions on certain broadcast and cable programming.[121] However, these rules were struck down by the U.S. Court of Appeals for the D.C. Circuit in November 2002, after the television broadcast and motion picture industries challenged the Commission's authority to require any video description on television.[122] In recent years, various attempts have been made to restore these video description mandates through federal legislation.

FCC Regulations

FCC rules implementing the captioning mandates created an elaborate schedule of deadlines that initially required 25 percent of all new, nonexempt programs to be captioned by January 2000 and increased this amount by an additional 25 percent every 2 years until January 2006, when 100 percent of all programming was required to contain captioning.[123] Thirty percent of older nonexempt programming, that is, programming first exhibited before the effective date of the FCC's rules, also had to be captioned by 2003, with this amount capping at 75 percent by 2008. Requirements for new, nonexempt Spanish-language programming followed a different schedule: 450 hours of captioned programming by 2001, 900 hours by 2004, 1,350 hours by 2007, and 100 percent of all such programming by 2010. Nonexempt Spanish-language programming first shown before the effective date of the FCC's rules had to provide captioning on 30 percent of its programs by 2005, with this amount increasing to 75 percent by 2012.

The FCC's captioning rules exempt all advertisements under 5 minutes, public service announcements under 10 minutes (unless they are federally funded or produced), programs shown between 2 a.m. and 6 a.m., locally produced instructional programming that is distributed to individual educational institutions, locally produced and distributed programs with limited repeat value (for example, parades and local school sports), nonvocal music, and programs in languages other than English or Spanish. In addition, captioning is not required for programming on new networks during their

---

[121]47 U.S.C. §713(f). *Video Description of Video Programming*, Report and Order, MM Dkt. No. 99-339, FCC 00-258, 15 FCC Rcd 15230 (2000), amended in part at Memorandum Opinion and Order on Reconsideration, FCC 01-7, 16 FCC Rcd 1251 (2001).

[122]*Motion Picture Association of America, Inc., et al. v. Federal Communications Commission*, et al., 309 F. 3d 796 (D.C. Cir. 2002)

[123]*Closed Captioning and Video Description of Video Programming, Implementation of Section 305 of the Telecommunications Act of 1996*, Report and Order, MM Dkt. No. 95-176, FCC 97-279, 13 FCC Rcd 3272 (August 22, 1997), amended in Order on Reconsideration, MM Dkt. No. 95-176, FCC 98-236, 13 FCC Rcd 19973 (October 2, 1998), codified at 47 C.F.R. §79.1 et seq.

first 4 years of operations or by programming providers with annual gross revenues under $3 million per year. Moreover, all providers are permitted to cap their captioning spending to 2 percent of their annual gross revenues.

All programs that have already been shown with captions and that are reexhibited on either the same channel or another channel must be shown with those captions intact unless the shows have been edited—whether or not the captioning schedules presented above have been met. Specific rules also exist for the provision of real-time captioning on newscasts. To save money, many local television stations caption their news with a method called the "electronic newsroom technique" (ENT). This technique converts the news scripts appearing over their teleprompters into live captions. However, precisely because it is prescribed, ENT often leaves out live information, including late-breaking stories, field interviews, and sports and weather updates. By contrast, real-time captions capture the entire audio track of a show's live program because the captions are exhibited simultaneously with the programming content. Current FCC rules require real-time captioning only on news programs exhibited by (1) the four major national broadcast networks (CBS, ABC, NBC, and Fox), (2) television stations affiliated with these four major networks in the top 25 television markets, and (3) national nonbroadcast networks (for example, cable) serving at least 50 percent of all households subscribing to television services. All other stations are permitted to use ENT for their news broadcasts.

In July 2004, concerns about a drop in captioning quality over recent years—largely caused by the proliferation of competitive captioning providers who may be compromising caption quality to win bids—prompted several national advocacy organizations representing people who are deaf and hard of hearing to submit a petition to the FCC requesting minimum standards of captioning quality, better enforcement of the existing captioning rules, and an expansion of the number of stations that must caption their local newscasts in real time.[124] This petition remains pending.

Emergency Captioning

In addition to the FCC's general captioning rules, in 2000, the Commission promulgated specific rules requiring visual and audio access to televised emergency programming.[125] Unlike the captioning mandates, these

---

[124]Petition for Rulemaking by Telecommunications for the Deaf, Inc., Consumer Advocacy Network, National Association of the Deaf, Self Help for Hard of Hearing People, Inc, and the Association of Late Deafened Adults, RM-11065 (July 23, 2004).

[125]*Closed Captioning and Video Description of Video Programming, Implementation of Section 305 of the Telecommunications Act of 1996, Accessibility of Emergency Programming*, Second Report and Order, MM Dkt. No. 95-176, FCC 00-136, 15 FCC Rcd 6615 (April 14, 2000), codified at 47 C.F.R. §79.2.

rules apply to all video programming distributors, including broadcasters, cable operators, and satellite television services, without exception. They require the provision of visual information—in the form of open or closed captions or other visual methods, such as crawls or scrolls that appear on the screen—whenever emergency information is televised. Emergency information that is provided in the video portion of a regularly scheduled newscast or an unscheduled programming break must also be described visually in the program's main audio track. If the emergency information is provided through a crawled or scrolled visual announcement during regular programming, an aural tone must be provided to alert people who have vision loss that there is an emergency and that they should turn to another source, such as a radio, for additional information.

The emergency access rules apply to weather disasters, such as tornadoes, hurricanes, earthquakes, and heavy snows; fires; civil disorders, such as toxic gas leaks and power failures; school closings; and all other televised information pertaining to the protection of life, health, safety, or property. Accessible information must include not only details about the events themselves but also how to respond to those events, including information about evacuations; emergency routes; road closures; shelters; and ways to obtain food, medical, and other relief assistance. Finally, the rules prohibit emergency information and closed captions from blocking one other. Over the past 2 years, the failure of several television stations to comply with these rules prompted the FCC to assess monetary forfeitures against television stations ranging from $8,000 to $25,000.[126]

Emergency Alert System

In addition to the mandates under Section 713 of the Communications Act described above, the FCC's emergency alert system (EAS) regulations require all cable providers serving 5,000 or more subscribers to provide EAS messages in both audio and visual formats on all channels.[127] While this provides an added layer of assurance that televised emergency information will be made accessible, these rules come into play only when EAS is triggered by the president of the United States to contact the viewing public during a national emergency or when local jurisdictions voluntarily use it

---

[126]For example, Notices of Apparent Liability were brought on February 23, 2005, against Channel 51 of San Diego, Inc.; KGTV of McGraw-Hill Broadcasting Company; and KFMB-TV of Midwest Television. On May 25, 2005, Notices were brought against Fox Television Stations, Licensee of WTTG-TV; ACC Licensee Inc., Licensee of WJLA-TV; and NBC Telemundo.

[127]47 C.F.R. §11.51. EAS is jointly administered by the FCC, the Federal Emergency Management Agency, and the National Oceanic and Atmospheric Administration's National Weather Service.

for the dissemination of information about weather and other emergencies that pose a threat to life and property. In addition, the visual information required to be presented as part of an EAS message need not be as comprehensive as that which is required under the FCC's televised emergency rules. These messages must contain information only about the originator, event, time period, and location of the EAS message and not all content that is provided aurally.

Cable systems serving fewer than 5,000 customers have the choice of either providing an EAS audio and visual message on all of their channels or an audio EAS message and a flashing video alert on all channels, together with a full EAS message on one programmed channel. Cable providers that choose the flashing alert option must make sure that the alerts flash on the television screen simultaneously with and for the same duration as the full-length EAS message. Information about which channel will contain the full audio and video message must be provided to viewers through billing statements and other public service announcements.

Individuals with Disabilities Education Act: Closed Captioning

In October 1959, the Office of Education, Bureau of Education for the Handicapped, of the U.S. Department of Health, Education, and Welfare initiated the Captioned Films for the Deaf program. Over the next two decades, this program authorized the production, acquisition, and distribution of captioned documentary, theatrical, and educational films and media equipment to deaf schools, clubs, and organizations across the United States.[128] In the 1970s and 1980s, it was the U.S. Department of Education that provided financial support for the development of Line 21 closed captioning and financed millions of dollars in discretionary grants for television captioning, pursuant to its authority under the Individuals with Disabilities Education Act (IDEA).[129] In the 1990s, these discretionary funds also became available for the provision of video description.

In the late-1990s, however, some members of Congress began to raise concerns about allowing the use of U.S. Department of Education money for what they perceived to be inappropriate television shows, such as *Baywatch* and *The Jerry Springer Show*. They succeeded in persuading their colleagues to amend IDEA to limit the distribution of closed captioning and video description grants to educational, news, and informational programs

---

[128]See e.g., P.L. 87-715 (September 28, 1962), P.L. 89-258 (October 19, 1965), P.L. 90-247 (January 2, 1968), and P.L. 91-61 (August 20, 1969).
[129]IDEA was first enacted in 1975 as the Education for All Handicapped Children Act. Its name was changed in 1990.

after September 2001.[130] In 2004, Congress again made changes to the scope of the closed-captioning and video description provisions, this time limiting funding to television programs that are "of educational value in the classroom setting to children with disabilities."[131] In addition, under these amendments, funding for video description and captioning is provided only when these services have not otherwise been provided by the program's producer or distributor or fully funded through other sources.

The 2004 amendments *did* provide the first federal funding for access to "new and emerging technologies," including "CDs, DVDs, video streaming and other forms of multimedia."[132] In addition, the new law establishes a system for the production of student textbooks in a standardized electronic file format called the National Instructional Materials Accessibility Standard, which can be used to convert books into accessible formats, including braille, large print, or electronic text.[133] This will go a long way toward ensuring that children who are blind or who have low vision will have access to information made available through textbooks and classroom materials at the same time that their fellow classmates receive such information. The American Printing House for the Blind will establish a National Instructional Materials Access Center to serve as a repository to receive, maintain, and distribute electronic copies of this instructional material.

POLICY IMPLICATIONS OF TECHNOLOGICAL CHANGE

In recent years, Americans have become increasingly reliant on digital and Internet technologies that have significantly changed the ways in which we communicate and receive information. Our society is slowly, but gradually, abandoning our reliance on the traditional telephone network in favor of high-speed broadband services that can simultaneously transport voice, data, and video all over a single network. These newer technologies already offer exceptional opportunities to enhance the independence and productivity of people with disabilities. Similarly, new and exciting television innovations, including interactive television services that are sent over high-speed computer networks to television set-top boxes or home computers, are beginning to allow viewers to use all types of devices to receive television programming.[134]

However, if history is any indicator, legislative and regulatory safe-

---

[130]This restriction was added by Section 687(c)(2) of the IDEA Amendments of 1987, P.L. 105-17, codified at 20 U.S.C. §1487.

[131]The Individuals with Disabilities Education Improvement Act, P.L. 108-446, Section 674 (c)(1)(A), codified at 47 U.S.C. §1474(c)(1)(A).

[132]20 U.S.C. §1474(c)(1)(B)(iii).

[133]20 U.S.C. §1474(e).

[134]See generally, Peltz Strauss, *A New Civil Right*: 241.

guards will be needed to ensure that these innovations are universally accessible to all Americans. Experience has shown that competitive pressures often make companies reluctant to invest in accessibility features perceived to have a small market with little or no profit. Recognizing this, in June 2007, the FCC took another step toward ensuring disability access to modern Internet-based technologies by adopting an order to extend the requirements of Section 225 (requiring telecommunications relay services) and Section 255 (requiring access to services and equipment) to providers and manufacturers of interconnected voice-over Internet Protocol services and equipment. This order completes two prior FCC inquires seeking ways to ensure disability access to broadband technologies.[135]

As the nation migrates away from legacy circuit-based technologies and analog television services, and transitions to more versatile and innovative IP-based communication and video programming technologies, disability advocates are looking to Congress to pass laws that will ensure that people with disabilities are not left behind. For example, in addition to proposing to extend various disability protections to IP-based services, bills introduced in 2006 contained a specific requirement for the FCC to report to Congress every two years on compliance with the accessibility provisions and the extent to which accessibility barriers still exist. In 2007, over 65 national and local organizations coalesced to form the Coalition of Organizations for Accessible Technology (COAT) to further legislative and regulatory efforts that will make this communications access a reality.[136]

One of the many advantages of IP-enabled products is that they largely rely on software-based solutions that make access for people with disabilities far easier to implement than was possible for many previous telecommunications technologies. Moreover, once features for people with disabilities are added to products and services, they typically benefit the general public, much in the way that closed captions—originally intended for use by people with hearing loss—are enjoyed by the mainstream public in bars, exercise facilities, and airports.

---

[135]See, e.g., *In the Matter of Appropriate Framework for Broadband Access to the Internet Over Wireline Facilities*, Notice of Proposed Rulemaking, CC Dkts. No. 02-33; 95-20; 98-10, FCC 02-42 (Feb. 15, 2002); *In the Matter of Inquiry Concerning High-Speed Access to the Internet Over Cable and Other Facilities, Appropriate Regulatory Treatment for Broadband Access to the Internet Over Cable Facilities*, Declaratory Ruling and Notice of Proposed Rulemaking, GN Dkt. No. 00-185; CS Dkt. No. 02-52, FCC 02-77 (March 15, 2002); *In the Matter of IP-Enabled Service*, Notice of Proposed Rulemaking, WC Dkt. No. 04-36, FCC 04-28 (March 10, 2004); *In the Matters of IP-Enabled Services, E9-1-1 Requirements for IP-Enabled Service Providers*, First Report and Order and Notice of Proposed Rulemaking, WC Dkts No. 04-36, 05-196, FCC 05-116 (June 3, 2005).

[136]See www.COATaccess.org.

CONCLUSION

Although the proposed legislation cited above will go a long way toward safeguarding access to the telecommunications and information technologies of the future, gaps and uncertainties still exist. For example, it is unclear whether the Television Decoder Circuitry Act's requirement for "television apparatus" to have captioning decoder capabilities applies to newer types of devices that can receive or display television programming, including cell phones; MP3 players; video recording devices; and stand-alone video media, such as home theaters. It is critical for this statute to be interpreted broadly or amended, lest deaf and hard-of-hearing consumers be denied access to the vast array of new video programming options available to the general public.

Similarly, although state equipment distribution programs have been very successful in distributing SCPE to hundreds of thousands of persons with disabilities across the United States, most of these programs limit their selections to wireline devices and fail to provide the wireless and Internet-based communication options that are now commonplace in mainstream society. In 2000, Missouri became the first state to make adaptive computer equipment used for access to the Internet and electronic mail available to its residents; others need to follow this example.

In addition, the Lifeline and Link-up programs, two universal service programs that help subsidize the cost of monthly telephone bills and first-time connections for low income subscribers, are available only for traditional telephone services. Many disability advocates believe that these should also be available to support the Internet-based services and equipment needed for communication by people with disabilities. For example, many deaf individuals have replaced their PSTN-based TTYs with video devices that they use to converse over broadband technologies. These individuals want the option of using universal service subsidies to help pay for their broadband service and equipment.

The agenda for communications access does not stop there: a plan for TTY users to migrate to the more modern text-based communications services needs to be developed to ensure that text is as reliable and interoperable as voice in emerging communications networks; firewalls imposed by businesses and government agencies need to be adjusted so that they do not block access by sign language users wishing to make video connections over broadband technologies; new digital products must offer multiple ways of controlling their operations so that soft button or graphic interfaces do not block access by people who cannot see; and accessible real-time solutions for emergency access in an Internet-based environment need to be devised and implemented. These and other accessibility needs must be addressed so that people with disabilities can be equal participants as our nation embarks on its newest technological revolution.

G

Transportation Patterns and Problems of People with Disabilities

*Sandra Rosenbloom**

INTRODUCTION

Transportation is an extremely important policy issue for those with disabilities. People with disabilities have consistently described how transportation barriers affect their lives in important ways. Over the last two decades the National Organization on Disability (NOD) has sponsored three successive Harris polls with people with disabilities, and respondents in each survey have reported that transportation issues are a crucial concern. In the last survey, undertaken in 2004, just under a third of those with disabilities reported that inadequate transportation was a problem for them; of those individuals, over half said it was a *major* problem. The more severe the disability of the respondent was, the more serious were the reported transportation problems (National Organization on Disability-Harris Interactive, 2004).

However, the policy debates over the local transportation needs of

---

*Professor of Planning, University of Arizona, Tucson.

these travelers often revolve around dichotomies that may be misleading—arguing over the role of buses compared with the role of paratransit,
for example. Moreover, these debates often focus on some topics at the
expense of other equally important issues. For example, there is a legitimate
concern about ensuring that people with disabilities receive the services
mandated by the 1990 Americans with Disabilities Act (ADA), but most
of the transportation needs of these travelers are not addressed at all by
the ADA. Colored by this perspective, many policy analyses ignore the fact
that most travelers with disabilities, as is true for travelers in the world at
large, make the majority of their trips in private vehicles and rely heavily on
walking to facilitate their use of all modes of travel. A narrow policy focus
tends to limit discussions of the barriers to both auto use and pedestrian
travel while slighting the connection between transportation programs and
other important policy initiatives, from land use planning to human and
medical service delivery.

To expand traditional discussions, this paper makes a clear distinction
between the kinds of transport services and facilities that are required by
regulations or law and those that are required to address the far larger mobility needs of most people with disabilities. This paper not only highlights
the value of understanding and enforcing the ADA (and related legislation)
but also indicates when and why policy discussions must go beyond a focus
on the ADA to address the full spectrum of the needs of travelers with disabilities. The paper also suggests that providing effective mobility options
for those with disabilities requires attention to a variety of interrelated
policy areas and service delivery models: from how, when, and where medical services are provided to the places where people are able to live.

This paper addresses local ground transportation; beyond its scope
are issues of air, sea, and intercity travel for people with disabilities. It has
three major sections. The following section gives an overview of the travel
patterns of people with disabilities, highlighting the problems that they
face with various modes of travel and the crucial role of both walking and
private vehicles in their mobility—whether or not they drive. The next major section, the third in this paper, examines the community transportation
resources provided to travelers with disabilities by public transportation
systems, other public and nonprofit agencies, and the private sector. The
final section suggests that more and better accessible transportation is a
necessary but not a sufficient resource for overcoming the multiple barriers
faced by most people with disabilities. Addressing the transportation needs
of such travelers requires active cooperation between transportation planners and those in a number of other policy and program arenas. Relevant
personnel range from educators to medical personnel, from employment
counselors to urban designers, and from housing remodelers to land use
planners.

THE TRAVEL PATTERNS OF PEOPLE WITH DISABILITIES

In 2000 just over 8 percent of those ages 5 to 20 years, 19.2 percent of those ages 21 to 64 years, and 41.9 percent of those ages 65 years and over reported some level of disability (U.S. Census Bureau, 2002). As is well known, the older people are, the more likely they are to report a disability and the more severe it is likely to be; for example, 40 percent of those ages 65 to 69 with a disability reported that their disability was severe, whereas over 60 percent of those ages 80 and over who reported a disability reported that their disability was severe (U.S. Census Bureau, 2005). Unfortunately, knowing that a person has a disability, even if it is severe, does not tell us whether that person faces significant mobility constraints. As a result, it is difficult to clearly link disability rates to specific mobility problems. For example, a significant number of people with disabilities so serious that they cannot walk far or use public transit can and do drive (Rosenbloom, 1982; OECD, 2001). On the other hand, some people have such severe disabilities that they cannot leave their houses without substantial assistance, which may mean that their transportation concerns are secondary to the other barriers they face.

Moreover, barriers to mobility have complicated causes. The 2004 NOD-Harris Interactive poll found that almost two-thirds of all the people with disabilities who reported major transportation problems had annual incomes below $35,000. For those with higher incomes, reported transportation problems dropped markedly, as did the differences in transportation problems between those with and without disabilities (National Organization on Disability-Harris Interactive, 2004 [computed from Table 6c]). Earlier work found the same patterns; both the U.S. Congressional Budget Office (U.S. CBO, 1979) and the U.S. Senate Select Committee on Aging (1970) concluded that almost all transportation problems among the elderly or those of any age with disabilities were related to income alone; reported transportation problems dropped drastically with rising income, even controlling for age, physical disability, and health status. Of course, income may well be related to the severity of personal disability but probably not in a linear fashion.

Overall, we have limited information on the travel patterns of people with disabilities. The data that we do have tend *not* to differentiate travel by the degree of severity of a person's disability, household income, driver's license possession, car ownership, and other significant variables that might affect mobility—such as sex and age. However, two major studies give us some background information: a 1994 disability supplement to the annual National Health Interview Survey (NHIS) and a 2002 congressionally mandated study undertaken by the Bureau of Transportation Statistics of the U.S. Department of Transportation. In addition, we have some useful data on the patterns of older drivers facing declining driving skills because of increasing illness or disability. These studies are discussed below.

Overall Travel Patterns

To develop policy-relevant data on disability, in 1994 four federal agencies jointly undertook a supplemental survey (NHIS-D) to the annual NHIS (NCHS, undated). Phase II of that supplement dealt with transportation (and other) concerns.[1] The NHIS-D asked detailed questions about the transportation needs and barriers among people with self-reported disabilities and impairments (U.S. National Center for Health Statistics, undated). The NHIS-D data show that 19 percent of adults under age 65 had problems in "getting around outside . . . home due to [their] impairment or health problem." The single most frequently cited reason was *difficulty in walking*; over 75 percent of those who said that they had difficulties getting around reported walking problems. The respondents were also questioned about other possible reasons for their difficulties in getting around (multiple responses were sought and permitted), but none was nearly as important: 13 percent reported *vision problems* and 10 percent reported *cognitive or mental problems*.

Two-thirds of NHIS-D respondents under age 65 who reported the existence of one or more disabling conditions drove a car every day or occasionally. Among the 29 percent who reported *never* driving, roughly 45 percent said that they did not drive because of their impairment or health problem. Among those who did drive, even if infrequently, less than 2 percent said that they needed or used a special vehicle or special equipment on their car to allow them to do so.

The dependency on the car may be related to the low level of public transit available to respondents (although cause and effect may be difficult to determine). Roughly a third of NHIS-D respondents said that there was no public transportation available in their area. But even among the majority who did report having transit, most said that they did not use it—although their health or disability was *not* the reason for nonuse. Over three-fourths of those who had public transit in their area said that they had not used it all during the past 12 months; only 6 percent reported using a regular bus, 1.3 percent a subway, and 0.9 percent an accessible bus at least once in the previous week. Only 16 percent of those respondents

---

[1] All data were calculated for this article from Section B, *Transportation*, of the 1994 Disability Phase II Adult Public Use File available on the website of the Centers for Disease Control and Prevention; the website also explains all sampling procedures, data handling, and variance estimation strategies. See http://wonder.cdc.gov/wonder/sci_data/surveys/nhis/type_txt/dfs94-b.htm.

who had not used available public transit reported that their failure to do so was related to their impairment or health problem.

Among those who ever used public transit, even if rarely, only 13 percent reported difficulty in doing so. Among the small number of those respondents who either had difficulty in using transit or could not use it because of their disability or health condition, the single most frequently cited problem was *difficulty in walking.* The second most frequently cited problem was *needing help from another person* (multiple responses were sought).

Roughly the same number of respondents reported the availability of other transportation alternatives—and they made slightly more use of them. Almost two-thirds of NHIS-D respondents reported that there were special bus, taxi, or van services for people with disabilities available in their area. The respondents most frequently mentioned services provided by the public transit authority but also identified programs offered by other governmental and private entities. Among those who did have such services in their area, only 10 percent reported using any of them at all in the last 12 months; only 1.2 percent had used such services at least once in the previous week. In fact, the respondents mentioned that they were almost twice as likely to use a regular taxi for which they had to pay full fare as a subsidized or special transportation option. Among the 90 percent who had not used special services, over 9 out of 10 explained that they had either not needed or not wanted to use the services. Although multiple responses were sought, few respondents gave additional reasons for their nonuse of specialized transport services.

In 2002 the U.S. Bureau of Transportation Statistics (BTS) undertook a congressionally mandated comparative study of the travel patterns of people of various ages with and without disabilities; BTS interviewed 5,019 people, of whom 2,321 reported having disabilities ranging from mild to severe.[2] The study found that people with disabilities traveled less and reported more mobility problems than those without disabilities. But some disabilities were so severe that people were unable or unwilling to leave their houses; almost 2 million people, or roughly 4 percent of those with a self-reported disability, were homebound—including 9 percent of those ages 65 and over. Although over two-thirds of those under age 65 left their homes almost daily, 7 percent of those under age 25, 15 percent of those ages 25 to 64, and over 25 percent of those ages 65 and over left their homes only once or twice a week (Sweeny, 2004, Table A1).

---

[2]The BTS study was undertaken by use of the computer-assisted telephone interviewing technique between July and September 2002. Survey weights were developed to reduce several sources of bias (nonresponse, no telephone in the household, etc). Full details on the weighting and variance estimation procedures are available in U.S. BTS (2003b).

On the other hand, the BTS study found that among those with disabilities of any severity, over 70 percent of those ages 25 to 64 and roughly 60 percent of those age 65 and over were currently drivers (Sweeny, 2004, Table A8) (driving status was attributed to those who reported driving; it was *not* based on licensing status). Only 13 percent of people with disabilities lived in a household without a car, and over 20 percent lived in a household with three or more cars (U.S. BTS, 2003a, Table 35). Table G-1 clearly indicates how dependent travelers of all ages were on a car, van, or truck, although the data do not indicate the frequency of use or the percentage of all trips taken by any travel mode. Over three-fourths of all travelers under age 65 and almost that share of those ages 65 and over rode in a car at least once in a month as either a driver or a passenger. Among those ages 25 to 64, over two-thirds drove a car at least once during that month.

Conversely, no more than one in five individuals ages 25 to 64 used general public transportation (public bus, subway, light right, or commuter rail) and only 8 percent of those over age 65 did. The figures were far lower for specialized and ADA paratransit use; no more than 10 percent of any cohort of people with disabilities used these modes in a month. On the other hand, walking was a major mode for travelers with self-reported disabilities of all ages. (If a traveler using a wheelchair traveled somewhere without using another mode [i.e., not in a bus, car, train, etc.] the trip was categorized as a walking trip.)

TABLE G-1 Travel Modes Used in the Past Month by People with Disabilities

Mode	Percentage of People		
	Under 25	25–64	65+
Personal vehicle (driver)	49.1	68.6	55.6
Personal vehicle (passenger)	89.6	77.5	70.5
Carpool, vanpool	28.7	8.8	3.6
Public bus	20.9	12.8	5.8
ADA paratransit	3.7	5.3	7.2
Other specialized services	2.6	4.0	2.9
Private or chartered bus	6.3	3.9	4.7
School bus	24.6	1.9	0.0
Subway/light rail/commuter rail	9.5	7.1	2.0
Taxicab	8.6	12.4	8.2
Electric wheelchair, scooter, golf cart	2.0	0.8	1.0
Bike	48.0	15.9	3.7
Walk	56.0	47.9	37.7
Other transportation	12.0	5.4	2.8

NOTE: Multiple responses were permitted; the sample sizes were very small.
SOURCE: Table A9, Sweeny (2004).

Auto use, often as the driver, was even higher for medical trips among all travelers with disabilities. Among those ages 25 to 64, for example, almost 9 out of 10 travelers reported using a personal vehicle to travel to the doctor and drove that vehicle almost 70 percent of the time. Less than 2 percent reported using ADA or other specialized paratransit to travel to a doctor, and no more than 4 percent took a public bus (Sweeny, 2004, Table A12). Dependence on a private vehicle was even higher among people with disabilities who were employed; over 80 percent used a private vehicle to commute, driving the vehicle in which they were riding roughly half the time. No one under age 25 and only 2 percent of those ages 25 to 64 used ADA or specialized paratransit services for their work trips; only 7 percent of those under age 25 and less than 6 percent of those ages 25 to 64 used public transport (Sweeny, 2004, Table A11).Table G-2 shows that being a driver did not fully explain the reliance on a private vehicle by people with disabilities. While drivers with disabilities were more reliant on the car than nondrivers, the dependency on the private vehicle by nondrivers is clear. These data were not published by age, and as in Table G-1, they do not indicate the percentage of trips taken by each mode or the frequency of modal use. Several patterns are obvious nonetheless. Almost every current driver drove at least once during the previous month. Moreover, drivers

TABLE G-2 Transportation Mode Used by Drivers and Nondrivers with Disabilities in the Past Month

	Percentage of People	
Mode	Current Drivers	Nondrivers
Personal vehicle (driver)	96.9	
Personal vehicle (passenger)	71.2	86.0
Carpool, vanpool	6.5	16.3
Public transit or city bus	5.0	26.0
Curb-to-curb ADA paratransit	2.0	12.6
Other specialized paratransit services	1.9	6.8
Private or chartered bus	3.2	5.8
School bus	2.6	3.4
Subway/light rail/commuter rail	4.0	10.6
Taxicab	5.8	21.9
Electric wheelchair, scooter, golf cart	5.3	6.9
Bike or pedal cycle	14.2	14.2
Walk, manual wheelchair, or scooter on sidewalks, crosswalks, intersections	48.2	40.2
Other	5.1	6.8

NOTE: Multiple responses were permitted; the sample sizes were very small.
SOURCE: Table 14 and Figure 4, U.S. BTS (2003a).

were substantially more likely to be either a driver or a passenger in a personal vehicle than to use buses, paratransit, or taxis.

Many drivers, however, did report that they also used a variety of
public transit modes, although nondrivers were more likely to report using
buses, specialized paratransit modes, and other alternatives. At the same
time, nondrivers with disabilities were remarkably reliant on the car—and
even more so if we add taxi use to the mix. Over 86 percent of nondrivers
were passengers in a car, 16 percent rode in a car- or vanpool, and almost
22 percent used a regular taxi during the previous month. In contrast, less
than 13 percent of nondrivers used ADA paratransit services and under 7
percent used other community paratransit services in that month.

The BTS also asked if respondents with disabilities needed help with
or had trouble getting needed transportation. Roughly 9 percent of those
under age 25, 14 percent of those ages 25 to 64, and 32 percent of those
ages 65 and over answered yes. The most frequent reasons for those trou-
bles were *having no car, having no or limited transportation,* and *having
no one on whom to depend* (multiple responses were permitted). Roughly
14 percent of those ages 25 to 64 and 7 percent of those ages 65 and over
said that they *didn't want to ask for help*; a somewhat smaller percentage
reported that their *equipment doesn't fit transportation* (unspecified) or
disability makes it hard to use (unspecified). Far fewer of those who said
that they needed help reported any difficulties with bus or taxi service or
fear of crime; 8 percent said that costs (unspecified) were too high (Sweeny,
2004, Table A7).

Overall, these studies show that people with disabilities do face important travel barriers, but not necessarily those on which the policy debates
have most centered. Roughly one-third of people with disabilities have no
public transportation or other transportation available to them, so the accessibility of those services is beside the point. At the same time, the rate
of use of these modes is not high among those people who do have such
services in their areas, and only a small percentage mention their disability or health status as the reason for nonuse. In fact, most travelers with
self-reported disabilities either drive themselves or take the majority of
their travel in private cars. The most significant transportation problems
mentioned (either overall or for the nonuse of public transit) are barriers in
the pedestrian environment, which far outnumber reported problems with
transit or paratransit modes (although they may well explain the lower rates
of use of those modes).

Driving and the Aging of Society

The data presented above make it clear how reliant people with disabilities of all ages are on the private car. However, we also know that

older people in every industrial country have become increasingly more dependent on the private car to maintain their mobility (ECMT, 1999; OECD, 2001; Rosenbloom and Stähl, 2003; Gagliardi et al., 2005). Older people make the majority of their trips in a car, and the vast majority of older people are licensed to drive; in fact, within two decades older drivers will constitute one in four drivers on U.S. highways (and will constitute substantially more drivers in states like Florida and Arizona) (Stutts, 2005; Herbel et al., 2006). Linked to this increased "automobility" is the growth of almost every indicator of travel among the elderly: trips made, miles traveled, and time spent in a vehicle (Hu and Reuscher, 2004), coupled with a dramatic decrease in the use of public transit. For example, the share of all trips taken by older people using public transit fell by half between 1995 and 2001 (Rosenbloom, 2004).

With the increasing number of older drivers, however, comes a growing concern with both safety and the mobility losses that will accompany driving cessation. Older drivers below age 80 have fewer crashes per capita than those ages 18 to 25 years; moreover, the per-capita crash rates among drivers over age 65 have dropped substantially over the last few decades (Evans, 1991; IIHS, 2000; Li et al., 2003; Dellinger et al., 2004; Stutts, 2005). However, many driving skills do diminish, on average, with age. Per exposure (miles driven), older drivers tend to have higher crash rates than middle-aged people (but they have crash rates roughly comparable to those of young drivers) (Ranney and Pulling, 1990; Evans, 1988; Johnson, 2003; O'Neil and Dobbs, 2004). In short, many of the rapidly increasing number of older people who have long relied on driving to meet their needs may face serious mobility problems as they as they age and experience increasing disability (Rosenbloom, 2006a).

It is important to note that a major reason for the lower per-capita crash rates among the younger cohorts of older people is that they simply drive less and less often in situations that they find risky. Many studies show that long before retirement people begin to self-regulate, that is, make changes in their travel patterns to accommodate a loss of driving skills or to react to problematic driving situations (De Raedt and Ponjaert-Kristoffersen, 2000; Lyman et al., 2001; West et al., 2003; Henderson, 2004; McKnight, 2003). As a 5-year longitudinal study of older drivers in Britain found,

> reduced driving is related to changes in health but the immediate factor in instigating these reductions is a decline in confidence in driving competence. That is, older drivers monitor their performance and react appropriately when they feel that their performance is becoming adversely affected by poor health, or for other reasons (Rabbitt et al., 2002, p. 1).

Moreover, Table G-3 shows that drivers with disabilities, regardless of age, impose more limitations on their driving than do those without dis-

TABLE G-3 Types of Driving Self-Regulation by People With and Without Disabilities

| | Percentage of People | |
Type of Self-Regulation	With Disabilities	Without Disabilities
Drive less in bad weather	66.3	49.8
Drive less often than before	64.5	32.2
Avoid driving during peak hours	58.0	42.0
Avoid busy roads and intersections	51.7	40.0
Avoid driving at night	51.5	25.8
Avoid driving distances >100 miles	47.2	21.9
Avoid high-speed highways	38.4	21.8
Avoid unfamiliar roads or places	38.0	27.5
Drive slower than speed limits	22.0	14.9
Avoid left-hand turns	11.4	8.4

NOTE: Multiple responses were permitted; the sample sizes were very small.
SOURCE: Table 37, U.S. BTS (2003a).

abilities. Among those with disabilities roughly two-thirds drive less in bad weather and less than they used to; over half avoid rush hour driving, busy roads and intersections, and night driving. Over a third avoid long distance driving, freeways, and unfamiliar places, roughly a fourth drive slower than the speed limit, and more than one in ten avoid left-turns.

Unfortunately, these kinds of self-regulatory behaviors, while perhaps increasing safety, may have significant impacts on mobility. Not all trips that have been postponed can be rescheduled; not all trips originally scheduled during peak hours or in the evening can be made at other times; not all routes avoided have alternative paths to the same locations. In short, the destinations to which it is easy to travel may not be good substitutes for those to which it is difficult or dangerous to travel (Rosenbloom, 2001, 2006a). Moreover, having the ability to choose to travel to more potential destinations generally signals greater mobility—and the reverse results in lower mobility. Thus older people and those with disabilities can suffer important reductions in mobility and access even if they continue to drive. While driving cessation may be the final blow for these travelers, they may have been losing mobility and independence for some time, and these losses should be recognized in policy discussions (Rosenbloom, 2001, 2006a; Rosenbloom and Winsten-Bartlett, 2002).

There is substantial evidence that the final loss of the ability to drive has a significant emotional component, above and beyond mobility losses. A 2003 study for the Department for Transport of the United Kingdom noted, "The main implications of no longer having access to a car are reductions in the choice of destinations, flexibility, and spontaneity of travel and *the psychological impact associated with the loss of independence"* (U.K. Department for Transport, 2003, p. 4, emphasis added).

Indeed, driving cessation, particularly among men, has been linked to serious depression and even suicide (Marottoli et al., 2000; Fonda et al., 2001; Johnson, 2003; Ragland et al., 2005). Thus it is easy to understand why many older drivers resist total driving cessatin for as long as possible (Shope, 2003).

At the same time, cause and effect are very difficult to untangle. It is not clear whether the disabilities that contribute to driving reduction or cessation also reduce the ability or desire to travel outside the home. The loss of independence may be multidimensional, and the actual ability to drive may not be the only issue to be addressed. In addition, the disabilities of older people (or of those who are younger) may have different implications for their use of different travel modes. For example, fairly old NHIS data showed that almost 40 percent of people of any age who were too disabled to use public transport actually drove a car (Rosenbloom, 1982); this percentage has likely increased over the last 25 years. In the 1994 NHIS-D, 50 percent more people reported that their impairments created difficulties in walking than reported that their impairments created problems in driving. A major European study commented,

> Older people who suffer from limitations related to health must often cease walking or using public transport before they are forced to cease driving. Approximately one-third of women over 80 years of age cannot use walking as a means of transport, but many with a license can still drive (OECD, 2001, p. 128).

It is for these reasons that policy analysts have suggested a variety of ways to enhance the driving of older people facing increasing disabilities. These include improving the roadway network in ways that respond to the special constraints of older drivers, developing aftermarket devices that can be installed on private vehicles to make driving easier (e.g., larger mirrors and swing-out seats), improving the vehicle itself (e.g., through the use of cruise control devices that help prevent rear-end collisions and lane drifting), providing appropriate driver reeducation and retraining programs, and developing car-sharing programs that allow older drivers and those with disabilities to give up their cars while still being able to drive occasionally (Staplin et al., 2001; Rosenbloom, 2005; Stutts, 2005; Herbel et al., 2006). In addition, there are similar vehicle options that make it easier for people with disabilities to ride as passengers in private vehicles (e.g., passenger-side swing-out seats, racks for wheelchairs and other mobility devices), and private vehicles accessible to those who cannot transfer from their wheelchairs). These policy options are central to all discussions of the mobility needs of people with disabilities, those both younger and older than age 65.

COMMUNITY TRANSPORTATION RESOURCES

This section has three subsections that describe the community transportation resources that exist or that should exist:

- The accessible transportation services and facilities that are or that should be provided by public transit operators
- Those that are or that should be provided by an array of public and private nonprofit organizations
- Those that are or that should be provided by the private sector in ordinary market interactions (e.g., on-street taxis and airport shuttles)

The discussions below have a dual focus: first, the obligations of these providers under ADA, and second, the much larger arena in which these operators could be providing services to enhance the mobility of those with disabilities.

Public Transportation Agencies

When the ADA was signed into law in July of 1990, it gave people with disabilities many of the same kind of rights that the Civil Rights Act of 1964 earlier gave to people of color.[3] Title II of the ADA specifically outlaws discrimination on the basis of disability in services, programs, and activities provided by public entities, including local transit operators. Public transit services owned or operated by a public entity (or provided under contract to a public entity by a private operator) must be accessible to individuals with disabilities, including those who use common wheelchairs, as the statute and regulations define accessibility for each mode. Transit operators are also required to ensure that both the pretravel and en route information provided by the system are available in a variety of accessible formats.

The ADA has clearly changed the landscape of public transit; as a national disability organization recently noted:

> As a consistent theme in most transit systems across the United States, the Americans with Disabilities Act of 1990 (ADA) has spawned great improvements. . . . As a result of the ADA, the past decade has brought about real improvements in access to transportation for people with disabilities, and access to public transportation has improved significantly since implementation of the ADA transportation provisions (NCD, 2005, pp. 13, 20).

---

[3]The ADA information summarized in this section comes largely from materials supplied on the website of the U.S. Access Board: http://www.access-board.gov.

There are many public transit modes: buses and trolley buses, heavy and light rail services, commuter rail, ferry boats, vanpools, and carpools. Each of these modes poses unique access and mobility problems for people with disabilities; there are ADA requirements for each mode, but there is also the potential for many modes to provide more mobility to people with disabilities than that mandated by the law. Of course, the significant cost implications cannot be ignored; as the National Council on Disability (NCD) notes (NCD, 2005), public transit is substantially underfunded in this country, and ADA mandates do not come with any additional funding so there is even less money for additional or nonmandated services. Yet the potential remains high for public transit to make a bigger and better contribution to the mobility of people with disabilities.

Heavy, Commuter, and Light Rail Systems

The ADA requires heavy and light rail systems to make some or all of their vehicles, stations, and transfer points fully accessible to people with disabilities. New systems must be fully accessible, as must be new purchases or new improvements on older systems (although there are some exceptions even on new systems). However, older systems are required to rebuild or retrofit only what are defined as *key stations* (for example, those with the most traffic or serving major activity centers). Moreover, older rail systems are required to make only a subset of their existing vehicles accessible to people with disabilities, although all new cars must be accessible. As with other travel modes, operators are required to provide accessible communications in many formats, including individual-stop announcements.

Today there are only 685 of these *key* stations in the United States; this number represents a fraction of the total number of rail stations in older systems. Disability advocates had hoped that the ADA regulations would require a larger number (or all) stations in older systems to be made accessible, but the costs were so high that the number of key stations was a political compromise (NCD, 2005). Clearly, then, the key station requirement, even if it is fully met, does not address the significant rail restrictions facing many travelers with disabilities in older systems, who can enter and exit the system only at a limited number of stations, not necessarily at their preferred origins and destinations; some trips cannot be made at all. As the National Council on Disability has noted, "train travel has improved greatly for people with disabilities, but the ADA's limited key station requirement has meant that some of the large, old East Coast rail systems in particular, have few accessible stations" (NCD, 2005, p. 14).

Key stations were to be accessible by 1993, but the deadlines have been extended by the U.S. Department of Transportation to 2013 for commuter rail and to 2023 for rapid and light rail systems. However, the Federal

Transit Administration (FTA) recently reported that "only" 96 key stations (14 percent) in 11 systems still fail to meet accessibility standards (NCD, 2005). Disability advocates, however, do not necessarily agree with the FTA assessment of how well some of those key stations actually meet the ADA requirements.

Continuing to meet ADA standards, even in newer rail systems, is an additional compliance problem; accessibility features—from way-finding devices for those with visual impairments to the mechanisms used to ensure level access into rail cars—require substantial maintenance. For example, over time, the horizontal and/or vertical gaps between the station/stop platform and the floor of the rail vehicle can become too great to allow level entry by a variety of travelers with disabilities without additional devices (such as manual or automated gap fillers, which themselves must be maintained and used properly). If these devices are not properly maintained, they cease to facilitate access by those with disabilities.

Finally, when new heavy or light rail systems or additional rail services are inaugurated, the transit system may decrease or reroute bus services to encourage rail ridership, often requiring modal transfers on trips people previously took without having to transfer. While some of these rerouted buses or the new rail services themselves may provide more or better service for people with disabilities, there is substantial evidence that such changes may in fact harm a large number of disadvantaged travelers from poor or minority communities who are more dependent on bus services. These situations have been the subject of many lawsuits across the United States (Rosenbloom, 1991, 2006b; Lee, 1997; Mann, 1997; TCRP, 1998c; Sanchez et al., 2003). To the extent that travelers with disabilities are members of such disadvantaged communities, they may, too, suffer mobility losses when bus services are reconfigured as rail services are expanded.

Buses

The ADA required public transit operators to purchase only accessible buses after August 1990; as a result over time all fleets should become totally accessible. Most accessible buses in the United States today are regular coaches which offer access by (1) lowering (kneeling) the entrance side of the bus by several inches so that those with difficulty with stairs will have a shorter first step up into the vehicle (particularly if they are boarding from a curb) and (2) providing mechanical lifts at an entrance to the bus for those who cannot climb stairs (including but not limited to those in wheelchairs). However, in 2002 the FTA announced that only 88 percent of all buses met the mandate; thus it is possible that today 5 to 10 percent of all buses in the United States are still not ADA accessible.

The more important ADA compliance issues today, however, are probably the maintenance and operation of accessible buses in service and the training given drivers to operate key accessibility devices. For much of the first decade after the passage of the ADA, the accessibility features of U.S. buses were still subject to substantial malfunctions. That often meant that travelers with handicaps were left waiting at a stop—or perhaps worse, stranded on a deployed lift that could be neither raised nor lowered. Even when a bus started the day with a functioning lift, however, lift problems could occur while the bus was in service.

There is substantial evidence that some drivers were afraid of disabling the bus once it was in service and so refused to cycle the lift at a stop. Or drivers who did not know how to cycle the lift refused to do so, telling a passenger waiting at a stop that the lift was not functional. Still other drivers were afraid that taking time to board a passenger with a disability would cause them to run behind schedule—although this rarely happens with well-maintained equipment, trained and experienced drivers (and/or passengers), and the use of proper scheduling algorithms (Rosenbloom, 1994; TCRP, 1998a). Other drivers would not "kneel" the bus unless a passenger knew to ask (even if system policy required kneeling at all stops). A substantial number would not allow travelers not using wheelchairs to board using the lift. In addition, driver failure to call out stops, as required by the law for travelers with visual impairments, has been a long-term compliance issue.

Many of these problems have lessened over time because of a combination of better equipment, improved maintenance, appropriate and timely driver training, and more serious management surveillance and response. However, passengers with disabilities have reported these same problems fairly recently in a number of systems, including Bi-State Transit (St. Louis), the Detroit Department of Transportation, MARTA (Atlanta), and the MBTA in Boston (NCD, 2005). Moreover, many systems have a significant number of very old buses with very old lift and securement systems that can no longer be repaired and that need to be replaced if the bus is kept in service.

The securement systems aboard buses also pose compliance problems (Zaworski and Hunter-Zaworski, 2006). The ADA requires that each vehicle have a minimum of two wheelchair securement areas and that these systems must accommodate "common wheelchairs." The regulations also require that drivers be trained to proficiency in the use of these devices. However, there are a variety of user, maintenance, and training problems with these systems. First, securement systems have traditionally had serious operational and maintenance issues; moreover, many drivers do not really know how to work them properly (TCRP, 2003d). While both the technology and driver training have improved over time, these issues remain a concern in many bus systems.

Second, an increasing number of people use very customized wheel-chairs that can test securement systems (Zaworski and Hunter-Zaworski, 2006). However, some systems have improved securement use even with unusual wheelchairs through the purchase of improved equipment and better driver training and surveillance. The Phoenix, Arizona, transit system has developed "kits" that wheelchair users can carry with them that show where on their chairs securement devices can be attached and/or that provide ways to appropriately extend the straps that are part of on-board securement systems. In addition, it is generally believed that the FTA has ruled that wheelchair securement is not mandatory if the user chooses to remain unsecured.

However, there are a host of ways in which bus systems could provide better mobility options for travelers with disabilities that go beyond the ADA mandates. Many of those have been identified and evaluated in a series of reports from the Transit Cooperative Research Program (TCRP). First is the need for a very different accessible bus (de Boer, 2004). The United States began requiring bus accessibility before the vehicle technology had advanced sufficiently (although it can be argued that the technology would not have improved in the absence of the ADA). While lowering the first step onto the bus (kneeling) can help some travelers and the lift can work well for those in wheelchairs (and perhaps others), neither option accommodates the full range of people with disabilities or their mobility devices (TCRP, 1994, 1998a).

In most circumstances, low-floor buses, widely available in Europe, would offer better access for many people and mobility aids, as well as for travelers with strollers, baby carriages, suitcases, or bulky packages (Aurbach, 2001; ECMT, 1999). From a curb, entry into a low-floor bus is almost level; even if the traveler enters the bus from the street, the first step onto the flat floor of the bus is (1) the only step required of the traveler and (2) much shorter than the first step on traditional coaches. Manual or powered ramps are available for those who cannot handle the much smaller horizontal and vertical gaps (TCRP, 1994, 1998b). However, low-floor buses have not been widely adopted in the United States. A 2002 TCRP study found that less that 9 percent of the U.S. bus fleet was composed of low-floor buses with ramps in 2002; while there are anecdotal accounts of widespread low-floor bus purchases, the TCRP study did not find a high level of low-floor bus purchases.

Second, studies of older people and those with disabilities strongly suggest the need to improve *traditional* transit services in several important ways (TCRP, 1997a,b, 1998b,c, 1999a,b, 2002a,b, 2003b; Rosenbloom, 2004). The majority of older people and some of those with disabilities want to travel at different times than most commuters; they need expanded routes and service hours, better schedule adherence, and improved and appropriate assistance from drivers. Some bus operators in the United States and abroad have increased ridership by operating smaller buses, allowing passengers to be closer to the driver, which often reduces the anxiety or fear felt by travelers with disabilities (TCRP, 1999b, 2002b). Some transit systems have been successful in replacing traditional bus routes with more carefully targeted community or neighborhood services whose schedules and routes are more focused on the specific needs of older travelers, even if they run only a few days a week (TCRP, 1997a, 1998c).

In addition, many studies show that almost all travelers seek better information on their travel options, both before they leave home and while they are en route (especially at transfer points) (TCRP, 1999a). Studies also show that many older people and those with disabilities who have never used a bus can benefit significantly from different kinds of transit familiarization and training sessions. In fact, several TCRP studies have shown significant and *continuing* transit ridership among older people and those with disabilities who were provided with targeted training—in some cases even if they were or had been drivers (TCRP, 1998c, 2002a). Finally, many people report being fearful about public transit use. For example, older people and those with disabilities have anxiety not only about crime but also about harassment. People also worry about falling while getting on or off a transit vehicle or while maneuvering to their seat when a bus is in motion. Transit operators need to address all these issues to provide meaningful service to a variety of travelers.

Third, several studies suggest that transit operators should consider providing a range of nontraditional services, from flexible routes and route deviation service to the kinds of service routes adopted successfully in Scandinavian countries and replicated to some degree in many Canadian and a few U.S. cities (TCRP, 2003c, 2004a,b; Rosenbloom, 2004, 2005; see Higgins and Cherrington [2005] for a more pessimistic assessment). Flexibly routed services are not without problems. Bus systems are not generally required to provide complementary paratransit parallel to flexibly routed services. Thus, it is possible for transit systems to use route deviation or flexible services to reduce their paratransit obligations, which might negatively affect those travelers with disabilities who could not use those flexible services. Overall, however, there is evidence that these kinds of services could provide some travelers with disabilities with better mobility options than they currently have (Rosenbloom, 1994, 1995; TCRP, 2004b).

Complementary Paratransit Services

The ADA requires public transit systems to also provide *complementary paratransit*—that is, special, demand-responsive transportation services—for people who are unable to board even an accessible bus or who do not have an accessible path to an accessible bus. Paratransit services are not required for those unable to access or use available rail services. Complementary paratransit services were clearly meant to provide only a safety net while transit systems became more accessible. However, many people have come to look upon them as a major transportation option; this is unfortunate, because these services are unlikely to be a significant part of the transportation resources of anybody except those with extremely serious disabilities. For those travelers, complementary paratransit services are a lifeline. However, ADA-required complementary paratransit services will play little role in the mobility patterns of the majority of travelers with disabilities because of the ways in which they are provided.

Transit operators must provide complementary paratransit services to eligible users in at least a 3/4-mile corridor paralleling their existing bus routes and during at least the same hours of service that those bus routes operate. Users may only be charged a fare equivalent to double the regular bus fare; and their requests for next-day services must be accommodated—which, depending on the hours of service, can be as little as 12 hours in advance. Systems are allowed but not required to provide same-day service; users must be allowed but are not required to request service 7 days in advance. Transit systems may not impose any restrictions on the type of trip taken. Most importantly, eligible travelers cannot be refused service on the basis of budget restrictions—that is, systems are not allowed to have capacity constraints, even if the costs of meeting the ADA standards are extremely high. The paratransit system may negotiate with riders, asking them to move their trips either an hour early or an hour later than their desired time of travel; otherwise, the system must provide all trips requested by eligible travelers within that time window.

Transit systems meet these mandates in a variety of ways, which often reflect the way they provided services before passage of the ADA, their experiences with the private paratransit providers in their service areas, and the outcomes of actual or threatened legal challenges. With respect to the last point, almost every major metropolitan transit operator has been sued by disability advocates and aggrieved riders over system failure to meet the ADA paratransit requirements. The transit systems of some cities, like that of Boston (MBTA), provide all paratransit services in their own vehicles with their own drivers or in dedicated contractor vehicles because of difficulties in the past with contract providers or regular taxi services. The Chicago Transit Authority provides some ADA paratransit services in system-owned vehicles, while some trips are served by contract providers and others by regular taxis called directly by users. The transit system of Austin, Texas (Capital Metro) provides some services in system-owned vehicles, usually to passengers who need accessible vehicles, and contracts with other private providers or taxi operators to serve passengers who can ride in sedans.

TABLE G-4 Complementary Paratransit Cost and Ridership Patterns for People With and Without Disabilities

System and City	Total Annual System Ridership[a] (in millions)	Annual Paratransit Ridership[a] (in millions)	Paratransit as a % of Total Ridership	Paratransit as a % of Operating Costs
Chicago (IL) Transit Authority	484,811	1,438	0.3	3.7
Los Angeles, CA[b]	428,504	1,904	0.4	8.2
MARTA (Atlanta, GA)	164,078	192	0.1	4.0
Kansas City (MO) Metro Transit	100,626	1,686	1.7	12.0
Tri-County Metro (Portland, OR)	91,186	782	0.9	7.4
Greater Cleveland, OH, RTA	60,094	317	0.5	6.5
Capital Metro Transit Authority (Austin, TX)	33,987	359	1.1	17.5
SUNTRAN (Tucson, AZ)	15,865	295	1.9	17.1
Hillsborough Area Regional Transit Authority (Tampa, FL)	9,815	14	0.1	4.5
Birmingham-Jefferson Co. Transit Authority (AL)	2,775	113	4.1	11.1

[a]Unlinked trips (e.g., having to transfer buses or transfer from a bus to a train on the way to work creates two unlinked trips; the more transfers the more unlinked trips created by just a one-way journey to work).

[b]Data are from four Los Angeles-area reports.

SOURCE: Computed for this study from the FTA 2004 National Transit Database.

Almost every system has found the complementary ADA paratransit requirements to be extremely costly because (1) they involve high ongoing operating costs and (2) there are limited opportunities for economies of scale. Paratransit tends to be expensive because it is difficult to group trips efficiently without making passengers ride or wait too long, miss their appointments, etc. The larger and lower density the paratransit service area is, the more difficult it is to carry many passengers in a vehicle per hour or mile of service; this substantially raises the cost of each trip provided. Moreover, passengers with serious disabilities tend to take longer to board and deboard, which also lowers productivity. As a result of these service features, the average one-way paratransit trip cost in the 50 largest U.S. transit agencies was $29.28 (calculated from unpublished data in FTA's 2004 National Transit Database). In other words, taking the average eligible traveler with disabilities to and from one doctor's visit would cost almost $60.

Table G-4 describes the 2004 cost and ridership data for 10 representative cities in the United States;[4] it shows that average trip costs are generally

---

[4]Some of these systems may be providing non-ADA paratransit services or may be allowing non-ADA-eligible riders (such as the elderly) to use their ADA-required services. The National Transit Database does not make this clear.

high. Indeed, total paratransit service expenses are a significant component of total transit system operating costs, even though paratransit riders are a small percentage of the total system ridership. Individual system costs for a one-way ADA-required paratransit trip ranged from a high of $47 in Cleveland, Ohio, to a low of $14 in Birmingham, Alabama; the average cost per one-way trip in the 10 cities was $30.81. Paratransit *riders* accounted for a low of 0.1 percent of the total system ridership in Atlanta to a high of 4.1 percent in Birmingham. However, paratransit service *costs* accounted for approximately 4 percent of total system operating costs in Chicago but over 17 percent of total system operating costs in Austin and Tucson, Arizona. For the 10 systems, the average percentage of total operating costs incurred to provide paratransit service was 9.2 percent for an average of 2 percent of the total system ridership. Even Birmingham, which had the lowest unit cost in the table, spent over 11 percent of its annual operating budget for the 4 percent of its ridership who used paratransit services.

Because of these costs many transit operators failed to even come close to meeting the ADA standards for at least a decade; for example, they routinely refused service for eligible travelers who called for next-day service and often gave preference to riders who made frequent recurrent trips (because they could be prescheduled). Although service has improved in most systems, sometimes as the result of lawsuits, a BTS study (U.S. BTS, 2003b) found that 53 percent of travelers with disabilities reported experiencing significant problems with ADA-required paratransit services, including the failure of the vehicle to show up during the permissible pickup window or even to show up at all. Over 40 percent reported the same problems for their return trips. About 6 percent said that service was not available when it was needed, and 4 percent said that they could not get through to make a reservation on the telephone.

Ironically, after 1990 many transit systems *initially* provided complementary paratransit service to travelers throughout their service area at a low fare because, prior to the implementation of ADA, they had been required to provide some paratransit services to the elderly and those with disabilities as a condition of federal funding. In general, most systems had previously provided fairly low levels of paratransit service; but at the same time, they tended not to be very strict about limiting eligibility and served a large area, often where they had no bus services at all (Rosenbloom, 1994). After the passage of the ADA, many systems kept those system parameters, for both practical and political reasons, in essence controlling costs by not meeting mandated service levels for those who were eligible for services under ADA.

However, as more systems have been required to actually provide ADA-mandated levels of service, the high costs have forced many systems to raise fares to the maximum allowed, restrict services to the minimum required, and adhere to very strict rider eligibility guidelines (TCRP, 1998a). As systems have cut paratransit coverage to the minimum, they have excluded a very large number of people with disabilities because so few live within or can travel to the minimum 3/4-mile corridors along an existing transit route to receive ADA-mandated paratransit service (Bogren, 1998; Rosenbloom, 2005).

Transit systems have also cut paratransit costs by implementing very strict, and even onerous, certification processes to determine paratransit eligibility for those who do live near (or can travel to) areas where bus services (and, thus, complementary paratransit) services are provided. A recent report by the National Center for Transit Research concludes that exceeding the minimum ADA requirements substantially increases ridership and, thus, costs (Thole and Harvey, 2005). While the report does not actually urge systems to cut service, raise fares, or increase the difficulty of becoming eligible for service, it makes clear the cost savings that will result from doing so. The report describes a number of transit systems that have managed to reduce their total paratransit ridership by instituting multistage and difficult eligibility procedures, raising fares to the maximum allowed, or cutting service quality (e.g., not allowing same-day service).

King County (Seattle, Washington), for example, changed its eligibility process to require a preapplication process and a telephone interview follow-up for all applicants. The county also substantially increased the number of applicants who were required to report in person for a functional evaluation at a medical center under contract to the transit operator (rather than accepting an evaluation from the rider's own doctor). As a result of these changes, the monthly rate of certification of new riders as eligible fell by half and the process removed the eligibility of 3,200 existing riders (Thole and Harvey, 2005). The NCD (2005) also describes a number of (different) systems that have undertaken restrictive actions and similar sharp reductions in the number of new or existing riders certified or recertified as eligible for paratransit service.

Clearly, these practices may result in decisions that discriminate against people genuinely eligible for paratransit services; the NCD has expressed concerns over this possibility (NCD, 2005). However, it is likely that a far larger number of potentially eligible travelers are simply discouraged from pursuing the complicated process at all; this problem is far more difficult to address. Moreover, many of those who are discouraged from applying for fear of being refused as well as those actually refused (re)certification may sometimes have serious disabilities but they just do not meet the strict requirements of the ADA for paratransit services. In short, the vast number of people with disabilities are already excluded from these services, many without being able to meet their mobility needs using public transit as it is currently delivered.

At the same time, the enormity of expanding paratransit service to provide rides to the vast number of people with disabilities is shown in Table G-5, which ultimately provides a very conservative estimate of the cost of expanding services to meet the needs of a wider range of people with disabilities. Table G-5 illustrates the costs of responding to the needs of people age 15 years and older with a severe disability in the major city served by each transit agency. The calculation assumes that only people with a severe disability are eligible for parastransit services under ADA. Indeed, some people with severe disabilities (as defined by the U.S. Census Bureau) may not meet the ADA criteria, while others with less serious disabilities may, but this is generally a reasonable and conservative estimate.

The calculations are conservative in another way; all of the agencies shown in Table G-5 serve a geographic area larger than the major city; these estimates, however, include only those who live in that large city. Matching the actual service area of each transit agency to census tracts to calculate the "real" number of potential riders is a task far beyond this paper, but doing so would simultaneously substantially increase the number of potential riders *and* significantly lower the average number of rides provided to all those aged 15 years and over with severe disabilities. In addition severe disabilities numbers were calculated using national rates by age but not by sex or race or ethnicity, which could well vary markedly by city. As a result these figures are only a gross, but conservative, calculation.

Table G-5 shows that only 1 of the 10 systems (that in Tampa, Florida) provides even one round trip *a year* to everyone with a severe disability in the large city in the center of its service area. The rest of the systems provide even less service to those with disabilities. In reality, most ADA-required complementary paratransit systems provide many trips to a few frequent riders, while they fail to serve the vast number of potentially eligible people or even those who have been certified as eligible. (Several studies have found that many people who become registered for the service never or rarely use it, probably because of its inherent limitations.) Building on these data, we can calculate that providing each person with a severe disability in the central city of each of the listed transit agency's service areas with one round trip per month would be staggeringly expensive. The Los Angeles regional transit operator, for example, currently spends over $68 million per year to provide ADA-mandated (and related) paratransit services; were it to offer only one round trip per month to everyone in the City of Los Angeles aged 15 years and over with a severe disability, the yearly cost would be $331 million or almost five times its current expenditures. If Los Angeles regional transit operator were to offer those travelers four round trips per month, the cost would be $1.3 billion annually.

These figures illustrate a number of points. First, they explain why so many local transit systems have failed to meet ADA complementary

TABLE G-5 Current Paratransit Service Coverage and Potential Expansion Costs

System and City	2004 Annual Paratransit Ridership[a] (in millions)	2004 Average Cost per Paratransit Ride[a]	Annual No. of Rides per Person Age 15+ with Severe Disabilities	2004 System Paratransit Costs (in millions)	Total Annual Cost to Provide One RT/Month to Each Person w/a Disability (in millions)
Chicago (IL) Transit Authority	1,438	$23.25	0.19	$33,428	$155,555
Los Angeles, CA[b]	1,904	$36.69	0.20	$68,843	$331,425
MARTA (Atlanta, GA)	192	$43.47	0.20	$8,338	$290,837
Kansas City (MO) Metro Transit	1,868	$24.74	0.03	$41,710	$28,264
Tri-County Metro (Portland, OR)	782	$19.90	0.07	$15,559	$27,394
Greater Cleveland (OH) RTA	317	$47.02	0.14	$14,887	$51,100
Capital Metro Transit Authority (Austin, TX)	359	$41.45	0.17	$14,867	$60,628
SUNTRAN (Tucson, AZ)	295	$21.82	0.17	$6,451	$26,541
Hillsborough Area Regional Transit Authority (Tampa, FL)	14	$35.94	2.44	$1,445	$29,472
Birmingham-Jefferson Co. Transit Authority (AL)	113	$13.84	0.89	$1,563	$33,458

[a]One ride is one *unlinked trip* (e.g., having to transfer buses or transfer from a bus to a train on the way to work creates two unlinked trips; the more transfers the more unlinked trips created by just a one-way journey to work).

[b]Data are from four Los Angeles-area reports.

SOURCE: Computed for this study from the FTA National Transit Database; 2003 American City Survey Data Profiles; and U.S. Census Bureau, 2005 (Table 1, Prevalence of Disability).

paratransit requirements and why, once they are forced to do so, they become extremely restrictive in their service parameters and eligibility. The figures also indicate how unlikely it is that most transit systems will expand their paratransit services beyond the minimum, even as the population of travelers with disabilities climbs, unless additional funding becomes available. Second, these figures suggest that policy makers must consider more cost-effective transportation measures for those who can use them, such as improving public transit services in the ways suggested above, while facilitating car use by those who do not live in areas where transit services can reasonably be provided. Third, these cost data also indicate the need to augment and strengthen the services of the other community transport providers that, by leveraging the resources of volunteers, can often provide less expensive (but still not cheap) paratransit services to many people with disabilities who are not eligible for ADA-mandated complementary para-transit services for a variety of reasons.

Other Community Providers and Obligations

Social and Human Service Agencies

Public transit systems are not the only agencies that provide transportation services to those with disabilities. A vast array of public and non-profit human, medical, and social service agencies provide transportation to people who use their programs or qualify for their services; the U.S. General Accounting Office (Siggerud, 2003; U.S. GAO, 2004) has identified 70 to 80 federal programs that allow state and local grantees to use grant funds for transportation services, most of which are provided to disad-vantaged people (but not necessarily those with disabilities). For example, the Job Access and Reverse Commute Program of the U.S. Department of Transportation has funded over 200 state and local recipients to provide transportation for disadvantaged people, including those with disabilities, to access job and job training sites. The Administration on Aging, as an-other example, allows its program funds to be used to provide transporta-tion services to older people. These social and human service agencies also have responsibilities under the ADA; they are not required to buy or own accessible vehicles, as long as their system, "when viewed in its entirety," provides the same level of service to those needing accessible vehicles as to its more general riders.

The Beverly Foundation annually undertakes a study of how what they call Supplemental Transportation Programs (STPs) for the elderly are orga-nized, managed, and financed across the United States; they have identified many exemplary service models. These range from transportation services that are provided entirely by volunteers in their own cars to systems that use paid drivers in system-owned vehicles, some of which are accessible to travelers using wheelchairs (The Beverly Foundation and the Community Transportation Association of America, 2005). In 2001 the Foundation designated 11 programs as Senior Transportation Action Response (STAR) award winners (Beverly Foundation, AAA Foundation for Traffic Safety, 2001).

However, the Beverly Foundation report shows that even exemplary systems vary widely in terms of the number of clients served, the accessibility of their vehicles, and overall costs. At one end of the spectrum, a STAR system on a Native American reservation (San Felipe, New Mexico) provided 34,000 one-way trips to 90 people at an average cost of 57 cents per one-way trip; it had no vehicles accessible to individuals with disabilities. At the other end of the spectrum, a system in Portland, Oregon (Ride Connections), provided almost 200,000 one-way trips to 7,000 people at an average cost of over $28 for each trip; it had some vehicles accessible to individuals with disabilities. If weighted by the number of trips made, the average exemplary STP cost was $20.31 per one-way trip (in 2002 dollars) because larger STP systems with more riders had much higher costs.

In fact, three of the STAR systems had costs roughly comparable to those of public transit operators, although they were generally operating with many volunteers, sometimes using their volunteers' cars. Gold Country Telecare (Grass Valley, California), Ride Connections (Portland, Oregon), and the Independent Transportation Network (ITN) (Westbrook, Maine) had average one-way trip costs that exceeded $27, even though all three (and particularly ITN) used some volunteer drivers. Of course, a number of variables may drive up costs; these providers serve large, low-density, or rural areas, which might mean that they must provide long and costly trips to distant medical and other facilities. The Gold County, California, system provided additional escort services, although the other two systems mentioned above did not. Ride Connection provided some services accessible to individuals with disabilities, which are generally more expensive. These systems may also face unique local or management challenges that may increase their expenditures.

However, while these systems are exemplary in their approaches to offering valuable mobility services for their older clients, it is clear that most of these 11 systems provide service to a small number of travelers. Moreover, the larger the system is, the higher the average costs are; many of the larger STAR systems had average costs equal to or only slightly less than those of large public transit agencies, even though all but one system used at least some volunteer drivers. These findings are consistent with those of other studies of social service agency transportation services (Siggerud, 2003; TCRP, 2004c). Moreover, a few of the 11 STAR systems do not appear to be in conformity with *their* obligations under ADA to provide the same level of transportation service to those needing accessible vehicles as they do to their more general riders. These data suggest, first, that even exemplary community services with substantial volunteer support can be expensive and, second, that it will require a very large number of such systems to meet the mobility needs of a growing population of disadvantaged travelers, particularly those with disabilities who need accessible vehicles.

Because these community-based transportation providers are so important to so many travelers—and have the potential to be even more important in the future—analysts have suggested a number of ways in which local communities might increase their number and effectiveness, reduce their costs, and ensure that they are able to offer services to those needing accessible vehicles. These suggestions include providing appropriate training to staff or volunteers in a variety of functional areas, from dispatching to dealing with the needs of travelers with significant disabilities. In addition, analysts have suggested ways to achieve cost savings through, for example, group purchase of insurance, vehicles, vehicle maintenance services, driver and dispatcher training, and computer dispatching programs (Ritter et al., 2002; Rosenbloom, 2005; The Beverly Foundation and the Community Transportation Association of America, 2005).

One approach to improving the delivery and lowering the cost of community-based transport services is *coordination* by encouraging or requiring active cooperation in some or all aspects of service delivery between and among the many transport providers in a community or region. Many small community transportation operators limit their services to a small number of agency clients, often restricting travel by trip purpose (medical or agency-related trips only), which results in the inefficient use of vehicles (and other facilities). This can clearly lead to high costs and, particularly in urban areas, substantial duplication and redundancies in service delivery (Siggerud, 2003; U.S. GAO, 2004). The conventional wisdom (Coordinating Council on Access and Mobility, 2000; Siggerud, 2003; U.S. GAO, 2004; TCRP, 2004c,d) is that community providers that are unwilling to cooperate with other providers in some or all aspects of transportation service delivery do so because they

- believe that their funding sources forbid them from cooperating with other providers;
- cannot figure out how to meet their financial and other reporting requirements if they provide services in different ways;
- do not understand their own cost and service patterns well enough to see how coordinating with other community providers could save them money or increase the quantity or quality of service that they provide to their clients;
- do not know about the coordination opportunities available in the community;
- do not have the skills or experience to attempt greater cooperation in service delivery or other operational areas; or
- want to "protect their turf."

Over the last 20 years there have been formal and informal efforts at both the national and the state levels to overcome these barriers through greater coordination among the federal agencies that fund transportation services, better information and training on a variety of the issues raised above, and the promotion of both voluntary and mandatory coordination programs. In the last few years there has been a flurry of executive and legislative activity at the national level. On February 1, 2001, President George W. Bush announced the New Freedom Initiative, designed to promote the full participation of people with disabilities in all areas of American life, including transportation. As part of its response, the U.S. Department of Transportation created an interagency working group to coordinate the many federal programs that fund transportation services for people with disabilities, produce a resource guide describing those programs, and develop examples of best practices in transportation service delivery that allow people with disabilities to get to work and job training.

In 2004 Presidential Executive Order 13330, the Coordination of Human Service Programs, created an independent interdepartmental Council on Access and Mobility to help reduce duplication among federally funded community transportation providers; increase the efficiency of their services; and expand the transportation access of a variety of disadvantaged travelers, including older people and those with disabilities. In 2006, the Safe, Accountable, Flexible, Efficient Transportation Equity Act (PL 109-59) went further and required local areas receiving funds for certain programs targeted at older people, those with disabilities, and poor people to prepare a plan for coordinating public transit and human service transportation in the area. Initial plans are required by 2007.

State and federal coordination efforts over the last three decades have helped many local providers to become more efficient and effective (TCRP, 2003a). Yet some analysts have noted that not all agencies that fail to coordinate with others are doing so for unacceptable reasons, and this may be most true for those providing service to travelers with disabilities. Some clients who need transportation may need more than just a ride (TCRP, 1997b, 2004c); many social agencies worry that without extra services some clients may choose not to travel or to use agency services at all (Rosenbloom and Warren, 1981; Rosenbloom, 1981). For example, some clients may need to be reminded several times of their appointments, helped with getting dressed or getting ready, encouraged to go to appointments or social events, etc.; without such additional assistance, they may miss or cancel their trips (McCray, 1998; Burke et al., 2004). Yet most organizations whose primary business is transportation are often unwilling or are unable to provide these additional services, at least without additional compensation (Carrasco, 2001; Griffin and Priddy, 2005).

In addition, not all areas have enough services to make major coordination efforts worthwhile; this may be particularly true in rural areas.

Some analysts have noted how difficult it is to set up and maintain effective coordinated programs without continuing financial assistance and leadership—as well as mandates—from regional or state agencies. The benefits of coordination are often diffused and are accompanied by some additional costs to the agencies involved, even if these additional costs occur only initially (Schlossberg, 2003, 2004). In short, while transportation coordination is clearly one way to help some community transport providers to become more efficient, it is not a panacea. Moreover, there are clearly instances in which coordination may lead to less mobility for travelers with disabilities.

Local Governments and the Pedestrian Environment

Most of the studies and surveys reported on in previous sections highlighted (1) the importance of walking to most travelers with disabilities and (2) how many barriers to mobility were created by problems in the pedestrian environment. However, improvements to pedestrian accessibility have lagged behind improvements to the rest of the transportation network, in part because no enforceable regulations for making the pedestrian (or public right-of-way) system accessible to travelers with either physical or visual impairments, or both, have been issued (although the U.S. Access Board has developed draft guidelines and has been working to improve industry standards for pedestrian facilities).

Most pedestrian facilities are built and maintained by local governments (or are required of developers in new areas by city or county subdivision ordinances). *If* these jurisdictions provide curb ramps, sidewalks, and/or bus stops, these elements must comply with the ADA. However, cities are not required to provide these pedestrian elements at any specific location if they do not exist. However, the ADA does require cities to undertake a program of providing access in their existing pedestrian facilities over time. Since almost 16 years have passed since the ADA requirements went into effect, many cities should have brought almost their entire pedestrian environments into compliance with the ADA.

Unfortunately, without enforceable standards, many communities have done the minimum. For example, they may provide some curb ramps and require all commercial and new residential developments to provide accessible sidewalks, but they rarely plan to substantially improve their existing sidewalks and bus stops if they can be viewed as accessible (and, arguably, in some cases, when they are not accessible). Moreover, many cities have been lax at properly maintaining the accessibility of the sidewalks and bus stops that do exist (repairing broken pavement or removing weeds and debris) or retrofitting built-up areas without sidewalks. They tend to be especially negligent about providing improvements critical to independent mobility by those with visual impairments, such as audible pedestrian signals at stoplights and detectable warnings at curb ramps.

However, in early 2004, the 9th Circuit Court of Appeals overturned a lower court ruling that allowed the city of Sacramento, California, to argue that people with disabilities could use special paratransit services if they lacked accessible sidewalks to bus or tram stops. In *Barden et al. v. Sacramento* (01-15744. DC No. CV 99-0497 MLS) the court ordered the city to address pedestrian barriers noting:

> [The ADA] reveals a general concern for the accessibility of public sidewalks, as well as a recognition that sidewalks fall within the ADA's coverage, and [the curb ramp requirement] would be meaningless if the sidewalks between the curb ramps were inaccessible. . . . Title II's prohibition of discrimination in the provision of public services applies to the maintenance of public sidewalks.

The court mandated a fairly draconian remedy, ordering Sacramento to spend a fifth of its annual transportation fund budget for up to 30 years to meet the accessibility needs of pedestrians. The U.S. Supreme Court refused to hear the city's appeal from the 9th Circuit; unless the Supreme Court accepts an appeal from another lower court and upholds the same standard, it is not clear how far-reaching this judicial decision will be.

In any case, the reality is that in many cities today people with disabilities lack an accessible route to an accessible transit facility. Because this situation has substantial mobility implications, several recent studies have suggested how communities can address deficiencies in their pedestrian networks to provide greater mobility for older people and those with disabilities, and these suggestions go beyond specific physical improvements. These suggestions begin, of course, by stressing the need to develop and maintain accessible pedestrian paths that link residential areas to one another and to commercial centers, as well as the need to provide access to transit facilities.

However, these studies and reports also stress enforcement, ensuring that cars are not parked in bus stops or on sidewalks and are not jutting out of driveways; using traffic-calming devices to lower traffic speeds and increase street attractiveness; and making both active and passive personal security efforts, that is, using police patrols (active) and design changes, enhanced lighting, and surveillance cameras (passive) to control on-street crime and harassment of pedestrians. Some studies have stressed the importance of using subdivision regulations and building codes to ensure the presence of accessible sidewalks in all *new* residential developments as well as commercial developments, while others have been concerned with *retrofitting existing* neighborhoods with accessible sidewalks and intersections, since so many older people are aging in place in older neighborhoods.

(Rosenbloom and Stähl, 2003; NCD, 2004; Kocera et al., 2005; Kihl et al., 2005; AARP, 2006; Herbel et al., 2006, Rosenbloom, 2005; Kochera and Bright, 2005–2006).

The Private Transportation Sector

Title III of the ADA has the same effect on private transportation providers (except airlines) that Title II has on public entities (airline access is covered under the 1986 Air Carriers Access Act, although the accessibility requirements are different). Title III does not require private providers, such as hotel and airport shuttle services, to purchase accessible transport vehicles, as long as they provide an equivalent level of service to those with disabilities as they provide to the general public. The extent to which these private providers have met their ADA mandates is open to debate; many had to be sued, sometimes several times, before they found ways to provide equivalent levels of service and/or bought at least some accessible vehicles.

The ADA also does not require private taxi operators to own or operate accessible taxis for ordinary on-street taxi service, as long as their vehicles carry less than eight passengers or are purchased used. However, taxi operators may not otherwise discriminate against those with disabilities—such as by charging additional fees for storing wheelchairs or refusing to carry service animals. Most cities regulate taxi services in their jurisdictions; under pressure from advocacy groups, many now require local taxi companies to own and operate a certain number of accessible taxis in ordinary private-pay street operations so that people with disabilities who cannot ride in regular sedans can simply call a taxi like everyone else. Most accessible taxis are aftermarket conversions of ordinary vans; as such, they can cost from $5,000 to $15,000 more than the sedans usually used as taxis. Some cities provide vehicles or other incentives to taxi companies or individual drivers to buy and operate accessible taxis.

However, the extent to which even taxis bought with public subsidies are actually available to people with disabilities for regular on-street or phone service is open to question. First, accessible taxi service can rarely be better than the ordinary service onto which it is added, and taxi services are poor in many communities. Second, in some cities with accessible vehicles, most are kept busy under contract to the ADA paratransit system. Third, in some cities accessible taxis have been found sitting at the airport and refusing requests for service from people with disabilities not at the airport because those taxis will often be called to the front of the taxi line, perhaps for a traveler with a disability but, more likely, for large groups traveling together or skiers or golfers with bulky equipment. Finally, most experts agree that providing taxi services to people who need special vehicles is generally less lucrative than providing ordinary services—independent of the cost of the vehicle—so some taxi drivers avoid passengers with disabilities even if they are operating an accessible taxi. In addition, passengers traveling with service animals often report that they are refused service (see a lengthy discussion of these issues in the report by NCD [2005]).

TRANSPORTATION AS PART OF A PACKAGE OF SOLUTIONS

The sections above have focused on ADA mandates in a variety of local transportation modes and the potential of these transportation modes to provide mobility for travelers with disabilities that is more frequent or better than that required by the ADA. This section focuses on the crucial nexus of direct transportation provision and a variety of other delivery systems for people with disabilities, highlighting the importance of seeing transportation services as inextricably linked to decisions made about many interrelated services and facilities—from how, where, and when medical services are provided to the strategies adopted by job training agencies.

Perhaps the most intractable issue in current debates is the tendency of those in every other substantive field from education to employment or from recreation to health care to assume that transportation deficiencies account for all or most of the underutilization of public and private services considered essential to the well-being of those with disabilities (see, for example, the work of Kenyon et al. [2003] and Lucas [2004]). In fact, substantial research shows that most people with disabilities face multiple barriers to both their mobility and their ability to get an education or a job or to access a range of public and private services from grocery stores to medical facilities. The causes of and solutions to these problems are complex; policy analysts must understand and address them in sophisticated ways that extend beyond public transit networks and, indeed, beyond transportation systems alone.

Of course, transportation problems are an important barrier to the mobility and access of those with disabilities. As the National Council on Disability has remarked,

> Some people who are willing and able to work cannot do so because of inadequate transportation. Others cannot shop, socialize, enjoy recreational or spiritual activities, or even leave their homes. And some individuals with disabilities who need medical services must live in institutions due solely to the lack of safe, reliable transportation to needed medical services (NCD, 2005, p. 13).

It is unlikely, however, that transportation is the only problem or barrier facing most people with disabilities. For example, a lack of accessible transportation may create barriers to employment; but the failure to obtain a meaningful job may also be the result of inadequate education and training, lack of experience, discrimination in the job market, or inadequate knowledge by employers about the kinds of reasonable accommodations that potential workers with disabilities require. Therefore, transportation services must be viewed and provided only as part of a package of supportive services and policies.

In the same vein, people with disabilities who lack accessible transportation may be unable to seek medical care in a timely way. Substantial research shows, however, that the "underutilization" of many kinds of medical and social services has a complicated variety of interrelated causes. Income and having health insurance (or Medicaid) are significant factors in service utilization; a 1996 study that used data from the 1987 Medical Expenditure Survey found that health status and having Medicaid benefits or private insurance were the most significant predictors of *home* health care (Kim, 1996). A 1997 study that used data from three national data sets on aging found that whether and how much older people used physicians and hospital services were consistently related to both their health status and having insurance (Miller et al., 1997).

A persistent research finding is that medical utilization rates differ significantly by race and ethnicity and that these differences are often independent of income or the availability of health insurance (Barnard and Pettigrew, 2003; Herbert et al., 2005; Jang et al., 2005; Welch et al., 2005). Roetzheim et al. (1999) attempted to explain the racial differences in the stage of the cancer when people were first diagnosed; the researchers found that neither insurance coverage nor socioeconomic status explained these racial differences. White-Means (1995) found that older African Americans were less likely to use emergency medical services than older white individuals with similar medical conditions and that these differences could not be explained by income or health status. White-Means (2000) also found clear racial differences in medical service utilization rates of people with disabilities that were not explained by socioeconomic variables. Wallace and colleagues (1998) observed that the "persistent effects of race/ethnicity [in medical service utilization] could be the result of culture, class, and/or discrimination." This suggests that the cost of medical services and the way in which they are both delivered and perceived by the intended recipients are as crucial as the lack of transportation resources in the failure to use medical services.

Other studies show that older people underutilize a range of services targeted to them for reasons ranging from a feeling that the services cannot really help to a concern about service costs, even when those costs are substantially subsidized (Takahashi and Smutny, 2001; Ku, 2005; Ness et al., 2005). There is even evidence that many people resist using special paratransit services because they fear being stigmatized or they do not believe that the services can or do meet their needs (Žakowska and Monterde, 2003; U.K. Department for Transport, Mobility and Social Inclusion Unit, 2006).

These findings still hold even when people *say* that transportation barriers prevent them from using medical or other services. Evashwick et al. (1984) concluded that when older people reported transportation difficulties, they were really reporting functional problems and not barriers to medical use. Rosenbloom (1978, 1982) suggested that older people reporting transportation barriers as the reason for the underutilization of medical services were using that reason to represent a bundle of problems, including an unwillingness to leave home, frustration with declining motor and other skills, an inability to pay for services, and unhappiness with the actual services offered, in addition to difficulty in accessing or obtaining transportation.

These observations are supported by early studies conducted for the U.S. Department of Transportation; when communities provided new medical and other transport services targeted at older people, ridership was almost entirely by people already making medical trips, presumably using a more problematic travel mode. That is, most new transport service users simply switched from whatever travel option that they had previously used to the new system, while very few of the people thought to be underutilizing services began to do so when they were provided with new transport options (Spear et al., 1978; Edelstein, 1979).

These findings may be linked to evidence that social and human service agencies must often provide more than just transportation to get their clients to leave home or use agency services (Burke et al., 2004). For example, McCray (1998) describes a special transport service in Detroit, Michigan, developed in response to the assumption that low-income pregnant women did not seek prenatal care because they lacked transportation. However, to actually get the intended riders to use the service, the female driver was required to offer incentives for the women to keep medical appointments, maintain records on the women's pregnancies, and offer prenatal and spousal abuse counseling on the bus.

Clearly, transportation difficulties add to the other burdens that many people with disabilities face, and they may be a significant component of these problems; but unless we understand their relationship to personal, community, and service delivery constraints, we are unlikely to address the mobility problems that these travelers face. The lack of appropriate and accessible transportation interacts with a range of personal and societal barriers to reduce a person's ability or willingness to leave home for a job, education, medical treatment, or socializing.

SUMMARY AND CONCLUSIONS

Research clearly shows that travelers with disabilities face multiple barriers in every mode of travel, although we lack good data by severity of impairment, income, automobile ownership, and a range of socioeconomic characteristics. People with disabilities travel less and report more mobility problems than those without disabilities; moreover, almost 2 million Americans report themselves to be homebound. At the same time, the barriers that these travelers face are not necessarily the ones that have gained the most traction in policy debates, particularly debates that center on ADA modal mandates. For example, one-third of people with disabilities have no public transit or ADA-mandated paratransit available to them. The other two-thirds—who have access to these services—rarely use them and generally do not blame their nonuse on their disability. In addition, the travel mode that created the largest barriers for people with disabilities was walking, a mode necessary for the successful use of all other modes, as well as personal mobility.

In contrast, most travelers with disabilities said that they used a car for most of their trips, the majority as the driver of that car. That finding may not be surprising, since (1) many people unable to walk or use public transit can and do drive, and (2) the car provides greater convenience and flexibility than other modes for those with disabilities, as well as the general public (and, arguably, more so for those with disabilities). The dependence on the car was especially striking among older people; this is cause for alarm, given that many (but certainly not all) older drivers will be unable to continue to safely drive as they age because of increasing impairments and/or disabilities. Many older people have long depended on the car to maintain their lifestyles and may face serious mobility problems if and when they must stop driving. For that reason many studies have suggested policies and programs to enhance the driving skills of older drivers as well as making the driving task more manageable (through vehicle and highway modifications, for example).

People with disabilities have three sources of community-based transport: accessible transit and paratransit services provided by public transit agencies, those provided by myriad social and human service agency providers as well as municipal organizations, and those provided by the private sector. Each of these sets of services faces important ADA accessibility mandates, which are being met to greater or less degrees. However, each mode also has the potential to provide additional mobility and access for travelers with disabilities if additional funding can be found.

While access and mobility on all these modes have increased substantially since the 1990 passage of the ADA, each mode has ADA compliance problems and poses other barriers for travelers with disabilities. Not all key stations on urban rail systems are yet accessible; even if they were, key stations are only a fraction of all stations in most urban rail systems. Almost all buses are accessible, but barriers to their use are posed by driver training and surveillance problems, as well as maintenance issues.

Complementary paratransit services are closer to meeting their mandates than they were in the past, but as costs have risen with compliance, many systems have reduced service to the minimum, raised fares to the maximum, and instituted rigorous certification processes that may have denied eligibility to people genuinely eligible while creating a chilling effect on others. Perhaps more important, the overwhelming majority of people with disabilities cannot use complementary paratransit services for a variety of reasons. This is in sharp contrast to a commonly held belief that such services are or could be an important part of the mobility of these travelers. The reality is that many people with disabilities who cannot use public transit will also be unable to use paratransit services.

Many regions host a wide variety of community-based transportation systems that provide an irreplaceable lifeline to the travelers with disabilities who can use them. However, while these systems all provide an invaluable service, many (certainly the larger) of these systems do so at costs not much cheaper than those charged by ADA paratransit providers, even though they use volunteer resources. More importantly, many provide limited services to a very small number of clients, often only for specific trip purposes. Moreover, some of the smaller community-based providers do not appear to be in conformity with their own ADA obligations to provide an equivalent level of service to travelers needing accessible vehicles. Overall, research suggests that we need to find ways to help some of these providers lower their costs and increase their effectiveness while expanding the number of community-based providers to meet the mobility needs of a growing population of disadvantaged travelers.

Significant improvements in the pedestrian network are also required because pedestrian barriers are the most frequently barriers cited by travelers with disabilities. All evidence suggests that ADA compliance with pedestrian (public right-of-way) systems may be low because we lack enforceable regulations in this area; as a result many people with disabilities lack an accessible route to an accessible bus stop. Research suggests the need to develop and maintain accessible and fully lit pedestrian paths while promoting greater enforcement of parking, safety, and security strategies.

Private transportation providers—including taxis and airport shuttles—have ADA mandates as well. Some evidence suggests, however, that these providers must be forced or given incentives to meet those mandates or to provide the levels of accessible services that are possible. While operators are not generally required to purchase and operate accessible taxis, many do so because of local regulations or local subsidies (or both). However, it is not clear that accessible taxis are providing the level of service for travelers with disabilities that they might.

Finally, all evidence suggests that transportation is a necessary but not a sufficient condition for the full access and mobility of travelers with disabilities. Transportation planners must work in cooperation with both the public and the private sectors and with professionals in a variety of disciplines and service delivery systems (doctors and medical facilities; educators and training facilities; employment counselors and job search programs; and a wide variety of human, medical, and social service agencies and providers) to address the access and mobility needs of a range of travelers with disabilities.

ACKNOWLEDGMENTS

I am grateful to Marilyn Field for her guidance, patience, and support and to Marilyn Golden, Disability Rights Education and Defense Fund, for being willing to share her extraordinary knowledge in these areas. I am also grateful to two anonymous reviewers for their trenchant comments. Of course, the errors that remain are entirely my responsibility.

REFERENCES

AARP (American Association of Retired Persons). 2006. *Reimagining America: AARP's Blueprint for the Future; How America Can Grow Old and Prosper.* Washington, DC: AARP.

Aurbach, G. 2001. Access to transportation systems for persons with reduced mobility: ways of improving the situation from an international perspective. *International Association of Traffic and Safety Sciences Research Journal* 25(1):6–11.

Barnard, H., and Pettigrew, N. 2003. *Delivering Benefits and Services for Black and Minority Ethnic Older People.* Research Report No. 201 of the U.K. Department for Work and Pensions. London, United Kingdom: Corporate Document Services.

The Beverly Foundation and the AAA Foundation for Traffic Safety. 2001. *Supplemental Transportation Programs for Seniors.* Washington, DC: AAA Traffic Safety Foundation.

The Beverly Foundation and the Community Transportation Association of America. 2005. *Innovations for Seniors: Public and Community Transit Services Respond to Special Needs.* [Online]. http://www.ctaa.org/ntrc/senior/innovations.pdf [accessed March 12, 2006.].

Bogren, S. 1998. You can get there from here. *Community Transportation* 16(3):10.

Burke, D., Black, K., and Pramanik, P. 2004. Community vans carry hope along with groceries. *In Transition* 12(Spring):16–19.

Carrasco, A. 2001. Has ADA turned transit properties into social service agencies? *Metro Magazine* 97(3):30–31.

Coordinating Council on Access and Mobility. 2000. *Planning Guidelines for Coordinated State and Local Specialized Transportation Services.* Washington, DC: U.S. Department of Health and Human Services and Federal Transit Administration, U.S. Department of Transportation.

de Boer, E. 2004. Introducing and sustaining accessible transport: social and physical challenges. In: *Transportation Research Record 1885*. Washington, DC: Transportation Research Board of the National Academies. Pp. 15–20.

Dellinger, A. M., Kresnow, M. J., White, D. D., and Shegal, M. 2004. Risk to self versus risk to others: how do older drivers compare to others on the road? *American Journal of Preventative Medicine* 26(3):217–221.

De Raedt, R., and Ponjaert-Kristoffersen, I. 2000. Can strategic and tactical compensation reduce crash risk in older drivers? *Age and Ageing* 29(6):517–521.

ECMT (European Conference of Ministers of Transport). 1999. *Transport and Ageing of the Population*. Economic Research Centre. Round Table 112. Paris, France: Organisation for Economic Cooperation and Development.

Edelstein, P. J. 1979. *Evaluation of the EASYRIDE Specialized Transportation Service*. U.S. Transportation Systems Center Evaluation Series. Final Report. Cambridge, MA: Transportation Systems Center.

Evans, L. 1988. Older driver involvement in fatal and severe traffic crashes. *Journal of Gerontology: Social Sciences* 43:S186–S193.

_____. 1991. Effects of sex and age. In: *Traffic Safety and the Driver*. New York, NY: Van Nostrand Reinhold. Pp. 19–43.

Evashwick, C., Rowe, G., Diehr, P., and Branch, L. 1984. Factors explaining the use of health care services by the elderly. *Health Services Research*. 19(3):357–382.

Fonda, S., Wallace, R. B., and Herzog, R. A. 2001. Changes in driving patterns and worsening depressive symptoms among older drivers. *Journals of Gerontology: Series B: Psychological Sciences and Social Sciences* 56B(6):S343–S351.

Gagliardi, C., Hirsiaho, N., Kucsera, C., et al. 2005. Background conditions for outdoor mobility in Finland, Germany, Hungary, Italy, and The Netherlands. In: Mollenkopf, H., Marcellini, F., Ruoppila, I., et al. (eds.) *Enhancing Mobility in Later Life*, Amsterdam: IOS Press. Pp. 11-42.

Griffin, J., and Priddy, D. A. 2005. Assessing paratransit eligibility under the Americans with Disabilities Act in the rehabilitation setting. *Archives of Physical Medicine and Rehabilitation* 86 (6):1267–1269.

Henderson, S. 2004. Driver and traffic safety in older adults: the visually impaired driver. *Topics in Geriatric Rehabilitation* 20(3):173–184.

Herbel, S., Rosenbloom, S., Stutts, J., and Welch, T. 2006. *The Impact of an Aging Population on Systems Planning and Investment Policies*. NCHRP Project 9-36, Task 50. Washington, DC: American Association of State Highway and Transportation Officials.

Herbert, P.L., Frick, K. D. S., Kane, R. L., and McBean, A. M. 2005. Causes of racial and ethnic differences in influenza vaccination rates among elderly Medicare beneficiaries. *Health Services Research* 40(2):517–537.

Higgins, L. L., and Cherrington, L. K. 2005. *Experience with Flex Route Transit Service in Texas*. Report SWUTC/05/1677148-1. College Station, TX: Texas Transportation Institute, Southwest Region University Transportation Center.

Hu, P. S., and Reuscher, T. R. 2004. *Summary of Travel Trends: 2001 National Household Travel Survey*. Oak Ridge, TN: Oak Ridge National Laboratories.

IIHS (Insurance Institute for Highway Safety). 2000. *Older Drivers up Close: They Aren't Dangerous Except to Themselves*. [Online]. www.iihs.org/safety_facts/fatality_facts/pdfs/olderpeople.pdf [accessed April 1, 2005].

Jang, Y., Kim, G., and Chiriboga, D. 2005. Health, healthcare utilization, and satisfaction with service: barriers and facilitators for older Korean Americans. *Journal of the American Geriatrics Society* 53(9):1613–1617.

Johnson, E. 2003. Transportation mobility and older drivers. *Journal of Gerontological Nursing* 29(4):34–41.

Kenyon, S., Rafferty, J., and Lyons, G. 2003. Social exclusion and transport in the UK: a role for virtual accessibility in the alleviation of mobility-related exclusion? *Journal of Social Policy* 32:317.

Kihl, M., Brennan, D., Gabhawala, N., List, J., and Mittal, P. 2005. *Livable Communities: An Evaluation Guide.* AARP Public Policy Institute. Tempe, AZ: Herberger Center for Design Excellence, Arizona State University.

Kim, S.Y. 1996. Home health care utilization patterns among the elderly. *Consumer Interests Annual* 42:225–227.

Kocera, A. Straight, A. K., and Guterbock, T. M. 2005. *Beyond 50.05: A Report to the Nation on Livable Communities: Creating Environments for Successful Aging.* AARP Public Policy Institute. Washington, DC: American Association of Retired Persons.

Kochera, A., and Bright, K. 2005–2006. Livable communities for older people. *Generations* 29(4 Winter):32–36.

Ku, L. 2005. *Effect of Increased Cost-Sharing in Medicaid: A Summary of Research Findings.* Washington, DC: Center on Budget and Policy Priorities. [Online]. www.cbpp.org/5-31-05health2.pdf [accessed March 23, 2006].

Lee, B. L. 1997. Civil rights and legal remedies: a plan of action. In: Bullard, R. D. and Johnson, G. S. (eds.), *Just Transportation: Dismantling Race and Class Barriers in Mobility.* Gabriola Island, British Columbia, Canada: New Society Publishers.

Li, G. H., Braver, E. R., and Chen, L. H. 2003. Fragility versus excessive crash involvement as determinants of high death rates per vehicle mile of travel among older drivers. *Accident Analysis and Prevention* 35(2):227–235.

Lucas, K. L. 2004. Introduction. In: Lucas, K. L. (ed.), *Running on Empty: Social Exclusion and Environmental Justice.* London, United Kingdom: Policy Press.

Lyman, J., McGwin, G., Jr., and Sims, R. V. 2001. Factors relating to driving difficulty and habits in older drivers. *Accident Analysis and Prevention* 33(3):413–421.

Mann, E. 1997. Confronting transit racism in Los Angeles. In: Bullard, R. D., and Johnson, G. S. (eds.), *Just Transportation: Dismantling Race and Class Barriers in Mobility.* Gabriola Island, British Columbia, Canada: New Society Publishers.

Marottoli, R., Mendes de Leon, C. F., Glass, T., Williams, C. S., Cooney, L. M., and Berkman, L. F. 2000. Consequences of driving cessation: decreased out-of-home activity levels. *Journals of Gerontology: Series B: Psychological Sciences and Social Sciences* 55B(6 Nov.):S334–S340.

McCray, T. 1998. Transporting the future: ITS and the Healthy Baby Service. *ITS Quarterly* 6(1):13–21.

McKnight, J. A. 2003. Freedom of the open road: driving and older adults. *Generations* 27(2):25–31.

Miller, B., and Campbell, R. T. 1997. Use of medical care by African American and white older persons; comparative analysis of three national data sets. *Journal of Gerontology; Series B: Psychology and Social Sciences* 52B(6):S325-336

National Organization on Disability-Harris Interactive. 2004. *N.O.D./Harris 2004 Survey of Americans with Disabilities.* Study No. 20835. Final Report. New York, NY: Harris Interactive.

NCD (National Council on Disability). 2004. *Livable Communities for Adults with Disabilities.* Washington, DC: NCD.

_____. 2005. *The Current State of Transportation for People with Disabilities in the United States.* Washington, DC: NCD.

NCHS (National Center for Health Statistics, Centers for Disease Control). Undated. *1994 National Health Interview Survey on Disability, Phase I and Phase II.* Survey and Data Collection Systems: National Health Interview Survey on Disability (NHIS-D). [Online]. http://www.cdc.gov/nchs/about/major/nhis_dis/nhisddes.htm [accessed December 7, 2006].

Ness, J., Cirillo, D. J., Weir, D. R., Nisly, N. L., and Wallace, R. B. 2005. Use of complementary medicine in older Americans: results from the Health and Retirement Study. *Gerontologist* 45(4):516–524.

OECD (Organisation for Economic Cooperation and Development). 2001. *Ageing and Transport: Mobility Needs and Safety Issues.* Paris, France: OECD.

O'Neill, D., and Dobbs, B. 2004. Age-related disease, mobility, and driving. In: *Transportation in an Aging Society: A Decade of Experience.* Conference Proceedings 17. Washington, DC: Transportation Research Board of the National Academies. Pp. 56–68.

Rabbitt, P., Carmichael, A., Shilling, V., and Sutcliffe, P. 2002. *Age, Health and Driving: Longitudinally Observed Changes in Reported General Health, in Mileage, Self-Rated Competence and in Attitudes of Drivers.* Basingstoke, United Kingdom: The University of Manchester and the AA Foundation for Road Safety Research.

Ragland, D. R, Satariano, W. A., and MacLeod, K. E. 2005. Driving cessation and increased depressive symptoms. *Journals of Gerontology: Series A: Biological Sciences and Medical Sciences* 60A(3):399–403.

Ranney, T. A., and Pulling, N. H. 1990. Performance difference on driving and laboratory tasks between drivers of different ages. *Journal of Gerontological Nursing* 10:12–15.

Ritter, A. S., Straight, A. K., and Evans, E. 2002. *Understanding Senior Transportation: Report and Analysis of a Survey of Consumers 50+.* AARP Public Policy Research Institute. Washington, DC: American Association of Retired Persons.

Roetzheim, R. G., Pal, N., Tennant, C., Voti, L., Ayanian, J. Z., Schwabe, A., and Krischer, J. P. 1999. Effects of health insurance and race on early detection of cancer. *Journal of the National Cancer Institute.* 91(16):1409–1421.

Rosenbloom, S. 1978. Transportation needs and social service utilization: a reassessment. *Traffic Quarterly* 32(3):333–348.

_____. 1981. Barriers to coordination: irrational or valid objections? In: *Transportation Research Record 818.* Washington, DC: Transportation Research Board, National Research Council. Pp. 33–39.

_____. 1982. Federal policies to increase the mobility of the elderly and the handicapped. *Journal of the American Planning Association* 48(3):335–350.

_____. 1991. *Reverse Commute Transportation; Emerging Provider Rules.* Final Report to the Federal Transit Administration (reprinted by US DOT Office of Technology Sharing).

_____. 1994. *How the ADA Affects Paratransit Operational Decisions.* Washington, DC: Federal Transit Administration.

_____. 1995. *Service Routes, Route Deviation, and General Public Paratransit.* Federal Transit Administration. Tucson, AZ: The Drachman Institute.

_____. 2001. Driving cessation among the elderly: when does it really happen and what impact does it have? In: *Transportation Research Record 1779.* Washington, DC: Transportation Research Board, National Research Council. Pp. 93–99.

_____. 2004. The mobility of the elderly: good news and bad news. In: *Transportation in an Aging Society: A Decade of Experience.* Conference Proceedings. Washington, DC: Transportation Research Board, National Research Council. Pp. 3–21.

_____. 2005. The mobility needs of older Americans. In: Katz, B., and Puentes, R. (eds.), *Taking the High Road: A Transportation Agenda for Strengthening Metropolitan Areas.* Washington, DC: Brookings Institution Press.

_____. 2006a. Is the driving experience of older women changing? Safety and mobility consequences over time. In: *Transportation Research Record 1956.* Washington, DC: Transportation Research Board of the National Academies. Pp. 127–132.

_____. 2006b. *Social Exclusion in Transportation in the United States: Lessons for Australia.* Department of Infrastructure. Melbourne, Australia: Department of Infrastructure.

Rosenbloom, S., and Stähl, A. 2003. Automobility among the elderly: the convergence of environmental, safety, mobility and community design issues. *European Journal of Transport and Infrastructure Research* 2(3–4):197–214.

Rosenbloom, S., and Warren, D. 1981. A comparison of two transportation brokerages: the lessons to be learned from Houston and Pittsburgh. In: *Transportation Research Record 830*. Washington, DC: Transportation Research Board, National Research Council. Pp. 7–15.

Rosenbloom, S., and Winsten-Bartlett, C. 2002. Asking the right question: understanding the travel needs of older women who do not drive. In: *Transportation Research Record 1803*. Washington, DC: Transportation Research Board, National Research Council. Pp. 78–82.

Sanchez, T. W., Stolz, R., and Ma, J. S. 2003. *Moving to Equity: Addressing the Inequitable Effects of Transportation Policies on Minorities*. A Joint Report of the Center for Community Change and The Civil Rights Project, Harvard University. [Online]. http://www.civilrightsproject.harvard.edu/research/transportation/MovingtoEquity.pdf [accessed February 6, 2005].

Schlossberg, M. 2003. Developing coordination policies for paratransit and the transportation disadvantaged. In: *Transportation Research Record 1841*. Washington, DC: Transportation Research Board, National Research Council. Pp. 73–80.

_____. 2004. Coordination as a strategy for serving the transportation disadvantaged: a comparative framework of local and state roles. *Public Works Management & Policy* 9(2):132–144.

Shope, J. T. 2003. What does giving up driving mean to older drivers and why is it so difficult? *Generations* 27(2):57–59.

Siggerud, K. 2003. *Transportation-Disadvantaged Populations: Many Federal Programs Fund Transportation Services, but Obstacles to Coordination Persist*. GAO Report GAO-03-698T. Washington, DC: U.S. General Accounting Office.

Spear, B. D., Page, E., Slavin, H., Hendrickson, C. 1978. Recent evidence from UMTA's Service and Methods Demonstration Program concerning the travel behavior of the elderly and handicapped. Staff paper. Cambridge, MA: Transportation Systems Center.

Staplin, L., Locco, K., Byington, S., and Harkey, D. 2001. *Highway Design Handbook for Older Drivers and Pedestrians*. Report No. FHWA-RD-01-103. Washington, DC: Federal Highway Administration.

Stutts, J. 2005. *Improving the Safety of Older Road Users*. National Cooperative Highway Research Program Synthesis of Highway Practice 348. Washington, DC: Transportation Research Board of the National Academies.

Sweeney, M. 2004. Travel patterns of older Americans with disabilities. Working Paper 2004-001-OAS. Washington, DC: U.S. Bureau of Transportation Statistics.

Takahashi, L. M., and Smutny, G. 2001. Explaining access to human services: the influence of descriptive and behavioral variables. *The Professional Geographer* 53(1):12–31.

TCRP (Transit Cooperative Research Program). 1994. *Low-Floor Transit Buses*. TCRP Synthesis of Transit Practice 2. Washington, DC: Transit Cooperative Research Program, Transportation Research Board, National Research Council.

_____. 1997a. *Guidebook for Attracting Paratransit Patrons to Fixed-Route Services*. TCRP Report 24. Washington, DC: Transit Cooperative Research Program, Transportation Research Board, National Research Council.

_____. 1997b. *Strategies to Assist Local Transportation Agencies in Becoming Mobility Managers*. TCRP Report 21. Washington, DC: Transit Cooperative Research Program, Transportation Research Board, National Research Council.

_____. 1998a. *ADA Paratransit Eligibility Certification Practices.* TCRP Synthesis of Transit Practice 30. Washington, DC: Transit Cooperative Research Program, Transportation Research Board, National Research Council.

_____. 1998b. *New Designs and Operating Experience with Low-Floor Buses.* TCRP Report 41. Washington, DC: Transit Cooperative Research Program, Transportation Research Board, National Research Council.

_____. 1998c. *Transit Markets of the Future: The Challenge of Change.* TCRP Report 28. Washington, DC: Transit Cooperative Research Program, Transportation Research Board, National Research Council.

_____. 1999a. *Passenger Information Services: A Guidebook for Transit Systems.* TCRP Report 45. Washington, DC: Transit Cooperative Research Program, Transportation Research Board, National Research Council.

_____. 1999b. *The Role of Transit Amenities and Vehicle Characteristics in Building Transit Ridership.* TCRP Report 46. Washington, DC: Transit Cooperative Research Program, Transportation Research Board, National Research Council.

_____. 2002a. *Improving Public Transit Options for Older Persons.* TCRP Report 82, Vol. 2. Washington, DC: Transit Cooperative Research Program, Transportation Research Board, National Research Council.

_____. 2002b. *The Use of Small Buses in Transit Service.* TCRP Synthesis of Transit Practice 41. Washington, DC: Transit Cooperative Research Program, Transportation Research Board, National Research Council.

_____. 2003a. *Economic Benefits of Coordinating Human Service Transportation and Transit Services.* TCRP Report 91. Washington, D.C.: Transit Cooperative Research Program, Transportation Research Board, National Research Council.

_____. 2003b. *Emerging New Paradigms: A Guide to Fundamental Change in Local Public Transportation Organizations.* TCRP Report 97. Washington, DC: Transit Cooperative Research Program, Transportation Research Board, National Research Council.

_____. 2003c. Bus routing and coverage. In: *Traveler Response to Transportation System Changes.* TCRP Report 95. Washington, DC: Transit Cooperative Research Program, Transportation Research Board, National Research Council.

_____. 2003d. *Use of Rear-Facing Position for Common Wheelchairs on Transit Buses.* TCRP Synthesis of Transit Practice 50. Washington, DC: Transit Cooperative Research Program, Transportation Research Board, National Research Council.

_____. 2004a. *Embracing Change in a Changing World.* TCRP Report 99. Washington, DC: Transit Cooperative Research Program, Transportation Research Board, National Research Council.

_____. 2004b. *Operational Experiences with Flexible Transit Services.* TCRP Synthesis of Transit Practice 53. Washington, DC: Transit Cooperative Research Program, Transportation Research Board, National Research Council.

_____. 2004c. *Strategies to Increase Coordination of Transportation Services for the Transportation Disadvantaged.* TCRP Report 105. Washington, DC: Transit Cooperative Research Program, Transportation Research Board, National Research Council.

_____. 2004d. *Toolkit for Rural Community Coordinated Transportation Services.* TCRP Report 101. Washington, DC: Transit Cooperative Research Program, Transportation Research Board, National Research Council.

Thole, C., and Harvey, F. 2005. *Update Methodology for ADA Demand Estimates: Lessons Learned.* National Center for Transit Research. Tampa, FL: Florida Department of Transportation.

U.K. Department for Transport. 2003. *Older People: Their Transport Needs and Requirements.* Main Report. [Online]. www.dft.gov.uk/stellent/groups/dft_mobility/documents/page/dft_mobility_506792.hcsp [accessed March 26, 2006].

U.K. Department for Transport, Mobility and Social Inclusion Unit. 2006. *Older Drivers and Driving Cessation*. Report No. UG535. London, United Kingdom: Corporate Document Services.

U.S. BTS (U.S. Bureau of Transportation Statistics). 2003a. *Freedom to Travel*. Report No. BTS03-08. Washington, DC: U.S. BTS.

_____. 2003b. *Transportation Availability and Use Study for Persons with Disabilities, 2002*. Washington, DC: U.S. BTS.

U.S. CBO (U.S. Congressional Budget Office). 1979. *Urban Transportation for Handicapped People: Alternative Federal Approaches*. Washington, DC: Government Printing Office.

U.S. Census Bureau. 2002. *U.S. Summary: 2000: Census 2000 Profile*. Economics and Statistics Administration. Report C2KPROF/00U.S. July Table DP-1 Profile of General Demographic Characteristics: 2000. Washington, DC: U.S. Census Bureau.

_____. 2005. Table 1 Prevalence of Disability by Age, Sex, Race and Hispanic Origin: 2002. Washington, DC: U.S. Census Bureau.

U.S. GAO (U.S. Government Accounting Office. 2004. *Transportation-Disadvantaged Seniors. Efforts to Enhance Senior Mobility Could Benefit from Additional Guidance and Information*. Report to the Chairman, Special Committee on Aging. U.S. Senate, August 2004. GAO-04-971.

U.S. Senate, Select Committee on Aging. 1970. *Older Americans and Transportation*. Washington, DC: Government Printing Office.

Wallace, S.P., Levy-Storms, L., Kington, R.S., Andersen, R.M. 1998. Persistence of Race and Ethnicity in the use of long-term care. *Journals of Gerontology: Series B: Psychological Sciences and Social* 53B(2):S104–S112.

Welch, L. C., Teno, J. M., and Mor, V. 2005. End-of-life care in black and white: race matters for medical care of dying patients and their families. *Journal of the American Geriatrics Society*. 53(7):1145–1153.

West, C. G., Gildengorin, G., Haegerstrom-Portnoy, G., Lott, L. A., Schneck, M. E., and Brabyn, J. A. 2003. Vision and driving self-regulation in older adults. *Journal of the American Geriatrics Society* 51(10):1348–1355.

White-Means, S. 1995. Conceptualizing race in economic models of medical utilization: a case study of community-based elders and the emergency room. *Health Services Research* 30(1):207–223.

_____. 2000. Racial patterns in disabled person's use of medical services. *The Journals of Gerontology* 55(2):S276–S291.

Žakowska, L., and Monterde I. B. H. 2003. *Results of Focus-Group Interviews and In-depth Interviews with Senior Citizens and Experts*. Deliverables D5 and D6, SIZE Project of the European Commission's Fifth Framework Programme. [Online]. www.size-project.at/results/SIZE_D5-6_complete.pdf [accessed March 9, 2007].

Zaworski, J. R, and Hunter-Zaworski, K. M. 2006. Wheelchair securement systems for urban transit vehicles: it's time to address the other side of the problem. Presented at 85th Annual Meeting of the Transportation Research Board. Washington, DC: Transportation Research Board of the National Academies.

H

Committee on Disability in America Biographical Sketches

Alan M. Jette, Ph.D., M.P.H., P.T. (*Chair*), directs the Health and Disability Research Institute at Boston University. He also serves as a professor of health policy and management at Boston University's School of Public Health. He was a member of the Institute of Medicine committee to review the Social Security Administration's disability decision process research (1998 to 2002), which conducted several workshops and produced several reports. His research emphases include late-life exercise; evaluation of treatment outcomes; and the measurement, epidemiology, and prevention of late-life disability. He has published more than 125 articles on these topics in the rehabilitation, geriatrics, and public health literature.

Elena M. Andresen, Ph.D., is a professor and chief of the Epidemiology Division, Department of Health Services Research, Management & Policy, at the University of Florida Health Sciences Center. She served on an Institute of Medicine committee tasked with developing an agenda for health outcomes research for elderly people and was a member of the Healthy People with Disabilities 2010 work group. With more than 60 publications, Dr.

561

Andresen's training and interests include health services research and the epidemiology of chronic disease. She has developed and taught graduate-level courses in disability and health. Her funded research includes topics on disability epidemiology, aging, and surveillance measures of health for use in policy and planning. Dr. Andresen is a member of the Society for Epidemiologic Research, the International Society for Quality of Life Research, the Academy for Health Services Research and Policy, the American College of Epidemiology, and the American Public Health Association.

Michael Chernew, Ph.D., is a professor in the Department of Health Care Policy at Harvard Medical School. One major area of Dr. Chernew's research focuses on assessing the impact of managed care on the health care marketplace, with an emphasis on examining the impact of managed care on health care cost growth and on the use of medical technology. He recently served on technical advisory panels for the Centers for Medicare and Medicaid Services that reviewed the assumptions used by Medicare actuaries to assess the financial status of the Medicare trust funds. In 1998, he was awarded the John D. Thompson Prize for Young Investigators by the Association of University Programs in Public Health. In 1999, he received the Alice S. Hersh Young Investigator Award from the Association of Health Services Research. Dr. Chernew is a research associate of the National Bureau of Economic Research, and he is on the editorial boards of *Health Services Research*, *Health Affairs*, and *Medical Care Research and Review*. His recent research has examined the economics of home health care and the growth of health care expenditures among Medicare beneficiaries with disabilities.

Dudley S. Childress, Ph.D., is a professor of biomedical engineering and of physical medicine and rehabilitation in the McCormick School of Engineering and the Feinberg School of Medicine, Northwestern University. He is director of the Northwestern University Rehabilitation Engineering Program and the Northwestern University Prosthetics Research Laboratory and is executive director of the Northwestern University Prosthetics and Orthotics Education Program. He is a member of the Institute of Medicine and served on the Committee on Assessing Rehabilitation Science and Engineering. Dr. Childress is the recipient of numerous honors and awards, including the Missouri Honor Award for Distinguished Service in Engineering and the Magnuson Award. He serves on the editorial board of the *Journal of Rehabilitation Research and Development* and has been a member of the Advisory Board, National Center for Medical Rehabilitation Research of the National Institutes of Health, and the National Research Advisory Council of the U.S. Department of Veterans Affairs. His research and development activities are concentrated in the areas of biomechanics; human walking;

artificial limbs; ambulation aids; and rehabilitation engineering, which involves the design and development of modern technological systems for amputees and other people with disabilities.

Vicki A. Freedman, Ph.D., is a professor of health systems and policy at the University of Medicine and Dentistry of New Jersey's School of Public Health. Dr. Freedman is a demographer and chronic disease epidemiologist with expertise in the measurement of disabilities in older populations. She has published extensively on the topics of population aging, disability, and long-term care, including several widely publicized articles on trends in late-life functioning. Her current research emphasizes interventions that can be used to prevent late-life disability decline, the socioeconomic and racial disparities in the incidence of late-life disabilities, the causes of late-life disability trends, and the role of assistive technology in ameliorating disability. She has served on more than a dozen national advisory panels for federal agencies, including the National Institute on Aging and the U.S. Department of Health and Human Services.

Patricia Hicks, M.D., is an associate professor in the Division of General Pediatrics in the Department of Pediatrics at the University of Texas Southwestern Medical School at Dallas and adjunct professor of law at Southern Methodist University. She is the director of the Residents' Continuity of Care Clinic in the residency training program, where she teaches residents and also cares for children with complex chronic health conditions and counsels and advises their families. Her teaching responsibilities include clinical ethics and a course in law, literature, and medicine. As a member of the hospital's Information Systems Committee, she is involved with projects related to electronic medical records and database organization and design for research, reporting, clinical decision support, and monitoring.

Lisa I. Iezzoni, M.D., M.Sc., is a professor of medicine at Harvard Medical School and associate director of the Institute for Health Policy, Massachusetts General Hospital. She is a member of the Institute of Medicine and has served on the Committee to Evaluate Measures of Health Benefits for Environmental, Health, and Safety Regulation; the Committee on Identifying Priority Areas for Quality Improvement; the Committee on Multiple Sclerosis; the Institutional Review Board Committee; and the Committee to Advise the National Library of Medicine on Information Center Services. Dr. Iezzoni has conducted numerous studies for the Agency for Healthcare Research and Quality, the Centers for Medicare and Medicaid Services, and private foundations on a variety of topics, including methods for predicting costs, clinical outcomes, and quality of care. She has worked extensively on risk adjustment and has edited *Risk Adjustment for Measuring Health*

Care Outcomes, now in its third edition (2003). She now studies health care quality and policy issues relating to people with disabilities, publishing *When Walking Fails* in 2003 and *More Than Ramps: A Guide to Improving Health Care Quality and Access for People with Disabilities*, coauthored with Bonnie L. O'Day, in 2006.

June Isaacson Kailes, M.S.W., L.C.S.W., is a disability policy consultant and serves as Associate Director and Adjunct Associate Professor at the Center for Disability Issues and the Health Professions at the Western University of Health Sciences. Her work focuses on health-related disability and aging issues as well as emergency plannng and response. Ms. Kailes works with a variety of managed care projects and government-related research projects as a consultant, trainer, writer, researcher, and policy analyst. These projects have included work with the Rehabilitation Research and Training Centers on Aging with a Disability, the National Center on Physical Activity and Disability, and the Rehabilitation Engineering Research Center on Accessible Medical Instrumentation. She teaches "Disability Competency in the Health Professions," an introductory course on disability issues for health professionals. It covers disability demographics, etiquette and communication, medical and social models of disability, quality of life, risk factors for disability, secondary conditions, compliance with the Americans with Disabilities Act, and other major disability-related public policy and ethical issues. As a presidential appointee to the United States Access Board from 1995 to 2003, Ms. Kailes served as its chair and vice chair. She is a frequent speaker at conferences, workshops, and seminars and has published widely on disability-related topics.

Laura Mosqueda, M.D., is a board-certified geriatrician and family physician. She is the director of geriatrics at the University of California, Irvine (UCI), School of Medicine, where she is also a professor of family medicine and holds the Ronald W. Reagan Endowed Chair in Geriatrics. As the director of geriatrics, she oversees both clinical and academic programs, including clinical care for seniors and adults with disabilities, research projects and grants, the education of health care professionals, and community outreach. In the clinical setting, Dr. Mosqueda implemented a multidisciplinary health assessment program for seniors and adults with disabilities and was instrumental in the development of the UCI Senior Health Center (SHC), an outpatient setting that caters to the special needs of seniors and adults with disabilities. As the medical director of SHC, she has an outpatient clinical practice specifically for seniors and adults with disabilities. For more than 10 years she was involved with the Rehabilitation Research and Training Center on Aging-Related Changes in Impairment for Persons Living with Physical Disabilities, a federally funded center headquartered at the Rancho

Los Amigos Medical Center in Downey, California. Additional research activities include a study on osteoporosis in adults with cerebral palsy and, more recently, a primary care initiative to improve access to care for adults with disabilities. Dr. Mosqueda coedited and contributed to a textbook entitled *Aging with a Disability: What the Clinician Needs to Know* (Johns Hopkins University Press, 2004). She is the founder of the Elder Abuse Forensic Center, which focuses on the abuse of elders and adults with disabilities. Areas of special interest include aging with a disability, dementia, abuse, and bioethics.

P. Hunter Peckham, Ph.D., is a professor of biomedical engineering and orthopedics at Case Western Reserve University. He also serves as director of the Functional Electrical Stimulation Center at the Louis Stokes Veterans Affairs Medical Center and director of orthopedic research for the Rehabilitation Engineering Center at MetroHealth Medical Center. He is a member of the National Academy of Engineering and serves on the Committee on Spinal Cord Injury: Strategies in a Search for a Cure. He is an expert in the areas of neural prostheses and the use of electrical stimulation of nerves to restore function in cases of central nervous system paralysis and holds multiple patents related to his work. Dr. Peckham is the recipient of numerous honors and awards for his innovative research, including the Paul B. Magnuson Award and the Food and Drug Administration Commissioner's Special Citation. In 2000, he was elected Engineer of the Year by *Design News*. In 1996–1997, he chaired the National Institutes of Health National Advisory Board to the National Center for Medical Rehabilitation Research.

James Marc Perrin, M.D., is director of the Division of General Pediatrics at the Massachusetts General Hospital for Children and the Massachusetts General Hospital Center for Child and Adolescent Health Policy and is a professor of pediatrics at Harvard Medical School. He has served on four Institute of Medicine committees, including the Committee on the Evaluation of Selected Federal Health Care Quality Activities, the Committee on Improving Quality in Long-Term Care, the Committee on Home-Based and Long-Term Care and Quality, and the Workshop on Maternal and Child Health Under Health Care Reform. For the American Academy of Pediatrics, Dr. Perrin chaired the Committee on Children with Disabilities and a committee to develop a practice guideline for attention deficit hyperactivity disorder. He is past president of the Ambulatory Pediatric Association (APA) and founding editor of the APA journal, *Ambulatory Pediatrics*. Dr. Perrin was a member of the Health Care Technology study section of the Agency for Health Care Policy and Research, the National Advisory Council for the Agency for Healthcare Research and Quality, and the National

Commission on Childhood Disability. He has also served as a consultant to the Social Security Administration on children's disability issues. He directs the Massachusetts General Hospital coordinating center for the Autism Treatment Network. His research has examined asthma, middle-ear disease, children's hospitalization, and childhood chronic illness and disabilities.

Margaret A. Turk, M.D., is a professor of physical medicine and rehabilitation at the State University of New York Upstate Medical University at Syracuse, with a joint appointment in the Department of Pediatrics. She is also medical director of rehabilitation services at St. Camillus Health and Rehabilitation Center. Dr. Turk serves as chair of the American Board of Physical Medicine and Rehabilitation. In addition to her clinical and administrative responsibilities, Dr. Turk is involved in rehabilitation research and has been funded by the Centers for Disease Control and Prevention over a 10-year period for projects related to secondary conditions of and health promotion for people with disabilities. Her publications and national and international presentations have been on pediatric rehabilitation, pediatric electrodiagnosis, tone management, adults with cerebral palsy, secondary conditions, health promotion in disability, and the health of women with disabilities. She participates with the New York State Department of Health Disability Prevention Program Working Group on Secondary Conditions, which she cochairs. She received the United Cerebral Palsy Research and Educational Foundation Isabelle and Leonard Goldenson Technology and Rehabilitation Award in 2004. She was recently appointed to the National Advisory Board on Medical Rehabilitation Research at the National Institutes of Health. She was a member of the Institute of Medicine committee that developed the report *Enabling America: Assessing the Role of Rehabilitation Science and Engineering* (National Academy Press, 1997).

Gregg Vanderheiden, Ph.D., is a professor of industrial engineering (human factors) at the University of Wisconsin–Madison. He directs the Trace Research and Development Center, which focuses on making standard information technologies and telecommunications systems more accessible and usable by people with disabilities. The Center has two Rehabilitation Engineering Research Center (RERC) grants from the National Institute for Disability and Rehabilitation Research (one for the Universal Interface and Information Technology Access RERC and the other for the Telecommunications Access RERC). Dr. Vanderheiden has worked with the computer industry to develop and build disability access features directly into their standard products. Interface features from Dr. Vanderheiden's research group are built into the MacOS, X-Windows for Unix, OS/2, and Microsoft Windows 95 through Vista operating systems. His work can also be found in the U.S. Postal Service's Automated Postal Systems and the new

Phoenix Airport cross-disability accessible information and paging system. His research interests focus on technology, human disability, and aging and include such specific topics as ergonomics, universal design, rehabilitation engineering, computer interface design, and augmentation of human functional capacities. He studies and develops standards for access to Web-based technologies, operating systems, and telecommunication systems. He served on the Toward an Every-Citizen Interface to the Nation's Information Infrastructure Steering Committee of the National Research Council.

John Whyte, M.D., Ph.D., is a physiatrist and experimental psychologist specializing in traumatic brain injury rehabilitation. He directs the Moss Rehabilitation Research Institute and is a professor of rehabilitation medicine at Thomas Jefferson University in Philadelphia. His research focuses on recovery from prolonged unconsciousness and attention deficits that result from traumatic brain injury. In addition, he has a long-standing interest in the special methodological challenges presented by rehabilitation research topics, including the definition of rehabilitation treatments and the measurement of treatment effects. His research has been funded by the National Institutes of Health (NIH), the National Institute on Disability and Rehabilitation Research, the Department of the Army, and a number of private foundations. He is the incoming president of the Association of Academic Physiatrists, former chair of the National Center for Medical Rehabilitation Research's Advisory Board, and principal investigator and program director for the Rehabilitation Medicine Scientist Training Program, an NIH-funded program to train physiatric researchers. He is the 2002 winner of the William Fields Caveness Award from the Brain Injury Association of America.

IOM Study Staff

Marilyn J. Field, Ph.D., study director, is a senior program officer at the Institute of Medicine (IOM). Her recent projects at IOM have examined postmarket surveillance of pediatric medical devices and clinical research involving children. Among earlier projects, she has directed three studies of the development and use of clinical practice guidelines, two studies of palliative and end-of-life care, and congressionally requested studies of employment-based health insurance and Medicare coverage of preventive and other services. Past positions include associate director of the Physician Payment Review Commission, executive director for Health Benefits Management at the Blue Cross and Blue Shield Association, and assistant professor of public administration at the Maxwell School of Citizenship and Public Affairs, Syracuse University. Her doctorate in political science is from the University of Michigan, Ann Arbor.

Afrah J. Ali is a senior program assistant at the Institute of Medicine. Prior to joining the Board on Health Sciences Policy, she held short-term positions in the National Academies' marketing and development departments and studied biology at Howard University. Ms. Ali has 7 years of integrated project management, executive administration, publishing, event planning, research, and marketing experience. Her previous positions include marketing specialist at Standard and Poor's E-marketing division in New York City.

Franklin Branch is a research assistant for the Board on Health Sciences Policy. Prior to joining the Institute of Medicine, he worked for the Adolescent Health Research Group at Johns Hopkins University and at the American Association of People with Disabilities. Mr. Branch graduated with a B.A. in psychology from the University of Michigan, Ann Arbor.

Index

O